ANALYZING AND CONCEPTUALIZING THE THEORETICAL FOUNDATIONS OF NURSING

Janice M. Morse, PhD (Nurs), PhD (Anthro), FCAHS, FAAN, is a professor and Barnes Presidential Chair, College of Nursing, University of Utah, Salt Lake City, and professor emeritus, University of Alberta, Edmonton, Canada. Her research contributions include the development of the Praxis Theory of Suffering and Comforting, the Morse Fall Scale (in use internationally), and the advancement of qualitative and mixed-method research. She has edited *Qualitative Health Research (QHR)* and *Global Qualitative Nursing Research,* and was founding editor of the *International Journal of Qualitative Methods (IJQM).* Her publications include *Compassionate Nursing, Principles of Mixed-Method Designs, Preventing Patient Falls* (Springer Publishing Company), and texts for several qualitative methods. In 1997, she founded the International Institute for Qualitative Methodology (IIQM), directing a network of eight international hubs and 115 universities, supporting training for QHR and mentoring qualitative researchers globally. She was the recipient of the fifth Sigma Theta Tau Episteme Award, an inductee of the Sigma Theta Tau Hall of Fame, and has received honorary doctorates from institutions in Australia and Canada.

ANALYZING AND CONCEPTUALIZING THE THEORETICAL FOUNDATIONS OF NURSING

Janice M. Morse, PhD (Nurs),
PhD (Anthro), FCAHS, FAAN

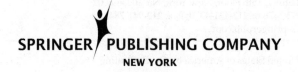

SPRINGER PUBLISHING COMPANY
NEW YORK

Springer Publishing Company, LLC
11 West 42nd Street
New York, NY 10036
www.springerpub.com

Acquisitions Editor: Joseph Morita
Production Editor: Kris Parrish
Composition: Exeter Premedia Services Private Ltd.

ISBN: 978-0-8261-6101-7
e-book ISBN: 978-0-8261-6102-4
Instructor's Manual ISBN: 978-0-8261-6103-1

Instructor's materials are available to qualified adopters by e-mailing textbook@springerpub.com.

16 17 18 19 20 / 5 4 3 2 1

The author and the publisher of this Work have made every effort to use sources believed to be reliable to provide information that is accurate and compatible with the standards generally accepted at the time of publication. Because medical science is continually advancing, our knowledge base continues to expand. Therefore, as new information becomes available, changes in procedures become necessary. We recommend that the reader always consult current research and specific institutional policies before performing any clinical procedure. The author and publisher shall not be liable for any special, consequential, or exemplary damages resulting, in whole or in part, from the readers' use of, or reliance on, the information contained in this book. The publisher has no responsibility for the persistence or accuracy of URLs for external or third-party Internet websites referred to in this publication and does not guarantee that any content on such websites is, or will remain, accurate or appropriate.

Library of Congress Cataloging-in-Publication Data

Names: Morse, Janice M.
Title: Analyzing and conceptualizing the theoretical foundations
   of nursing / Janice M. Morse.
Description: New York, NY : Springer Publishing Company, LLC, [2016] |
   Includes bibliographical references and index.
Identifiers: LCCN 2016004889| ISBN 9780826161017 | ISBN 9780826161024 (e-book)
Subjects: | MESH: Nursing Theory | Nursing Research | Concept Formation
Classification: LCC RT81.5 | NLM WY 86 | DDC 610.73072—dc23
LC record available at http://lccn.loc.gov/2016004889

Special discounts on bulk quantities of our books are available to corporations, professional associations, pharmaceutical companies, health care organizations, and other qualifying groups. If you are interested in a custom book, including chapters from more than one of our titles, we can provide that service as well.

For details, please contact:
Special Sales Department, Springer Publishing Company, LLC
11 West 42nd Street, 15th Floor, New York, NY 10036-8002
Phone: 877-687-7476 or 212-431-4370; Fax: 212-941-7842
E-mail: sales@springerpub.com

Printed in the United States of America by Gasch Printing.

For Bob

CONTENTS

SECTION III: EMERGING CONCEPTS

SECTION VI: MIXED- AND MULTIPLE-METHOD APPROACHES

SECTION VII: THE QUANTITATIVE MINDFRAME

SECTION IX: TOWARD THEORY-BASED INTERVENTIONS

CONTRIBUTORS

Tina L. Bloom, PhD, MPH, RN, is an assistant professor at the University of Missouri Sinclair School of Nursing, Columbia, Missouri.

Laura Bohannan, PhD (1922–2002), conducted fieldwork with the Tiv tribe of southeastern Nigeria from 1949 to 1953. Under the name Elenore Smith Bowen, she also wrote *Return to Laughter* (1954, Victor Gollancz, London). She served as editor of the *American Anthropologist* for 1970 to 1973.

Joan L. Bottorff, PhD, RN, FCAHS, FAAN, is a professor in the School of Nursing, Faculty of Health and Social Development at the University of British Columbia, Canada, and professorial fellow in the Faculty of Health Sciences at Australian Catholic University, Australia.

Patricia L. Eldershaw, PhD (sociology), RN, is a lecturer in behavioral sciences at the University of Maine, Presque Isle, and a charge nurse with the Maine's Veteran's Home rehabilitation unit. She is currently pursuing a master's degree in nursing education with a focus on end-of-life care of veterans.

Deborah Finfgeld-Connett, PhD, RN, FAAN, is a professor at the Sinclair School of Nursing, University of Missouri, Missouri.

Joanne M. Hall, PhD (Nurs), RN, FAAN, is a professor in the College of Nursing at the University of Tennessee, Knoxville.

Judith E. Hupcey, EdD, FAAN, is a professor and associate dean for graduate education and research in the College of Nursing at the Pennsylvania State University, University Park, Pennsylvania.

E. Diane Johnson, MLS, is assistant director of information services and resources at the University of Missouri J. Otto Lottes Health Sciences Library, Columbia, Missouri.

Kristy K. Martyn, PhD, CPNP-PC, FAAN, is a professor, assistant dean of clinical advancement, and director of the doctor of nursing practice program at Emory University Nell Hodgson Woodruff School of Nursing.

Kim Martz, PhD, RN, is an associate professor at Boise State University School of Nursing in Boise, Idaho.

Janice M. Morse, PhD (Nurs), PhD (Anthro), FCAHS, FAAN, is a professor and presidential endowed chair at the University of Utah College of Nursing; professor emeritus, University of Alberta, Canada; and holds an honorary appointment at the University of Bournemouth, England.

Charlotte Pooler, PhD (Nurs), RN, is a clinician scientist with the Edmonton Zone of Alberta Health Services, Canada, and a member of the faculty of nursing, University of Alberta, Canada.

Stephanie Richardson, PhD, RN, is a professor at the Rocky Mountain University of Health Professionals, where she is also the program director for graduate nursing programs.

Shirley M. Solberg, PhD, RN, is professor emeritus, Memorial University, St. John's, Newfoundland, Canada.

Judith A. Spiers, PhD, RN, is an associate professor of the faculty of nursing, University of Alberta, Canada.

Terrie Vann-Ward PhD, APN, FNP-BC, GNP-BC, is a practitioner, teacher, and consultant with Behavioral Medical Associates in the Chicago area.

Kathryn Weaver, PhD, RN, is an associate professor at the University of New Brunswick, Fredericton, New Brunswick, Canada.

PREFACE

WHAT TO EXPECT (AND NOT TO EXPECT) FROM THIS TEXTBOOK

This Book Is For . . .

This textbook is intended for graduate students who are beginning their master's or doctoral programs. It is intended to provide an overview of the components and structure of theory as they are used to inform and develop nursing knowledge, as well as the types and uses of theory in nursing research and practice. It is intended to assist you to become a scholar, an excellent researcher, and a wise and smart clinician.

This textbook is about how to understand and critique concepts relevant to nursing, appreciate and use mid-range theory, and become an informed consumer, applying theory to practice. Theories in nursing have expanded in recent years to become much more than traditional frameworks and theories that emerged in the 1970s, 1980s, and 1990s. Rather, this book addresses most types of theory as they are actually used in nursing research and practice. We discuss how to develop concepts and mid-range theory using qualitative research methods, merge mid-range theories to develop scope, and move toward certainty—with evidence for practice. We address the construction of frameworks for quantitative inquiry, explore theory built from mixed-method design, and examine how theory develops inquiry toward practice-based evidence. Each approach to concepts or theory is preceded by a description of the methodological approach, followed by examples that use that particular approach to concept or theory development.

Exploring the Contents

This textbook provides you with the foundational skills to become an excellent scholar and researcher. The book is divided into 10 sections, each addressing a distinct area of inquiry and each with a different use or application for theory. But there is a progressive theme to these sections, so the text will be easier to follow if you start at the beginning and move forward. There are useful practice exercises accompanying each chapter. For instructors, Stephanie Richardson and Janice M. Morse have prepared an excellent

Instructor's Manual, which expands these exercises for the entire class. **Qualified instructors may obtain access to ancillary materials by contacting textbook@springerpub.com.**

Let us consider the contents of this textbook. Section I, "Desperately Seeking Theory," sets the stage. Chapter 1, "The Fringes of Knowledge," addresses several important concepts: the interrelationship between scholarship and research, the values of nursing, the role of perception, the friction between the art and the science of nursing, and between research and scholarship. The next chapters contribute to the understanding of perspective and reality. Chapter 2, "Where We Came From," summarizes traditional nursing theories and frameworks—but this is only a summary; if you want to know details about any particular theory, please read the original works. Chapter 3, by Laura Bohannan, uses various interpretations of *Hamlet* to remind us that perspective is culturally bound, and is only perspective. Chapter 4 addresses how theory focuses (or links) research, data, and practice; "Orientation 101" (Chapter 5) consists of definitions essential to the comprehension of subsequent chapters. Finally, in Chapter 6, "The Battlefield of Knowledge," we explore the different approaches to inquiry. Rather than considering induction–deduction as complementary strategies, we find that they have become competitive perspectives.

Section II, "All About Concepts," provides the tools for understanding concepts. Types of concepts, along with their anatomy and physiology, are described in Chapter 7. Chapter 8 summarizes the major methods for development of concepts, and Chapter 9 discusses inductive–deductive pitfalls. In Chapter 10, Judith Spiers tells us how to avoid the "pink elephant syndrome," or the invalid attribution of data in concept identification.

Section III, "Emerging Concepts," shows that we still have some distance to go to in understanding nursing concepts, and begins with a "map for approaching concept development." This part of the text deals with research methods for identifying concepts, and how to study and build them. Research methods described include qualitative methods for concept development (Chapter 12), concept identification (Chapter 13), building concepts from data (Chapter 14), building concepts using structured interviewing techniques (Chapter 15), and the prototypical method for concept development (Chapter 16).

Section IV, "Partially Developed Concepts," provides several research methods for developing concepts and moving them toward maturity. Pragmatic utility uses the literature as data (the method is described in Chapter 17 and examples are presented in Chapter 18). Other methods use qualitative inquiry research interviews to elicit the components of the concepts or for concept comparison. Judith Hupcey presents the example of cultural cohesion in social support and discusses disciplinary differences in trust in Chapter 19; Eldershaw and Morse compare self-transcendence and self-reformulation in Chapter 20. Our goal is to provide you with the skills to develop strong, insightful, rigorous, and useful concepts, and in doing so, will move our discipline forward. The examples here use completed studies, but the underlying message is that there is still plenty of space for you to explore and to make a real contribution.

Next, in Section V, "Toward Mid-Range Theory," you are provided with examples of the development of mid-range theory from more mature concepts. Nursing theory must be clinically useful, for application in practice and as practice-based evidence. Our examples include Kathryn Weaver's development of ethical sensitivity (Chapter 21) and a methodological chapter on processes of mid-range theory and theory construction by linking and ordering concepts (Chapter 22). Chapter 23 addresses the significance of "making theory useful," and in the last chapter of this part (Chapter 24), Janice Morse and Charlotte Pooler present an example of useful theory, including the conceptualization on modes of releasing suffering in women as they receive the results of biopsies for breast cancer.

Section VI presents "Mixed and Multiple Method Approaches" for theory development. In Chapter 25, Janice Morse describes theoretical frameworks for mixed-method research, and in Chapter 26, Joan Bottorff provides an example of mixed methods, by describing nurses' patterns of attending. She qualitatively identifies the patterns, and then, by conducting confirmatory factor analysis, develops a model of attending in the nurse–patient relationship.

In Section VII, "The Quantitative Mindframe," the use of concepts, operationalization, and construction of theoretical frameworks as a basis for quantitative inquiry is introduced in Chapter 27. Then, in Chapter 28, Shirley M. Solberg describes the social determinants of health as an expanded framework, linking it to strategies for research and policy and its possibilities for nursing.

Section VIII, "Building a Mature Theoretical Base," moves the researcher toward certainty with "meta-techniques." Chapter 29 is an introduction to methods. Deborah Finfgeld-Connett illustrates meta-techniques, using two examples: nursing presence (Chapter 30) and homelessness (Chapter 31). Meta-synthesis builds certainty by synthesizing theories using meta-synthesis and meta-analysis, as described in Chapter 32. In the last chapter (Chapter 33), the Illness-Constellation Model (Morse & Johnson, 1991), is presented. In this research project, six grounded theories of various illnesses and experiences relevant to nursing are used to build a theory of illness.

Section IX, "Toward Theory-Based Interventions," introduces theories developed from and for practice that have an expanded area of scope, called *theoretical coalescence* (Chapter 34). These theories are usually linked laterally, thereby increasing the scope of inquiry, and two examples of applied theories are presented: the Praxis Theory of Suffering (Chapter 35) and the Praxis Theory of Comfort and Comforting (Chapter 37). Chapter 38, by Joanne Hall, is "The Theory of Becoming Resolute: Guiding Mental Health Practice With Survivors of Maltreatment." This theory also has clear clinical implications for survival, called "becoming resolute."

Finally, Section X consists of "The Myth of a Theory Base" (Chapter 39), calling for nurses to attend to dissemination and practice-based evidence. Finally, in the Postface, we address the problem of dissemination of the developing theory base of nursing, with a call for a (r)evolution in nursing.

Becoming a Scholar

As you progress through the chapters of this book, you will realize the essential and diverse uses of theory, both in our everyday lives and in our research, while at the same time learning to become a critical thinker. Our goal in the use of this textbook is that students learn to conceptualize, appreciate, and use theory.

Pessimistic?

> *Nursing seems to be suffering in its quest for a scientific foundation. Like the mythological Danaids who kept filling their jars with water only to have it leak through the holes, nursing finds its search for scientific underpinnings as elusive as the liquid.*
>
> —*Jean Watson (1981, p. 413)*

Although it has been almost four decades since Jean Watson wrote her insightful words about nursing's theoretical base, and since then we have done a few important things as fast as we can, her words still ring true and make us a little uncomfortable. I ask that we revalue nursing concepts and theory development, the way we teach them and expect them to be used. We must work together with our quantitative colleagues—who need this same understanding of theory. Mixed methods provide one way to overcome this barrier, but there are other ways. Some are embarrassingly simple; others are not so easy, requiring a change of values, practice, and policy.

For instance, in this book, I challenge some assumptions about the literature: "old" literature (defined as more than 5 or 10 years, or whatever cut-off) is often considered "expired" —that is, a period considered not worth searching in the databases or of reading, and if cited, is an indication that the work is outdated. This "rule," perhaps coming from medicine and hard sciences, is not true for social science behavioral research, which is still very pertinent to our understanding of the concepts we will explore. This means that when you are searching the literature, I expect you to conduct your literature searches as far back as you need to go. *Behavioral descriptions do not expire. We must acknowledge and cite the seminal efforts to develop behavioral concepts and to grasp our conceptual foundations.* Nursing has not yet learned to be respectful of the ideas and research of those who have come before, and we can ill afford unnecessary replication and reinventing. As I age, I am frustrated with our tendency to ignore, do-over, repeat, rediscover, unknowingly replicate, and reinvent work that is languishing in the library.

Next, I ask for a more global and less segmented approach to concept and theory development and research, between research theory and the theory of practice; and between theory for practice and concept and theory development.

Concept and theory development is not something that is "done" somewhere at the beginning of the doctoral program and checked off—it should permeate all our programs in the baccalaureate and graduate levels. It should be something that lives both within us and in our research and practice, even below our level of awareness. It should make us better scholars, better researchers, better nurses, and wiser people.

Where to Place This Textbook on Your Bookshelf

Should this book be classified as a textbook about nursing theory or as a research textbook? One indicator of the uniqueness of the approach to theory in this book is the dilemma of "where to file it." It is a research book about theory; our goal for this textbook is to teach critical thinking and provide skills to enhance the understanding of the structure of nursing knowledge. It is intended for use at the beginning of programs for graduate nurses, before they begin their research courses.

This textbook is not a compendium of, nor an analysis of, what are known as traditional nursing theories; there are already many books that do that. Neither is this book a research text in the usual sense, and it is not meant to replace qualitative, quantitative, or mixed-method research texts.

This textbook is foundational in that it will facilitate students learning to conceptualize, appreciate theory, and, we hope, enjoy learning. It will give students the skills to access the essence of nursing—the parts that have been out of reach for too long. And it will, we hope, enable them, as the next generation, to create a strong and relevant theoretical base for nursing.

Janice M. Morse

REFERENCES

Morse, J. M., & Johnson, J. (1991). *The illness experience: Dimensions of suffering.* Newbury Park, CA: Sage. Retrieved from http://goo.gl/6va9Ql

Watson, J. (1981). Nursing's scientific quest. *Nursing Outlook, 29*(7), 413–416.

ACKNOWLEDGMENTS

I have a lot of people to thank for their assistance over the years. The credit for the development of my thinking—for agreement, disagreement, even tolerance—over the course of more than 30 years goes to my professors, students, patients, and research participants, who taught, haunted, challenged, and jarred my thinking.

To my colleagues in research, both collaborators and students: I know we learned and grew from our collaborative efforts, including the technical arts of researching, thinking, and writing, and that, for me, was an unexpected bonus. I thank you for your assistance and enthusiasm, your excitement at seeing emergence, and your enduring support. Your contribution is acknowledged and endures in citations and reference lists everywhere.

Special thanks go to my colleagues beyond nursing, who tolerated and patiently explained alternative approaches, concepts, and theories. Special thanks go to Carl Mitcham, who unstintingly shifted his perspective from philosophy, ethics, and engineering to nursing, effluvia, and the agony of living—patiently, and without even sniggering.

Writing this book required special help. I thank the Ida May "Dotty" Barnes, RN, and D. Keith Barnes, MD, Presidential Endowed Chair, University of Utah College of Nursing, for the time to write. Thanks to Tracii Haynes for her vital (and cheery) assistance, and to students from my theory classes and my faculty friends, both near and far, for their advice and support. Particular admiration goes to the authors of sections and chapters in this book, for their knowledge, skills, speed-writing, patience, and flexibility. I thank Mary McFarland, Eccles Health Science Library, for her support and skill, and Mitch Allen for his astute advice. Thanks to my supporters, Lauren Clark, Nancy Allen, Stephanie Richardson, and Joanne Singleton, for keeping me sane, and for their fine contributions both to this book and to my life. To my husband, Bob, for his careful attention to my often-jumbled sentences, and his astute listening ear: Thank you.

SECTION I

DESPERATELY SEEKING THEORY

I'm taking a research class, and as a final project we need to develop a research study. I have pretty much everything I need: question, sample, environment, review of lit, all of that. What I don't have is a theory to use as the "framework" for my study. I'm not sure how to go about finding it.

How do your programs present this? Are you provided with a list of theories, as a suggestion? Are there lists out there, which can at least be used as a jumping off point?

Part of my frustration is that I feel like I'm ready to write this project . . . and rather than look for a theoretical framework that helps my project, I'm now looking for a theoretical framework that *fits* my project. It's an exercise, not true assistance. Oh, and while I actually like a lot of aspects of research, I really despise theory. Probably doesn't help matters.

—Bluegrass, RN[1] (October 18, 2010)

---

[1] Retrieved from http://goo.gl/lSoH5a January 10, 2014.

Janice M. Morse   1

THE FRINGES OF KNOWLEDGE

> *If I go out into nature, into the unknown, to the fringes of knowledge,*
> *everything seems mixed up and contradictory, illogical and incoherent.*
> *This is what research does; it smoothes out contradiction and makes*
> *things simple, logical and coherent.*
> —Szent-Gyorgi (1972, p. 966)

"Research" and "scholarship" form two keystones of the faculty role. "Teaching" and "service" are the other two interrelated components,[1] but the main worry of a faculty member in 2016 is meeting criteria of "research-and-scholarship" in order to be tenured, promoted, and keep one's job teaching, researching, and scholarship-ing.

The reason for this anxiety is complex. First, *doing research* requires that one "come up" with a project that is reasonably unique, that will make an applied contribution, is fundable and publishable, and is, at the same time, interesting enough to hold one's attention for 1 to 2 years. These are all components over which a person has little, if any, control—especially the funding criterion. However, there is a disjuncture: Whereas we teach research endlessly in the classroom, particularly at the doctoral level, in classes to develop research skills (i.e., mostly research design and statistics), classes for "scholarship" are missing—unless one makes a rather difficult argument that such content is integrated throughout the program.

I asked students what the difference was between research and scholarship. How were they interrelated? They agreed that they were connected and astutely pointed out the research could be technical, structured; scholarship more creative.

"Can you do one without the other?" I asked.

"No," they said. "Scholarship is crucial for the development of the idea; for recognizing the implications and application of the research."

---

[1] Rosenthal et al. (1994).

My next question was: "Why is 'research' apparently more valued by universities and the public, than is 'scholarship'?"

Students:

> Research has a pay line, if funded, grants make the university happy, and if it's applied research, the pay line is in the form of a potential patent. Scholarship may have a minor pay line, indirectly, in the form of royalties.[2]

By this time I was feeling uncomfortable; were we so transparent that new graduate students could see our problems? Since when did academic research become a business? Scholarship appeared to be an essential skill—necessary for research; yet it did not have equal monetary reward and was not formally taught.

"How do you learn to become a scholar, if it is not taught?"

No answer.

This book is an attempt to fill this gap. In this book we discuss the theoretical foundations of nursing—how we find, develop, and use concepts and theory; how concepts and theory form the basis of research and how they are used and applied clinically. Most importantly, I hope the book will teach "how to think" and "how we think" as health care researchers and as professionals. I hope it will be the beginnings of appreciating scholarship, and revaluing it in nursing—for without it our research is a rote exercise, and we will be stymied as a profession, dogpaddling at the Olympics.

But scholarship *is* becoming valued, although rather awkwardly. The Magnet® designation to improve nursing[3] has required that philosophies of nursing and frameworks for practice be applied at the institutional level. But frameworks are selected by hospitals (or rather by nurses working in those institutions) and now used to organize our practice—those that were primarily developed in the 1970s and 1980s, and philosophies developed since the 1990s. Examples of frameworks for nursing care from the 1970s were Orem's Self-Care Model (first published in 1971, followed by at least five editions since that time [Denyes, Orem, & Bekel, 2001; Orem, 1980, 1985, 1991, 1995]), Roy's Adaptation Model (1970, 1988, 2009a, 2009b, 2011a, 2011b; Roy & Andrews, 1999; Roy, Wetsell, & Federickson, 2009), Leininger's Sunrise Model (Leininger, 1978, 1995), Leininger's Culture Care Theory, (1981, 1988, 1995, 2002), and, more recently, Kolcaba's Theory of Comfort (Kolcaba,

---

[2] Missing from the students' rationale of the pay line of scholarship, was "dissemination." While dissemination is usually treated as a research function, it is actually a function of scholarship. In Chapter 39, I discuss how, to be disseminated, an article must be read, understood, recognized as useful, and most of all, *liked*.

[3] The Magnet Recognition Program, organized by the American Nurses Credentialing Center, provides credentials to institutions for "quality patient care, nursing excellence and innovations in professional Nursing practice" (see www.nursecredentialing.org/Magnet/ProgramOverview.aspx).

2003; Kolcaba, Tilton, & Drouin, 2006). Examples of philosophies of care[4] are Parse's Human Becoming Theory (Parse, 1981, 1992, 1996, 1998, 1999, 2001) that posits quality of life from each person's own perspective as the goal of nursing practice, and Watson's Transpersonal Caring Relationships, which are used to guide our practice (Watson, 1985, 1988, 1999, 2000, 2002, 2006, 2007, 2008, 2009).

Although these conceptual modes or frameworks and philosophies have been used in research (e.g., Roy, 2014) and practice (e.g., Parker, 2010), they do not directly prescribe nursing interventions, but rather provide a way to conceptually organize or to guide caregiving. On the other hand, more specific concepts, models, and mid-range theories derived from qualitative research, wasting away in libraries and in journals, are still separated from patient care by the infamous research–practice "gap."[5] These models and mid-range theories are usually developed from detailed observations essential for directing patient-centered care: from interviews, stories of care from patients, nurses, or relatives, but they are considered too specific to guide comprehensive policies necessary for institutional use. This research, for instance, is directed to particular patient groups (patients with diabetes, or who have had a stroke, or are learning to breastfeed) or problems (experiencing immobility, a loss, or living in an abusive relationship). At the same time, quantitative theories, mainly directed toward improving technical, procedural aspects of care, are being tested, revised, and sometimes applied in practice. This research may compare and evaluate procedures, and make recommendations, thus contributing to evidence-based care.

Although the need for excellent, useful patient-centered theory remains an urgent requirement for the provision of care, nursing's theoretical foundation continues to be weak. The art of nursing suffers. We have little to build upon, and little that separates our theory from social science theory in general. We still use concepts borrowed from sociology, anthropology, public health, or other disciplines. These are concepts that fit our caregiving mission poorly, discounting important aspects of the patient experience, such as intimacy and dependency, and theories that appear stagnant and static in our fast-paced, flexible, and rapidly changing discipline.

THE SCIENCE OF THE ART

Nursing is a fascinating profession. Everyone agrees it is essential at the societal and individual levels. Everyone agrees it is a rewarding and satisfying

---

[4] Parse's work and Watson's work are regarded and evaluated as theories, but I am arguing they are *used* as philosophies, providing beliefs and values that less directly guide practice.

[5] The research–practice gap refers to the non-utilization of research in the clinical arena (see Squires et al., 2011).

profession. Yet no one[6] can be certain about how nursing *works*—what good nursing is—or even agree on a definition of nursing.

Now, this is a common problem in science: I study patient falls, and no one can produce a valid and comprehensive definition of a *fall* either, but we will not solve that problem in this book.[7] Nevertheless, there is a huge difference between defining an event (a fall) and something as important, essential, and comprehensive as a *nurse* and *nursing*. And as many have noted, not being able to articulate what a nurse—or nursing—is and does, cripples our professional identify (Summers & Summers, 2010).

But, there is worse. We cannot agree about what a nurse *does*, and how we attempt to determine this is impeded by our profession's value placed upon "real" science; we fund studies on particular nursing care problems (usually physiological or technical), but ignore our largest and most significant problems (such as how to endure illness, of noncompliance, and what it means to be ill).

We do not have a clear understanding of the nursing phenomenon associated with our nursing practice. In the 1980s, we conducted time-and-motion studies, trying to get at this question (e.g., see Giovannetti, 1978); now we have moved toward demonstrating nursing competency by measuring inputs and outputs, indicators of morbidity at the population level[8] (Aiken et al., 2012) leaving the internal, daily caring, unexamined. Can we be satisfied with the nurse–patient relationship, integral to our profession, as being described as "intuitive" (Benner, 1984, 2004; Benner & Tanner, 1984; Benner, Tanner, & Chesla, 1996/2009)?

We know, of course, that nursing is distinct from medicine and that we have a different focus, different concerns, and different practices, yet we have difficulties even with understanding the everyday phenomena that we handle. Pain is an excellent example of a nursing phenomenon that we do not approach comprehensively from the nursing perspective. Even the evaluation of pain using a 1 to 10 rating is the butt of jokes.[9]

Drugs for the alleviation of pain are primarily the purview of pharmacy and medicine, although even this line is blurring.[10] Administering pain medication is largely within the scope of nursing (but usually under the prescriptive privilege of medicine), but analgesics are not the only way to alleviate pain. Nonpharmaceutical methods of alleviating pain are important and

---

[6] No one? Try asking a patient!

[7] A recent study by Simon, Klaus, Gajewski, and Dinton (2013) explored the definition of patient falls by asking a large sample of nurses how they defined a fall, seeking agreement. Yet all of these nurses had been taught how a fall was defined in their safety program and in nursing school—so that this study was not actually defining a fall, merely tautologically what nurses had actually been taught. This "posttest" design is not uncommon in research.

[8] I am thinking of the work of Aitken, who showed differences in patient outcomes by level of education of the nurses (Aiken, Clarke, Cheung, Sloane, & Silber, 2003; Aiken et al., 2011; Sermeus et al., 2011).

[9] "My doggie has a broken molar. The vet scored her 2 out of 5 on a chronic pain scale."

[10] "I did so clean her teeth—Does anyone study the shames of caregiving?"

within the purview of nursing, yet they are poorly integrated into our practice, seldom listed in our nursing notes, and poorly researched. And even if we knew such techniques, if we do not have time to do them, then they are lost to our profession.[11]

Nursing becomes impotent.

Rest and sleep is another example of an everyday nursing care problem that is poorly addressed by nursing. Even Florence Nightingale made a case for the patient to "be in the best positions for nature to heal" (Nightingale, 1860/1969), yet we continue to wake patients, shine lights in their faces while they sleep, permit a noisy environment during the day (as well as night), and keep patients busy with examinations, tests, visitors, and other poorly coordinated events during their short hospitalization. In this noisiness we do not schedule or provide for daytime rest periods. No time to heal.

We do not practice what we know.

We spend little time observing patients, and little time learning what it is like to be a patient, to be in pain, facing loss, facing death. If we understood these things, the mechanisms of how they worked, and the impact on our patients as persons, our interventions would be on target, our intervention "kit sets" would increase many fold, and we could truly make our care evidence-based and our outcomes appropriate.

We could stop guessing.

If we developed our concepts, we would have a consistent language that explained nursing phenomena. It would give us a language, so we would be able to understand and communicate about our practice, both to ourselves and to others. Research would be consistent, on target, and would take a giant leap forward.[12]

Which of our concepts are underdeveloped? Even our major ones: No one suggests that the nurse's role is not important. We are an integral part of caring and the maintenance of health—at least half of the equation. Yet the term "caring" is ambiguous, and lacks precision. We do not fully grasp how the caring interaction works; if we did, we would be a step closer to understanding what we do, would do it more deliberately, and would even demonstrate evidence and efficacy.

We cannot develop a profession from the "fringes of knowledge." But before becoming too discouraged, let us take stock of our assets. We are advantaged by having a discipline that is well established, so that we are not developing our knowledge base from scratch. Thus it seems reasonable that if we analyze the care nursing actually provides in the moment, then we will be able to describe, to articulate, to classify, and to identify concepts and to develop nursing-specific theories. We will be able to understand the

---

[11] "Hmmmm. The shames in caregiving??? How come no one writes about that? Another hole in the literature . . ."

[12] "But there is a lot in the caregiving literature about guilt!"

mechanisms of nursing care and identify our outcomes. We will develop as a profession.

EXPLORING THE FRINGES: THE CLINICAL UTILITY OF CONCEPT INQUIRY

Why do we care? Qualitative inquiry has assumed the role of describing nursing care. But qualitative inquiry has produced compartmentalized studies; these are generally isolated units that do not build on one another. Even qualitative researchers, who cite one another in their literature reviews and discussions, insist on developing their studies entirely inductively, from scratch, and naming their categories, themes, concepts, and theories by creating their own emic labels. *Emic labels* refers to those names that are terms generally used by the participants and derived from data that are particular to each study. Some qualitative researchers using emic labels do not take the time, or care, to go the additional step and compare their findings with other qualitative researchers' findings or the concepts already described in the literature. The result is that our literature is cluttered with similar concepts and processes with various names and results in something that I have labeled as "theoretical congestion" (Morse, 2000). This keeps our research close to data, and does not result in the development of a set of useful concepts, enable abstraction, generalization, the incremental building of theory—or even enabled confirmation of others' findings by our colleagues. The fact that we must work inductively does not excuse us—researchers can avoid deductive threats to validity when using the work of others (or one's own prior work), by building within scaffolds (i.e., creating dense detail within the frame of another's work) or on skeletons (i.e., the using the work of others as a foundation; Morse & Mitcham, 2002). Neither do recent efforts at qualitative meta-syntheses facilitate the type of concept formation and theory building that is needed.[13]

We desperately need good concepts: concepts for and about nursing. These are concepts that can be understood *in use*: concepts that would clarify our practice. We desperately need pertinent, solid, and valid operational definitions building consistent quantitative concepts; we need excellent pertinent nursing theory that will guide our practice in the institution and at the bedside.

THE ESSENTIALNESS OF EXAMINING OUR PRACTICE

"You study *that!*" This comment of disbelief was from a quantitative researcher who had dropped into my office to see what qualitative research

---

[13] Q: "What is the difference between guilt and shame?"

was all about. At that particular moment, I was analyzing a video of trauma care, with all its apparent confusion and noise from everyone speaking at once, crowded around the gurney. I dissected the scene for him, explaining the roles of each person and what I call the channels of communication—who is talking to whom. I explained the focus of my study, the nurse and the patient; how they used the loudest of all of the channels of communication—and that their voices could be easily be heard over the top of the noise. As the patient screamed, my guest shrugged, made a face, and quickly left.

Undoubtedly such scenes of providing urgent care appear chaotic to those unfamiliar with trauma care—but to trauma nurses, the confusion is not an issue when describing their roles or responsibilities. They understand some of their actions, what they actually do and why. I am not talking about taking blood pressures, or recording, or other established and formalized technical tasks, but rather, how nurses interact and help patients through the assessment and treatments, how they assist patients to maintain control, how they manage the environment—even controlling the panic and shouting of the physicians—and how they keep care paced and prevent multiple procedures being done at the same time to various parts of the patient's body. Nurses new to the trauma care told me that they "watched experienced nurses 'like a hawk'" for at least a year—not to learn technical procedures, but to learn how to "manage" patients. They were especially concerned about patients who could not be considered responsible for their own behaviors: patients in agony, inebriated, mentally ill, or patients who fought care and fought off caregivers.

But if we observe carefully, or interview nurses, asking them to tell us about their interventions, their emotions, and other components of care that cannot always be observed, we find that nurses have complex cognitive responses and do much that is not described in textbooks or taught in the classroom—or reported in the media.

Once I asked emergency room (ER) nurses if I could come and observe how they comforted patients, and they told me: "Sure you can come, but we do not have time to comfort patients." I came, observed, and classified their actions into categories of comforting.

Some of these were:

- Talking patients through agonizing pain
- Keeping the normal/keeping things cool
- Keeping the doctors on track
- Bringing in the relatives (see Box 1.1)

Then I met with the nurses to present my results. They were stunned: "Yes we do *do* all of those things, but they are not part of our work." I told them those undocumented tasks were lifesaving, critical for excellent care, and critical for the smooth, rapid conduct of the resuscitation.

> **BOX 1.1. DESCRIPTIONS OF COMFORTING STRATEGIES ROUTINELY USED BY EMERGENCY NURSES**
>
> **Talking patients through agonizing pain:** Later I studied "talking through" with speech communication specialist Adele Proctor, describing the *comfort talk register* (CTR; Morse & Proctor, 1998; Proctor, Morse, & Khonsari, 1996). I am convinced that when pain is overwhelming, the nurses' use of the CTR is lifesaving.
>
> **Keeping the normal/keeping things cool:** Nurses deliberately control panic behaviors of the patient and the physicians. (One nurse deliberately sang during the trauma.) Nurses constantly monitor the environment and the patient, while the physicians focus on the puzzle of diagnosis.
>
> **Keeping the doctors on track:** Nurses remind physicians when the patient last had analgesic, when it is time to move the patient for a scan or to intensive care unit (ICU), and so forth.
>
> **Bringing in the relatives:** Nurses are very aware of relatives waiting outside and offer them support, and bring them in to see their injured relatives. During this time, nurses are vigilant, watching the relatives in case they become emotionally overwhelmed, and even collapse.

Describing what nurses actually do is the most urgent task of nursing research, and is discussed often in this text.[14]

But description in itself is not enough. We need to develop concepts and theories from those descriptions; we need to operationalize those concepts and theories, and move this content into our texts, to the classroom, to nursing research, and then back into nursing. We need to develop and test theories. Once we do this, nurses will be able to be paid for all that they do, workload calculations may be corrected, care improved, and nurses may be taught comprehensively, and nursing research will move forward in giant steps.

Who will do this describing and theorizing?

You will.

You will do it as a student; you will do it in the classroom, you will do it as a researcher; you will do it as become a published author.

If we are to develop and to test theories, describing and theorizing is an essential, continuous and ongoing activity, and it is the responsibility of us all.

But before we move forward to the "how" let us explore the role of values in what we see and do, as a foundation for the concepts we select to study and the theories we develop. We then discuss the role of conceptual inquiry and theory in nursing as it is related to the development of the nursing profession.

WHY DO WE HAVE TO KNOW?

Already I have discussed how developing the theoretical foundations of nursing will facilitate the education of our nurses, our research, and our

---

[14] ANS: "Guilt is not cleaning the teeth at all; shame is merely doing a poor job of brushing."

practice. But what I have also tried to communicate is that exploring the implicit components of nursing is not easy. (If it were easy, it would have already been done.) It is difficult because of the nature of nursing itself and the way the art of nursing works.

How the Art of Nursing Works

Nursing has many characteristics that make it a unique profession. There is no question that the therapeutic part of the nursing occurs between the nurse and the patient, yet we sequentially replace each other around the clock and day by day. Despite this, nurses still manage to work effectively, even with patients whom they have not seen before. Three characteristics, co-occurring, make nursing both complex and unique.

Reading the Patient

First, "reading the patient" is the speed at which nurses make implicit and explicit judgments. We see a patient walk into the ER, and nurses must approach that person with the correct affect, with minimal information, whether the person is angry, distraught, in despair, in acute pain, or confused or inebriated. Nurses walk into a patient's room, find the patient in acute distress, and must respond to the distress before they know exactly the circumstances causing the distress. This they do by *reading the patient's cues* and adjusting their responses to the patient's cues of distress. This implicit part of nursing is learned by experience, as a part of becoming an expert nurse, and forms a critical part of the nurse–patient interaction.

These same rapid responses occur as the nurse observes the patient's condition: for signs of shock; indices of pain or discomfort; or signs of improvement, relief, or comfort. And, the nurse makes her judgment while doing other tasks.

Multitasking

The second significant characteristic is that the nurse is rarely doing one task at a time. While a nurse is greeting the patient, he or she is also assessing, identifying needs, and prioritizing care. While they are taking a blood pressure, they are also noting other signs—the condition and temperature of the skin, odor of the breadth, while asking if the patient slept well.

Relationship Building

Nurses know that technically perfect care can be provided to a mannequin—yet this care is not good nursing care. For good care to occur there must be a relationship between the nurse and the patient. Both must trust each another—patients trust the nurse to watch over them while they sleep, or are in declining illness, or as they die. Correspondingly, patients will do their part: following instructions, reporting new symptoms, and swallowing their pills.

THE ROLE OF VALUES IN DEVELOPING KNOWLEDGE

Currently, as a profession, we are moving rapidly toward a research and evidence-based practice—focusing on care practices that are supposedly true, right, and proven. But let us for a moment step back, behind those truths, and talk about our assumptions, our beliefs, and our values that determine our profession, our roles in society, and even how we think.

Facts and Values

Only a part of what we see in the world may be considered facts. Facts are "hard," concrete, and real, usually stable (unchanging) and may be replicated from one time to another, from one place to another, and from one person to another. Facts may be verified, proven, tested, and demonstrated, and are validated by directly comparing the description with the actual entity. Only some components of nursing fit this model.

Our reality is subjective. Nursing is a human, interpersonal profession. What we see in our interactions with others is based on a combination of our values and beliefs, our cultural perspective, and our opinions and perceptions. Thus, despite accuracy in measurement, even what those measures mean is subject to interpretation. This subjectivity may be an advantage or a disadvantage. It advantages nursing, for instance, if our values are considered beneficial and support nursing, such as basing our practice on the value of caring. On the other hand it may be harmful, if we believe, for instance, that pain must be tolerated (rather than relieved or alleviated); then we will not be providing analgesics when we should be, and so forth. And these two values, caring and refusing the right to pain relief, may occur concurrently.

Values and beliefs provide us with a particular way of seeing our practice in a certain way. They may blind us, bias us, or stigmatize our perspective. Alternatively, they may direct our practice in a positive way: these values may be convictions that drive us—as they drove Florence Nightingale to provide care in Crimea or Margaret Sanger to provide contraceptive care in the 1930s—or they may misguide us or harm our profession. For instance the belief that caring was a privilege, prerogative, or even the obligation of women, kept our salaries low, that caring was "good," a "natural" part of women's roles and even that we would "get our reward in heaven." In childbirth, values sometimes placed pain "as a lesson," for instance to teach unwed women chastity, and may have resulted in few analgesics provided during labor. This differential perspective of values toward various ethnic groups or socioeconomic classes may have resulted in differential care, with better care for some groups, and with poor immigrants or Black people receiving inferior care.

TO DO 1.1. IS IT GOOD TO CARE?

Something to think about: We believe that caring is "good," but this value may be contradicted by other actions. Watch Steven King's (1990) film *Misery.* Observe and document the caring behaviors of nurse Annie Wilkes. Think about her role, her behaviors, and her underlying affect. Nurses have found themselves in precarious positions because of their caregiving skills—such as working in prisoner of war camps. Discuss the relationship between care and kindness and from the patient's perspective, if *kindness* or *caring* is the more important value to the nurse–patient relationship, is more essential, and could make a greater difference. Consider other situations that make the value of kindness and care (or caring) contradictory.

Perceptions of Reality

Our perception of the world (or our worldview) determines our emotional responses, what we believe is right, and our actions: how we live on a daily basis. It determines our behavior: how we organize our day, how we move through events, how we make the most of opportunities, how we resolve problems, and how these differ from one another. Our perceptions may show one setting as a normal event whereas the same setting might appear to another person as a frightening and confusing affair. We know this from the first day of school as a child, from moving to a new city, from taking a driving test, and from starting the first day of the graduate theory class.

It is our perception of the subjective world that makes research difficult. In order to conduct research, to obtain consistency, validity, and reliability, we must all be talking about the same phenomenon, using the same definitions, from the same perspective. We must be clear, consistent, and able to describe exactly what we mean. Even so, it is disconcerting to realize that despite such precautions and precision, we may be wrong.

THE RISE OF NURSING RESEARCH AND THE USE OF FRAMEWORKS AND MODELS

Since the time of Nightingale, research has been an integral part of the nursing profession. Note how I have worded this—as a part of the nursing profession, not necessarily a part of nursing practice. Nursing traditionally has been a profession based on priorities and principles, on techniques and habits, rules and regulations; on the appearances of cleanliness, rather than knowledge derived from research. Moving research into nursing practice has been the challenge to nursing for many decades, and it is only since nursing has made a concerted effort, through the evidence-based nursing movement (Melnyk & Fineout-Overholt, 2011), that there has been a deliberate and policy-based effort to actually use research clinically.

TO DO 1.2. RESEARCH EVIDENCE AS A HOLY GRAIL

My practice area is the prevention of patient falls. We know that one of the difficulties for older adults is poor eyesight and glare from polished floors.

Look at your institution, and see how sunlight bounces along the corridors.

Why is the floor shiny? It has something to do with the association of the concepts of "shine" and "clean," and shiny *meaning*, or indicating, clean. Yet the association between shine and cleanliness is a moot relationship, because floor polish now comes in matt finishes, and costs exactly the same as polish with a shiny finish—so it is not a cost issue. It is the *value* of the shine to the institution, and valuing the shine over patient safety.

Have you ever tried to get the housekeeping department to change their polish? One manager pulled himself up to his full height: "Where is the evidence?" he asked.

"In *Gray's Anatomy* of the eye," I replied, equally glibly.

The shiny floor remained.

DISCUSS

Do we need an experimental study of corridors, comparing *shiny* with *matt* finishes, and measuring slips and falls (a relatively rare event) to demonstrate something that is so obvious? I have more to do with my time—yet without a golden *p* value, change will not occur.

Why do we value research results?

Why do we rely on policy changes, rather than instigating such a change?

REFERENCES

Aiken, L. H., Cimiotti, J. P., Sloane, D. M., Smith, H. L., Flynn, L., & Neff, D. F. (2011). The effects of nurse staffing and nurse education on patient deaths in hospitals with different nurse work environments. *Medical Care, 49*(12), 1047–1053. doi:10.1097/MLR.0b013e3182330b6e

Aiken, L. H., Clarke, S. P., Cheung, R. B., Sloane, D. M., & Silber, J. H. (2003). Educational levels of hospital nurses and surgical patient mortality. *The Journal of the American Medical Association, 290*(12), 1617–1623. doi:10.1001/jama.290.12.1617

Aiken, L. H., Sermeus, W., Van den Heede, K., Sloane, D. M., Busse, R., McKee, M., . . . Kutney-Lee, A. (2012). Patient safety, satisfaction, and quality of hospital care: Cross sectional surveys of nurses and patients in 12 countries in Europe and the United States. *British Medical Journal, 344*, e1717. doi:10.1136/bmj.e1717

Benner, P. (1984). *From novice to expert: Excellence and power in clinical nursing practice*. Menlo Park, CA: Addison-Wesley.

Benner, P. (2004). Using the Dreyfus model of skill acquisition to describe and interpret skill acquisition and clinical judgment in nursing practice and education. *Bulletin of Science, Technology & Society, 24*(3), 188–199. doi:10.1177/0270467604265061

Benner, P., & Tanner, C. (1984). How nurses use intuition. *American Journal of Nursing, 87*(1), 23–31.

Benner, P., Tanner, C. A., & Chesla, C. A. (1996/2009). *Expertise in nursing practice: Caring, clinical judgment and ethics*. New York, NY: Springer Publishing.

Denyes, M. J., Orem, D. E., & Bekel, G. (2001). Self-care: A foundational science. *Nursing Science Quarterly, 14*(1), 48–54.

Giovannetti, P. (1978). *Patient classification systems in nursing: A description and analysis* (Vol. 4). Hyattsville, MD: Department of Health, Education, and Welfare, Public Health Service, Health Resources Administration, Bureau of Health Manpower, Division of Nursing.

Kolcaba, K. (2003). *Comfort theory and practice: A vision for holistic health care*. New York, NY: Springer Publishing.

Kolcaba, K., Tilton, C., & Drouin, C. (2006). Comfort theory: A unifying framework to enhance the practice environment. *Journal of Nursing Administration, 36*(11), 538–544.

Leininger, M. M. (1978). *Transcultural nursing: Concepts, theories and practices*. New York, NY: John Wiley & Sons.

Leininger, M. M. (1981). Cross-cultural hypothetical functions of caring and nursing care. In M. M. Leininger (Ed.), *Caring: An essential human need* (pp. 133–143). Thorofare, NJ: Slack.

Leininger, M. M. (1988). Leininger's theory of nursing: Culture care diversity and universality. *Nursing Science Quarterly, 1*(4), 151–160.

Leininger, M. M. (1995). Overview of Leininger's culture care theory. In M. Leininger (Ed.), *Transcultural nursing concepts, theories, research & practices* (2nd ed., pp. 93–112). New York, NY: McGraw-Hill. College Custom Series.

Leininger, M. M. (2002). Culture care theory: A major contribution to advance transcultural nursing knowledge and practices. *Journal of Transcultural Nursing, 13*(3), 189–192.

Melnyk, B. M., & Fineout-Overholt, E. (Eds.). (2011). *Evidence-based practice in nursing and healthcare*. Philadelphia, PA: Wolters Kluwer Health.

Morse, J. M. (2000). Theoretical congestion [Editorial]. *Qualitative Health Research, 10*(6), 715–716.

Morse, J. M., & Mitcham, C. (2002). Exploring qualitatively-derived concepts: Inductive-deductive pitfalls. In J. M. Morse, J. E. Hupcey, J. Penrod, J. A. Spiers, C. Pooler, & C. Mitcham. (2002). Issues in validity: Behavioral concepts, their derivation and interpretation. *International Journal of Qualitative Methods, 1*(4), Article 3. Retrieved from http://ijq.sagepub.com/content/1/4/28.full.pdf+html

Morse, J. M., & Proctor, A. (1998). Maintaining patient endurance: The comfort work of trauma nurses. *Clinical Nursing Research, 7*(3), 250–274.

Nicoilaides, S., Reiner, R., Scheinman, R., & Stott, J. (Producers), & Reiner, R. (Director). (1990). *Misery* [Motion picture]. United States: Columbia Pictures.

Nightingale, F. (1860/1969). *Notes on Nursing: What it is and what it is not*. New York, NY: Dover.

Orem, D. E. (1980). *Nursing: Concepts of practice* (2nd ed.). New York, NY: McGraw-Hill.

Orem, D. E. (1985). *Nursing: Concepts of practice* (3rd ed.). Chevy Chase, MD: McGraw-Hill.

Orem, D. E. (1991). *Nursing: Concepts of practice* (4th ed.). St. Louis, MO: Mosby.

Orem, D. E. (1995). *Nursing: Concepts of practice* (5th ed.). St. Louis, MO: Mosby.

Parker, M. E. (2010). *Nursing theories & nursing practice*. Philadelphia, PA: F. A. Davis.

Parse, R. R. (1981). *Man-living-health: A theory of nursing*. New York, NY: Wiley.

Parse, R. R. (1992). Human becoming: Parse's theory of nursing. *Nursing Science Quarterly, 5*(1), 35–42.

Parse, R. R. (1996). The human becoming theory: Challenges in practice and research. *Nursing Science Quarterly, 9*(2), 55–60.

Parse, R. R. (1998). *The human becoming school of thought: A perspective for nurses and other health professionals*. Thousand Oaks, CA: Sage.

Parse, R. R. (1999). *Illuminations: The human becoming theory in practice and research*. Burlington, MA: Jones & Bartlett Learning.

Parse, R. R. (2001). Rosemary Rizzo Parse: The human becoming school of thought. In M. Parker (Ed.), *Nursing theories and nursing practice* (pp. 227–238). Philadelphia, PA: F.A. Davis.

Proctor, A., Morse, J. M., & Khonsari, E. S. (1996). Sounds of comfort in the trauma center: How nurses talk to patients in pain. *Social Science & Medicine, 42*(12), 1669–1680. doi:10.1016/0277-9536(95)00298-7

Rosenthal, J. T., Cogan, M. L., Marshall, R., Meiland, J. W., Wion, P. K., & Molotsky, I. F. (1994). The work of faculty-expectations, priorities, and rewards. *Academe-Bulletin of the AAUP, 80*(1), 35–48.

Roy, C. (1970). Adaptation: A conceptual framework for nursing. *Nursing Outlook, 18*(3), 42–48.

Roy, C. (1988). An explication of the philosophical assumptions of the Roy adaptation model. *Nursing Science Quarterly, 1*(1), 26–34.

Roy, C. (2009a). *The Roy adaptation model* (3rd ed.). Upper Saddle River, NJ: Pearson.

Roy, C. (2009b). *The Roy adaptation model* (3rd ed.). Upper Saddle River, NJ: Pearson.

Roy, C. (2011a). Research based on the Roy adaptation model: Last 25 years. *Nursing Science Quarterly, 24*(4), 312–320.

Roy, C. (2011b). Extending the Roy adaptation model to meet changing global needs. *Nursing Science Quarterly, 24*(4), 345–351.

Roy, C. (2014). *Generating middle range theory: From evidence to practice*. New York, NY: Springer Publishing.

Roy, C., & Andrews, H. A. (1999). *The Roy adaptation model* (2nd ed.). Stanford, CT: Appleton & Lange.

Roy, C., Whetsell, M. V., & Frederickson, K. (2009). The Roy adaptation model and research global perspective. *Nursing Science Quarterly, 22*(3), 209–211.

Sermeus, W., Aiken, L. H., Van den Heede, K., Rafferty, A. M., Griffiths, P., Moreno-Casbas, M. T., . . . Brzostek, T. (2011). Nurse forecasting in Europe (RN4CAST): Rationale, design and methodology. *BMC Nursing, 10*(1), 6–10.

Simon, M., Klaus, S., Gajewski, B. J., & Dinton, N. (2013). Agreement of fall classification among staff in U.S. hospitals. *Nursing Research, 62*(2), 74–81. doi:10.1097/NNR.0b013e31827bf8c9

Squires, J. E., Hutchinson, A. M., Boström, A. M., O'Rourke, H. M., Cobban, S. J., & Estabrooks, C. A. (2011). To what extent do nurses use research in clinical practice? A systematic review. *Implementation Science, 6*(1), 21. doi:10.1186/1748-5908-6-21

Summers, S., & Summers, H. J. (2010). *Saving Lives: Why the media's portrayal of nurses puts us all at risk.* New York, NY: Kaplan.

Szent-Gyorgyi, A. (1972). Dionysians and Apollonians. *Science, 176*(4038), 966.

Watson, J. (1985). *Nursing: Human science and human care.* New York, NY: Appleton-Century-Crofts.

Watson, J. (1988). *Nursing: Human science and human care: A theory of nursing.* New York, NY: National League for Nursing.

Watson, J. (1999). *Nursing: Human science and human care.* New York, NY: NLN/Jones & Bartlett.

Watson, J. (2000). Leading via caring-healing: The fourfold way toward transformative leadership. *Nursing Administration Quarterly, 25*(1), 1–6.

Watson, J. (2002). Intentionality and caring-healing consciousness: A practice of transpersonal nursing. *Holistic Nursing Practice, 16*(4), 12–19.

Watson, J. (2006). Caring theory as an ethical guide to administrative and clinical practices. *Nursing Administration Quarterly, 30*(1), 48–55.

Watson, J. (2007). Watson s theory of human caring and subjective living experiences: Carative factors/caritas processes as a disciplinary guide to the professional nursing practice. *Texto & Contexto-Enfermagem, 16*(1), 129–135.

Watson, J. (2008). *Nursing: The philosophy and science and caring* (Rev ed.). Boulder, CO: University Press of Colorado.

Watson, J. (2009). Caring science and human caring theory: Transforming personal and professional practices of nursing and health care. *Journal of Health and Human Services Administration, 31*(4), 466–482.

Janice M. Morse

2

WHERE WE CAME FROM

I have a confession—and an apology—to make. Once, in 1982, the director of nursing at a Canadian hospital decided to implement a nursing theory to guide nursing practice uniformly throughout the hospital. It was decided, using the principles of democracy, to let the nurses select the theory. Workshops were held describing the two main contenders, Orem's and Roy's theories, and nurses campaigned for their preferences. Signs appeared everywhere, and nurses wore buttons stating their favorite. (I wore both, of course. I still have mine somewhere.) After a certain period of time, elections were held, and nurses voted.

I cannot remember which theory "won" or, more importantly, if there was any subsequent change in care. But I can remember how scornful I was of the process. "Selecting a theory for care is not a political process," I said. Did they not understand that, if these theories worked, we would be able to see the difference in nursing care according to the theory selected? Did they not realize that by observing care, we should be able to identify an Orem nurse or a Roy nurse by their style of nursing? And, to my knowledge, because we could not do that, why are we bothering with all this performance? Besides, I muttered, the theory one uses should be in context, according to patient needs, nursing assessment, and patient preferences—it cannot be legislated carte blanche.

But I did not see it then as an opportunity to conduct research.

Now, almost, 30 years later, this is happening again, and on a much grander scale. For Magnet® hospital certification, staff select and implement a theory or framework to guide care within the hospital. Older and wiser, I hold my breath and hold my tongue. And watch.

CHASING NURSING THEORY

> *The topic of theory development has been addressed by nursing leaders since Flexner's definition of a profession appeared in the 1920s. Since that time nursing leaders have been attempting to determine whether or not nursing did indeed have a unique and identifiable body of knowledge.*
>
> —Johnson (1978, p. v)

In the past century, from about the 1960s, nursing leaders began to realize that in order for it to be a profession in its own right, nursing must be distinct from other disciplines, and they needed to delineate the role of nursing, as a distinct body of nursing knowledge. To attain this, nursing must be cohesively contained within a single nursing paradigm, with its own nursing theory or theories. They recognized that nursing must invest in science and develop a practice based on scientific principles. The result was a determined movement, decades long, to develop the discipline of nursing.[1]

Nursing needed leaders with vision, committed nurse theorists to create the theory (or theories), scientists to develop it, and educators to teach it. The key was to develop the theoretical base for nursing, and many components of this plan had to be conducted simultaneously. It was recognized that they needed nurse theorists to create the theory, nurse scientists to test the theory, journals and texts to communicate the theory, nurse educators to teach the theory, and nurses to use the theory for patient care and to develop practice.

In the following 30 years, many theories were created. Consider these theories, which I call *traditional nursing theories*, as they were envisioned and created by experienced nurses and academics of the past century. Although some theories may have been stimulated by observations from clinical practice, with few exceptions, they were not generally derived from research.

A timeline showing the major nursing theories or models is listed in Figure 2.1. The date preceding the author's name is the reference date indicating the major work. As these theories were developed over a period of time, the date in square brackets is the date of the first (or last) publication of the theory by the author. References are provided in Appendix 2.1.

THE NEED FOR NURSING THEORY

In the 1970s, the rush to develop nursing theory began in earnest. Some of these theories were very abstract; the theory by Martha Rogers (1970) was the

---

[1] A glossary of terms is provided in Chapter 5.

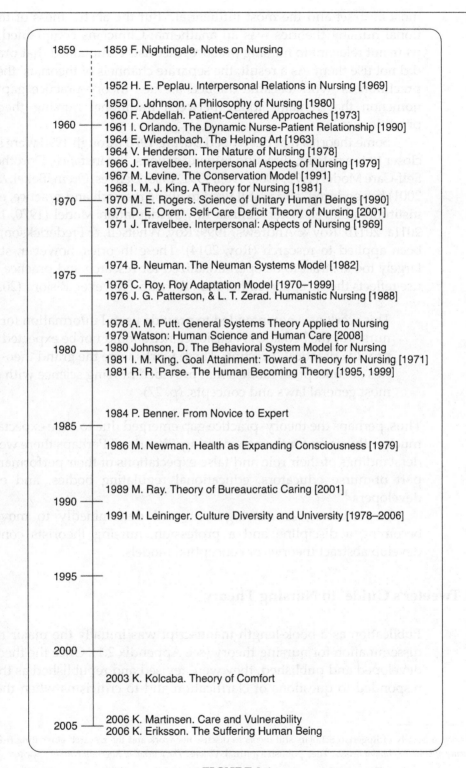

1859	1859 F. Nightingale. Notes on Nursing
	1952 H. E. Peplau. Interpersonal Relations in Nursing [1969]
	1959 D. Johnson. A Philosophy of Nursing [1980]
	1960 F. Abdellah. Patient-Centered Approaches [1973]
1960	1961 I. Orlando. The Dynamic Nurse-Patient Relationship [1990]
	1964 E. Wiedenbach. The Helping Art [1963]
	1964 V. Henderson. The Nature of Nursing [1978]
	1966 J. Travelbee. Interpersonal Aspects of Nursing [1979]
	1967 M. Levine. The Conservation Model [1991]
	1968 I. M. J. King. A Theory for Nursing [1981]
1970	1970 M. E. Rogers. Science of Unitary Human Beings [1990]
	1971 D. E. Orem. Self-Care Deficit Theory of Nursing [2001]
	1971 J. Travelbee. Interpersonal: Aspects of Nursing [1969]
	1974 B. Neuman. The Neuman Systems Model [1982]
1975	
	1976 C. Roy. Roy Adaptation Model [1970–1999]
	1976 J. G. Patterson, & L. T. Zerad. Humanistic Nursing [1988]
	1978 A. M. Putt. General Systems Theory Applied to Nursing
	1979 Watson: Human Science and Human Care [2008]
1980	1980 Johnson, D. The Behavioral System Model for Nursing
	1981 I. M. King. Goal Attainment: Toward a Theory for Nursing [1971]
	1981 R. R. Parse. The Human Becoming Theory [1995, 1999]
1985	1984 P. Benner. From Novice to Expert
	1986 M. Newman. Health as Expanding Consciousness [1979]
1990	1989 M. Ray. Theory of Bureaucratic Caring [2001]
	1991 M. Leininger. Culture Diversity and University [1978–2006]
1995	
2000	
	2003 K. Kolcaba. Theory of Comfort
2005	2006 K. Martinsen. Care and Vulnerability
	2006 K. Eriksson. The Suffering Human Being

FIGURE 2.1

Timeline showing introduction of traditional nursing theories.

most abstract and the most influential.[2] But the abstractness of these traditional nursing theories was an anathema: Clinicians complained that they were not relevant to nursing practice; theorists complained that practitioners did not use them. As a result, the separate channels of theorists' theories and practitioners' work became dubbed as the "theory–practice gap"—a phenomenon that remains today between traditional nursing theorists and practitioners.

Some theories that developed during 1970 through 1990 were somewhat closer to the patient, directing nursing actions. For instance, Dorothea Orem's Self-Care Model (1971, 1980, 1985, 1991, 1995; Denyes, Orem, Bekel, & SozWiss, 2001) has endured, and is still used to guide research and practice, even at the institutional level. Sister Callista Roy's Adaptation Model (1970, 1988, 2009, 2011a, 2011b; Roy & Andrews, 1999; Roy, Whetsell, & Frederickson, 2009) has been applied to research (Roy, 2014). These theories, however, still remain largely too abstract to be operationalized for research and practice, and their use reflects the exception rather than the rule. However, Risjord (2010) notes:

> This work was not intended to provide useful information for nurses at the bedside . . . Basic science should not be expected to provide practical direction. These works were the grand theories or conceptual models that provided nursing science with its most general laws and concepts. (p. 27)

Thus, perhaps the theory–practice gap emerged due to false expectations, too much enthusiasm for the new nursing "theories." Perhaps there were misunderstandings of their role and false expectations of their performance on the part of nurse educators, educational regulating bodies, and even their developers.[3]

Nevertheless, as nursing continued determinedly to move toward becoming a discipline and a profession, nursing theorists continued to develop abstract theories or conceptual models.

A Tweeter's Guide[4] to Nursing Theory

Publication as a book-length manuscript was initially the major method of dissemination for nursing theory (see Appendix 2.1). Once the theories were developed and published, they were revised and republished as the authors responded to questions of clarification and to criticisms when the theories

---

[2] Today, a Society of Rogerian Scholars still meets to discuss her work and the research emanating from the theory *Science of Unitary Human Beings*. They publish a journal, *Visions: The Journal of Rogerian Nursing Science*.

[3] What do you think Florence Nightingale's intent was in 1860, when she wrote *Notes on Nursing: What It Is and What It Is Not*?

[4] Tweeter: An active user of the website Twitter.

were implemented in practice or used in research. Alternatively, journal articles were used for the dissemination of nursing theory, and these articles were often updates or minor modifications of the theory. Of necessity, these articles were shorter and lacking essential details about the major theory. In particular, some journals have made significant contributions to nursing theory, especially *Advances in Nursing Science,* and later, *Nursing Science Quarterly* (Meleis, 2012).

In the past 20 years, these theory books have been replaced with edited books that devote a chapter to each theorist's theory, sometimes presented by the theorists themselves, and sometimes by another person familiar their work (e.g., Alligood & Marriner-Torney, 2010; McEwan & Wills, 2014). However, this literature lacks the scientific debate and criticism of nursing theory in these books and nursing journals—something that would normally occur in other disciplines (Paley, 2006)—and this lack ultimately stymied the development and testing of the theories.

Another more recent development in dissemination of these theories is the websites that have appeared, which list skeletal summaries of most of the major theories. For instance, these sites provide only the major concepts, propositions, categories, and so forth in point form for each theory.[5] Although these summaries are convenient for nurses needing to grasp an overview of each theory, they do not provide a full understanding. We have reached the ultimate reduction of the substance of nursing theory.

The Development of Core Nursing Metaparadigmatic Concepts

Nursing was still concerned about developing a unique domain, which Hardy (1978) described as presenting a general orientation that "holds a commitment and consensus of the scientists of a particular discipline" (p. 39). Attempting to reach consensus on what was nursing, in 1972, the National League for Nursing (NLN) Council of Baccalaureate and Higher Degree Programs in Nursing stated that nursing curricula should be based on a conceptual framework. Yura and Torres surveyed 50 accredited programs from 1972 to 1973 in order to identify "concepts used by the majority" (Yura & Torres, 1975, p. 2). Four central concepts (man, society, health, and nursing) were identified by these researchers (Torres & Yura, 1975) as a curriculum framework to organize and give "clarity and direction to the program's philosophy, so that it can be clearly developed into courses and learning experiences" (p. 8). These central concepts were intended to link the philosophy,

---

[5] Some of the websites summarizing traditional nursing theories are:
Current Nursing: Open Access Nursing Research and Review Articles: http://goo.gl/ubTfJh
Nursing Theory JCHS Library (Jefferson College; a link to nurse theorists' websites) http://goo.gl/VgOk3P
Clayton State University: Nursing Theory: http://goo.gl/N3i3Q4
Roseman University of Health Sciences: Nursing Theory Websites: http://goo.gl/we2g4n
Cox Health: Nursing Theories and Theorists: www.coxhealth.com/body.cfm?id=4964

program objectives, "statements of terminal behaviors" (outcome objectives), and "design learning experiences" (p. 7). These four concepts were later championed by Fawcett (1978, 1984, 2000, 2005, Fawcett & DeSanto-Madeya, 2013) as the "metaparadigm of nursing" with the labels modified to *person, environment, health,* and *nursing*.

Regarding research, even Fawcett & Hayes (1983) noted that conceptual frameworks are "indirectly tested by research" (p. 200). The problem was that nursing, as a discipline, forgot the tentative nature of the metaparadigmatic concepts. They were treated as "compulsory" through accreditation bodies, adopted by faculty as a criterion of disciplinary relevance, and used for evaluation of curriculum frameworks and models:

> How are the four essential concepts of nursing explicated in the model?
> How is person defined and described?
> How is environment defined and described?
> How is health defined? How are wellness and illness differentiated?
> How is nursing defined? What is the goal of nursing? How is the nursing process described? (Fawcett, 1980, p. 12; also see, Fawcett, 1993, p. 36)

Yet, there were other problems: although the metaparadigm concepts consisted of the most abstract concepts that a discipline might use, the four selected were so abstract that they are not unique to nursing (Cody, 1996), with of course, the exception of "nursing." Risjord (2010) noted that Fawcett's approach to developing a metaparadigm to unify nursing was an approach akin to mid-century philosophers' received view.

Were these four propositions helpful to theory development? In 2006 Paley writes:

> Here are four words—person, environment, health, and nursing—which just sit there, inert, like four garden gnomes. They say nothing, they do nothing. They make no claims, express no thoughts, represent no beliefs or assumptions. They just are. (p. 277)

However, I disagree with Paley's assertion that "they do nothing." Because early nursing theories and research were required to address these four metaparadigmatic concepts and propositions explicitly, Paley's question should be: Did they do *harm?* Fawcett (1978) argued that these four essential units made theory "readily identified as *nursing theories*" (p. 26, italics in the original). The metaparadigmatic concepts bounded nursing theory by demanding their presence and thereby dictating the level of the theory produced. For instance, if a nursing study were to explore patient pressure ulcers, and at one level a research project, perhaps linking in-bed movement with pressure ulcers, this may easily accommodate the bounds of the four concepts; but at another level, perhaps a research project exploring pressure ulcer formation at the cellular level, this would not encompass all four concepts, and would be considered as "not nursing research."

> It may be argued that a theory dealing with only one, two, or
> even three of the essential units of nursing is not, in fact, a
> nursing theory, especially if the unit *nursing* is not included.
> (Fawcett, 1978, p. 26)

With the wisdom of hindsight, we cannot imagine the ways in which this requirement stunted the growth for nursing. Neither could we imagine how limited the portfolio of National Institute of Nursing Research (NINR) might be, should these metaparadigmatic concepts become criteria for the guiding and funding of nursing research today.

Nevertheless, theories were evaluated according to their definition and description of these metaparadigmatic concepts (Fawcett & DeSanto-Madeya, 2013), regardless of the level, the function of the theory, and the scope actually required by the theory per se.

Fawcett's notion of theory development is deductive—that "the testability of grand theory is met when the grand theory has led to the generation of one of more middle-range theories" (Fawcett & DeSanto-Madeya, 2013, p. 314). But this is not the way nursing conceptual frameworks and theories were actually used in nursing: They were taught as fact in education and used as criteria for program accreditation, and applied carte blanche at the institutional level in practice. Researchers did not test theories and trial one theory against another, so that they may be modified and improved over time (Morse, 1996; Paley, 2006).

Thus, these four concepts gave direction to nursing science, but even the intended cohesiveness of focusing them for the development of nursing science was lost; authors were free to define these concepts accordingly. Phillips (2006) asks: if "each model and theory has a different philosophical and theoretical foundation, [and] nurses who use them have different realities of nursing, how are these differences related to what constitutes nursing science?" (p. 43). Even the term "nursing" was considered ambiguous and overutilized. One solution to this awkward term was to use nursing as a noun, not a verb, as the central concept, as suggested by Paterson and Zderad (1976) and endorsed by Reed (1996/2013).[6]

Elsewhere, I argued that the compulsory use of the metaparadigmatic concepts forced nursing theory to an inappropriate level of abstraction and to a level that diluted its relevance for clinical practice (Morse, 1996). For a low-level theory, incorporating the metaphysical concepts becomes a task of

---

[6] Are you a nursologist?

describing the obvious, which is usually unnecessary, or irrelevant, to the level of theory. Yet without these definitions, the theory did not meet the criteria for evaluation of a nursing theory; it did not pass inspection regardless of the quality and contribution of the remaining content. Some graduate programs even insisted that dissertations, in order to be considered *nursing* research, must include a nursing framework or theory (Morse, 1996). I trust nursing has now moved beyond this stage.

THE NEED FOR NURSE SCIENTISTS

The nurse scientist program was introduced in the late 1960s, with the goal of developing research and doctoral education in nursing, by the Division of Nursing, Bureau of Health Resources Development, U.S. Department of Health, Education, and Welfare (Bourgeois, 1975). Initially, federal funding was provided for nurses to obtain their doctorates in other disciplines, with the intention they would return to nursing following graduation, and build doctoral programs in nursing and contribute to research in nursing. Most did, but they also brought theories and research methods from those disciplines back into nursing, so that nursing research developed, at least in part, with a borrowed theoretical base.

Yet, the need for nursing research was acute; but it happened relatively slowly. For the large part, with the exceptions of those who obtained their doctorates in anthropology, the first nursing research was quantitative, and often focused on nurse and nursing education.

THE NEED FOR NURSING CONCEPTS

There are several conceptualizations about the relationship of concepts and theories. The earliest descriptions were that concepts enabled full descriptions of phenomena useful to nursing. For instance, Peplau (1952) introduced the term "empathy" into nursing to describe the natural process by which maternal emotions are transmitted to infants. Carl Rogers was invited to keynote at the American Nurses Association (ANA) conventions in 1957 on the essential characteristics of a therapeutic relationship, and this initiated interest in empathy in nursing. Gunter (1962) continued to cite Rogers's postulates directly, substituting "patient" for "client" to illustrate the applicability of the model for psychiatric nursing, counseling techniques, and later in nursing as a whole. During this period, Hildegard Peplau continued writing on therapeutic communication and theory, not only in the psychiatric nurse–patient interaction (1952, 1962), but also in general nurse–patient relationships (1997), and developing the concepts of anxiety (1963) and loneliness (1955) into nursing. Her work began a revolution into recognizing the need for concept development. The Nursing Concept Development Group (1973) later developed into methods of concept development (e.g., Norris, 1982), and texts appeared such as those by Walker and Avant (1983) and others (see Rodgers & Knafl, 1993, 2000). Books providing analyses of concepts also began to appear (e.g., Norris, 1982; Roberts, 1976).

MID-RANGE AND SITUATION-SPECIFIC THEORIES

In contrast to deductive theory that was constructed by identifying the domain and then the relevant concepts and their definitions, the inductive mode of theory development was first to identify the concepts, which were used as the "building blocks of theory" (Hardy, 1974; Walker & Avant, 2011, p. 59). Although this is considered a poor analogy (Paley, [1996, p. 577], prefers "niches"), it is clear that understanding concepts is critical to the development of disciplinary knowledge and to theory development. Inductive theory construction was conceived as consisting of the relevant concepts of various degrees of abstraction, starting with the context, and with linkages, building up to the domain.

The meaning of concepts depends on how they are used both in the context and in theory; concepts may change over time, and broadly with the context, so that concept analysis is not a time-limited goal for a discipline. Concept analysis must be taken seriously, as a research task.

Introducing the Patient

From the early 1980s with the gradual inroads of qualitative research, pushed by Glaser and Strauss and their students at University of California at San Francisco (UCSF), both a substantive area and the method of grounded theory developed (Glaser & Strauss, 1967), initiating the rise of mid-range (or middle-range[7]) theory (Swartz, 2009). The research group bought the patient forward as a *person* by writing a series of monographs of mid-range theories of dying (Strauss & Glaser, 1970; Strauss et al., 1984), and the comfort work of nurses (1984). For instance, Jennie Quint (later Benoliel) conducted a study of dying, *The Nurse and the Dying Patient,* in 1967, which had a profound effect on nursing education and practice. Grounded theories were often directly linked to patient care, to nursing problems, and as applicable to care. Much of the research from the UCSF research group has influenced the course of nursing and illness theory, and that has an influence, which continues today (Swartz, 2009).

---

[7] The term mid-range theory is less cumbersome than Merton's term "middle-range" or research developed according to a "practical purpose" (1949, p. 174).

The Rise of Mid-Range Theory as a Therapeutic Tool

From the mid-1980s, as qualitative method courses became increasingly adopted into nursing programs and qualitative methods were adapted to clinical research, the relevance for patient care immediately became apparent. In addition to the numerous mid-range theories developed using grounded theory, and other qualitative methods were used to develop nursing mid-range theory. In 1979, Germain published the first monograph-length ethnography conducted in a clinical setting, and phenomenology was used to elicit patient responses to illness (for example, see, Morse, Bottorff, & Hutchinson, 1995).

While these methods continue to be refined and developed, for instance, ethnography now consists of institutional ethnography, or critical ethnography, as well as the various other types (such as community-based participatory research [CBPR] and even autoethnography), our understanding of the experiential aspects of health and illness has also developed. Mid-range theories now comprise a large body of scholarship, and examples appear in this book. However, the last step, application of these models for the use by clinicians and the directing of practice, is still developing.

In 1999, Im and Meleis introduced *situation-specific theory*, which was connected to context, at a low level of abstract, encompassed diversity, of limited generalizations, but linked theory and practice. It was intended to build a solid nursing base of research that is relevant to practice.

THE NEED FOR NURSE EDUCATORS

Despite the criticisms of traditional nursing theory, these theories, frameworks for organizing nursing practice and nursing approaches to care, were (and still are in some nursing programs) highly influential in nursing education. Therefore, recognizing the importance of the adoption of nursing theory, from the mid-1970s to the mid-1990s, all nurses were taught about these theories in their undergraduate and graduate nursing programs. They were included in many types of courses, from the introduction to nursing, and "nursing theory" courses became established core components of the curriculum (however, it is interesting that these courses were not a part of the research curricula), and were not used by expert practitioners.

> . . . most expert practitioners abandon explicit adherence to a conceptual framework once they have systematized their thinking and, thereafter, adapt their decision-making processes. Because of this, models in pure form exist only in nursing curricula (the strategy for training neophytes) and in the theoretical communities of the model builders. If we accept this view of their contribution, models then become the means to systematic

reasoning rather than its end, and a mutually agreed upon definition of the profession becomes the common language for effective communication among and between nurses. (Thorne et al., 1998, p. 1266)

All nurses were taught about substance of the major nursing theories. Some programs organized their curriculum around nursing theories, so that nurses were very familiar with traditional nursing theory by the time they graduated. Nurses knew if they attended an Orem program or if their school was based on Roy. They were taught the structure of the theories and their intent to guide practice. It is important to note that many of the nurse theorists were not clinicians, but were academics, largely responsible for nurse educational programs and teaching.

However, when nurses commenced clinical practice, they were disillusioned about the application of the theories to practice. These traditional nursing theories were too abstract (Risjord, 2010); the language of the theories was not the language of patient care (Paley, 2006); and the gap between theory and practice was very wide.

In 1995, Levine made an impassioned plea for the revision of these theories:

> Skeptics who question the validity and relevance of nursing theory in the nursing curriculum demonstrate the failure to persuade nursing of the importance of theory. Attempts to justify theory by forcing its use in contexts where it barely fits have contributed to the increasing disenchantment . . . it is misused and misunderstood. (p. 11)

But theories continued to be developed in even more abstract and obtuse language. Mason, the editor of the *American Journal of Nursing*, wrote in 1999:

> Say "nursing science" to many nurses and they'll roll their eyes, remembering the seemingly useless theory and research courses they've sat through. And it's true: Theory and research have too often been irrelevant to the daily practice of nurses. So who, other than researchers and academics, should care about the state of our science? (p. 7)

Nurses were taught how to evaluate theory, but these evaluations were primarily concerned with the structure of the theory, and only in part about the content. Graduate students were taught that all nursing theories must contain Fawcett's (1984) four metaparadigmatic concepts, as these theories defined nursing, delineated nursing's domain, purpose, or mission, and some theories described the role of the nurse in relation to patient needs and/or nurse–patient interactions. Yet at the same time, these concepts kept nursing theories at a particular level of abstraction, so that they could not be readily applied to practice or used clinically, and only one of the concepts (nursing, of course) was unique to nursing.

Nevertheless, nursing graduate students continued to be urged to include a nursing theory in their dissertations, believing that without such content it was not a *nursing* study (Morse, 1996).[8] Often such theories were tacked on as an afterthought and not integrated into the study at all (Downs, 1994).

THE PERFORMANCE AND PRODUCTS OF NURSE RESEARCHERS

The increase in nurse scientists in the United States occurred relatively rapidly in the 1900s. By 1980 there were 10 doctoral programs in the United States, and with funding for nursing research from the National Institutes of Health (NIH) National Center for Nursing Research (later the NINR).

Despite their expected role for "testing" traditional theories, various problems such as the abstractness of these theories, the difficulty in operationalization, and the needs for basic clinical research pulled nurse researchers in a different direction, away from traditional nursing theory—not away from theory—all of their research used theory in some form or another. But, it was not traditional nursing theory.

Yet, the extensive research conducted by these researchers was extremely important for the development of clinical practice, as well as establishing nurses as scientists. Donaldson (2000) identified *breakthrough* research as "knowledge that transcends the discipline of origin" and adopted by other health professional disciplines seeking "scientific evidence as a basis for practice" (p. 248). She was interested in knowledge that related to "experience, health status or behavior" of "intact humans" (as opposed to cellular or organ systems, or animal research). While these nurse researchers collaborated across disciplines, the research maintained a nursing perspective. The major areas in which breakthroughs occurred were:

- Person and family health
- Pain management
- Neonatal and young child development
- Research utilization
- Dementia care
- Site transitional care
- Health and violence
- Women's health
- Psychobiological health

---

[8] Fortunately, nursing has outgrown this idea.

In acknowledgment of the influence and contributions of nursing research programs funded by NINR, major projects are listed in Box 2.1. Note that these were largely quantitative research with clinical outcomes. Although they provided evidence to change or improve nursing care, they did not contribute to nursing theory as it was perceived and defined by the nurse theorists.

BOX 2.1. ACCOMPLISHMENTS OF EXTRAMURAL RESEARCH PROGRAMS OF NINR-FUNDED RESEARCHERS

1994: *Dr. Loretta Sweet Jemmott* tested several gender-appropriate, culturally sensitive interventions on hard-to-reach vulnerable populations and significantly reduced sexual risk behaviors for HIV. Her "Be Proud! Be Responsible!" intervention became the Centers for Disease Control and Prevention's model curricula.

1998: *Dr. Joanne Harrell*, building on research that showed risk for cardiovascular disease can begin at an early age, demonstrated that a specially designed classroom educational program for elementary school children could significantly lower their cholesterol levels in just 8 weeks.

Dr. Nancy Bergstrom, in a multisite study, tested the Braden scale for risk of pressure sores and found its predictive capability accurate. The scale is now widely used in nursing homes and hospitals.

1999: *Dr. Mary Naylor* demonstrated that transitional care from hospital to home could significantly improve the health of older adult patients and substantially reduce patient days in hospitals, hospital readmissions, and health care costs.

Dr. Jon Levine established that gender plays a key role in pain relief, in which women obtained satisfactory relief from kappa opioids whereas men received little benefit.

2002: *Dr. Linda Aiken* demonstrated that hospital working conditions and adequacy of nurse staffing per patient can affect patients' recovery and that in hospitals where nurses have lower patient workloads, patients have substantially lower mortality rates.

2003: *Dr. Martha Hill* found that interventions conducted at the community level by a multidisciplinary health care team reduced high blood pressure in young inner city African American males, who are typically underserved by the health care system. Culturally sensitive, successful interventions can be conducted for vulnerable populations and can help reduce health care disparities.

2006: *Dr. Bernadette Melnyk* demonstrated that her Creating Opportunities for Parent Empowerment (COPE) program, which aims to support the parents of premature infants, resulted in improved knowledge and parenting behaviors, decreased parental stress, and shortened length of neonatal intensive care unit (NICU) stays by about four days, reducing health care costs associated with premature births by about $4,800 per infant.

2007: *Dr. J. Randall Curtis* and collaborators reported that an intervention to improve communication between intensive care unit (ICU) clinicians and family members of dying patients significantly reduced feelings of stress, anxiety, depression, and other symptoms of posttraumatic stress disorder in the family members for up to 3 months after the loss of their loved one.

2009: *Dr. Pamela Mitchell* reported that a behavioral intervention called Living Well with Stroke reduced the incidence of depression in stroke survivors, both immediately after treatment for stroke and at a 1-year follow-up.

Adapted from NINR (n.d.).

Thus, nurse researchers were most productive, but were conducting research in a different space from the traditional nursing theory movement. And they were contributing directly to health, to nursing practice, and to patient care at the bedside.

Traditional Nursing Theories Used as a *Philosophy* for Care

Nursing philosophies teach us how to *think*, how to approach nursing, and somehow to interact and care for the patient. Recognizing the importance in philosophy for nursing, in the mid-1990s, Kikuchi and Simmons developed the Institute for Nursing Philosophy at the University of Alberta, training doctoral and postdoctoral students, holding an annual conference, and publishing texts. These authors were attempting to address values and ethics as a foundation for nursing practice (Kikuchi, 1997). The link with traditional nursing theory was essential, and in 1999 the journal *Nursing Philosophy* was launched, along with the International Society of Nursing Philosophy.

What is the difference between qualitative inquiry and philosophical inquiry? Pesut & Johnson (2008) argue it is in the "authority"—in qualitative research it is held within data (i.e., the participant's experiences); in philosophy it is the philosopher's experience and philosophical analysis. Philosophical analysis in nursing research focuses on three "strands": (a) philosophical ideas focusing on identifying and analyzing basic presuppositions of nursing discourse (including nursing models); (b) philosophical problems (epistemology and ethics in nursing), and (c) critically analyzing nursing theory using a philosophical lens (Edwards, 2001; Kikuchi 1997; Pesut & Johnson, 2008).

These traditional theories are conceptual models that are actively used clinically to provide a nursing perspective toward care, and are still developing, as previously noted, fostered by the Magnet® organization's requirements. Examples are Martha Rogers's (1970), Theory of Unitary Human Beings and Margaret Newman's (1979, 1986) Health as Expanding Consciousness. Rosemarie Rizzo Parse's (1992, 1996, 1998, 2001) Theory of Human Becoming and Jean Watson's Philosophy and Science of Transpersonal Care (1999, 2000, 2008; Watson & Smith, 2002) provide an approach to nursing practice. Importantly, in the past decade, some of these theories have been brought to the bedside and demonstrated relevance for administration. Examples of frameworks for nursing practice are Leininger's Culture Care Theory of Diversity and Universality and the Sunrise Model (1991) and Ray's Theory of Bureaucratic Caring (2001). Both have large categories that frame the way we approach nursing, research, and scholarship, but are not intended to closely direct patient care; they do not provide instructions for providing care that is pragmatically useful in day-to-day caregiving. Some of these theories have been published as book-length works and have made an enduring impact (e.g., Paterson & Zderad, 1976), and some even exist beyond the horizon of American nursing—in Scandinavia (Eriksson, 2006) and Kati Martinsen (Alvsvag, 2006), and Kyung Rim Shin (1997, 2001) in Korea. In Canada, Margaret Campbell (1987) developed the "UBC Model for Nursing" and Moyra Allen developed the "McGill Model" (Gottlieb & Rowat, 1987; Thorne, 2011). Both models were used as a base for curricula at both universities respectively, but these theories have not been adopted in the United States.

NURSING THEORY FOR DIRECTING NURSING ACTIONS FOR PATIENT CARE

Sometimes called *practice theories*, these theories are intended to direct nursing action and nursing care. Examples of such theories are Sister Callista Roy's Adaptation Model (1970, 2009); Dorothea Orem's Self-Care Deficit Theory (1971; Denyes, Orem, Bekel, & SozWiss, 2001); Myra Levine's Conservation Model (1966, 1996); Immogene King's (1971, 2007) Interacting Systems Model; and Dorothy Johnson's (1980) Behavioral System Model.

Fueled by the requirements of the Magnet program (American Nurses Credentialing Center[9]), some nurse theorists have made their theory available for adoption by institutions so that care will be consistent at all levels from policy to beside care. For instance, Parse's (1998) Theory of Human Becoming implemented in Sunnybrook Hospital, Toronto, and later expanding to other hospitals in Ontario and Saskatchewan, Canada, as Human Becoming 80-20 (Bournes & Ferguson-Paré, 2007), Kolcaba's Theory of Comfort (Kolcaba, 2003; Kolcaba, Tilton, & Drouin, 2006); and Watson's (2006) Theory of Caring, are now used institution-wide in many hospitals in the United States.

THE GAP REMAINS

Although the gap between these nursing theories and research (primarily evaluation) is closing, nursing theory is still taught as a topic that is separate from the research courses in the nursing doctoral curriculum. Today we find ourselves in three parallel positions on theory:

* Quantitative researchers are increasingly developing, using, and testing nursing theory—both basic and applied theory, as applicable to nursing practice. They are developing theory that has a nursing focus, but also theory that interacts or intercepts with theory from allied disciplines. There is no reason for nursing not to use these additional theories from allied disciplines, and indeed it will be a hallmark of maturity

---

[9] http://www.nursecredentialing.org/FunctionalCategory/AboutANCC/Headlines/MagnetRecognitionProgramintheNews.html

once other disciplines start using theories that were developed in nursing. The evidence-based practice movement (Melnyk & Fineout-Overholt, 2011) is making a strong contribution to practice, which will eventually meet and contribute to quantitative theory development. In addition, qualitative methods will contribute to practice-based evidence (Leeman & Sandelowski, 2012).

- Qualitative researchers continue to develop mid-range theories and situation-specific theories and to create broader theories and also ways to apply qualitative theory to practice. Researchers are also exploring ways to integrate qualitative theory with quantitative in mixed-method designs. Recognizing that our theoretical base still needs and will continue to need development, concept analysis continues, and methods to do this task are improving.
- Nursing theorists continue to develop theory, although, as Figure 2.1 shows, this is occurring at a slower pace. Nursing theory is still taught as a topic that is separate from the research courses in the doctoral curricula.

DID WE FORGET?

> *. . . placing emphasis upon the conceptual portion of the phrase "the conceptual structure of knowledge" clearly focuses upon the thought processes involved. The outcomes, in the beginning at least, are theoretical constructs or sets of conventions created by the theorist. Note that I said created because they are not "givens" or predetermined by nature but are relatively arbitrary inventions of a human being.*
>
> —Jeanne S. Berthold (1968, p. 196)

WHERE ARE WE NOW?

There Is a Torrent of These Theories Being Developed Today

Nursing research no longer uses the traditional nursing metaparadigm as a framework; nurse researchers are free to construct the most appropriate model or theory that meets their needs.

Mark Risjord (2010) considered that the relevance gap was created by some kind of "philosophical illusion." The early nurse theorists made a mistake ("a distortion of the scientific enterprise"). Theory using basic sciences was "out of touch with the needs of practice." Risjord's (2010) solution is to correct the philosophy, by "reconceptualizing theory, methods and professional values," building on the work already completed, thereby closing the relevance gap, "not with new kinds of science, but with new kinds of philosophy" (p. 222). But it seems that, if nurse researchers do not use traditional nursing theory, rewriting philosophy for the relationship between nursing and nursing theory will not correct the problem.

> The problem is not adapting nursing theories to practice.
>
> The problem is not practice adopting nursing theory.
>
> We must recognize the king has no clothes.

Traditional nursing theory is in a domain that is separate from the research courses in the nursing doctoral curriculum, and has little impact on nursing practice. Therefore, the problem is not philosophical; rather, it appears that the problem is with educators and what they teach nursing undergraduates, master's students, and doctoral students.

Traditional nursing theory is ingrained in the introductory class: "This is what nursing is; this is how it is defined, and this is nursing theory."

Let us teach what theory *is* as it is being used in nursing research today:

- How it is formulated
- How it is used in nursing research
- How it can subsequently be used in practice.

Let us teach what theory is for nursing practice:

- Let us develop situation-producing theory
- Let us develop mid-range theory
- And even formulate and respect practice-based evidence

Then, theory will not be an abstract, "created" theory, but will contain data and be linked to other theories. The infamous theory–practice gap will simply go away.

We will recognize that theory used in research is derived for the research project according to the needs of the project.

We will recognize that research develops or modifies that theory according to the results of the research project.

We will recognize that when theory is introduced into practice according to the context of practice, it guides actions, is versatile, and is relevant to the particular problem in hand. The theory is tested and again modified. And so on, ad infinitum. This integration is what this book is about:

- Nursing theory for nursing knowledge
- Nursing theory for nursing research
- Nursing research for nursing practice
- Building the conceptual basis of nursing

> *Nursing theory is a part of nursing research, and research segues right into nursing practice. This phenomenon is not a phase with a distinct beginning and end, nor is it a helix with separate components.*
> —Stephanie Richardson (Personal Communication, 2015)

Educators may ask:

"But what will we teach in the introductory classes?"

Think on these things:

- Let us teach critical, abstract, and pragmatic thinking.
- Let us develop philosophical inquiry for nursing.
- Let us learn the structure of concepts and how they are developed, so we may develop meaningful concepts, modified as concepts change, and learn what we know.
- Let us learn the nature and use of appropriate theory and use theory.
- Let us become smart practitioners, learning from wise educators.

Then, *if* we do learn traditional nursing theories, let us understand them within their historical context:

How they were intended to be used over time,
What they achieved, and
Let us respect them for their role in the development of nursing.

... and then, let us move on.

WHERE ARE WE GOING?

TO DO 2.1. FILL IN THE BLANK

TO DO 2.2. TAKE A BREAK AND THINK ABOUT THIS

Pull up a comfy chair and read Chapter 3, "Seeing What We Know," for thinking about this account will be much more fun, and more meaningful, than listening to me.

"Seeing What We Know," is based on Laura Bohannan's (1956) article "Shakespeare in the Bush," an account of the *Tiv's* interpretation of the story of *Hamlet*. Enough said. This is a "time-out"—a space to read and reflect. It is included to illustrate the significance of cultural values and beliefs, how we perceive the world, others' interactions, and how we are perceived. It affects what we see and how we respond. The story illustrates the power of culture and the lens culture places on our perceptions, values, and worldview.

REFERENCES

Alligood, M. R., Marriner-Torney, A. (2010). *Nursing theorists and their work*. Maryland Heights, MO: Mosby Elsevier.

Alvsvag, H. (2006). Philosophy of caring: Kari Martinsen. In A. M. Tomey & M. E. Alligood (Eds.), *Nursing theorists and their work* (6th ed., pp. 167–190). St. Louis, MO: Mosby.

Berthold, J. S. (1968). Prologue. Symposium on theory development in nursing. *Nursing Research, 17*(3), 196–197.

Bourgeois, M. J. (1975). The special nurse research fellow: Characteristics and recent trends. *Nursing Research, 24*(3), 184–188.

Bournes, D. A., & Ferguson-Paré, M. (2007). Human becoming and 80/20: An innovative professional development model for nurses. *Nursing Science Quarterly, 20*(3), 237–253.

Campbell, M. A. (1987). *The UBC model for nursing: Directions for practice*. Vancouver, British Columbia: University of British Columbia.

Cody, W. K. (1996). Drowning in eclecticism. *Nursing Science Quarterly, 9*(3), 86–88.

Denyes, M. J., Orem, D. E., Bekel, G., & SozWiss, G. (2001). Self-care: A foundational science. *Nursing Science Quarterly, 14*(1), 48–54.

Donaldson, S. K. (2000). Breakthroughs in scientific research: The discipline of nursing, 1960–1999. *Annual Review of Nursing Research, 18*(1), 247–311.

Downs, F. (1994). Hitching the research wagon to theory. *Nursing Research, 43*, 195.

Edwards, S. D. (2001). *Philosophy of Nursing: An Introduction*. New York, NY: Palgrave.

Eriksson, K. (2006). *The suffering human being*. Chicago, IL: Nordic Studies.

Fawcett, J. (1978). The "what" of theory development (pp. 17–33). In *Theory development: What, why and how?* New York, NY: National League for Nursing, Publication No. 15-1708.

Fawcett, J. (1980). A framework for analysis and evaluation of conceptual models of nursing. *Nurse Educator, 5*(6), 10–14.

Fawcett, J. (1984). The metaparadigm of nursing: Present status and future refinements. *Image: Journal of Nursing Scholarship, XVI*(3), 84–87.

Fawcett, J., (1993). *Analysis and evaluation of nursing theories*. Philadelphia, PA: F. A. Davis.

Fawcett, J. (2000). *Contemporary nursing knowledge: Analysis and evaluation of nursing models and theories*. Philadelphia, PA: F. A. Davis.

Fawcett, J. (2005). *Contemporary nursing knowledge: Analysis and evaluation of nursing models and theories* (2nd ed.). Philadelphia, PA: F. A. Davis.

Fawcett, J., & DeSanto-Madeya, S. (2013). *Contemporary nursing knowledge: Analysis an evaluation of nursing models and theories* (3rd ed.). Philadelphia, PA: F. A. Davis.

Fawcett, J., & Hayes, E. (1983). Using conceptual frameworks in nursing practice and research. In M. B. White (Ed.), *Curriculum development from a nursing model: The crisis theory framework* (pp. 195–212). New York, NY: Springer Publishing Company.

Glaser, B. S., & Strauss, A. (1967). *The discovery of grounded theory. Strategies for qualitative research*. New York, NY: Aldine Transaction.

Gottlieb, L., & Rowat, K. (1987). The McGill model of nursing: A practice-derived model. *Advances in Nursing Science, 9*(4), 51–56.

Gunter, L. M. (1962). Notes on a theoretical framework for nursing research. *Nursing Research, 11*(4), 219–222.

Hardy, M. E. (1974). Theories: Components, development, evaluation. *Nursing Research, 23*, 100–107.

Hardy, M. E. (1978). Evaluating nursing theory. In *Theory development: What, why, how?* (p. 75). New York, NY: National League for Nursing, Publication No. 15-1708.

Im, E.-O., & Meleis, A. I. (1999). Situation-specific theories: Philosophical roots, properties, and approach. *Advances in Nursing Science, 22*(2), 11–24.

Johnson, D. E. (1978). State of the art of theory development in nursing. In *Theory development: What, why, how?* (pp. 1–10). New York, NY: National League for Nursing, Publication No. 15-1708.

Johnson, D. E. (1980). The behavioral system model for nursing. In J. P. Riehl & C. Roy (Eds.), *Conceptual models for nursing practice* (pp. 207–216). New York, NY: Appleton-Century-Crofts.

Kikuchi, J. F. (1997). Clarifying the nature of conceptualizations about nursing. *The Canadian Journal of Nursing Research, 29*(1), 97–110.

King, I. M. (1971). *Toward a theory for nursing: General concepts of human behavior*. New York, NY; Wiley.

King, I. M. (2007). King's conceptual system, theory of goal attainment, and transaction process in the 21st century. *Nursing Science Quarterly, 20*, 109–111.

Kolcaba, K. (2003). *Comfort theory and practice: A vision for holistic health care*. New York, NY: Springer Publishing.

Kolcaba, K., Tilton, C., & Drouin, C. (2006). Comfort theory: A unifying framework to enhance the practice environment. *Journal of Nursing Administration, 36*(11), 538–544.

Leeman, J., & Sandelowski, M. (2012). Practice-based evidence and qualitative inquiry. *Journal of Nursing Scholarship, 44*(2), 171–179. doi:10.1111/j.1547-5069.2012.01449.x

Leininger, M. (1991). *Culture care and diversity: A theory of nursing*. New York, NY: National League for Nursing.

Levine, M. E. (1995). The rhetoric of nursing theory. *Image Journal of Nursing Scholarship 27*(1), 11–17.

Mason, D. (1999). Nursing science: Who cares? [Editorial]. *American Journal of Nursing, 99*(12), 7.

McEwan, M., & Wills, E. M. (2014). *Theoretical basis for nursing* (4th ed.). Philadelphia, PA: Lippincott Williams & Wilkins.

Meleis, A. I. (2012). *Theoretical nursing: Development and progress* (5th ed.). Philadelphia, PA: Wolters Kluwer Health/Lippincott Williams & Wilkins.

Melnyk, B. M., & Fineout-Overholt, E. (Eds.). (2011). *Evidence-based practice in nursing and healthcare*. Philadelphia, PA: Wolters Kluwer Health.

Merton, R. K. (1949). The role of applied social science in the formation of policy: A research memorandum. *Philosophy of Science, 16*(3), 161–181.

Morse, J. M. (1996). Nursing theory: Sense and sensibility. *Nursing Inquiry, 3*(2), 74–82.

Morse, J. M., Bottorff, J. L., & Hutchinson, S. (1995). The paradox of comfort. *Nursing Research, 44*(1), 14–19.

National Institute of Nursing Research. (n.d.). *Important events in NINR history*. Retrieved from http://www.nih.gov/about-nih/what-we-do/nih-almanac/national-institute-nursing -research-ninr

Newman, M. (1979). *Theory development in nursing*. Philadelphia, PA: F.A. Davis.

Newman, M. (1986). *Heath as expanding consciousness*. St. Louis, MO: Mosby.

Norris, C. (1982). *Concept clarification in nursing*. Rockville, MD: Aspen.

Nursing Development Conference Group. (1973). *Concept formalization in nursing process and product*. Boston, MA: Little, Brown.

Orem, D. E. (1971). *Nursing: Concepts of practice*. New York, NY: McGraw-Hill.

Orem, D. E. (1980). *Nursing: Concepts of practice* (2nd ed.). New York, NY: McGraw-Hill.

Orem, D. E. (1985). *Nursing Concepts of practice* (3rd ed.). Chevy Chase, MD: McGraw-Hill.

Orem, D. E. (1991). *Nursing: Concepts of practice* (4th ed.). St. Louis, MO: Mosby.

Orem, D. E. (1995). *Nursing: Concepts of practice* (5th ed.). New York, NY: CV Mosby.

Paley, J. (1996). How not to clarify concepts. *Journal of Advanced Nursing, 24*, 572–578.

Paley, J. (2006). Nursing theorists and their work [Book review]. *Nursing Philosophy, 7*(4), 275–280.

Parse, R. R. (1992). Human becoming: Parse's theory of nursing. *Nursing Science Quarterly, 5*(1), 35–42.

Parse, R. R. (1996). The human becoming theory: Challenges in practice and research. *Nursing Science Quarterly, 9*(2), 55–60.

Parse, R. R. (1998). *The human becoming school of thought: A perspective for nurses and other health professionals*. Thousand Oaks, CA: Sage.

Parse, R. R. (2001). Rosemary Rizzo Parse: The human becoming school of thought. In M. Parker (Ed.), *Nursing theories and nursing practice* (pp. 227–238). Philadelphia, PA: F.A. Davis.

Paterson, J. G., & Zderad, L. T. (1976). *Humanistic nursing.* New York, NY: John Wiley & Sons.

Peplau, H. E. (1952). Interpersonal relations in nursing. *The American Journal of Nursing, 52*(6), 765.

Peplau, H. E. (1955). Loneliness. *The American Journal of Nursing, 55*(12), 1476–1481.

Peplau, H. E. (1962). Interpersonal techniques: The crux of psychiatric nursing. *The American Journal of Nursing, 62*(6), 50–54.

Peplau, H. E. (1963). A working definition of anxiety. In S. F. Burd & M. A. Marshall (Eds.), *Some clinical approaches to psychiatric nursing* (323–327). Toronto, Canada: Macmillan.

Peplau, H. E. (1997). Peplau's theory of interpersonal relations. *Nursing Science Quarterly, 10*(4), 162–167.

Pesut, B., & Johnson, J. (2008). Reinstating the 'Queen': Understanding philosophical inquiry in nursing. *Journal of Advanced Nursing, 61*(1), 115–121.

Phillips, J. (2006). What constitutes nursing science? In. W. K. Cody (Ed.), *Philosophical and theoretical perspective for advanced nursing* (4th ed., pp. 43–50). Boston, MA. Jones & Bartlett.

Quint, J. (1967). *The nurse and the dying patient.* New York, NY: Macmillan.

Ray, M. A. (2001). The theory of bureaucratic caring. In. M. Parker (Ed.), *Nursing theory and nursing practice* (pp. 421–444). Philadelphia, PA: F. A. Davis.

Reed, P. G. (1996). Transcendence: Formulating nursing perspectives. *Nursing Science Quarterly, 9*(1), 1–4.

Risjord, M. (2010). *Nursing knowledge: Science, practice, and philosophy.* Oxford, UK: Wiley-Blackwell.

Roberts, S. L. (1976). *Behavioral concepts and the critically ill patient.* Englewood Cliffs, NJ: Prentice-Hall.

Rodgers, B. L., & Knafl, K. A. (1993). *Concept development: Foundations, techniques and applications.* Philadelphia, PA: Saunders.

Rodgers, B. L., & Knafl, K. A. (2000). Concept analysis: An evolutionary view. In B. L. Rodgers & K. A. Knafl (Eds.), *Concept development in nursing* (2nd ed., pp. 77–117), Philadelphia, PA: Saunders.

Rogers, M. (1970). *An introduction to the theoretical basis of nursing.* Philadelphia, PA: F. A. Davis.

Roy, C. (1970). Adaptation: A conceptual framework for nursing. *Nursing Outlook, 18*(3), 42–48.

Roy, C. (1988). An explication of the philosophical assumptions of the Roy adaptation model. *Nursing Science Quarterly, 1*(1), 26–34.

Roy, C. (2009). *The Roy adaptation model* (3rd ed.). Upper Saddle River, NJ: Pearson.

Roy, C. (2011a). Research based on the Roy adaptation model: Last 25 years. *Nursing Science Quarterly, 24*(4), 312–320.

Roy, C. (2011b). Extending the Roy adaptation model to meet changing global needs. *Nursing Science Quarterly, 24*(4), 345–351.

Roy, C. (2014). *Generating middle range theory: From evidence to practice.* New York, NY: Springer Publishing.

Roy, C., & Andrews, H. A. (1999). *The Roy adaptation model* (2nd ed.). Stanford, CT: Appleton & Lange.

Roy, C., Whetsell, M. V., & Frederickson, K. (2009). The Roy adaptation model and research: Global perspective. *Nursing Science Quarterly, 22*(3), 209–211.

Shin, K. (1997). A study for the development of Korean nursing theory: A humanistic approach based on Shinhyung, Naekyungpyun in Dongeuibogam. *The Journal of Korean Nursing Academy, 27*(1), 141–155.

Shin, K. (2001). Developing perspectives on Korean nursing theory: The influences of Taoism. *Nursing Science Quarterly, 14*(4), 346–353.

Strauss, A. L., Corbin, J., Fagerhaugh, S., Glaser, B. G., Maines, D., Suczek, B., & Wiener, C. L. (1984). *Chronic illness and the quality of life.* St. Louis, MO: Mosby.

Strauss, A. L., & Glaser, B. G. (1970). *Anguish: A case history of a dying trajectory.* Mill valley, CA: Sociology Press.

Swartz, A. (2009). The mouse that roared. Doctoral program in Sociology celebrated 40 years. *Science of Caring, 21*(2): 22–25

Thorne, S. (2011). Theoretical issues in nursing. In J. C. Ross-Kerr & M. J. Wood (Eds.), *Canadian Nursing: Issues and Perspectives* (5th ed., pp. 85–194). Toronto, Canada: Elsevier.

Thorne, S., Canam, C., Dahinten, S., Hall, W., Henderson, A., & Kirkham, S. R. (1998). Nursing's metaparadigm concepts: Disimpacting the debates. *Journal of Advanced Nursing, 27*(6), 1257–1268.

Walker, L. O., & Avant, K. C. (1983). *Strategies for theory construction in nursing* (1st ed). Norwalk, CT: Appleton-Century-Crofts.

Walker, L. O. & Avant, K. C. (2011). *Strategies for theory construction in nursing* (5th ed). Upper Saddle River, NJ: Prentice Hall.

Watson, J. (1999). *Nursing: Human science and human care.* New York, NY: National League for Nursing/Jones & Bartlett.

Watson, J. (2000). Leading via caring-healing: The fourfold way toward transformative leadership. *Nursing Administration Quarterly, 25*(1), 1–6.

Watson, J. (2006). Caring theory as an ethical guide to administrative and clinical practices. *Nursing Administration Quarterly, 30*(1), 48–55.

Watson, J. (2008). *Nursing: The philosophy and science and caring* (Rev. ed.). Boulder, CO: University Press of Colorado.

Watson, J., & Smith, M. C. (2002). Caring science and the science of unitary human beings: A trans-theoretical discourse for nursing knowledge development. *Journal of Advanced Nursing, 37*(5), 452–461.

Yura, H., & Torres, G. (1975). Today's conceptual framework within baccalaureate nursing programs. In *Faculty-curriculum development, part III: Conceptual framework—Its meaning and function* (pp. 17–25). New York, NY: National League for Nursing.

APPENDIX 2.1

Abdellah, F. G., Beland, I. I., Martin, A., & Matneney, R. V. (1961). *Patient-centered approaches to nursing*. New York, NY: Macmillan.

Abdellah, F. G., Beland, I. I., Martin, A., & Matheny, R. V. (1973). *New directions in patient-centered nursing: Guidelines for systems of service, education, and research.* New York, NY: Macmillan.

Benner, P. (1984). *From novice to expert.* Menlo Park, CA: Addison-Wesley.

Denyes, M. J., Orem, D. E., & Bekel, G. (2001). Self-care: A foundational science. *Nursing Science Quarterly, 14*(1), 48–54.

Eriksson, K. (2006). *The suffering human being.* Chicago, IL: Nordic Studies.

Henderson, V. (1964). The nature of nursing. *American Journal of Nursing, 64*(8), 62–68.

Henderson, V. (1966). *The nature of nursing.* New York, NY: Macmillan.

Henderson, V. (1978). The concept of nursing. *Journal of Advanced Nursing, 3*(2), 113–130.

Johnson, D. E. (1959). A philosophy of nursing. *Nursing Outlook, 61*(11), 63–66.

Johnson, D. E. (1980). The behavioral system model for nursing. In J. Riehl & C. Roy (Eds.), *Conceptual models for nursing practice* (2nd ed.). New York, NY: Appleton-Century-Crofts.

King, I. M. (1971). *Toward a theory for nursing: General concepts of human behavior.* New York, NY: John Wiley & Sons.

King, I. M. (2007). King's conceptual system, theory of goal attainment, and transaction process in the 21st century. *Nursing Science Quarterly, 20,* 109–111.

Kolcaba, K. (2003). *Comfort theory and practice: A vision for holistic health care.* New York, NY: Springer Publishing.

Leininger, M. M. (1978). *Transcultural nursing: Concepts, theories and practices.* New York, NY: John Wiley & Sons.

Leininger, M. M. (1991). *Culture care diversity and universality: A theory of nursing.* New York, NY: National League for Nursing.

Leininger, M. M., & McFarland, M. R. (Eds.). (2006). *Culture care diversity and universality: A worldwide nursing theory.* Burlington, MA: Jones & Bartlett Learning.

Levine, M. E. (1967). The four conservation principles of nursing. *Nursing Forum, 5,* 45–49.

Levine, M. E. (1991). The conservation principles: A model for health. In K. Schaefer & J. Pond (Eds.), *Levine's conservation models: A framework for nursing practice* (pp. 1–11). Philadelphia, PA: F. A. Davis.

Martinsen, K. (2006). *Care and vulnerability.* Oslo, Norway: Akribe.

Neuman, B. M. (1974). The Betty Neuman health care systems model: A total person approach to patient problems. In J. P. Riehl & C. Roy (Eds.), *Conceptual models for nursing practice.* New York, NY: Appleton-Century-Crofts

Neuman, B. M. (1982). *The Neuman systems model: Application to nursing education and practice.* Norwalk, CT: Appleton-Century-Crofts.

Newman, M. (1979). *Theory development in nursing.* Philadelphia, PA: F. A. Davis.

Newman, M. A. (1986). *Health as expanding consciousness.* St. Louis, MO: Mosby.

Nightingale, F. (1992). *Notes on nursing* [Reprint of 1859 edition]. Philadelphia, PA: J. B. Lippincott.

Orem, D. E. (1971). *Nursing: Concept of practice.* New York, NY: McGraw-Hill.

Orem, D. E. (1980). *Nursing: Concept of practice* (2nd ed.). New York, NY: McGraw-Hill.

Orem, D. E. (1985). *Nursing: Concept of practice* (3rd ed.). New York, NY: McGraw-Hill.

Orem, D. E. (1991). *Nursing: Concept of practice* (4th ed.). St. Louis, MO: C.V. Mosby.

Orem, D. E. (1995). *Nursing: Concept of practice* (5th ed.). St. Louis, MO: C.V. Mosby.

Orem, D. E. (2001). *Nursing: Concept of practice* (6th ed.). St. Louis, MO: C.V. Mosby.

Orem, D. E., & Taylor, S. G. (1986). Orem's general theory of nursing. In P. Winstead-Fry (Ed.). *Case studies in nursing theory* (pp. 37–71). New York, NY: National League for Nursing, Publication No. 15–2152.

Orem, D. E., Taylor, S. G., & Renpenning, K. M. (2001). *Nursing: Concepts of practice.* (6th ed.). St. Louis, MO: Mosby.

Orlando, I. (1961). *The dynamic nurse-patient relationship.* New York, NY: G.P. Putnam's Sons.

Orlando, I. (1990). *The dynamic nurse-patient relationship.* New York, NY: National League for Nursing, Publication No. 15–2341.

Parse, R. R. (1981). *Man-living-health: A theory of nursing,* New York, NY: John Wiley & Sons.

Parse, R. R. (1995). *Illuminations: The human becoming theory in practice and research.* New York, NY: National League for Nursing, Publication No. 15–2670.

Parse, R. R. (1998). *The human becoming school of thought.* Thousand Oaks, CA: Sage

Parse, R. R. (1999). *Illuminations: The human becoming theory in practice and research.* Burlington, MA: Jones & Bartlett Learning.

Paterson, J. G., & Zderad, L. T. (1976). *Humanistic nursing.* New York, NY: John Wiley & Sons.

Paterson, J. G., & Zderad, L. T. (1988). *Humanistic nursing* (pp. i–iv, 1–129). New York, NY: National League for Nursing, Publication No. 41–2218.

Peplau, H. E. (1952). *Interpersonal relations in nursing.* New York, NY: G.P. Putnam's Sons.

Peplau, H. E. (1991). *Interpersonal relations in nursing: A conceptual frame of reference for psychodynamic nursing.* New York, NY: Springer Publishing. (Original work published 1952.)

Putt, A. M. (1978). *General systems theory applied to nursing.* Boston, MA: Little, Brown.

Ray, M. (1989). The theory of bureaucratic caring for nursing practice in the organization culture. *Nursing Administration Quarterly, 13*(2), 31–42.

Ray, M. E. (2001). The theory of bureaucratic caring. In M. Parker (Ed.), *Nursing theories and nursing practice* (pp. 422–431). Philadelphia, PA: F. A. Davis.

Rogers, M. E. (1970). *An introduction to the theoretical basis of nursing.* Philadelphia, PA: F.A. Davis.

Rogers, M. E. (1990). *Nursing: Science of unitary, irreducible, and human beings*: Update 1990. National League for Nursing, Publicaion No. 15-2285.

Roy, C. (1970). Adaptation: A conceptual framework for nursing. *Nursing Outlook, 18*(3), 42–45.

Roy, C. (1976). *Introduction to nursing: An adaptation model*. Englewood Cliffs, NJ: Prentice-Hall.

Roy, C. (1981). *Introduction to nursing: An adaptation model*. Englewood Cliffs, NJ: Prentice-Hall.

Roy, C. (1984). *Introduction to nursing: An adaptation model* (2nd ed.). Englewood Cliffs, NJ: Prentice-Hall.

Roy, C., & Andrews, H. A. (1999). *The Roy adaptation model* (2nd ed.). Norwalk, CT: Appleton & Lange.

Roy, C., & Roberts, S. L. (1981). *Theory construction in nursing: An adaptation model*. Englewood Cliffs, NJ: Prentice-Hall.

Travelbee, J. (1966). *Interpersonal aspects of nursing*. Philadelphia, PA: F. A. Davis.

Travelbee, J. (1971). *Interpersonal aspects of nursing* (2nd ed.). Philadelphia, PA: F. A. Davis.

Travelbee, J., & Doona, M. E. (1979). *Intervention in psychiatric nursing*. Philadelphia, PA: F. A. Davis.

Watson, J. (1979). *Nursing: The philosophy and science of caring*. Boston, MA: Little, Brown.

Watson, J. (1985). *Nursing: Human science and human care*. Norwalk, CT: Appleton-Century-Crofts.

Watson, J. (1988). *Nursing: Human science and human care—A theory of nursing*. New York, NY: National League for Nursing, Publication No. 15–2236

Watson, J. (1994). *Applying the art and science of human caring* (No. 42). New York, NY: National League for Nursing.

Watson, J. (1999). *Nursing: Human science and human care: A theory of nursing* (No. 15). Burlington, MA: Jones & Bartlett Learning.

Watson, J. (2008). *Nursing: The philosophy and science of caring* (Rev. ed.). Boulder, CO: University Press of Colorado.

Weidenbach, E. (1963). The helping art of nursing. *American Journal of Nursing, 63*(11), 54–57.

Weidenbach, E. (1964). *Clinical Nursing: A helping art*. New York, NY: Springer-Verlag.

Laura Bohannan

3

SEEING WHAT WE KNOW: KNOWING WHAT WE SEE

> *Once there were five peas in one pod; the peas were green and the pod was green, and so they believed that the whole world was green—and that was absolutely right!*
>
> —Hans Christian Andersen (n.d.)

This short story was written one wet day by an anthropologist, Laura Bohannan, who was doing fieldwork with the Tiv in Africa. It was her turn to tell a story, and she chose Shakespeare's Hamlet. *The Tiv's interpretation of the story illustrates the power of cultural differences—even linguistic nonequivalence—and how terms acquire different meanings when translated. The trick, in concept analysis, is to be able to uncover and identify nuances of meaning of terms that are different, but have the same label.*

SHAKESPEARE IN THE BUSH

Laura Bohannan[1]

Just before I left Oxford for the Tiv in West Africa, conversation turned to the season at Stratford. "You Americans," said a friend, "often have difficulty with Shakespeare. He was, after all, a very English poet, and one can easily misinterpret the universal by misunderstanding the particular."

I protested that human nature is pretty much the same the whole world over; at least the general plot and motivation of the greater tragedies would always be clear—everywhere—although some details of custom might have

---

[1] Bohannan (1956).

to be explained and difficulties of translation might produce other slight changes. To end an argument we could not conclude, my friend gave me a copy of *Hamlet* to study in the African bush: It would, he hoped, lift my mind above its primitive surroundings, and possibly I might, by prolonged meditation, achieve the grace of correct interpretation.

It was my second field trip to that African tribe, and I thought myself ready to live in one of its remote sections—an area difficult to cross even on foot. I eventually settled on the hillock of a very knowledgeable old man, the head of a homestead of some 140 people, all of whom were either his close relatives or their wives and children. Like the other elders of the vicinity, the old man spent most of his time performing ceremonies seldom seen these days in the more accessible parts of the tribe. I was delighted. Soon there would be 3 months of enforced isolation and leisure, between the harvest that takes place just before the rising of the swamps and the clearing of new farms when the water goes down. Then, I thought, they would have even more time to perform ceremonies and explain them to me.

I was quite mistaken. Most of the ceremonies demanded the presence of elders from several homesteads. As the swamps rose, the old men found it too difficult to walk from one homestead to the next, and the ceremonies gradually ceased. As the swamps rose even higher, all activities but one came to an end. The women brewed beer from maize and millet. Men, women, and children sat on their hillocks and drank it.

People began to drink at dawn. By mid-morning, the whole homestead was singing, dancing, and drumming. When it rained, people had to sit inside their huts: There, they drank and sang or they drank and told stories. In any case, by noon or before, I either had to join the party or retire to my own hut and my books. "One does not discuss serious matters when there is beer. Come, drink with us." Since I lacked their capacity for the thick native beer, I spent more and more time with *Hamlet*.

Before the end of the second month, grace descended on me. I was quite sure that *Hamlet* had only one possible interpretation, and that one universally obvious.

Early every morning, in the hope of having some serious talk before the beer party, I used to call on the old man at his reception hut—a circle of posts supporting a thatched roof above a low mud wall to keep out wind and rain. One day I crawled through the low doorway and found most of the men of the homestead sitting huddled in their ragged clothes on stools, low plank beds, and reclining chairs, warming themselves against the chill of the rain around a smoky fire. In the center were three pots of beer. The party had started.

The old man greeted me cordially, "Sit down and drink." I accepted a large calabash full of beer, poured some into a small drinking gourd, and tossed it down. Then I poured some more into the same gourd for the man second in seniority to my host before I handed my calabash over to a young man for further distribution. Important people should not ladle beer themselves.

"It is better like this," the old man said looking at me approvingly and plucking at the thatch that had caught in my hair. "You should sit and drink with us more often. Your servants tell me that when you are not with us, you sit inside your hut looking at a paper."

The old man was acquainted with four kinds of "papers": tax receipts, bride price receipts, court fee receipts, and letters. The messenger who brought him letters from the chief used them mainly as a badge of office, for he always knew what was in them and *told* the old man. Personal letters for the few who had relatives in the government or mission stations were kept until someone went to a large market where there was a letter writer and reader. Since my arrival, letters were brought to me to read. A few men also brought me bride price receipts, privately, with requests to change the figures to a higher sum. I found moral arguments were of no avail, since in-laws are fair game, and the technical hazards of forgery difficult to explain to an illiterate people. I do not wish them to think me silly enough to look at any such papers for days on end, and I hastily explained that my "paper" was one of the "things of long ago" of my country.

"Ah," said the old man, "Tell us."

I protested that I was not a storyteller. Storytelling is a skilled art among them; their standards are high and the audiences critical—and vocal in their criticism. I protested in vain. This morning they wanted to hear a story while they drank. They threatened to tell me no more stories until I told them one of mine. Finally, the old man promised that no one would criticize my style, "for we know you are struggling with our language." "But," put in one of the elders, "you must explain what we do not understand, as we do when we tell you our stories." Realizing that here was my chance to prove *Hamlet* universally intelligible, I agreed.

The old man handed me some more beer to help me on with my storytelling. Men filled their long wooden pipes and knocked coals from the fire to place in the pipe bowls; then, puffing contentedly, they sat back to listen. I began in the proper style, "Not yesterday, not yesterday, but long ago, a thing occurred. One night three men were keeping watch outside the homestead of the great chief, when suddenly they saw the former chief approach them."

"Why was he no longer chief?"

"He was dead," I explained. "That is why they were troubled and afraid when they saw him."

"Impossible," began one of the elders, handing his pipe on to his neighbor, who interrupted, "Of course it wasn't the dead chief; it was an omen sent by a witch. Go on."

Slightly shaken, I continued. "One of these three was a man who knew things"—the closest translation for scholar, but unfortunately it also meant witch. The second elder looked triumphantly at the first. "So he spoke to the dead chief saying, 'Tell us what we must do so you may rest in your grave,' but the dead chief did not answer. He vanished, and they could see him no more. Then the man who knew things—his name was Horatio—said this event was the affair of the dead chief's son, Hamlet."

There was a general shaking of heads round the circle. "Had the dead chief no living brothers? Or was this son the chief?"

"No," I replied. "That is, he had one living brother who became the chief when the elder brother died."

The old men muttered: such omens were matters for chiefs and elders, not for youngsters; no good could come of going behind a chief's back: clearly Horatio was not a man who knew things.

"Yes, he was," I insisted, shooing a chicken away from my beer. "In our country the son is next to the father. The dead chief's younger brother had become the great chief. He had also married his elder brother's widow only about a month after the funeral."

"He did well," the old man beamed and announced to the others, "I told you that if we knew more about Europeans, we would find they really were very like us. In our country also," he added to me, "the younger brother marries the elder brother's widow and becomes the father of his children. Now, if your uncle, who married your widowed mother, is your father's full brother, then he will be a real father to you. Did Hamlet's father and uncle have one mother?"

His question barely penetrated my mind; I was too upset and thrown too far off balance by having one of the most important elements of *Hamlet* knocked straight out of the picture. Rather uncertainly, I said that I thought they had the same mother, but I was not sure—the story did not say. The old man told me severely that these genealogical details made all the difference and when I got home I must ask the elders about it. He shouted out the door to one of his younger wives to bring his goatskin bag.

Determined to save what I could of the mother motif, I took a deep breath and began again. "The son Hamlet was very sad because his mother had married again so quickly. There was no need for her to do so, and it is our custom for a widow not to go to her next husband until she has mourned for 2 years."

"Two years is too long," objected the wife who had appeared with the old man's battered goatskin bag. "Who will hoe your farms for you while you have no husband?"

"Hamlet," I retorted without thinking, "was old enough to hoe his mother's farms himself. There was no need for her to remarry." No one looked convinced. I gave up. "His mother and the great chief told Hamlet not to be sad, for the great chief himself would be a father to Hamlet. Furthermore, Hamlet would be the next chief; therefore he must stay to learn the things of a chief. Hamlet agreed to remain, and all the rest went off to drink beer."

While I paused, perplexed at how to render Hamlet's disgusted soliloquy to an audience convinced that Claudius and Gertrude had behaved in the best possible manner, one of the younger men asked me who had married the other wives of the dead chief.

"He had no other wives," I told him.

"But a chief must have many wives! How else can he brew beer and prepare food for all his guests?"

I said firmly that in our country even chiefs had only one wife, that they had servants to do their work and that they paid them from tax money.

It was better, they returned for a chief to have many wives and sons who would help him hoe his farms and feed his people; then everyone loved the chief who gave much and took nothing—taxes were a bad thing.

I agreed with the last comment, but for the rest fell back on their favorite way of fobbing off my questions. "That is the way it is done, so that is how we do it."

I decided to skip the soliloquy. Even if Claudius was here thought quite right to marry his brother's widow, there remained the poison motif, and I knew they would disapprove of fratricide. More hopefully I resumed, "That night Hamlet kept watch with the three who had seen his dead father. The dead chief again appeared, and although the others were afraid, Hamlet followed his dead father off to one side. When they were alone, Hamlet's dead father spoke."

"Omens can't talk!" the old man was emphatic.

"Hamlet's dead father wasn't an omen; seeing him might have been an omen, but he was not." My audience looked confused as I sounded. "It *was* Hamlet's dead father. It was a thing we call a 'ghost'," I had to use the English word, for unlike many of the neighboring tribes, these people did not believe in the survival after death of any individuating part of the personality.

"What is a 'ghost'? An omen?"

"No, a 'ghost' is someone who is dead but who walks around and can talk, and people can hear him and see him but not touch him."

They objected. "One can touch zombies."

"No, no! It was not a dead body the witches had animated to sacrifice and eat. No one else made Hamlet's dead father walk. He did it himself."

"Dead men can't walk," protested my audience as one man.

I was quite willing to compromise. "A 'ghost' is the dead man's shadow."

But again they objected. "Dead men cast no shadows."

"They do in my country," I snapped.

The old man quelled the babble of disbelief that arose immediately and told me with that insincere but courteous agreement one extends to the fancies of the young, ignorant, and superstitious, "No doubt in your country the dead can also walk without being zombies." From the depths of his bag he produced a withered fragment of kola nut, bit off one end to show it was not poisoned, and handed me the rest as a peace offering.

"Anyhow," I resumed, "Hamlet's dead father said that his own brother, the one who became chief, had poisoned him. He wanted Hamlet to avenge him. Hamlet believed this in his heart, for he did not like his father's brother."

I took another swallow of beer. "In the country of the great chief, living in the same homestead, for it was a very large one, was an important elder who was often with the chief to advise and help him. His name was Polonius. Hamlet was courting his daughter, but her father and her brother . . . [I cast hastily about for some tribal analogy] warned her not to let Hamlet visit her when she was alone on her farm, for he would be a great chief and so could not marry her."

"Why not?" asked the wife, who had settled down on the edge of the old man's chair. He frowned at her for asking stupid questions and growled, "They lived in the same homestead."

"That was not the reason," I informed them. "Polonius was a stranger who lived in the homestead because he helped the chief, not because he was a relative."

"Then why couldn't Hamlet marry her?"

"He could have," I explained, "but Polonius didn't think he would. After all, Hamlet was a man of great importance who ought to marry a chief's daughter, for in his country a man could have only one wife. Polonius was afraid that if Hamlet made love to his daughter, then no one else would give a high price for her."

"That might be true," remarked one of the shrewder elders, "but a chief's son would give his mistress's father enough presents and patronage to more than make up the difference. Polonius sounds like a fool to me."

"Many people think he was," I agreed. "Meanwhile Polonius sent his son Laertes off to Paris to learn the things of that country, for it was the homestead of a very great chief indeed. Because he was afraid that Laertes might waste a lot of money on beer and women and gambling, or get into trouble by fighting, he sent one of his servants to Paris secretly, to spy out what Laertes was doing."

"One day Hamlet came upon Polonius's daughter Ophelia. He behaved so oddly he frightened her. Indeed"—I was fumbling for words to express the dubious quality of Hamlet's madness—"the chief and many others had also noticed that when Hamlet talked one could understand the words but not what they meant. Many people thought that he had become mad." My audience suddenly became much more attentive. "The great chief wanted to know what was wrong with Hamlet, so he sent for two of Hamlet's age mates [school friends would have taken a long explanation] to talk to Hamlet and find out what troubled his heart. Hamlet, seeing that they had been bribed by the chief to betray him, told them nothing. Polonius, however, insisted that Hamlet was mad because he had been forbidden to see Ophelia, whom he loved."

"Why," inquired a bewildered voice, "should anyone bewitch Hamlet on that account?"

"Bewitch him?"

"Yes, only witchcraft can make anyone mad, unless, of course, one sees the beings that lurk in the forest."

I stopped being a storyteller, took out my notebook, and demanded to be told more about these two causes of madness. Even while they spoke and I jotted notes, I tried to calculate the effect of this new factor on the lot. Hamlet had not been exposed to the beings that lurked in the forests. Only his relatives in the male line could bewitch him. Barring relatives not mentioned by Shakespeare, it had to be Claudius who was attempting to harm him. And, of course it was.

For the moment I staved off questions by saying that the great chief also refused to believe Hamlet was mad for love of Ophelia and nothing else. He was sure that something much more important was troubling Hamlet's heart.

"Now Hamlet's age mates," I continued, "had brought with them a famous storyteller. Hamlet decided to have this man tell the chief and all his homestead a story about a man who had poisoned his brother because he desired his brother's wife and wished to be chief himself. Hamlet was sure the great chief could not hear the story without making a sign if he was indeed guilty, and then he would discover whether his dead father had told him the truth."

The old man interrupted, with deep cunning, "Why should a father lie to his son?" he asked.

I hedged: "Hamlet wasn't sure that it really was his dead father." It was impossible to say anything, in that language, about devil-inspired visions.

"You mean," he said, "it actually was an omen, and he knew witches sometimes send false ones. Hamlet was a fool not to go to one skilled in reading omens and divining the truth in the first place. A man-who-sees-the-truth could have told him how his father died, if he really had been poisoned, and if there was witchcraft in it; then Hamlet could have called the elders to settle the matter."

The shrewd elder ventured to disagree. "Because his father's brother was a great chief, one-who-sees-the-truth might therefore have been afraid to tell it. I think it was for that reason that a friend of Hamlet's father—a witch and an elder—sent an omen so his friend's son would know. Was the omen true?"

"Yes," I said, abandoning ghosts and the devil; a witch-sent omen it would have to be. "It was true, for when the storyteller was telling his tale before all the homestead, the great chief rose in fear. Afraid that Hamlet knew his secret he planned to have him killed."

The stage set of the next bit presented some difficulties for translation. I began cautiously. "The great chief told Hamlet's mother to find out from her son what he knew. But because a woman's children are always first in her heart, he had the important elder Polonius hide behind a cloth that hung against the wall of Hamlet's mother's sleeping hut. Hamlet started to scold his mother for what she had done."

There was a shocked murmur from everyone; a man should never scold his mother.

"She called out in fear, and Polonius moved behind the cloth. Shouting, 'A rat!' Hamlet took his machete and slashed through the cloth." I paused for dramatic effect. "He had killed Polonius!"

The old men looked at each other in supreme disgust. "That Polonius truly was a fool and a man who knew nothing! What child would not know enough to shout, 'It's me!'" With a pang, I remembered that these people are ardent hunters, always armed with bow, arrow, and machete; at the first rustle in the grass, an arrow is aimed and ready, and the hunter shouts "Game!" If no human voice answers immediately the arrow speeds on its way. Like a good hunter Hamlet had shouted, "A rat!"

I rushed in to save Polonius's reputation. "Polonius did speak. Hamlet heard him. But he thought it was the chief and wished to kill him to avenge his father. He had meant to kill him earlier in the evening . . . " I broke down, unable to describe to these pagans, who had no belief in individual afterlife, the difference between dying at one's prayers and dying "unhousell'd, disappointed, unaneled."

This time I had shocked my audience seriously. "For a man to raise his hand against his father's brother and the one who has become his father—that is a terrible thing. The elders ought to let such a man be bewitched."

I nibbled at my kola nut in some perplexity, then pointed out that after all the man had killed Hamlet's father.

"No," pronounced the old man, speaking less to me than to the young men sitting behind the elders. "If your father's brother has killed your father, you must appeal to your father's age mates; they may avenge him. No man may use violence against his senior relatives." Another thought struck him. "But if his father's brother had indeed been wicked enough to bewitch Hamlet and make him mad, that would be a good story indeed, for it would be his own fault that Hamlet, being mad, no longer had any sense and thus was ready to kill his father's brother."

There was a murmur of applause. *Hamlet* was again a good story to them, but it no longer seemed quite the same story to me. As I thought over the coming complications of plot and motive, I lost my courage and decided to skim over dangerous ground quickly.

"The great chief," I went on, "was not sorry that Hamlet had killed Polonius. It gave him a reason to send Hamlet away, with his two treacherous age mates, with letters to a chief of a far country, saying that Hamlet should be killed. But Hamlet changed the writing on their papers, so that the chief killed his age mates instead." I encountered a reproachful glare from one of the men whom I had told undetectable forgery was not merely immoral but beyond human skill. I looked the other way.

"Before Hamlet could return, Laertes came back for his father's funeral. The great chief told him Hamlet had killed Polonius. Laertes swore to kill

Hamlet because of this, and because his sister Ophelia, hearing her father had been killed by the man she loved, went mad and drowned in the river."

"Have you already forgotten what we told you?" The old man was reproachful. "One cannot take vengeance on a madman; Hamlet killed Polonius in his madness. As for the girl, she not only went mad, she was drowned. Only witches can make people drown. Water itself can't hurt anything. It is merely something one drinks and bathes in."

I began to get cross. "If you don't like the story, I'll stop."

The old man made soothing noises and poured me some more beer.

"You tell the story well, and we are listening. But it is clear that the elders of your country have never told you what the story really means. No, don't interrupt! We believe you when you say your marriage customs are different, or your clothes and weapons. But people are the same everywhere; therefore, there are always witches and it is we, the elders, who know how witches work. We told you it was the great chief who wished to kill Hamlet, and now your own words have proved us right. Who were Ophelia's male relatives?"

"There were only her father and her brother." *Hamlet* was clearly out of my hands.

"There must have been many more; this also you must ask of your elders when you get back to your country. From what you tell us, since Polonius was dead, it must have been Laertes who killed Ophelia, although I do not see the reason for it."

We had emptied one pot of beer, and the old men argued the point with slightly tipsy interest. Finally, one of them demanded of me, "What did the servant of Polonius say on his return?"

With difficulty I recollected Reynaldo and his missions. "I don't think he did return before Polonius was killed."

"Listen," said the elder, "and I will tell you how it was and how your story will go, then you may tell me if I am right. Polonius knew his son would get into trouble, and so he did. He had many fines to pay for fighting, and debts from gambling. But he had only two ways of getting money quickly. One was to marry off his sister at once, but it is difficult to find a man who will marry a woman desired by the son of the chief. For if the chief's heir commits adultery with your wife, what can you do? Only a fool calls a case against a man who will someday be his judge. Therefore Laertes had to take the second way: He killed his sister by witchcraft, drowning her so he could secretly sell her body to the witches."

I raised an objection. "They found her body and buried it. Indeed Laertes jumped into the grave to see his sister once more—so, you see, the body was truly there. Hamlet, who had just come back, jumped in after him."

"What did I tell you?" The elder appealed to the others. "Laertes was up to no good with his sister's body. Hamlet prevented him, because the chief's heir, like a chief, does not wish any other man to grow rich and powerful. Laertes would be angry, because he would have killed his sister without benefit to himself. In our country he would try to kill Hamlet for that reason. Is this not what happened?"

"More or less," I admitted. "When the great chief found Hamlet was still alive, he encouraged Laertes to try to kill Hamlet and arranged a fight with machetes between them. In the fight both the young men were wounded to death. Hamlet's mother drank the poisoned beer that the chief meant for Hamlet in case he won the fight. When he saw his mother die of poison, Hamlet, dying, managed to kill his father's brother with his machete."

"You see, I was right!" exclaimed the elder.

"That was a very good story," added the old man, "and you told it with very few mistakes. The poison Hamlet's mother drank was obviously meant for the survivor of the fight, whichever it was. If Laertes had won, the great chief would have poisoned him, for no one would know that he arranged Hamlet's death. Then, too, he need not fear Laertes's witchcraft; it takes a strong heart to kill one's only sister by witchcraft."

"Sometime," concluded the old man, gathering his ragged toga about him, "you must tell us some more stories of your country. We, who are elders, will instruct you in their true meaning, so that when you return to your own land your elders will see that you have not been sitting in the bush, but among those who know things and who have taught you wisdom."

REFERENCES

Andersen, H. C. (n.d.) *"Fem fra en Ærtebælg"* (J. Jersholt, Trans.). Retrieved from http://www.andersen.sdu.dk/vaerk/hersholt/FivePeasFromAPod_e.html

Bohannan, L. (1956). Shakespeare in the bush. *Natural History, 75,* 28–33.

Janice M. Morse

4

INCORPORATING THEORY INTO PRACTICE RESEARCH

> *Repression as the theory of neurosis served as the ground for which a
> number of revolutionary movements to gain freedom originated. The
> Victorian outlook on manners and the self-containment of past decades
> have not become expressionism at any cost. But while we all believe
> that more people are not mentally healthier because they "express"
> themselves, this has yet to be proven.*
>
> —Burton (1974, p. 14)

The biologist and Nobel Laureate, Szent-Györgyi (1972), once said that in order to be a great researcher, one must think of a groundbreaking approach to familiar problems that everyone sees. In nursing, this begins with an understanding of the theory–practice–research link, or relationship between theory, research, and practice. The theory–practice–research link was discussed in detail by nurse researchers and theorists in the early 1980s. As a result of these discussions, several landmark articles were written. These acclaimed articles are still in use in doctoral theory courses, and are often unquestioned and unchallenged. Since then, we have grown evolved, and developed as a profession, and we should now reconsider our approach to this vital and foundational topic, as the process of deciding what to research, and which perspective to adopt, and how to re-explore the topic, is of paramount importance (Beck, 2016). Here, I examine the relationships between how we perceive clinical problems, or what I call theoretical perspectives considered pertinent to those problems; ensuing research methods; and the influence of various research products as they are applied to nursing practice. This article is based on a plenary address I prepared for a summit intended to discuss new directions for the research agenda in the area of urinary incontinence.

This article illustrates how theoretical frameworks may be applied to that substantive area, through various lenses, but I believe that the points made here may be applicable to nursing research's agenda as a whole.

We should be cognizant of these sometimes conflicting perspectives in our daily interactions, especially as they relate to determining what research will or will not be funded. These conflicts prioritize which problems are considered important and are subsequently researched. By prioritizing one problem over another, conflicts may arise during patient care, in the classroom, and in private meetings of granting agencies. Newspapers may also cover these conflicts, and they may be brought to light during government allocation meetings and in response to special interest groups and lobbyists.

In nursing, our subdiscipline drives what we identify as meaningful research topics, and what we consider as standard modes of inquiry, as data, and as realistic outcomes. Perspectives on such matters are diverse within our profession and vary based on what our view of nursing is, what theories we have been taught, and the role we believe the political agenda should play in resolving these clinical problems. Even though we believe in holism, we fractionate our profession into subdisciplines. Subdisciplines enable us to care for the entire person, but simultaneously our bio-psycho-socio mandate makes nursing one of the most eclectic of all the medical disciplines. For instance, a nurse administrator will likely have different research interests than a home health nurse or a nurse who specializes in women's health. Similarly, the research interests of a nurse with pathophysiological interests will likely differ from a qualitative nurse researcher concerned with experience and perception, and so on. It is important we study these diverse perspectives from the theories that emanate from them and make them part of our awareness and our consideration.

SCENARIO

To help us better understand these perspectives, let us create a scenario upon which to focus our discussion. In this scenario, Hagar is an elderly woman with deteriorating health. A few months prior to this exchange, Hagar moved in with her son, Marvin, and his wife, Doris. Doris is the primary caregiver who is struggling to continue caring for Hagar in their home. Because Hagar's health continues to decline, Marvin and Doris decide they must place her in a nursing home:

> He [Marvin] stands there awkwardly, his hands held out. Doris sidles up to him, nudges his ribs with a brown rayon elbow.
>
> "Go on now, Marv. You promised."

Marvin clears his throat, swallows, but fails to speak.

"Stop fidgeting, Marvin, for heaven's sake. I can't bear people who fidget. What is it?"

"Doris and me, we've been thinking—" His voice peters out, goes thin as shadows, vanishes. Then, in a gunfire burst of words, "She can't look after you any longer, Mother. She's not been well herself. The lifting—it's too much. She just can't do it—"

"Not to mention the disturbed nights—" Doris prompts.

"Yes, the nights. She's up and down a dozen times and never gets a decent sleep. You need professional care, Mother—a nurse who'll see to everything. You'd be much happier, yourself, as well—"

"More comfortable," Doris says. "We've been to Silverthreads Home, Mother, and it's really cozy. You'd love it, once you got used to it."

I can only gaze as though hypnotized. My fingers pleat my dress.

"A nurse—why should I need a nurse?"

Doris darts forward, her face not soft and flabby now, but peering earnestly. She gesticulates, as though she could convince me by this trembling of her hands.

"They're young and strong, and it's their business. They know how to lift a person. And all the other things—the beds—"

"What of the beds?" My voice is austere, but for some reason my hands are unsteady on the squeezed silk of the dress. Doris reddens, glances at Marvin. He shrugs, abandoning her to her own judgment.

"You've wet your sheets," she says, "nearly every night these past few months. It makes a lot of laundry, and we haven't been able to afford the automatic washer yet."

Appalled, I search her face.

"That's a lie. I never did any such thing. You are making it up. I know your ways. Just so you'll have some reason for putting me away."

She grimaces, an unappealing look, and I see that she is nearly in tears.

"I guess maybe I shouldn't have told you," she says. "It's not a nice thing to be told. But we're not blaming you. We never said it was your fault. You can't help—"

"Please!"

My head is lowered, as I flee their scrutiny, but I cannot move, and now I see that in the entire house, mine, there is no concealment. How is it that all these years I fancied violation meant an attack upon the flesh?

How is it that I never knew about the sheets? How could I not have noticed?

"I'm sorry," Doris mumbles, perhaps wanting to make it totally unendurable, or perhaps only blundering, having to wait another thirty years or so before she can know. (Laurence, 1966, pp. 73–74)

NURSING PERSPECTIVES

Let me introduce you to four of my fictional colleagues:

Emily

Emily primarily studies the epidemiology of incontinence in older adults. Most recently, she has undertaken a population study of types of incontinence. Her *quantitative* research is well published, and many of her articles have appeared in *Applied Nursing Research* and in *The Gerontologist*. She is considered by her colleagues to conduct meticulous research using complex models. Emily is most interested in identifying patterns of incontinence and occurrences of complications among older adults with diabetes. She completed her master's in nursing in 1982 and her PhD in 1997.

Chelsea

Chelsea specializes in gerontological nursing, and her research of at-home caregiving for older adults has appeared in *Qualitative Health Research* (QHR) and *Global Qualitative Nursing Research*. Her most prominent study was an ethnography of at-home familial care of insulin-dependent older adults with incontinence. This study was funded by a grant from the university where she is on faculty. She has a PhD, and has a reputation with her peers to be an expert in qualitative methods. She has refined and published many of these innovative techniques because of the number of grants she has obtained using these methods.

Joanne

Joanne is a 55-year-old nurse clinician at a large metropolitan hospital. She graduated from the hospital school of nursing and has her diploma hanging in a prominent location in her office. A decade later, when her children were in high school, she completed her baccalaureate in nursing. She is passionate about patient home care, with a particular interest in patients with incontinence. She is respected by her peers and described as a methodical and clinical expert. The latter is largely due to her many years in the field and her efforts to stay abreast of new topics. She attends numerous conferences on aging, especially those related to patient care, and subscribes to the *American Journal of Nursing*.

Megan

As a nurse physiologist, Megan is primarily concerned with the neuromechanisms of bladder control in older adults with diabetes. She is a focused individual who earned her PhD in 2000 at the age of 27. Her research commonly involves rats, and she conducted most of her work during her postdoctoral program on diabetic kidney disease through the biomechanisms of bladder control. Her studies are typically well-funded by the National Institutes of Health, and she primarily publishes in *Diabetes* and the *Journal of Physiological Nursing*.

DIALOGUE

While having coffee together, Megan tells them about Hagar's family and they begin to discuss our scenario.

"I think before any interventions could be made, we'd need to study the root cause of Hagar's diabetes incontinence and associated physiological conditions that may be contributing to her uncontrolled diabetes," says Megan. "If we can study and control those factors, Hagar might be able to stay at home longer. Without an understanding of the physiological mechanisms of her problem we can't truly address any of their concerns."

"And who is going to pay for you to do this research?" asked Emily. "Furthermore, who is going to pay for any of these interventions that emerge from your study? Knowing the root cause or associated conditions is less important, but first we need to know how widespread this problem is. Thousands upon thousands of older adults may be afflicted with incontinence. And," Emily continued, "do these patients even have a support system or family member willing and able to provide care for them?"

"I think you're both missing the bigger picture," Joanne interrupted. "These are people who need solutions right now, not years from now when your studies and analyses have been completed. It's clear that improved home care would benefit them most, and will benefit them right now in this situation. Yes, we need to know what's causing the incontinence in order to prevent it, but Doris needs the support of nurses who visit on a regular basis and can provide basic, practical help. Someone who can help her navigate all that is involved in Hagar's care."

"Joanne makes a valid point," says Chelsea. "Nurse researchers sometimes get so wrapped up in the bigger picture that we forget there are many immediate scenarios that, although they pose interesting and important research problems, primarily need immediate solutions. However, this doesn't even begin to take into account what the afflicted person's emotional responses are. Very little is known about how a family responds to and endures this diagnosis on an emotional level. Symptoms, as Doris told us, are sometimes severe and jarring. Just like in Hagar's case, sometimes the elderly person doesn't know or can't accept that he or she is incontinent—or even realize that it occurs, especially at night. What happens when her family tells her?"

This discussion sheds light on the idea that we all bring different *theoretical frames* to the discussions of care and research. The term *theoretical frame* should be used to refer to one's perspective on his or her research program. A theoretical frame encompasses more than "perspective"; it also includes the epistemology of research, the stages of the research program, and the projected outcomes and applications.

Theoretical frames create differences in *how a person applies a theory*. Examples of this can be seen in how theory and research designs interact with one another, which approaches and methods we deem significant, and how we identify and value the outcomes of our research, including determining our research *goals*. All of these vary. Theoretical frames encompass how *we determine something as fact* and play a role in what we consider as valid or invalid.

Variances and clashes in *theoretical frames*, as we have seen illustrated in the conversation about Hagar's story, define what form *theory* is and what it *does*. It shapes how a particular outlook influences the structure and role of research. Theory also helps us define the focus or topic of our research. Although similar to a theoretical frame, an applied theory is more personal and more narrow in scope than a paradigm. A paradigm is a lens through which we view the world and, for our purposes, conduct research. Once an individual subscribes to a paradigm, it seems to be very difficult, if not impossible, for a researcher to change. The labels provided by paradigms are so enduring that the entire scope of a researcher's work is usually consistent with his or her paradigm. This, unfortunately, means paradigms often divide groups of researchers. Even researchers who focus on a single topic may engage in "paradigmatic wars" with other researchers who subscribe to a different paradigm. No matter what *theoretical frame* you subscribe to, a paradigm provides a subtle and permeating perspective.

We can also see how each nurse within the same discipline interprets the same story differently, and others may not share the same *theoretical frame*. In this discussion, we clearly see how theoretical frames shape each nurse's ideas of which topics they deem important, researchable, fundable, and useful.

In their responses to Hagar's story, we see the manifestation of all these concepts. The theoretical frames that were formed by each nurse during her training and education within her respective subdiscipline, practice, and personal interest shape her concerns, her voice, and ultimately drive her research agenda. Contrary to what you and these nurses might think about incontinence, it is evident that differences in these theoretical frames are at the center of their disagreement. And although Joanne is correct reminding us that there are still people like Hagar who have persistent and immediate problems and these patients must remain at the center of these conflicts, there exists a need to discuss theory.

This brings us to the quintessence of science in nursing research. I believe nursing has not invested enough time or resources into the development of the foundational concepts and theories of our profession. This lack of agreement around theoretical principles agendas breeds a grave epistemological problem. This work was started in 1979 by a collection of nurse scholars who began exploring concepts important to nursing (Carlson, 1970; Nursing Development Conference Group, 1973). I believe their work was eclipsed by the development of abstract nursing theories and nursing frameworks for practice. Since there were not strong qualitative skills in place to challenge, modify, or support these abstract theories and frameworks, the profession, for the most part, continued, accepted, and implemented them. As is often seen when theoretical frames collide, the small emerging group[1] did not have the resources they needed to continue their significant work. Instead, nurses interested in concepts explored what the larger group determined as the "research priority," which happened to be implementing theoretical frameworks into nursing education and prioritizing quantitative inquiry.

I ask if we have failed to further their important legacy. Not many researchers are funded to explore nursing's theoretical foundations, and we, as a profession, do not seem to make this a priority. Prioritizing research through funding speaks to the problem that deems some theories and research questions are more credible, and thus more worthy of research funding, than other research. This has substantial consequences in all disciplines of research, because by investing in those topics that are considered more important, or more orthodox, other topics do not receive funding.

But the conversation continued:

"Our processes of generalization, or how we prioritize data sources, theories, and the varying degrees of certainty we have about different theories

---

[1] See Carlson (1970) and Nursing Development Conference Group (1973).

speaks volumes about our training within each of our disciplines" said Emily. "Each discipline teaches that some theory is more reliable than others, which translates into which theories will get research funding and attention and which ones will not."

"For years my patients have complained of physical pain at times of loss," said Joanne. "But until a neuropsychologist showed through functional magnetic resonance imaging (fMRI) that hurt feelings provide similar neural correlates to physical pain, not many people took them, or me, seriously."[2]

This is a prime example of how the hierarchy in nursing prioritizes "hard" sciences over "softer" ones. In Joanne's example, the patient reports are not seen as reliable sources of data because they are "subjective." Therefore, any theories developed from these accounts (such as the theory that bereavement may manifest as physical pain) were not taken seriously. It was not until a "harder" science, such as neuropsychology, showed this to be true that the profession took these observations more seriously and, in doing so, may finally implement better interventions (Cassell, 2002; Diamond, 1987).

"I think our research agenda should look at ways to reduce the suffering of the diabetic and use a quality of life measure," Emily said.

"How can you have any clue if their suffering has decreased without first defining what suffering is?" exclaimed Chelsea. "Once you do that, you'll be able to determine if you have reduced suffering."

As a qualitative researcher, Chelsea's framework means she is most interested in understanding the phenomenon of diabetes and defining its characteristics as a concept. Questions that Chelsea would likely be interested in include a definition of the nature of suffering in older adults with diabetes, and determining if there is a relationship between the quality of life and suffering. She might also plan to link her study of concepts, such as internalized shame, to modified behavior. As a smart qualitative researcher, she understands the importance of systematically expanding her research to the conceptual and theoretical levels. Chelsea also knows that to study internal shame from incontinence will require a broader study of behaviors linked to such concepts as isolation. Her theoretical frame keeps Chelsea from being able to delimit the research problem simply, which she would consider a threat to validity.

Emily senses this and jumps in. "Theories are what focus quantitative research. It is theory that tells researchers what to include, how to define it."

"Precisely, but recall that Burton (1974) tells us that theories are also political and by including one piece of data, you're excluding another," Chelsea added.

"And anyway, not all theories are sound," says Megan. "Most of the time, I feel like theory isn't at all the intended outcome of my research."

---

[2] Eisenberger, Lieberman, and Williamson (2003).

"Many of the theories we subscribe to in nursing were not created methodically. Take Leventhal[3] for example—he developed the Health Belief Model by sequentially describing 17 studies that theoretically derived that model over 30 years. First he used his own perspectives. Then he allowed his nurse to add her point of view, and over the course of 20 years, he systematically modified his instrument using quantitative methods with different groups of people. He expressed that he really needed to consult with colleagues, but he wasn't sure how."

Moving from an atheoretical basis directly to quantitative inquiry has been exhaustively documented and discussed. This is at the heart of our epistemological problems in nursing, and even though funding and manpower are now available for researchers to backtrack and pursue the basic inquiries needed to recreate the theoretical basis of our profession, very little progress has been made. It is clear that the National Institute of Nursing Research (NINR) should prioritize this task, but there does not seem to be any urgency within our community to undertake this important task.

"I didn't know that about Leventhal's model, but doesn't it seem that sometimes theory may be wrong?" said Joanne innocently.

Emily laughed, *"Just ask anyone following a fad diet"* (Foster et al., 2003; Hart, Greenwood, & Truby, 2003).

Theory can also be misguided in a multitude of ways. One of the most common ways is called *making conceptual leaps*. This is the practice of linking indicators in the data too haphazardly to concepts that are also very abstract or to concepts that have been slovenly created. Quantitative researchers are taught this early on and often (correlation does not necessarily equal causation), but, unfortunately, qualitative researchers commonly make conceptual leaps. Qualitative researchers are obliged to apply existing knowledge as it emerges from the data (this is sometimes called incorporating "official concepts"), but they should also be cognizant of these concepts in the real world, and be careful when generalizing during data analysis.

Concepts and theories exist in a varied and conceptual place. Some are hyperlocalized to data with a very narrow scope, and others, like classes of behavior, may be very broad and generally applied. Still, there may be other theories and concepts that have a broad scope, are widely applied, but may be very specific under certain circumstances. Take, for example, Selye (1976). Selye was discouraged when he recognized that the physiological stress response could be triggered by almost any stressor. Another example is to describe suffering as a behavioral response to bereavement or psychological assault (Morse, 2001). I call these *horizontal concepts*. They are common, usually very abstract, often have wide-reaching applications, and are exceedingly useful. They enable researchers to classify behaviors or responses within various contexts. In nursing, these might emerge as *shame, coping, urgency,* and many more.

---

[3] Leventhal (1993, January 12).

You may ask, "Do we really need to question the concept of urgency?" Many within our profession have a solid idea of what urgency is, but there are different types of urgency, and perhaps these manifest themselves in different ways. Because of this, patients may have different experiences of urgency, which may cause them to use different language to describe their experience. By inquiring about the linguistic possibilities of this phenomenon, we may be able to identify certain speech patterns or even particular phrases that could be used during the diagnostic process. Many researchers have noted that we lack language for certain topics that people find hard to talk about. I suggest that we, as a profession, search interviews for, and analyze metaphors (Johnson, 1987; Lakeoff & Johnson, 1980; Ortny, 1998) that may help us develop, a language that allows us to describe these concepts in a uniform way, similar to Melzack's (1987) revolutionary work on pain descriptors.

After all this discussion, you may question the necessity of theory altogether, and perhaps believe there are cases in which research does not require a theory at all. However, when analyzing the values and perspectives of seemingly atheoretical research, we are bound to find remnants of the researcher's theoretical frame. This gives rise to the notion that when theory is not deliberately used, our research is less useful, has less power, and cannot be applied as widely. However, the opposite of applying a theory to data which does not quite fit is also true and equally problematic. In nursing, this approach is commonly employed by sorting data into categories such as physical, psychological, social, and environmental. Reducing data to such simple terms does little to advance our discipline's research and practice initiatives. Theory is, after all, a tool, and just as a research method is a tool to uncover knowledge, so is theory.

DISCUSSION

Concerted efforts to find new paradigms or new approaches to research have the power to raise awareness of hidden problems. It is my sincerest hope that you will undertake basic research when the problem demands it, but will also be confident enough to recognize sound theory and apply it to each problem, viewing it as a multifactorial one that demands a multifaceted approach in which examination of all possible angles will be employed. Try to remember Megan, Joanne, Emily, and Chelsea and their varying perspectives, be they social science, psychology, phenomenology, or others. Although researchers do not often devote time to identifying new research paradigms, we remain much resolved in our desire to petition for research funding to further this cause. Recognize that clinical needs often drive the areas of scientific research that thrive and evolve and, in doing so, exclude and stymie others. Know that it is in research-funding organizations that scientists with varied worldviews engage in conversations like the one between Megan, Joanne, Emily, and Chelsea when they determine which projects to fund or not fund. Unfortunately, funding may still be a political process, with the majority of funds being allocated to those disciplines higher up in a given discipline's hierarchy, a hierarchy that, in some cases, may even be determined on the basis of the researcher's affiliations. To invert this hierarchy, we should make attempts to direct the course of research programs by publishing requests for applications (RFAs). Doing so may provoke vital research results, but could also produce "instant experts," who happen to prepare an excellent proposal, but may not have the most experience or methodological expertise to actually conduct the necessary work. On a national level, it is imperative that we cultivate the maximum number of scientists we can reasonably support. It is a value statement frequently motivated by political agenda, to provide targeted support to applied or basic research. We elevate those topics we decide to support, be it breast cancer, HIV/AIDS, suffering, or incontinence, and ignore those topics that are not awarded funding. Our approach as a discipline and as individuals should be to shed light on and award those teams undertaking multidisciplinary approaches, those with multisite research teams or simply principal investigators with small research staff. The current trend of targeting research funding to particular problems, which may be determined by current fads, denies funding to other areas and marginalizes excellent, albeit less "fashionable" research. Although these scientists are working with fewer resources than their counterparts and may not be valued by current standards, history has shown us that some of the most significant, landmark work is often conducted under such conditions, only to be revered many years, or even decades, later.

REFERENCES

Beck, C. T. (2016). *Developing a program of research*. New York, NY: Springer Publishing Company.

Burton, A. (1974). The nature of personality theory. In A. Burton (Ed.), *Operational theories of personality* (pp. 1–19). New York, NY: Brunner/Mazel.

Carlson, C. C. (1970). *Behavioral concepts and nursing interventions*. Philadelphia, PA: Lippincott.

Cassell, J. (2002). Perturbing the system: "hard science," "soft science," and social science: The anxiety and madness of method. *Human Organization, 61*(2), 177–185.

Diamond, J. M. (1987). Soft sciences are often harder than hard sciences. *Discover, 8*(8), 34–39.

Eisenberger, N., Lieberman, M., & Williamson, K. D. (2003). Does rejection hurt? An fMRI study of social exclusion. *Science, 302*, 290–292.

Foster, G. D., Wyatt, H. R., Hill, J. O., McGuckin, B. G., Brill, C., Mohammed, B. S., . . . Klein, S. (2003). A randomized trial of a low-carbohydrate diet for obesity. *New England Journal of Medicine, 348*(21), 2082–2090.

Hart, K., Greenwood, H., & Truby, H. (2003). Pound for pound? Comparing the costs incurred by subjects following four commercially available weight loss programmes. *Journal of Human Nutrition & Dietetics, 16*(5), 365.

Johnson, M. (1987). *The body in the mind: The bodily basis of meaning, imagination and reason.* Chicago, IL: University of Chicago Press.

Lakeoff, G., & Johnson, M. (1980). *Metaphors we live by.* Chicago, IL: University of Chicago Press.

Laurence, M. (1966). *The stone angel.* Toronto, ON: McClelland & Stewart.

Leventhal, H. (1993, January 12). *The study of illness cognition from thought to action at the biobehavioral interface* [videotape]. Colloquium, Gerontology Center, The Pennsylvania State University, Old Main, State College, PA.

Melzack, R. (1987). The short-form McGill pain questionnaire. *Pain, 30*(2), 191–197.

Morse, J. M. (2001). Toward a praxis theory of suffering. *Advances in Nursing Science, 24*(1), 47–59.

Nursing Development Conference Group. (1973). *Concept formalization in nursing: Processes and product.* Boston, MA: Little, Brown.

Ortny, A. (1998). *Metaphor and thought* (2nd ed.). Cambridge, UK: Cambridge University Press.

Selye, H. (1976). *The stress of life.* Boston, MA: Butterworths.

Szent-Györgyi, A. (1972). Dionysians and Apollonians. *Science, 176*(4038), 966.

ORIENTATION 101: DEFINITIONS AND OTHER ESSENTIAL EXTRANEOUS NOTES

> *"When I use a word," Humpty Dumpty said in rather a scornful tone, "it means just what I choose it to mean—neither more nor less."*
>
> *"The question is," said Alice, "whether you can make words mean so many different things."*
>
> *"The question is," said Humpty Dumpty, "which is to be master— that's all."*
>
> —Lewis Carroll, *Through the Looking Glass* (1871/2015)

Before we go any further, let us make it clear about what we are talking about, and briefly define concepts, frameworks, theories, philosophical underpinnings, paradigms, components, and parts of all these, so that by the end of this book, we will know exactly the structure of knowledge and the role of each.

PARADIGM

A paradigm is a worldview of science, a perspective that is generally accepted as true. Paradigms encompass widely accepted theories and determine which facts are "knowledge claims." "They structure future research: determining which facts are theoretically salient; defining what constitutes a paradox and what questions urgently need to be examined and what kinds of evidence are considered meaningful" (Geddes, 2010, p. 7). Seven major scientific revolutions have involved substantial conceptual change: those of Copernicus, Newton, Einstein, Darwin, the development of quantum theory, and the theory of plate tectonics (Thagard, 1999, p. 51).

Paradigms fall (or fail) sometimes because of their own internal contradictions, and their inability to deal with inconvenient facts thrown up by the world . . . They may be "overthrown by well organized, coherent, mobilized oppositions" and when this happens, a period of chaos and contention follows (Geddes, 2010, p. 6).

This means that paradigms are very hard to identify when you are living them. But once society moves on, they are easy to spot. Let us interrupt this chapter by looking at a paradigm: the diseases caused by masturbation.

TO DO 5.1. MEET A PARADIGM

Find and read Engelhardt (1974).

Engelhardt's article is important because the underlying theory on which the research is based is clearly inaccurate today, with our 20–20 hindsight. In this case, those who believed in the causative links between insanity and madness, had a theory, a research design, and an intervention—all of which were shown to be inaccurate.

A paradigm is often considered a global perspective, that is generally accepted and relatively abstract and generalizable. For instance, the current paradigm about obesity is that people are responsible for their weight, can lose weight if they "work at it" if given enough incentive, and that diet and inadequate exercise are the primary causes of obesity. This perspective may change over time (i.e., a paradigm shift) as we learn more about the complexities of obesity.

Philosophy

Philosophy deals with systems of ideas, beliefs, values, opinions, or principles based on an overall understanding of the system of existence and the universe. It deals with a basic set of principles of the discipline and logical reasoning. A philosophical system provides a particular view or outlook. Moral philosophy deals with principles of human behavior and ethics.

Philosophy enables one to theorize, explain, reason, or argue for a particular position. *Epistemology* is the nature and scope of knowledge; *ontology* is the study of the nature of being and becoming, existence or reality.

Phenomenon

· A phenomenon is a collection of behaviors, occurrences, or experiences that are observable or recordable. Phenomena are not as well understood or developed as a concept. Sometimes they are labeled, but often not well defined nor are the characteristics well described.

Further, a phenomenon may be a behavior that is recognizable, but has not been analyzed to describe the process, nor developed into a concept or sub-concepts. The sub-concepts contained within the phenomenon are not specifically identified, and the researchers have not analyzed "what is going on."

Assumption

Assumptions are the taken-for-granted, underlying, suppositions. They may form the premise underlying the theory or research.

Domains

A domain is an area of study, or the scope of the topic or phenomenon.

Model

A model is a "simplified representation of a process. Its purpose is to illuminate a basic logic underlying a process that might not be perceptible from observation of the entire complicated reality overlaid, as all reality is, with multitudinous irrelevant details" (Geddes, 2010, p. 32). A model may be a schematic (diagrammed) or a scaled physical representation. A model should illuminate the process that had not been evident before; it aids in communication.

Concepts

There are many definitions of "concept." A concept is *a mental image*, a "conceptualization" of a thing, a collection of behaviors, or an idea. It is a representation of reality in one's mind.

A concept must have the following components:

- *A label*: we must name it to know what we are talking about.
- *A definition*: The definition must be clear, and one that we may recognize. The label and the definition are generally agreed upon, and allows us to communicate with others.

- *Attributes*—or characteristics of the concept. These are present in every instant of the concept, and they make the concept what it *is*. It was an Aristotelian rule that all attributes must be present in every case in order to identify the concept, although some philosophers believe that this is not necessary. They believe that the presence of *most* of the attributes is adequate for the concept to be identified.

Let us start with an easy example. If I speak of a table, we envision a piece of furniture with a flat top and legs of a height that allow you to sit at the table. Tables usually have four legs, but some may have only one (e.g., a pedestal table). And other tables, such as a conference table, may have more than four legs. But the flat top and the legs are the attributes of a table.

Now, a table is used to put things on, but if we have a table in our article, it is a structure for us to put things "on" or into—we have borrowed one of the attributes from a table as a piece of furniture, and used it to name a tool for our writing. Or we may have a tabletop mountain, that is, a mountain with a flat top, borrowing the attribute of the flat tabletop to describe the top of the mountain. Note we are using the attribute to conceptualize—in the mental image sense—not as an attribute of components of articles or of mountains.

Therefore, it is the attributes that make the concept the concept. Although that all must be present in the concept, these attributes may be present in different "strengths," and this makes for different forms and uses of a concept. In one type of the concept, some of the attributes may be stronger than the others, and this pattern may differ in other types of the concept.

- All concepts have a boundary, that is, a limit beyond which the concept is no longer an example of that particular concept. Near the boundary, the attributes become weak or when another concept overlaps, the attributes of the second overlapping concept are shared with other concepts, so that it may be difficult to recognize which attributes belong to which concept. For this reason, researchers analyzing concepts always begin their study examining the clearest, purest, and most represented example of the concept they can find.
- *Antecedents:* Antecedents are conditions that precede the concept and give rise to the concept. For example, attraction may be an antecedent to love.
- *Outcomes:* In addition, all behavioral concepts have outcomes, or behaviors that consistently follow the occurrence of the concept.

We have types of concepts, according to their function, or what they describe. *Behavioral concepts* are concepts that refer to collections of behaviors that have been given a name.

Lay concepts are developed in everyday life in the course of conversation. First, they are introduced as slang terms, as trade names, or simply given a name; then as their use becomes more common, familiar, and everyday, they are eventually formally adopted into the dictionary. You may think of any number of new concepts around the areas of computers, cell phones, and software (or ways they are used), that may not yet be in the dictionary. These *lay concepts* reveal the dynamic nature of language, of ideas, of changing society, and so forth.

Scientific concepts are developed in the course of science as scientific definitions, or terms that are needed in order to conduct research. These are introduced into the scientific literature deliberately and cautiously, at the same time introduced with a label, formal definition, attributes, and boundaries.

But language is dynamic and fluid. As lay concepts become more important to science, they are "developed," usually through qualitative inquiry, and then used as scientific concepts in research. Qualitative researchers develop detailed descriptions of the concept in context, identify the attributes, explore forms of the concepts, refine the definitions, and describe the boundaries, antecedents, and outcomes. Alternatively, this may be done with the use of the literature or philosophical inquiry. Think of articles developing such lay concepts as comfort or privacy, over the past few years.

On the other hand, as scientific concepts become increasingly used on a daily basis in the everyday context, they may "move" from the science to the lay lexicon. For instance, *social support* is one of these concepts—developed in science and now used in everyday language. Social support does not yet appear in the dictionary, but I have no doubt it will within the next 10 years.

Concepts appear in various forms—some are very close to the data, quite narrow in scope, and represent quite specific things. Other are more abstract ("higher level") and very broad in scope, and may encompass other, more local, concepts. For instance, *suffering* is a broad concept, encompassing the lower level concepts such as bereavement, grief, sorrow, and despair. Concept may be horizontal, encompassing a large number of concepts. *Stress* is an example of a horizontal concept, which may be applied to metals or bridges, to physical exercise, or to emotions. Incidentally, stress is a concept that was once in the lay lexicon and moved to the scientific.

Another interesting thing about concepts is that they cluster, and we call the concepts that are similar to—but not exactly the same as—the first concept, *allied concepts*. Allied concepts may share some of the attributes of the first concept, but not all. They may overlap with the first concept, near the boundary where the attributes are weak. Two concepts may also merge, changing the nature of both original concepts (e.g., when hope "seeps in" to emotional suffering, it changes the nature of suffering to form the reformulated self in the *Praxis*

Theory of Suffering [Morse, 2011, Chapter 35, this volume]). Finally, the attributes within a concept may vary in strength, giving the concept a different appearance, but really the concept remains the same, but in a stronger or weaker form. For instance, a "strong" form of hope, may be referred to as "high hopes" by lay persons, or even as "false hopes," is still a form of the concept hope.

TO DO 5.2. IS NO HOPE A TYPE OF HOPE?

1. If a person is a "no hoper"—that is, one for whom we have no hope that he or she will ever succeed in life—is this absence of hope that we have for this person a form or type of hope? Argue your answer.

Theoretical Framework

A framework, often called a *theoretical framework,* is a representation of what a researcher thinks is happening in reality. It is really a way of organizing concepts or variables (for quantitative research) or showing data collection points, focus, and even data collection strategies, for a qualitative project. It shows the scope of the project, the components (usually concepts), and the relationship of the various concepts in the framework. A theoretical framework consists of concepts and phenomena and their linkages, necessary to explain a research or clinical problem, with the purpose of communicating the data plan to the reader. As does a model, the framework illustrates the process that will be researched, or the process of care that will be provided.

Theory

A theory differs from a framework in that its purpose is to both communicate the data collection plan and to test the hypothesized model and relationships between the concepts. A theory is therefore a system of concepts describing a topic or process. Hypotheses tentatively suggest relationships between these concepts, and the relationships between the concepts tested. Once a theory is proven, it is no longer a theory, but a fact.

Theory usually consists of interrelated concepts about a particular topic. Quantitative researchers usually diagram their theory with the concepts in "balloons" and lines illustrating the hypothesized linkages and types of relationships (positive or negative, and the p value) between the concepts (see Chapter 27).

Quantitative theories may be developed from the literature, using (even combining) the work of others, from previous research, or from the results of qualitative inquiry. Theories vary in their degrees of conjecture or supposition. Quantitative theories show how each variable will be measured, and as quantitative theories are tested, they may be subsequently modified, until the researcher is satisfied that they are reasonable approximations of what is going on in reality.

In qualitative inquiry, the theory is the outcome of the research. If qualitative researchers use a diagram to illustrate the theory with the position and interrelationship of the concepts, it is usually drawn with the concepts closer together, even overlapping. Qualitatively derived theory is "tested" or verified during the process of construction (Meadows & Morse, 2001). Qualitative methods demand that each small advance on the theory is tested—replicated—before proceeding. Therefore, qualitative theory *approaches* certainty, and it is not usually intended to be tested as a whole. Indeed, testing may be a fruitless task, for the reason that qualitative inquiry was used in the first place because there was no measure of the concepts available, and this deficiency remains, even in the presence of the theory.

Theories differ in their level of abstraction, or distance from the data. *Descriptive theory* depicts very local action, close to the context; *grand theories* are highly abstract and broad in scope, accounting for large areas of phenomena. They usually include a formal organization of abstract concepts.

Mid-range (or middle-range) theory lies between descriptive and grand theory. Mid-range theory is less abstract and more clearly delineated to a particular domain or context, than grand theory. They usually have developed concepts that are linked to clinical phenomena, and are therefore applied and linked to practice. These levels of theory are on a continuum, and mid-range theory may approach a descriptive theory. The previously mentioned mid-range theory may provide insights from nursing: how to negotiate care, provide hope, and so forth; at a higher level, it may be useful for understanding communities and poverty, or aspects of culture and health, and so forth.

Context

A context is place or setting in which a phenomenon occurs. The context may have a profound influence on the concept, influencing its form and function.

Can a concept be separated from its context? The process of making the concept abstract is a process of *decontextualization*, or removing or stripping the context. This is a process of abstraction, and it is by removing the context that generalization occurs in qualitative inquiry. Once the concept is applied to a new setting a process of *recontextualization* is put in place.

Induction

Induction is the cognitive process of working, or thinking, from the data through processes of categorization, synthesis, and abstraction. It is reasoning from the particular to the general, from the data to synthesized statements about the data, to more abstract, generalized statements. The commonalities within instances are identified to form sets or groups and these are then combined as larger components. Induction is the primary cognitive mode used in qualitative analysis.

Deduction

Deduction is reasoning from the general, by developing propositions from variables and confirming these with data. Deduction is the primary cognitive mode used in quantitative analysis.

Abstraction

Abstraction is the extraction of the idea or observation from the context or concrete instance to the concept itself. Abstract ideas become more generalizable because they are not linked to a particular context.

TO DO 5.3. ASSIGNED BEDTIME READING

Through the Looking Glass
   "You are sad," the Knight said in an anxious tone: "let me sing you a song to comfort you."
   "Is it very long?" Alice asked, for she had heard a good deal of poetry that day. "It's long," said the Knight, "but it's very, *very* beautiful. Everybody that hears me sing it—either it brings the *tears* into their eyes, or else—"
   "Or else what?" said Alice, for the Knight had made a sudden pause.
   "Or else it doesn't, you know. The name of the song is called '*Haddocks' Eyes*'."
   "Oh, that's the name of the song, is it?" Alice said, trying to feel interested.
   "No, you don't understand," the Knight said, looking a little vexed. "That's what the name is *called*. The name really *is* '*The Aged Aged Man*'."
   "Then I ought to have said 'That's what the *song* is called'?" Alice corrected herself.
   "No, you oughtn't: that's quite another thing! The *song* is called '*Ways and Means*': but that's only what it's *called*, you know!"
   "Well, what *is* the song, then?" said Alice, who was by this time completely bewildered.
   "I was coming to that," the Knight said. "The song really *is* '*A-sitting On a Gate*': and the tune's my own invention." (Carroll, 1871/2015, Chapter 8)

REFERENCES

Carroll, L. (2015). *Through the looking glass, and what Alice found there*. London, UK: Macmillan. (Originally published 1871)

Engelhardt, H. T., Jr. (1974). The disease of masturbation: Values and the concept of disease. *Bulletin of the History of Medicine, 48*, 234–248.

Geddes, B. (2010). *Paradigms and sand castles: Theory building and research design in comparative politics*. Ann Arbor, MI: University of Michigan.

Meadows, L., & Morse, J. M. (2001). Constructing evidence within the qualitative project. In J. M. Morse, J. Swanson, & A. Kuzel (Eds.), *The nature of evidence in qualitative inquiry* (pp. 187–200). Newbury Park, CA: Sage.

Morse, J. M. (2011). The Praxis Theory of Suffering. In J. B. Butts & K. L. Rich (Eds.), *Philosophies and theories in advanced nursing practice* (pp. 569–602). Burlington, MA: Jones & Bartlett.

Thagard, P. (1999). *How scientists explain disease*. Princeton, NJ: Princeton University.

Janice M. Morse

6

THE BATTLEFIELD OF KNOWLEDGE: DIFFERENT PURPOSES, DIFFERENT APPROACHES

> *"It's a bird." "It's a plane." "It's Superman!"*
> —Maxwell and Duchovny (1939)

As our perception of something changes, and we see the "thing" more clearly, so our understanding of whatever the thing is, also changes. The "thing" itself does not change, of course, just our understanding, or perception of it.

Our perceptions are manipulated by various mechanisms. The one you experienced when you read Bohannan's "Shakespeare in the Bush" (Chapter 3) was a cultural frame. Our culture indoctrinates us from the earliest age, providing us with sets of values and beliefs, and sets of ways to view the world. Our own culture connects us by groups but also divides us by race, nationality, gender, occupational group, religion, age, politics, and economic status. You can name any of these demographic divides by characteristics that sort us as "like me" and "not like me." But it is also true that culture separates us from others. As we learned from the Tiv, culture gives us all the confidence of believing that we alone are *right*.

Research has an equal set of such frames—frames that provide us with different approaches of seeing the phenomenon we are researching. And with the equal force of a belief, some regard these frames as correct and incorrect, right and wrong, and worthy or not worthy of teaching, funding, publishing, and using the results.

But we hope we are wiser than our colleagues who divide. We see these frames, these alternative ways of seeing and doing research, as alternative tools with different purposes, different goals, and different outcomes. Considering the selections, the onus is on you to recognize the difference, and to select the correct "frame" for your task in hand.

For decades, debates have argued over the objectivity of science, but for the purposes of this book we will assume that no research is value-free. Even the selection of your topic is something that has come to your attention as "being interesting," "being in need of research," or even "important to understand." But, the trick when doing research is to be able to recognize one's values, beliefs, culture, background, and interests that have led to your present position. Whether one approaches research objectively and supposedly without bias, or subjectively, with the need to access the phenomenon subjectively overriding objective technique, one may come to understand one's own lens with which one views reality.

A *lens* is the broad perspective that one overlays a problem, providing a paradigmatic perspective on the way you see the world.[1] For example, the perspective of feminism may adjust your gaze to give your research a particular agenda: you may passionately believe that your research will improve the status of women, will bring the plight of women to the attention of others, and so forth, so that your research, either objectively or subjectively conducted, will allow you to view the world from the perspective of a feminist, and to ask research questions that will explore the plight of women.

Another such lens may be adherence to *culture* as a framework, so that all of your research explores cultural beliefs and practices, differences in behaviors, health and illnesses, and so forth. One may write as an *ecologist*, considering environmental concerns; or as a *humanist*, focusing on the plight of the poor. One may adhere to the writings of a particular *theorist* (and, for instance, be considered a Marxist), or have a *perspective*, such as feminism, or *a theoretical stance*, such as the social determinants of health.[2]

These perspectives often follow disciplines, and as a result are closely tied to the set of concepts of interest. For instance, if you are a nurse physiologist, you will be interested in the physiological concepts and theories that address physiological processes such as homeostasis. If you are interested in gerontological nursing, you may be interested in concepts concerned with aging. Someone who is interested in the nurse–patient interaction may have a list of concepts that includes:

- Concepts important for the nurse and the patient: trust, respect, privacy, and dignity
- Concepts important for the nurse: acknowledgment, empathy, sympathy, commiserations, condolence, compassion, reflective listening, being with, and presence
- Concepts important for the patient: hope, dignity, suffering, sorrow, grief, and despair

---

[1] Q: What is the difference between a paradigm and a theoretical lens?

[2] ANS: A paradigm may be used as a theoretical lens—or not (e.g., it may be used without the researcher's awareness). A theoretical lens may be smaller than a paradigm—or not. So they may be the same—or not.

Concepts that are associated with a single topic are usually called "concept families." They may be separate, addressing different aspects of your topic, overlapping, addressing related areas of your concept as allied concepts, or competing concepts addressing the same phenomena.

TO DO 6.1. CONCEPT FAMILIES

1. Make a table of *concept families* in your area of interest (practice or research topic).
2. Indicate which of these are lay concepts and which of these are scientific concepts.

INDUCTIVE APPROACHES TO CONCEPT DEVELOPMENT

Induction

Induction is usually, but not always, associated with qualitative research. Induction is the cognitive process of working, thinking "up" from the data through processes of categorization, synthesis, and abstraction. It begins with seeking and identifying commonalities in pieces of data, and forming categories of common data. The researcher then looks for characteristics *within* each category and differences *between* categories, and from this develops concepts, identifies the relationships between categories, and thus develops theory. As such, induction is the primary mode of thinking in developing qualitative theory.

Role in Inquiry

Is induction value-free? Do researchers who use inductive inference work from a "blank slate?" The answer is, "no." Qualitative research is usually conducted within a particular paradigm or even a frame that gives the research perspective. Ideally, with an inductive approach, the researcher puts aside all presumptions and commences inquiry from these data allowing the categories to be developed and be incrementally built, rather than using preconceived categories. The categories are built by looking for patterns as provided in the data by participant's interviews and observations, rather than the investigator's—or the literature's—a priori notions and conceptualizations.

If the researcher has a preconceived framework, assumptions of paradigmatic view, this creates the agenda for conducting research or may rise even to affecting the question being asked. For instance, a researcher may have a social justice lens for his or her research program. However, the research should then attempt to bracket all assumptions, and approach the

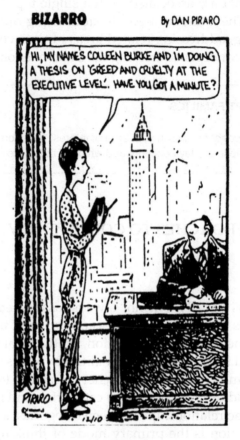

FIGURE 6.1
The value of induction.
Reprinted by permission of Daniel Piraro.

researcher with a neutral stance. If the researcher retains the underlying perspective and uses it in the data collection and analysis, this should be done consciously, to prevent untoward bias in the research. An example of using a preconceived notion is shown in the cartoon (Figure 6.1) in which Colleen Burke considered the executive approach as one of "greed and cruelty." In this case, not only is her perspective forming her questions and presupposing her findings, she will also find it difficult to recruit executives into her study, for being "greedy and cruel" are not desirable states, especially for successful executives.

Using Frameworks in Qualitative Inquiry

Although valuing induction, qualitative inquiry does not take place in a vacuum, or from a "blank slate." However, to begin qualitative research from a theoretical perspective may be dangerous, for one may use the theoretical frame to either consciously or unconsciously prove a certain point or position. For this reason, phenomenologists document all that they know about the topic before starting, and then try to begin their study by putting these assumptions aside, a process called *bracketing* in phenomenology (van Manen, 1990, 2014).

Even when researching relatively harmless, or value-free, topics, the consent process itself may interfere with induction. The consent form contains a description of the study (or even the title), which informs the participants about the study, and the interviews are therefore slanted toward this topic (or concept), rather than emerging more or less spontaneously (Morse, 2008).

Do qualitative studies use theoretical frameworks? This is rather a contentious issue, as the framework itself may circumscribe investigation, prematurely restricting the boundaries and becoming a source of invalidity. Consider if from the framework you developed a checklist. This means you were working deductively. In this case, does the researcher discover anything new? No—at worst, the data collection form restricts inquiry to checking frequencies in each preidentified item. The answer is to keep such frameworks removed from the data and to use them with care. For this reason, qualitative inquiry does not use forced choice questionnaires. Frequently, with semistructured questionnaires, the researcher identifies all questions that should be asked within a certain domain, but does not know enough about the responses to make the questionnaire fixed choice. So, even semistructured questionnaires may constrict the inquiry by limiting and overly guiding the participant's responses.[3] Nevertheless, because the domain is restricted by the questions *asked*, the researcher must be careful to obtain an adequately large sample—or again validity is threatened.

Theoretical Contexts

Contextual frameworks are different from theoretical frameworks, as they encompass the proposed study making an argument for its significance, placing it in context. They are used to justify the research questions or to establish a context for the study—usually one that is larger than the actual study. Once, I wanted to study gift giving in hospitals (I also discuss the results of this study in Chapter 15). I wrote a straightforward proposal, but it was denied by the funding agency. I was informed that the topic was trivial and insignificant. I am not certain that was the whole story, for gifts given to nurses seem to cause embarrassment to the administration, believing that nurses are in a position to inappropriately solicit such gifts, and nursing organizations and hospitals have rules prohibiting nurses from accepting gifts. Despite this, gifts still come. Why?

---

[3] Why? Think this one through yourself.

In the resubmission, I created a contextual framework, trying to show the significance of the study. I argued:

> Caring for patients frequently requires intensely personal and intimate tasks to be performed by nurses. In their professional role, nurses are relative strangers to the patients, yet are responsible for providing support for patients in their most distressing moments, such as when they are in pain or facing the fear of death. Nurses also provide patients with such care or treatment as assisting with bedpans, bathing or catheterization, that would in other circumstances be considered "shameful" and private to the patients. Although these procedures are expected and routine nursing tasks, they rarely become expected and accepted by the patients themselves. Patients frequently apologize and express shame at the "work" being created by the loss of bodily control.

> Nurses work for the hospital, yet they give care to the patient. I argue that this situation creates an imbalance in the nurse–patient relationship. It creates a loss of power, dependency and passivity within the patient, and a feeling of being obligated to reciprocate for the care given. Chapman (1976, 1980), Dowd (1975) and Kayser-Jones (1979, 1981) note that reciprocity is an essential part of the therapeutic process, although, ironically, the practice is discouraged in health care. As the nurse's employer considers that the nurse has already been reimbursed adequately in the form of salary, and recognizes the more powerful position of the nurse and the potential for exploitation, administrative policy frequently is such as to prohibit gift giving. I suggest that such a policy inhibits patient recovery and that the constant refusal results in a double-bind situation for nurses. The nurses are placed in a situation whereby they must choose between accepting or refusing the gift. The former involves breaking hospital rules with the subsequent feeling of guilt and the possibility of reprimand; the latter violates social norms (i.e., it is considered rude) and may be construed as rejecting the patient. Finally, although this must be investigated further, the lack of a direct patient-nurse reward system may foster burnout in nurses. (Morse, 1989, pp. 33–34)

Note that by using this theoretical context I was not intending to study the "imbalance" in the nurse–patient relationship or the outcomes if this gift relationship was interrupted. The framework is larger than the study, but I placed it in context and showed its significance.

Theoretical Frameworks

If qualitative research is supposed to be inductive, why does a researcher even consider using theoretical frameworks in the proposal? In quantitative inquiry, theoretical frameworks are established at the beginning of the study. They are intended to broadly guide inquiry, to provide parameters that scope the study, to justify its significance, and to fit it within current theory or practice. Despite the qualitative researcher's need to work inductively, and Glaser's (1978) admonition that qualitative researchers need not go to the library before starting their study, researchers always need to know the literature. Researchers must be familiar with the major concepts, theories, and findings of others that are relevant to their project. They need to justify their project, explain their theoretical orientation, and what assumptions and concepts they are using. This assists fieldwork and analysis, for when researchers begin analysis and see something, they will recognize it, know what it is for, and how it has been previously described. Then they may compare their data by sliding their analysis over the descriptions of the well-established contexts and see if they are adding something new or disagreeing with the standard conceptualization. This is preferable to finding themselves in the position of the middle management team in *The Restaurant at the End of the Universe* (Adams, 1980) who, 10,000 years after they were ejected into space and rediscovered the wheel, were still holding meetings to decide what color it should be.

If you are using phenomenology and wish to bracket this theoretical knowledge,[4] then do so, but remember that phenomenological methods take the perspective of phenomenological concepts and incorporate the perspective of the other—and the literature—into phenomenological analyses. In other words, the literature is incorporated during the process of analysis; it is not ignored (or bracketed out) altogether.

Note that this use of theory in research is the most important difference between qualitative and quantitative researchers. In quantitative research, the theory is established at the beginning of the proposal to build the model to be tested in the research and to justify the selections of concepts for theory testing. Then, during the actual conduct of the research, the theory is put aside—that is what control groups are for—to prevent bias. Once results are obtained they are then placed in the context of the original theory. In qualitative inquiry, the theory may run right through the research process, and give meaning to the analysis and the results.

---

[4] "Bracketing" is deliberately partitioning off what is known about, or what you think (or hope) you will find in a phenomenological study.

Qualitative Concepts

In this book we will primarily discuss developing concepts using qualitative inquiry. As described in Chapter 12, nursing as a discipline skipped over this stage in its development. We do not have the long monographs that gave anthropology and sociology their theoretical bases in the 1960s and 1970s. Qualitative researchers are usually interested in lay concepts, developed inductively from everyday language using qualitative inquiry. Using qualitative inquiry, lay concepts are identified and defined, their attributes located and described, and their boundaries located. In addition, their *role* is identified, meaning how these concepts are used. Concepts have antecedents (i.e., conditions that lead to the concept), and outcomes (i.e., conditions that result from the concept) are described. Here we describe the development of hope (Chapter 16) and privacy (Chapter 12).

Occasionally, a concept may be developed that does not have a label or name in the lay lexicon. Empathy was new to nursing in 1956 when Carl Rogers introduced it in a keynote at the American Nurses Association (ANA) Convention (Rogers, 1956). It was therefore originally a scientific concept.

When studying empathy in trauma care, we had data "left over" that did not fit the definition of empathy as defined in the literature. Is this another new concept? These data referred to the sharing of physical pain. Pain experienced by a person was similarly reported to be experienced by those who *observed* the person in pain. This we developed inductively from data and labeled *compathy* (see Chapter 13).

Developing Qualitative Theory

Qualitative theory is developed using two major processes: (a) via inquiry directly from data and (b) by using concepts developed in previous studies.

Developing Theory From Data

Because qualitative theory is developed inductively from data, first and foremost, researchers must collect adequate and appropriate data about their particular topic. These data must be rich, detailed, and saturated. Once one has the data transcribed, the procedure is to code data by highlighting important words and phrases and making summary comments about the data in the margin. At this time one may also begin to make memos (that is, theoretical comments) into the transcription itself. Keep these memos separate from the actual transcript by using upper case letters.

The second operation is to sort data into categories or themes. Categories are developed usually by creating separate "bins" (I use separate files) and placing the copied segments into separate files that must have initially been given very broad labels. (Remember to label each segment with participant number and page number.) For example, a study may have an emerging category called "support." Once these categories have adequate data in them they may be subsequently subdivided into smaller subcategories.

Using a theme requires a different operation. Themes run right through the data and are more difficult to identify. For example, in a study, a theme may be "fear of dying." Such themes are identified by examining data paragraph by paragraph and sentence by sentence. Use the footnote feature in your software to make notes about each segment of data to record your insights. Once you have been right through your transcript (and this is the trick) change footnotes to endnotes and there, at the end of the article, you will find a list of your comments. From these the theme, or themes, within the data may be identified and described.

Asking Analytic Questions

Asking analytic questions of the data is the most important operation in analysis. Data does not analyze itself; neither do themes and concepts "emerge from data." Processes of analysis occur only with cognitive work, insight and intuition, and with sound knowledge of the literature. These skills enable the researcher to recognize and develop important and significant themes from data.

Categories may then be developed into concepts (and in this book we will describe these processes in detail). Identifying concepts from themes is more difficult, because the themes are less easily demarcated—this means their boundaries are more difficult to recognize—and their attributes are less easily located within the process of theming.

As the concepts and themes develop, so does the qualitative theory as the concepts mature, and their role and interrelationships are recognized. If the process is frustrating and the theory is obscure, and the researcher finds him- or herself unable to think conceptually (students call this "the stage of babbling"), explaining one's data to others or holding a seminar may help. Essential components for a seminar are three or four friends willing to listen, a white board for diagramming, a recorder, and oatmeal raisin cookies. The researcher is not permitted to use notes but rather to tell participants about his or her data. This process enables the student to synthesize, to link data, to compare and contrast examples, and usually, after 2 or 3 hours, the theory is constructed. The recorder is essential, for often the student will say something brilliant without realizing, have to be stopped, the recorder rewound and replayed, and the student commended. Of course, this step in analysis is appreciated. The role of the friends is to ask analytical questions, identify gaps, and perhaps suggest "outside" literature.

Developing Theory From Concepts

Sometimes qualitative researchers begin inquiry from a position of partial development of the concept. Perhaps they have already conducted a study on the concept and wish to continue, or another researcher—or many researchers—have done extensive work on the topic and the researcher has the confidence in their work to use it as a foundation, and continue from there. In these cases, the researcher may use the prior work as a foundation, building up the conceptual structure in areas in which investigation is strong, and use it as a *skeleton*. Then subsequent research builds on the skeleton to provide additional detail (as "flesh on the bones"). Alternatively, the researcher may use it as a *scaffold*, as a boundary, and fill in the missing details. These will be discussed further in Chapter 9.

DEDUCTIVE APPROACHES TO CONCEPT DEVELOPMENT

Deduction is the development of concepts and theories to meet a need in a research program where there is a gap. Researchers must have (a) a profound knowledge of the area, (b) available literature, (c) available theories and concepts, and (d) a process of being able to logically associate and correlate variables that will result in a hypothesis to answer a research question. Quantitative theory does not arise out of nowhere: the cognitive work in developing a quantitative proposal is not a process that may be circumvented.

Developing Quantitative Concepts

Quantitative concepts are called *scientific concepts*, in that they are constructed according to the needs of the research program, using the logic of science and the scientific literature. Concepts are developed from a scientific need, a name for a process, or created. These concepts are defined carefully, and an operational definition developed. The operational definition identifies the variables in the study, and how they will be measured. For instance, a quantitative concept may be created by the researcher developing a definition, defining attributes (in this case, the variables) and boundaries, according to the needs of his or her research program. These quantitatively developed concepts are usually proposed to the scientific community only after a means to measure the concept has been developed, administered, and data to support the concept as available at the time of publication.[5] In social science, measurement is usually in the form of an instrument—a scale or test that supports or illustrates the presence and utility of the concept.

---

[5] Wow—Q: Does this mean that qualitative concepts aren't scientific?

Validity is usually determined *concurrently*. Concurrent validity is obtained by the simultaneous administration of an established instrument, one that is already developed that measures an allied concept, and then the results are compared for similarities and differences. If data do not support the new concept, the researcher deliberately makes adjustments to the concept, revises the data collection instrument accordingly, and the researcher repeats the process of testing the new concepts against other quantitative concepts. Once reasonable results are obtained, the researcher introduces the concept to the scientific community by publishing the findings.

Quantification and Testing

Quantitative theories are theories in the richest sense: They originate as simply conjectures, and the goal of quantitative inquiry is to test and validate these theories.

In order for these theories to be tested, an essential criterion is that each of the concepts in the theory must be measurable. Therefore, in quantitative inquiry, a great deal of effort is given to the development and testing of instruments such as psychological tests, developing adequate surveys, and even physiological instrumentation. The quality of quantitative inquiry depends on the reliability and validity of its measurement. If a concept cannot be measured or if an item in a questionnaire cannot be developed to quantitative standards, then qualitative inquiry must be used. For the testing of quantitative theories, research design may be descriptive, quasiexperimental, or experimental, with appropriate statistics used according to the design and goals of inquiry.[6]

DEVELOPING QUANTITATIVE MODELS AND THEORIES

Developing Theory Through a Research Program

As this process of developing and testing theory proceeds, quantitative researchers subsequently refine their measurements, their measurement instruments and procedures, or move their research from one population to another, sequentially testing and refining their theory.[7] Using this feedback model, science progresses. For example, in a 1993 address, Howard Leventhal (1993) described his research program as consisting of 17 studies conducted over a period of 30 years, with each study systematically modifying a

---

[6] Of course, qualitatively derived concepts, identified through interviews or observations, are not necessarily *lay* concepts—they may be new. The process of concept development makes them scientific.

[7] These qualitative concepts that we are worrying about have not been developed for measurement—they are new knowledge. Lauren Clark thinks this is a new category of concepts!

deductively derived model. Briefly, his first study (testing a theoretical framework derived from his own experience, and which was not subsequently supported by data) was a theoretical model for the way fear and fear messages affect the adoption of new behaviors. Next, Leventhal demonstrated the importance of exposing the patient to a combination of threat messages and an action plan. This study led to a series of studies on the influence of preparation (e.g., explanation and a suggested plan of action on patient experiences and the amount of distress experienced). From this, he developed studies in the 1970s on the effect of concrete information cues and abstract notions on coping with people in pain. He then explored individual differences and self-regulation, showing the influence of age and negativity on treatment compliance. Next, he determined that age was not a process variable.

After describing three decades of research, which deductively established his theory, at the end of his talk he concluded that he would "really like to go and talk to those folk [his subjects]," but he "didn't know how [to]." Perhaps, developing his Health Belief Model qualitatively would have resulted in a more truncated and productive research career.

Developing Theory by Organizing Quantitative Concepts

The most common way to create a quantitative theory is by developing a theoretical framework for quantitative study by organizing established quantitative concepts according to their relationship to each other, usually in a formation that determines causality. These concepts are usually well established, have been used in other research, and have measurement instruments with validity and reliability statistics and normative values. Examples of concepts usually used in nursing research are such concepts as social support and caring.

Essential to the building of quantitative theory is the selection of concepts to be used as variables in the theoretical model. Such variables must not only be an excellent analytic fit for your purposes but also must have rigorous measurement tools available. By analytic fit, the concept must be defined and operationalized to also meet the needs of your study.

ABDUCTION

Abductive inference involves both inductive and deductive processes. Usually an idea, insight, or even a hypothesis is developed from data inductively; it is then tested deductively and, if supported, the inquiry moves forward to the next step. Thus, the overall direction of inquiry is inductive, with the deductive processes providing intermediate confirmation. Think of it as gaining an insight (inductive), then checking it out with others (deductive), and moving forward conceptually in this stepwise fashion.

THE COMPLEMENTARY RELATIONSHIP BETWEEN QUALITATIVE AND QUANTITATIVE KNOWLEDGE

Ideally, when we complete qualitative inquiry or begin quantitative inquiry, we know what something *means*: It is well described, the phenomena will be defined, concepts will be richly described and developed, and there is concept development or even appropriate theory, enabling the development of measurement, quantitative instrument development, and theory testing research.

However, research does not always proceed in such an orderly fashion. A part of the problem is that some quantitative researchers may not know how to conduct qualitative inquiry, and develop instruments from their own experiences within their practice area, they may be too impatient to conduct the necessary basic qualitative research, not realizing the foundation needed before embarking on quantitative inquiry, and so forth. Qualitative researchers themselves may not create an adequate foundation. They may have an inadequate sample or use poor techniques that invalidate or limit their project, or they may not have continued inquiry long enough to develop adequate concepts and theory. Both excellent qualitative and quantitative inquiry is essential.

The four cells in Figure 6.2 (*a, b, c*, and *d*) illustrate the four conditions required to develop quantitative measures. These conditions are arbitrary but, in health care, they are often considered conditions that are (a) poorly described and lack an understanding of causation and (b) lack adequate measurement (i.e., diagnostic tests are not available)—and therefore not treated. They are may be classified as psychosomatic conditions, such as fibromyalgia, chronic fatigue syndrome, migraines, and so forth.

Cell *a*: Description Is Adequate; Measurement Possible

In Figure 6. 2a, fever is used as an example of a condition that is both well understood (well described) and for which measurement has been developed. The meaning—physiology of a fever has been identified, and we can measure the severity of the fever quantitatively using a thermometer. In this case, both the theory *and* the quantitative measures for the concept have been well developed. This is an ideal situation, for the qualitative and quantitative knowledge provides understanding and the quantitative measure is reliable and valid. Research and clinical application may further develop.

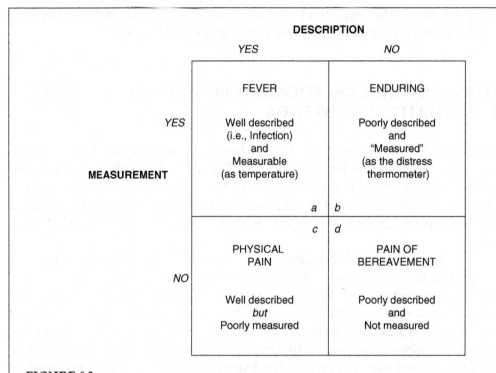

FIGURE 6.2
Relationship between qualitative and quantitative phenomena according to the relationship between, and the development of, *description* and *measurement*, for four phenomena.

Cell *b*: Description Is Lacking; Measurement Present

In the second cell (top right) we have a concept (enduring) about which little is known and does not appear extensively as a concept in the academic literature. I have selected enduring as the example. It is a lay concept, that is, one that is used in everyday language, is defined in the dictionary, yet the behavioral indices are only now being identified and described.

This lack of development of a concept causes difficulties in the literature. Consider the case of breast cancer. Clinicians noted that some patients undergoing diagnosis for breast cancer were distraught and others devoid of emotions. They labeled this behavior as "passive coping" (Pieterse et al., 2007) and as a "negative emotional expression" (Iwamitsu, Shimoda, & Abe, 2005), yet these clinicians, from their own perspective, thought all patients should be emotionally distressed. Yet qualitative inquiry shows that when women suppressed the expected signs of distress, that is, enduring, so they could "get through" the experience, they fulfill their roles as mother and employees. Further, if they manifest distress, this would signal to others the seriousness of their suspected illness. Thus, by understanding this context, enduring must be a healthy response. Unaware of the Praxis Theory of Suffering (Morse, 2011), which describes enduring behaviors, oncologists moved directly into measurement. The Distress Thermometer (Mitchell, 2007) is now administered to these women to try to quantify their distress—distress that has no apparent behavioral correlates as "distress." Thus we have an example in which a measure is being used without a solid theoretical foundation—an essential criterion for validity.

Cell *c*: Meaning Is Adequate; Measurement Inadequate

In cell *c*, we use the example of pain—a physical sensation that has been adequately described (see Melzack, 1975, for listing of the types of sensory, affective, and evaluative pain descriptors). However, pain researchers have been stymied by the lack of a measurement tool to quantify pain intensity, type, and duration. Clinicians have developed a workaround by using a scale from 1 to 10 (1 being in no pain at all and 10 being in the worst imaginable pain) but the validity of the unidimensionality of the scale is questioned. Patients teach each other—"if you want something for pain, tell the nurse your pain is a '7'." Without solid theory link to measurement, research is weak at best.

Cell *d*: Meaning Is Inadequate; Measurement Absent

In the last cell both meaning and measurement are lacking. The examples that fall in this cell are usually unexplained phenomena. As an example, I have chosen chest pain or the pain that accompanies bereavement. But, of course, as science comes to "believe" the frequent patient reports of such pain, they will eventually start to attend to the phenomenon, to describe it carefully, and then look for indices that may be measured (see Eisenberger, 2012).

Knowledge is constantly developing, and we are continually being enlightened about phenomena—which are first described qualitatively and eventually measured quantitatively. However, it should be clear that without clear definitions, excellent description, and good concepts (i.e., qualitative inquiry), quantitative inquiry may be invalid, measuring the unknown, poorly understood, or "missing its mark." This results in confusion, with two concepts sharing the same name, or misconstruing what they represent. Science stumbles.

TO DO 6.2. LEVELS OF KNOWLEDGE DEVELOPMENT

Create your own chart with four cells and place in each cell examples that fit into the various levels of knowledge development.

LAST THOUGHTS

In this chapter, I reviewed the different ways of thinking when developing qualitative and quantitative concepts. This chapter is called "The Battlefield of Knowledge." Why? Why do we now see these two approaches as complementary?

ADDITIONAL READING

Thorne, S., Joachim, G., Paterson, B., & Ganam, C. (2002). Influence of the researcher frame on qualitatively-driven health science knowledge. *International Journal of Qualitative Methods, 1*(1), 1–34.

REFERENCES

Adams, D. (1980). *Restaurant at the end of the universe.* New York, NY: Macmillan.

Chapman, C. M. (1976). The rights and responsibilities of nurses and patients. *Journal of Advanced Nursing, 1,* 111–127.

Chapman, C. M. (1980). The rights and responsibilities of nurses and patients. *Journal of Advanced Nursing, 5,* 127–134.

Dowd, J. J. (1975). Aging as exchange: A prefact to theory. *Journal of Gerontology, 30*(5), 584–594.

Eisenberger, N. I. (2012). The pain of social disconnection: Examining the shared neural underpinnings of physical and social pain. *Nature Reviews Neuroscience, 13*(6), 421–434.

Glaser, B. G. (1978). *Theoretical sensitivity.* Mill Creek, CA: Sociology Press.

Iwamitsu, Y., Shimoda, K., Abe, H., & Okawa, M. (2005). Anxiety, emotional suppression, and psychological distress before and after breast cancer diagnosis. *Psychosomatics, 46*(1), 19–24.

Kayser-Jones, J. (1979). Care of the institutionalized aged in Scotland and the United States: A comparative study. *Western Journal of Nursing Research, 1*(3), 190–200.

Kayser-Jones, J. (1981). *Old, alone and neglected: Care of the aged in Scotland and the United States.* Berkley, CA: University of California.

Leventhal, H. (1993, January 12). *The study of illness cognition from thought to action at the biobehavioral interface* [videotape]. (Available from Colloquium, Gerontology Center, The Pennsylvania State University, PA.)

Melzack, R. (1975). The McGill Pain Questionnaire: Major properties and scoring methods. *Pain, 1*(3), 277–299.

Mitchell, A. J. (2007). Pooled results from 38 analyses of the accuracy of distress thermometer and other ultra-short methods of detecting cancer-related mood disorders. *Journal of Clinical Oncology, 25,* 4670–4681. doi:10.1200/JCO.2006.10.0438

Morse, J. M. (1989). Gift-giving in the patient-nurse relationship: Reciprocity for care? *Canadian Journal of Nursing Research, 21*(1), 33–46.

Morse, J. M. (2008). Does informed consent interfere with induction? [Editorial]. *Qualitative Health Research, 18*(4), 439–440. doi:10.1177/1049732307313614

Morse, J. M. (2011). The Praxis Theory of Suffering. In J. B. Butts & K. L. Rich (Eds.), *Philosophies and theories in advanced nursing practice* (pp. 569–602). Burlington, MA: Jones & Bartlett.

Pieterse, K., van Dooren, S., Seynaeve, C., Nartels, C. C. M., Rinsburger, A. J., de Koning, H. J., . . . Duivenvoorden, H. J. (2007). Passive coping and psychological distress in women adhering to regular beast cancer surveillance. *Psycho-Oncology, 16,* 851–858.

Rogers, C. (1956). A counseling approach to human problems. *American Journal of Nursing, 56,* 994–997.

van Manen, M. (1990). *Researching the lived experience: Human science for an action sensitive pedagogy.* London, ON, Canada: University of Western Ontario Press.

van Manen, M. (2014). *Phenomenology of practice: Meaning-giving methods in phenomenological research and writing.* Walnut Creek, CA: Left Coast Press.

SECTION II

ALL ABOUT CONCEPTS

THE CONCEPTUALIZATION OF CONCEPTS

Student (S):	*I have been struggling trying to find criteria for evaluating a concept. Do you have any suggestions?*
Philosopher (P):	*You can't do that: A concept just is.*
S:	*Then, how do you know if it is any good?*
P:	*You have to link it—or delink it with other concepts. Concepts are always woven into a fabric of understanding. They're a package deal.*
S:	*Oh, that sounds like theory?*
P:	*Yes. Concepts are not isolated entities: they are embedded in reality—or a perception of reality.*
S:	*But some concepts have different meanings. How do we know which conceptualization is right?*
P:	*Who cares? It depends on the linkages. That is what makes life interesting.*
	What are meanings anyway? Psychologists call it perception; *anthropologists call it the* cultural conception of reality; *sociologists call it the* construction of meaning; *and religious studies call it* faith.
S:	*What do philosophers call it?*
P:	*Stupid. Or pointless.*
S:	*But researchers try to operationalize concepts.*
P:	*Keeping them busy, isn't it?*
S:	*Hey, I get to ask the questions. Now, how does one know which conceptualization is* **best**?
P:	*Don't be such a pragmatist. Best for what? Concepts are neither true nor false It's propositions that link (and delink) concepts that have "truth" value.*
S:	*How can I be clear about the meaning of a concept?*
P:	*By weaving it into a web of other concepts. Logicians aim to do this via principles of rational argument, but this doesn't always work—in everyday contexts, humans can be notoriously irrational. Linguists study speech in context as a means to understand cognition, but that is restricted because our classification of things changes overtime, as things themselves change.*
S:	*What would you do?*

P: *Think about it.*
S: *Do concepts emerge?*
P: *Sure. They come and go with fads and fancy. They develop, disappear, and change their names. And new ones are introduced.*
S: *How?*
P: *Through experience and reflecting on experience. By identifying a void. By describing—by using thick description. Why am I telling **you** this? And by linking with other concepts.*
S: *How much description is enough to make a concept?*
P: *Just convince me—a concept just is.*
S: *Well, how do I know when I have a new concept?*
P: *Enough to convince me that it is, that it has come to be.*
S: *Well, what is a concept?*
P: *Now, that's an interesting question . . .*

—Janice Morse and Carl Mitcham

Janice M. Morse

7

CONCEPTS IN CONTEXT

> *. . . the important innovations in social science are conceptual, a way of seeing the social world, and that the most important innovations that matter will be at that level.*
>
> —Michael Agar (2011, p. 18)

We learned in Chapter 1 that concepts were important components of science, and that concepts relevant to nursing were in urgent need of development. It is ironical that developing concepts is the one part of our research programs that, at least in nursing, is not directly supported by funding agencies. In Chapter 2, we reviewed the development of traditional nursing theory in nursing thus far, their contributions, and their limitations. In this chapter, we examine context and how concepts emerge within contexts. We commence with a brief overview of the components of concepts, work through a very simple example using our own general knowledge, and then revisit all of the components in greater depth.

How do you know a concept when you see one?

Suddenly we have reached the point at which you need to know every-thing at once. You need to know what a concept is, and how it is structured, what it has to do with the context, how it sorts and guides nursing knowl-edge, how it links with theory and enables us to move forward, further devel-oping nursing knowledge.

WHAT IS CONTEXT?

Context is the setting in which the behavior(s) of interest, or phenomenon, occurs. It is simply the environment and circumstances—and sometimes the participants—in which the behavior or action occurs. The context should have standard features that are present in every setting where the action of interest takes place. Think of it as the "container" for the phenomenon in which you are interested or perhaps as the setting on the stage and the "actors" involved in a particular scene. Each scene has particular features that enable certain behaviors, which may be evident in persons in the setting and which allow certain other behaviors to occur.

Phenomenon of Interest

A phenomenon is an incident, an event, or a collection of behaviors that occurs within a particular context. The phenomenon may consist of patterned behavior and reoccurring behavior; it may contain a concept or several concepts, or even be a concept in itself. It may be a one-time incident, or a random or coincidental occurrence. Thus, we think of a phenomenon as simply clusters of behaviors that occur within a particular context. These behaviors may be patterned, run sequentially, or occur haphazardly. They may consist of a single concept; multiple, unrelated concepts; or allied (similar, related) concepts that are not exactly the same as the first concept, and differ in some important way. These context-bound concepts contain various amounts of "noise" (i.e., random actions that are not integral to the concept). At this point in our inquiry, we usually select and focus on a "phenomenon of interest" to study.

Just because it is a phenomenon with a recurring pattern of behavior, does not mean that it is (or contains) a concept. The behavior that interests you may not have been developed into a concept—or even given a name. Douglas Adams has an example of such a phenomenon: "the vaguely uncomfortable feeling that you get from sitting on a seat which is warm from somebody else's bottom" (Adams, 2002, p. 11). This concept is silent: It has not been given a label, nor is even spoken about very often.

One more point: Concepts may occur at various levels of abstraction from the data from microanalytical concepts that are very close to the data and which explain these data in detail. Or, we may find a broad concept that is relatively abstract and removed from the data, has a broad level of explanation, and may even encompass several lower level concepts.

What is meant by "encompassing several levels of concepts?" A good high-level concept may encompass lower level concepts, which are more particular, closer to the data, or further subdivide our main concept. Compare this with a broader concept that may extend laterally and encompass several more tightly integrated concepts existing at approximately the same level of abstraction. These concepts may even be "types of" the main concept. For instance, "interaction" may be the primary, broad concept, and types of interactions (such as, "intimate interaction" or "argumentative interaction") the concepts encompassed within the concept of interaction.

WHAT IS A CONCEPT?

> *CHORUS*
> A concept is a mental image, a "conceptualization" of a thing, a collection of behaviors, or an idea. It is a representation of reality in one's mind. It is abstract. The concept may be the image in its entirety—or an image of some of the characteristics of the actual thing. In an empirical sense, definitions are neither true nor false, but only a basic descriptor for the phenomenon.
>
> A concept needs a *label*, or name—we must identify what we are talking about—and it must have a generally accepted definition. This is important, because a concept allows us to communicate with others. And a concept must have attributes, that is, characteristics that are common to every instance of a particular concept. It is, therefore, the attributes that define the concept—that make the concept what it *is*. However, these attributes may be present in different "strengths" and this patterning leads to different forms and uses of a concept.
>
> Each concept has a *boundary*—a limit beyond which a case is no longer an example of that particular concept. Near the boundary, the attributes become weak or are shared with other concepts, and become difficult to recognize.
>
> Concepts have *antecedents,* or conditions that precede and give rise to the concept. All behavioral concepts have outcomes—behaviors that necessarily follow the occurrence of the concept of interest.

Let us start with an easy example that illustrates a concept and its components and functions:

If I speak of a table, we envision a piece of furniture with a flat top and legs that allow you to sit comfortably at the table. Tables usually have four legs, but this is not always so. Some, such as a table with a pedestal, may have only one, and other tables, such a conference table, may have more than four legs. The flat top and the legs are the attributes of a table, as they are present in all instances.

Now, a table is used to put things on. But we may have a table in our article. In this case it is a frame for us to put things "on" or into—we have borrowed one of the attributes from furniture, and use it to name a tool for our writing. Or we may have a tabletop mountain, that is, a mountain with a flat top, borrowing that attribute of the tabletop to describe the top of the mountain. Note we are using the attribute as a concept—in the mental image sense—not as an attribute of components of articles or of mountains.

Where do concepts come from? They are developed in everyday life in the course of conversation. These we call *lay concepts*. Often, new concepts are developed as slang or as trade names. Eventually, as their use becomes more common and familiar, these names are formally adopted into the dictionary. You may think of any number of new concepts concerning computers, cell phones, and software (or the ways they are used) that may not yet have a definition. These lay concepts reveal the dynamic nature of language, of ideas, of changing society, and so forth. We will discuss this further, later in this chapter.

Another type of concept is *scientific concepts*, which are developed in the course of science as operational definitions, or terms that are needed to conduct research. These are introduced into the scientific literature deliberately and cautiously, along with a formal definition.

But language is dynamic and fluid. As lay concepts become more important to science, they are "developed," usually through qualitative inquiry, and then used as scientific concepts in research. Qualitative researchers develop detailed descriptions of a concept in context; they identify its attributes, explore its forms, refine its definitions, and describe its boundaries, antecedents, and outcomes. Alternatively, this may be done using the literature or via philosophical inquiry. Think of the number of articles developing such lay concepts as caring or trust over the past few years.

Scientific concepts become increasingly used on a daily basis; in the everyday context, they may "move" from the scientific to the lay lexicon. For instance, *social support* is one of these concepts—developed in science and now used in everyday language.

Concepts appear in various forms—some are very close to the data, quite narrow in scope, and referring to specific things. Others are more abstract ("higher level") and very broad in scope, encompassing other more local concepts. For instance, suffering is a broad concept, encompassing the lower level concepts of bereavement, grief, sorrow, and despair. A concept may be horizontal, encompassing a large number of concepts. *Stress* is an example of a horizontal concept; that may be applied to metals or bridges (as a deforming force), to physical exercise (as its high levels negatively affect the individual), or to emotions (when the individual cannot conceal them). Incidentally, stress is a concept that was once in the lay lexicon, and later moved into the scientific arena.

Another interesting thing about concepts is that they cluster, and we call the concepts that are similar to—but not the same as—the first concept, *allied concepts*. Allied concepts may share some of the attributes as the first concept, but not all. They may overlap with the first concept, near the boundary where the attributes are weak. Two concepts may also merge, changing the nature of both original concepts (for instance, when hope "seeps in" to emotional suffering, it changes the nature of suffering to form the reformulated self in the *Praxis Theory of Suffering* [Morse, 2011]). Finally, the attributes within a concept may vary in strength, giving the concept a different appearance, but really the concept remains the same, only just in a stronger or weaker form. For instance, a strong form of hope, referred to as "high hopes" by lay persons or even as "false hopes," is still a type of the concept of hope.

TO DO 7.1. BUILD A LIST OF CONCEPTS THAT ARE ENCOMPASSED UNDER THE CONCEPT OF SUFFERING

Consider, which of these concepts are scientific concepts and which are lay concepts? Which are transitioning from lay to scientific? Or from scientific to lay? Create it as a three-column chart.

BEHAVIORAL CONCEPTS

When communicating about behavior we largely use *behavioral concepts*— terms that have been given to a set of behaviors, terms that are used by others, and that others recognize, therefore, enabling us to communicate.

As with all concepts, behavioral concepts must be defined, and the definition must be shared and common to others. Language provides an essential basis for our descriptions of phenomena and the communication of these concepts, but that is only a part of the game. Context may vary the meaning, and as meaning is developed *in use*. However, scientific concepts used professionally may be discipline-specific. Therefore, it is our responsibility, as nurses, to identify nursing phenomena and from those phenomena, to create and define concepts relevant to our practice, that is, scientific concepts. We need to build pertinent explanatory theory that will enable us to perceive and understand patient behavior in a consistent way so that care may be targeted, compassionate, therapeutic, and so that interventions will be evidence-based. We need concepts that are of interest to nursing, that explain nursing, and that allow us to communicate nursing. We need solid theory, not only to explain patient behaviors and necessary nursing care, but which also will enable us to test and expand our interventions. This way, our discipline will mature, and our care will become optimal, effective, and efficient.

Lay Concepts

A lay (everyday) concept is something that refers to a "thing" or a behavior with particular attributes: The concept may be simple or complex; it may be close to reality, or abstract; it may be narrow and particular, or broad and encompass other concepts. Lay concepts are in the common lexicon; they are used in everyday discourse; and they are not fixed—new cases may appear, old cases fade and disappear.

Definitions for lay concepts may sometimes be found in the dictionary, but as such definitions do not usually provide any information about the properties (attributes) of the item. Dictionaries are rather a crude tool for discerning concepts. Dictionary meanings, providing lay definitions, are usually semantically ambiguous; they describe by providing the base from which a meaning may be derived within the context of a sentence. The purpose of the dictionary is to define words, not to develop concepts. If information about a concept that you are interested in cannot be found in the nursing literature, an encyclopedia may be a better source.

The dictionary meanings and labels are inadequate and superficial because they include only minimal descriptors. Think of a lemon: it has a particular shape, color, taste, and flesh—those we will call defining attributes. Now look up *lemon* the dictionary: the dictionary definitions are: (a) yellow or green citrus fruit; (b) tree that bears lemons; (c) pale yellow color; (d) defective product.

Lay behavioral concepts are integral to language, but are often not developed adequately for professional use in nursing practice or for scientific use in research. A lay definition is inadequate for the use of the concept in clinical nursing, and it is the role of qualitative inquiry to investigate and develop the concept, hence helping to develop the theoretical foundations of nursing. An example of a lay concept that is developing is trust; this concept is now increasingly appearing in the nursing research literature and maturing into a scientific concept (Hupcey, Penrod, Morse, & Mitcham, 2001). Therefore, the correspondence between the definition and the defining attributes of the concept is one of logic and fit. This means there may be "better" or "poorer" examples of the definitions. Recall that observing the concept usually derives definitions. If they are not based on observation (i.e., on reality), the likelihood that the concept is meaningful (that it contains attributes and has relationships) is considerably impaired. The concept name is always standardized—for lay concepts, standardization occurs from use in everyday speech; these terms (labels) are usually used consistently in language.

One more example: Although there is general agreement about the definition, the dictionary definition is usually inadequate for use within a discipline for professional purposes. For instance, if we look at the definition of *privacy* (meaning 3 in the dictionary is: "A private or personal matter" [Determinant, 2014, p. 2359], we do not learn anything that we did not know, and the definition is not useful clinically. It does not tell us what kind of information is private, and therefore should not be shared. On the other hand, we may think about the differences between privacy and secrecy when, in Downton Abbey (Fellowes, 2010, Season 1) a lady's maid was found to be hiding a typewriter on the top of her closet. There was a general inquiry in the household about why she was hiding it and keeping it a secret. Anna, a fellow maid, said, "She is not keeping it secret, she is keeping it private: there is a difference."

TO DO 7.2. RELATIONSHIPS AND DIFFERENCES

Consider: What is the difference in relationship between private and secret?
List the characteristics of each concept, private and secret.

Techniques of developing and assessing concepts are discussed throughout this book. Once a concept is developed qualitatively, quantitative research may then explore the concept in use, and further develop and confirm its correlates and theoretical applications.

Scientific Concepts

A *scientific* concept is one that is developed by a researcher and is defined and labeled as an operational definition in the process of doing science. Scientific concepts are therefore standardized by the researcher who developed the operational definition, as the concept was created, introduced, or "invented."

The concept meaning of scientific concepts is fixed by the operational definition that clearly indicates which instances are to be considered within the class of the concept and which are not. Therefore, scientific concepts are clear and concise. Except for a few instances, scientific concepts are significant or meaningful only when they have referents. That is, there are phenomena in the real world that correspond to their definition—in philosophical terms, their class is not empty. Most of the physiological concepts in nursing are scientific concepts. They are stable and used consistently, having been tested using the scientific process of debate and consensus.

Therefore, scientific definitions are not usually found in the dictionary (at least initially); you may have better luck searching in an encyclopedia or online in *Wikipedia*.

The names of scientific concepts are simply labels. Although they are the purview of the person first suggesting or creating the concept, their definitions may be challenged or modified in subsequent investigation. Problems occur when they are overtly used as originally proposed, but deviate from the original meaning in the conduct of research. Hupcey's (1998a, 1998b; see Chapter 19) analysis of the original definition of social support, is an excellent example of such unnoticed, undocumented transition, in which the actual definitions continued to be used by researchers, but the operationalization of the concept changed over time, until it no longer matched the definition.

In this way, scientific concepts are formulated for research purposes according to the needs of the scientist's research. Concept definitions are specific, precise, and do not usually exist in ordinary language until they have been transferred there through general use, and eventually becoming a part of the general lexicon of common speech.

Comparing Scientific and Lay Concepts

Unfortunately, the distinction between scientific and lay concepts is not always clear, and this results in several problems. First, occasionally scientists use definitions that are ambiguous. The same concept label may be shared for a scientific and an ordinary language lay concept, yet, implicitly or explicitly, the scientists or lay persons use different definitions for the concept. *Care* is such a concept: In everyday language we talk about "caring for you," which may mean "feelings of affection" or "looking after," as in "caring for my baby." The scientific meaning of the term "care" refers to professional care, as in the nurse–patient relationship of "providing care."

Second, not all definitions created by scientists are "good" definitions in that they have not clearly defined their concepts. In these situations, as the frequency of use of the concepts increases, these concepts become "muddled." Clarity is lost, and confusion abounds.

A further problem is that the language of science is not always particular to science: Scientists often use labels of lay concepts to designate their scientific concepts. This is commonplace when the researcher wants to explore patient experiences, for example, as it directly links experience as perceived and experienced by the patient, to those of interest to the researcher; qualitative methods are then useful. When terms from ordinary language are used to designate scientific concepts, the scientific definition may be clear and fixed, but this definition may or may not resemble the dictionary definition. Unless the concept is clearly defined in each context, the use of concept labels shared between science and ordinary language may cause much confusion.

Another condition for the concept to be meaningful is that it must have relations with other concepts. Indeed, a concept can only be used in a theory if relationships with other concepts are suggested or actually exist. Scientists choose or define concepts in such a way that relevant relationships are likely to exist. Further, concepts used in disciplines such as nursing are meaningful only if they provide labels for the phenomena of concern to the profession.

In the provision of nursing care, we are generally interested in *behavioral concepts*, which refer to a cluster of behaviors, labeled and defined. These may be lay concepts, referred to as psychosocial concepts, such as *dignity* or *dependence*, emotional states, such as anxiety, or scientific concepts such as *social support*, or physiological concepts such as *electrolyte balance.*

Concepts that originate from science, even those with operational definitions, are also dynamic and initially not usually stable. As a scientific term becomes increasingly communicated, it becomes known, accepted into, and used in everyday speech, and it takes on a dual existence as both a lay and a scientific term. Thus, pyrexia, a scientific term, may be found in Oxford Dictionaries (2014, p. 2430), and *fever,* its roughly equivalent lay term, may both be found in medical texts.

THE STRUCTURE OF CONCEPTS

If a concept is simply a mental image, how could it possibly have a *structure*? This "structure" is simply a framework conceived to organize the essential components of a concept. This framework and components consist of what we metaphorically call the *anatomy* of the concept (i.e., the label, definitions, and the antecedent, boundary, attributes or characteristics, and the outcomes) and the *physiology*, that is, how the concept functions within different contexts and situations, and in the presence of other concepts.

THE "ANATOMY" OF CONCEPTS

When talking about the anatomy of concepts, we are referring to their structures: their labels, definitions, attributes, boundaries, antecedents, and outcomes. That is, we are referring to the perceived constituents, structures, or components that we use to describe the collections of behaviors that make up the concept. To summarize, the antecedents are the conditions that must exist to give rise to the concept; the boundary delineates what is and is not a part of the concept; the antecedents are the characteristics that are present in all cases of the concept, and the consequences are the outcomes. We also include the definition and the concept label as a part of the concept when evaluating its anatomy.

Concept Labels

To make things a little more complicated, concepts are not actual entities. Rather, they are names for ideas—for instance, labels for ideas and even images for what behaviors we consider that occur together and signify a particular purpose. Concepts do not exist in empirical reality; only their referents do, that is, the concepts refer to representations of behaviors that signify the attributes that cluster or co-occur, and form the concept. Concepts, by definition, are abstractions of reality; they are not concrete entities in themselves. They are labels for clusters of behaviors that have common characteristics, which we call *attributes*.

Antecedents

Antecedents are the conditions that always precede the concept and give rise to the concept; without these conditions and circumstances—and behavioral response—the concept could not occur. The antecedent may be described relatively abstractly. Although antecedents may be directly linked to a particular type of context, it is not always the case that antecedents are tied to the particular setting being explored. For instance, in order to *hope*, there *must be* and *always is*, something to hope against. It is a perceived threat to the self. The concept of hope commences when the person perceives the threat and then hopes against that threat (hopes that it will not occur), and begins to plan for alternative actions to avoid the threat (Morse & Doberneck, 1995, p. 278).

Attributes

Identifying the attributes of the concepts expands our understanding and raises the level of abstraction to include all instances of the concept. The label given to the characteristics changes form as they are rewritten and *decontextualized* as formal attributes. For instance, references to local conditions are removed and they are made more general, and they are succinctly formatted so that they apply to all contexts. Thus, decontextualization is the stripping of the local features attached to the attributes, and the identification and retention of the features that are present in all instances of the concept in any context. Think of it as identifying the "bones," the essential features, without any particular "noise" associated with a certain situation or setting.

This is the first step in abstraction, and the first step in making the concept generalizable. The most common way to move from characteristics to attributes is to decontextualize by comparing the concept in different settings. In context #1, list the characteristics of the concept. Then do the same in a second context or situation, in the third context, and so forth. Once you have listed the characteristics of the same concept in each setting, examine your chart: Those features that are common to all contexts or settings are probably the attributes of the concept. Those features that appear in one or two settings are local features. It is this process of identifying attributes that enables abstraction. Once abstracted, the attributes (and therefore the concept) are not tied to any particular setting, context, or circumstance.

At the center of the concept, the attributes are the strongest, and these may provide the optimal exemplar of a particular concept, as a clear and undisputed example (see Figure 7.1). But as we move toward the boundary of the concept, these characteristics become weaker, and the attributes of other allied or similar concepts may be present, causing analytic confusion.

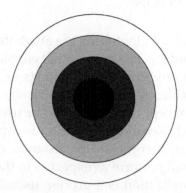

FIGURE 7.1
The attributes are strongest/clearest at the center of the concept and weakest at the boundary.

One last point: Remember that the attributes may not be equally strong in all settings—they just have to be present. And it is variation in the strength of different attributes that gives the concept its different form or pattern. Traditionally, the concepts are weakest near the boundary.

Boundaries

Boundaries determine when a concept is or is not an example of a certain concept. Cases located near the boundary of the concepts are weaker than examples near the center, and as these examples approach the boundary, their attributes become weak, they may contain noise and are therefore more difficult to study and analyze, and may be shared with neighboring concepts. Therefore qualitative researchers always commence inquiry by studying the best example that can be located.

When *all* of the attributes are no longer present in the concept, and the concept meets or overlaps with other concepts, *boundary* of the concept forms. Boundaries do not often occur as sharply delineated "marks," and often the boundaries are fuzzy, with some ambiguity occurring. Ask yourself: Is this an example of this concept or not?

Consequences

Consequences are, of course, the outcome of the concept. In the hope example, the outcome would be realization of the hoped-for goal. The concept of hope may not always result in the hoped-for outcome (we have dashed hopes, lost hopes) and the process of hoping may have to be repeated, another goal hoped for, or one's fate (i.e., the threat) accepted.

RECONTEXTUALIZATION

Recall the process of identifying the attributes of the concepts is called *decontextualization*, and it is this process that enables the concept to become abstract and relevant to any number of contexts or situations. This is an important process that enables *qualitative generalization* of our concepts and theories.

Before a concept can be adopted or used in a second setting, it must be recontextualized. Recontextualization is a process of determining *fit* of the concept to the new context—for instance, determining if the attributes are pertinent and will perform as expected in the new setting (Figure 7.2).

Recontextualization is a process usually arising from the host context. One problem limiting the adoption of concepts and theories is that literature searches are often conducted by context rather than by concepts. For instance, Mary Applegate conducted a good study on the concept of privacy (Applegate & Morse, 1994; see Chapter 12). Although the study was conducted as ethnography in a nursing home, her major finding was that the type of relationships between the nurse and the patient determines whether or not privacy norms were respected. When the nurse and the patient viewed one another as friends or even as strangers, the norms of privacy were respected; all of the privacy violations occurred when they viewed one another as objects.

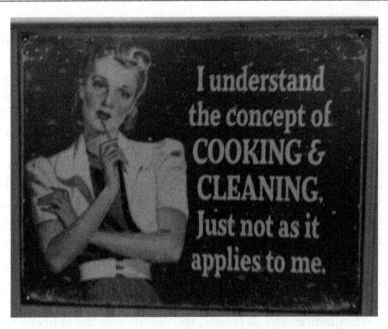

FIGURE 7.2
Failed recontextualization.

Such insights into the concept of privacy were decontextualized from the nursing home setting and are strong enough to be applicable to any total institution. They would be applicable to a hospital, prison, or school—anywhere there is a problem of privacy not being respected and others have access to the person. Understanding such generalization, or transference, is important—those wishing to use the findings should *search the databases by concept* and *not* by participants/setting/context/situation used in the original research. It is the abstract concept (or theory) that contains the principles or holds the key for the program you wish to adopt. Recontextualize those concepts or theories by applying them to your context.

Allied Concepts

Allied concepts are those concepts that closely resemble each other, and may even share some of the attributes, but they are different and separate concepts in their own right. For instance, the concepts *secret* and *private*, mentioned earlier in this chapter, are allied concepts. Exploring their similarities and differences of their attributes will reveal how they differ by an important characteristic.

Allied concepts are important: As reality is not categorical, but continuous, at some point you will have to make a decision about whether a certain case is a part of this group of concepts or belongs to a different group. Allied concepts provide linkages to other concepts—rather like a bridge—by sharing an attribute with the other concept. The allied concept differs from the first concept because it has other attributes that are *not* present in the first concept. Nevertheless the shared attribute serves as a linkage between the two concepts, and this is essential for building models and theories and for understanding transitions. They enable us to model change and variation in concepts.

Can allied concepts compete?

Sometimes they do compete, particularly when they have not been carefully dissected.

Competing Concepts

If two allied concepts have different labels and similar or slightly different definitions, the researcher has to decide whether a single concept is actually involved and simply has two names, or if two concepts are involved and are different referents, deserving different names and different definitions.

To complicate matters further, often concepts overlap, sharing some or even most of their attributes, but not all, thereby being *competing concepts*. In this instance, the concepts may refer to two slightly differing concepts or to two concepts referring to slightly different manifestations of the same concept.

TO DO 7.3. COMPETING OR ALLIED CONCEPTS?

Ask those around you: Is wishing the same as hoping? How are they the same and how are they different?

THE "PHYSIOLOGY" OF CONCEPTS

The "physiology" of concepts refers to the way they act and interact in different contexts (changing their strength and impact), how their attributes change in strength and in relationship to one another, thus changing the form of the concept. For instance, think again of hope. We may be able to identify different types of hope: high hopes, false hopes, misdirected hopes, and so forth. But consider hopeless or no hope: are they forms of hope? Is the absence of hope a form of hope? I do not know.

But I do know that it is useful to nurses or to psychologists to classify "no help" as the "baseline" of hope, for it directs a plan of care.

In a trajectory, concepts may change in form as the context changes, as they come in contact with other concepts; may interact, combine, divide, or split. If you consider concepts to be more than merely a label, and view them as dynamic, you can see them function in changing as context changes, thus acting as a low-level theory.

Of course, in any context there is more than one concept. These concepts may interact, and at the boundaries, share attributes. Boundaries may be sharply delineated or "fuzzy," and merge into a second concept. This concept may be similar to the first concept, differing in some, but not all attributes, or differ entirely from the first concept.

TYPES OF CONCEPTS

Concepts vary in two ways: (a) level of abstraction (i.e., how closely they are linked to data or have been inferred from the context) and (b) the scope of the concept (i.e., how broadly or how much of the context they encompass). These two aspects may vary with the concept's use or application—for instance, it may also vary because of the nature of the concept itself, and be programmed into its definition.

Levels of Abstraction

The level of abstraction of both lay and scientific concepts may arise from the nature of the concept itself—from necessity of what it represents. The lower

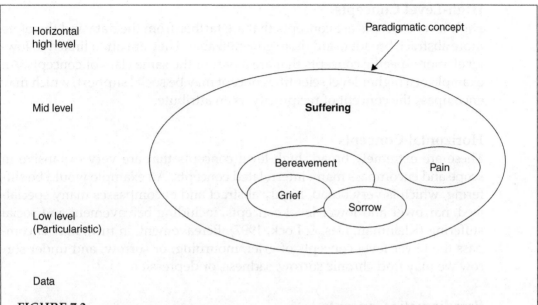

FIGURE 7.3
Relationship between paradigmatic concepts and lower level concepts.
Source: Morse, J. M. (2004). Constructing qualitatively-derived theory: Concept construction and concept typologies. *Qualitative Health Research*, 14(10), 1387–1395.

the level of a concept, the closer it is to the data (i.e., to reality) and the more grounded its position in theory (Figure 7.3). In lower level concepts, the attributes of the concept are more easily observed and there is less confusion about the definition and the attributes themselves.

Low-Level Concepts
Low-level concepts create the linkages between the context and the concept, and again between the context and higher level concepts. The lowest level of concepts is particular concepts. They are derived directly from data and remain close to the phenomena they represent. As such, these concepts are local, and narrow in scope, and hence might have restricted application to other contexts and to new situations and refer to a particular set of behaviors. They have limited application and are not widely generalizable. An example of such a concept may be sorrow. (As we discuss later, it is these linkages that are crucial for assessing the adequacy of the theory.) Because low-level concepts are *low level*, they are generally specific and delimited in *scope*.

Mid-Level Concepts
Mid-level concepts are generally specialized to a particular phenomenon. For instance, grief and bereavement are generally applied to the emotional responses to loss associated with death.

High-Level Concepts

High-level concepts are concepts that are farther from the data and therefore more abstract, broader, and more generalizable. They are often linked to low-level, more specific concepts that are a part of the same class of concepts. An example of a higher level scientific concept may be social support, which may encompass the concept of reciprocity as an attribute.

Horizontal Concepts

These are extremely broad, high-level concepts that are very expansive in scope and encompass many interrelated concepts. An example would be suffering, which is very broad, highly abstract and encompasses many specialized, narrower and lower level concepts, including bereavement and social suffering (Kleinman, Das, & Lock, 1997). Bereavement, in turn, may encompass the lower level concepts of grief, mourning, or sorrow; and under sorrow we may find chronic sorrow, sadness, or depression.

Paradigmatic Concepts

Paradigmatic concepts are scientific concepts of a very high level of abstraction that are applied deductively to a cluster of concepts or a developing theory. The concept is placed on to the emerging theoretical scheme, so there is not a direct link from the paradigmatic concepts developing the theory. An example of such a paradigmatic concept is "cultural safety" (Ramsden, 1993). But, Anderson et al. (2003) noted that cultural safety was *interpretive*, and had to be inferred:

> In the conceptual phase and planning of the research, we had thought it possible to identify and name "culturally safe" and "culturally unsafe practices." In fact, in our initial attempts to code the data, we developed a category for cultural safety. Paradigmatic concepts are applied deductively rather than emerging from the data. Suggesting an assumed transparency of the concept . . . The quandary for us was that cultural safety did not announce itself in the transcripts—it was not a "thing" that could be "found," *but became interpretative work on our part* . . . As we reexamined the data to get a handle on the concept of cultural safety, it became evident that *any* code category could illuminate the concept, depending on *our interpretation.* (Anderson et al., 2003, pp. 204, 206)

TO DO 7.4. IS THE "EPIDEMIC OF OBESITY" A PARADIGM?

Argue:
The epidemic of obesity in the United States is caused by gluttony.

Therefore, positioning the categories under the rubric of cultural safety was meeting the researcher's political agenda, rather than inductively deriving the concept (Morse, 2004). Other concepts may be substituted for cultural safety—cultural competence (Canales & Bowers, 2001), for instance, or even more abstractly, trust or social support. Of course, the level of abstraction could become very abstract, and the concepts may be all encompassing and therefore so abstract as to be meaningless or to introduce error through misattribution of the concept. Looking in the other direction, the concept closest to the data may be a part of a more abstract concept. For instance, sorrow may be a part of bereavement, which in turn is a part of suffering.

Let us talk more about ordering concepts in a conceptual hierarchy.

Determining the Conceptual Hierarchy

The ordering of concepts to one another depends on the focus of the research—that is, which concept you are focusing on—and the fact that your model is malleable, changeable, and shifting. Even the presence or absence of concepts within such a hierarchy depends on the concept you are targeting, the

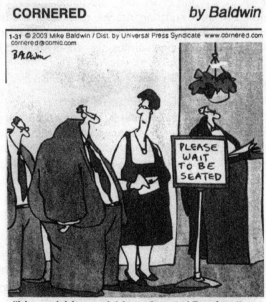

FIGURE 7.4
Misapplication of a high-level concept to a local context.
Reprinted by permission of Mike Baldwin.

context, and the purpose of the research. It depends on the values and beliefs of the researcher (who is in the driver's seat) and on quality of the data (information, literature) used to create the model.

We need hierarchies of concepts, developed both linguistically and logically. Linguistics allows us to describe a particular context with particular features. Logic allows us to generalize when we need to use a high-level concept. Look at Baldwin's (2003) cartoon (Figure 7.4)—and you will see the problems with application of a high-level concept—in this case "global economic slowdown"—to a local context, or the delay in being seated in a restaurant.

Changing your focus, or selecting a different concept to target, would reorder your concept hierarchy. You may produce a different chart, and a different ordering of concepts, and even different concepts within the model itself. And as we have begun to talk about the linkages of concepts and models, we are working our way toward developing theory.

TO DO 7.5. ORDERING CONCEPTS

List the concepts that are types of suffering that you created, each on a small sticky note.

Now create a hierarchy, placing those that are least general (or most specific) at the bottom of the page and those that are more general at the top of the page.

Examine the linkages in the chart you have made ordering the concepts encompassed beneath the high-level concept of suffering. Are you clear about the relationship between the concepts, that is, which concepts are a part of larger concepts? Did you include pain?

How do we know that pain is beneath the concept of suffering? There is a linguistic test to determine position.

Ask: Can one suffer pain? Yes.
         Can one pain suffering? NO

Therefore, as pain is suffered, and may inherently be a part of suffering, it should be on your chart.

But to complicate things further, if you are studying **pain**, *focusing on pain itself*, you may reorder your chart, putting pain at the highest level. Then suffering may appear below pain, on the side, as an *emotional reaction* to pain.

Linkages

Link is the term describing the association or hypothetical connection between the higher level concept and the lower level concept or vice versa—the association between the lower level theory and the more abstract concept. *Linkage* is also the term that denotes a connection between the context and the concept or vice versa. Of course, *data* is the term for indicators of the concept used within the context that enables measurement or description, and these may be textual or numerical.

APPROACHES TO UNDERSTANDING CONCEPTS

Important note: There are three perspectives on the attributes of concepts. *The classical perspective* (Laurence & Margolis, 1999) states that concepts using the same label must have all of the same attributes. That is, if we have a concept called "trust" and define the concept in a particular way, identify the attributes, and so forth, then all instances of the concept of trust should all have the same attributes. Now, these attributes may be of different strengths, but they must all be present in the concept for it to be considered an example of (in this case) trust.

The second perspective, the *neoclassical theory of concepts*, states that *most* of the attributes (but not all) must be present for the concept to be an example of a particular concept (Wittgenstein, 1953/1968; Laurence & Margolis, 1999). Thus it is considered to be partial, looking at family resemblances, and necessary, graded and typical conditions. An example of such a concept is depression. According to the *Diagnostic and Statistical Manual of Mental Disorders* (4th ed.; DSM-5; American Psychiatric Association, 2013), there are eight symptoms ("attributes") listed for depression, yet to be diagnosed with depression, the person needs to present with only five (and any five) of those eight symptoms. I prefer the more precise classical requirement for concept, and that will be used in this text.

The third perspective is the *Prototype Theory of Concepts* (Laurence & Margolis, 1999, p. 28), which states that attributes may be identified by categorizing an instance (a "best example") or an exemplar, and extending to "statistical prominent properties" around which the class of examples clusters (Roche, 1978). This model does not consider if the attributes co-occur, but if they probably co-occur. The study of hope at the end of this chapter is an example of this approach, using only the first phase, the categorization of the exemplar.

THE CONTRIBUTION OF CONCEPTS

What do concepts *do?*

First of all they allow us to communicate. As *names* for sets of abstract ideas, it is important to realize that concepts per se do not exist as an entity. They are created. Lay concepts are created in social interaction, and by informal agreement about meaning. Over time these meanings become more established. As previously noted, concepts are malleable—new concepts arise, become accepted, or may change form. They could expand and incorporate new dimensions and attributes, or may become old fashioned and no longer used.

Scientific concepts may also change meaning or be used in a different way; although they are developed from research as operational definitions, with a fixed meaning, they may retain the original, formal meaning, yet be used differently.

Concepts also transition from scientific to lay concepts as they become increasingly used in everyday life and as the public becomes more aware of science. Lay concepts form a large part of the art of nursing: touch, caring, comfort, listening, dignity, privacy. Some of these have been explored and developed so they can be used in nursing science, but many have not.

Lay concepts also move into the scientific lexicon, as the lay concepts are refined and their attributes identified, usually through qualitative inquiry. This is a tremendous need in nursing research, in particular in areas where the basis of nursing care is subjective.

Thagard (1992) clearly delineated the role of concepts in both everyday life and in science:

1. Categorization: It enables us to place similar entities into classes, thereby clustering allied concepts, and giving the class a name.
2. By linking and sorting examples into classes, it enables learning through examples.
3. By working from the concept to the case, it enables recognitions and aids memory.
4. In the research processes such linkages from the concept to the particular allow for inference, explanation, problem solving, generalization, and analogical inference.
5. The increased understanding about the components of concepts facilitates problem solving and explanation.
6. Understanding a phenomenon enables the recognition of new examples, thereby enabling generalization.
7. Knowledge about a phenomenon permits reasoning using identified similarities.
8. Understanding achieved from prior conceptual knowledge provides comprehension, and the expression and communication of these ideas.

FRAMEWORKS AND MODELS

It is time to differentiate a concept from a framework, sometimes called a *theoretical framework*. A framework is a representation of what a researcher thinks is happening in reality. It is really a way of organizing variables (for quantitative research) or showing data collection points, focus, and even data collection strategies, for a qualitative project. It shows the scope of the project and the relationship of the various components of the framework. As the framework is a representation of reality, so is a model a representation of an actual thing, usually reduced in size, to show how the original works. The framework may be described in text, and the model is a schematic representation of the framework; the purpose of both is to communicate the perceived structure to the reader.[1]

THEORY

A theory differs from the framework: it is more formalized, and usually incorporates the findings from earlier research (in the case of quantitative theory) or is derived from research (as in the case of qualitative inquiry). Theory incorporates concepts within its structure, in that its purpose is to communicate the perceived structure and the relationships within the theory, for the data collection plan, and also to test the hypothesized model and relationships. Theory is therefore suggested tentatively or as conjecture, until it convinces (as in the case of qualitatively derived theory) or is proven or demonstrated (as in the case of theory for quantitative testing). Of course, a theory may be "dethroned" or modified as new facts are uncovered. But if a qualitative theory convinces, or quantitative theory is tested, it becomes fact and is no longer a theory—except by habit or naming convention.

Theory usually consists of interrelated concepts. Qualitative researchers, if they use a diagram, illustrate the concepts close together and the relationship to the other concepts spatially (see Figure 7.5a). Quantitative researchers usually diagram their theory with the concepts in "balloons" and with lines illustrating the hypothesized linkages and types of relationships (positive or negative) between the concepts (see Figure 7.5b). While different in form, both of these diagrams actually show the same depiction of reality, separated (abstracted) from the context. Note that the concepts in both models may be the same—in the quantitative model they have been separated to allow for the linkages to be seen and the relationship values inserted on the lines.

Nevertheless, for both of these diagrams, you can see the significance of concepts in both qualitative and quantitative theory. But the most interesting thing is that both of these models, the qualitative and the quantitative, may represent the same context—they are merely diagrammed differently.

Some call concepts the "building blocks" of theory (Chinn & Kramer, 2011), recognizing that concepts are the substance of theory. If the relevant and necessary concepts for nursing are not available or not adequately developed for quantification of the theory, it is easy to see how the dearth of

---

[1] Frameworks may also be very abstract, resembling grand theory, as we classified in Leininger and Roy's theory (or as Fawcett [1980] classified as a conceptual model.) Such frameworks may be so abstract that they may be used to structure policy, as Solberg discusses in Chapter 28 with the social determinants of health.

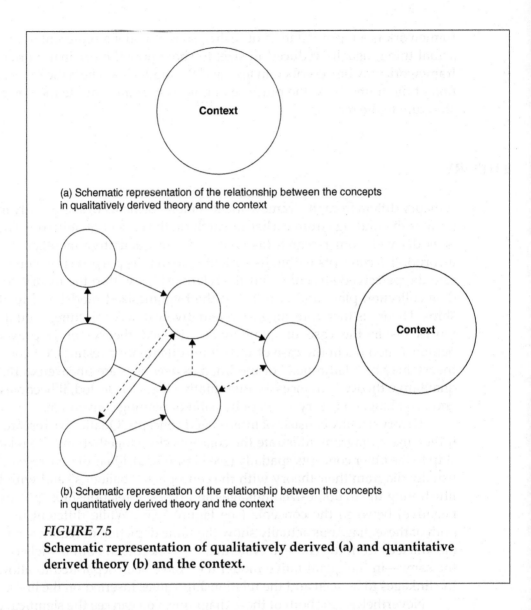

(a) Schematic representation of the relationship between the concepts in qualitatively derived theory and the context

(b) Schematic representation of the relationship between the concepts in quantitatively derived theory and the context

FIGURE 7.5

Schematic representation of qualitatively derived (a) and quantitative derived theory (b) and the context.

appropriate concepts in nursing is concerning. It is also easy to see the significance of concept development methods and the significance of qualitative inquiry for concept identification.

Theories may be developed from the literature, using—even combining—the work of others from previous research, or from the results of qualitative inquiry. Theories vary in their degrees of conjecture or supposition. Quantitative theories show how each variable will be measured and, as quantitative theories are tested, they may be subsequently modified and retested, until the researcher is satisfied that they are a reasonable approximation to what is going on in reality.

Qualitatively derived theory is verified ("tested") during the process of construction (Meadows & Morse, 2001). Qualitative methods demand that each small advance on the theory be tested—replicated—before proceeding. Therefore, since a qualitative theory approaches certainty, there should be no need for it to be tested as a whole. Indeed, paradoxically, testing is a fruitless task: the reason that qualitative inquiry was used in the first place was simply because the researcher did not have enough information available to know what concepts were involved in the phenomenon, or there were no instruments available to measure the concepts. These deficiencies remain, even in the presence of the developed qualitatively derived theory, until quantitative instrument development is achieved.

Often qualitatively derived theories, most often mid-range theories, are used clinically to enhance the nurse's gaze or to illustrate the rationale and actions that will produce certain clinical outcomes. They also differ in their level of abstraction—sometimes suggesting very local action, close to the context; other times they may be abstract, high-level theories. The previously mentioned mid-range theory may provide insights from nursing regarding how to negotiate care, provide hope, and so forth, with higher level theory useful for understanding communities and poverty, or aspects of culture and health, and so forth.

LAST WORDS

Your task is to understand the structure and form of concepts, what they do and cannot do, and what their role is in knowledge development. Most importantly, it is to appreciate that they are *constructed* socially, through use, through perception, and through language. Lay concepts are shared culturally; scientific concepts are shared prescriptively—but may change definition deliberately as science develops, or silently, as they are used.

Developing concepts from phenomena gives order to chaos, enables communication, and provides the structure for inquiry and the development of theory. The structure of concepts may appear rigid, but it is a form that has developed to expedite knowledge development and generalization. The form of the attributes enables decontextualization, or the removal of the concept from its original context, and its application to all instances of the particular conditions identified by the definitions and concept label. Appreciating the "strength" of the attributes allows for the recognitions of "types" of the concept, and the mode of linking with attributes from other concepts permits the investigations of trajectories and change, of complex models, and the construction of theory. Identifying the boundaries delimits inquiry to particular conditions, as does recognizing the antecedents and consequences.

Does this mean that once a concept is identified, it is "fixed," cemented, and we move on? No, of course not. Concepts are malleable, and change as knowledge evolves.

REFERENCES

Adams, D. (2002). *The salmon of doubt*. New York, NY: Macmillan.

Agar, M. (2011). *Method to my madness*. Michael Agar Ethnoworks LLC. Retrieved from http://www.ethknoworks.com

American Psychiatric Association. (2013). *Diagnostic and statistical manual of mental disorders DSM-5*. (5th ed.). Arlington, VA: Author.

Anderson, J., Perry, A., Blue, C., Browne, A., Henderson, A., Khan, K. B., . . . Smye V. (2003). "Rewriting" cultural safely within the postcolonial and postnational feminist project. *Advances in Nursing Science, 26*(3), 196–214. doi:10.1097/00012272-200307000-00005

Applegate, M., & Morse, J. M. (1994). Personal privacy and interaction patterns in a nursing home. *Journal of Aging Studies, 8*(4), 413–434. doi:10.1016/0890-4065(94)90012-4

Baldwin, M. (2003). *Cornered*. Universal Press. Retrieved from http://www.universaluclick.com

Chinn, P. L., & Kramer, M. K. (2011). *Integrated theory and knowledge development in nursing* (8th ed.). St. Louis, MO: Mosby.

Canales, K. K., & Bowers, B. J. (2001). Expanding conceptualizations of culturally competent care. *Journal of Advanced Nursing, 36*(1), 102–111. doi:10.1046/j.1365-2648.2001.01947.x

Determinant. (2014). *Oxford English dictionary* [Online]. Retrieved from http://www.oxford dictionaries.com/definition/english/determinant

Fawcett, J. (1980). A framework for analysis and evaluation of conceptual models of nursing. *Nurse Educator, 5*(6), 10–14.

Fellowes, J. (2010). *Downton Abbey* (UK Edition). United Kingdom: PBS/Carnival Film & Television.

Hupcey, J. E. (1998a). Social support: Assessing conceptual coherence. *Qualitative Heath Research, 8,* 304–318.

Hupcey, J. E. (1998b). Clarifying the social support theory-research linkage. *Journal of Advanced Nursing, 27,* 1231–1241.

Hupcey, J., Penrod, J., Morse, J. M., & Mitcham, C. (2001). An exploration of the advancement of the concept of trust. *Journal of Advanced Nursing, 36*(2), 282–293.

Kleinman, A., Das, V., & Lock, M. (1997). *Social suffering*. San Francisco, CA: University of California.

Laurence, S., & Margolis, E. (1999). Concepts and cognitive science. In E. Margolis & S. Laurence (Eds.), *Concepts: Core readings* (pp. 3–82). Cambridge, MA: MIT Press.

Meadows, L., & Morse, J. M. (2001). Constructing evidence within the qualitative project. In J. M. Morse, J. Swanson, & A. Kuzel (Eds.), *The nature of evidence in qualitative inquiry* (pp. 187–200). Newbury Park, CA: Sage.

Morse, J. M. (2004). Constructing qualitatively-derived theory: Concept construction and concept typologies. *Qualitative Health Research, 14*(10), 1387–1395.

Morse, J. M. (2011). The Praxis Theory of Suffering. In J. B. Butts & K. L. Rich (Eds.), *Philosophies and theories in advanced nursing practice* (pp. 569–602). Burlington, MA: Jones & Bartlett.

Morse, J. M., & Doberneck, B. M. (1995). Delineating the concept of hope. *Image: Journal of Nursing Scholarship, 27*(4), 277–285.

Ramsden, I. (1993). Kawa Whakaruruhau—Cultural safety in nursing education in Aotearoa (New Zealand). *Nursing Praxis in New Zealand, 8*(3), 4–10.

Roche, E. (1978). Principles of categorization. In E. Roche & B. Lloyd (Eds.), *Cognition and categorization* (pp. 27–28). Hillside, NJ: Erlbaum.

Thagard, P. (1992). *Conceptual revolutions.* Princeton, NJ: Princeton University Press.

Wittgenstein, L. (1953/1968). *Philosophical investigations* (3rd ed.). Oxford, UK: Blackwell.

Janice M. Morse

8

SUMMARY OF MAJOR METHODS FOR EXPLORING CONCEPTS

> *"Anything worth doing, is worth doing properly . . ."*
> —Bob's mother (personal communication)

Important concepts that contribute to the discipline, to theory development, and to understanding, must be developed using solid methods and optimal information as data. The goal is to develop the best possible concepts in order to contribute to theory, research, and the discipline. In this book, the major methods of concept analysis are reviewed. These methods may be classified as philosophical, meta-analytic, and those using qualitative inquiry or a combination of data sources.

PHILOSOPHICAL METHODS FOR CONCEPT ANALYSIS

Philosophical methods, based on the work of Wittgenstein, use logic, reflection, reviews of the literature, and created exemplars (as cases) for the development of concepts. This is the most frequently used approach for concept development. Perhaps because of the clarity in the description of the method, the fact that there is a need for the collection of data (and the institutional review board [IRB] application and approval), the work may be easily completed as a class assignment. However, the method has been criticized: Results are predictable, and lack depth and insight. Of greatest concern, the most common finding at the completion of the studies is that "further investigation is required," indicating that the method does not achieve its original aim of actually "developing" the concept.

Walker and Avant (1983, 2011)

In 1963, John Wilson, a British high school teacher, published a small book describing a straightforward method of concept analysis for high school students, based on the work of Wittgenstein. This method used an 11-step process which, in 1983, Walker and Avant further simplified and published as eight steps, to be used iteratively:

1. Select a concept.
2. Determine the aims or purposes of the concept.
3. Identify all uses of the concept that you can discover.
4. Determine the defining attributes.
5. Identify a model case.
6. Identify borderline, related, contrary, invented, and illegitimate cases.
7. Identify antecedents and consequences.
8. Define empirical referents. (Walker & Avant, 2011, p. 160)

Details for conducting each step are provided in their text. Briefly, the method is "an analysis of the [selected] descriptive word" as it is "used in language coupled with an explanation of how it is "like and not like other related terms or words" (p. 158). Walker and Avant (2011) are concerned with the actual and possible uses of the words that convey conceptual meanings (p. 158). By doing so, they hoped to "break the concept into its simpler elements" to "determine its internal structure" (p. 158). Data are obtained from dictionaries, thesauruses, literature, and so forth, to "identify as many uses of the word as possible" including the "ordinary and scientific uses," and "keeping in mind the purpose of your work." Instructions are vague, but the student has access to many examples.

Defining the attributes extends from these definitions and uses of the word. Model cases are prototypical cases that may come from the literature, experience, or "even constructed by you," and demonstrates "all instances of the attributes" (Walker & Avant, 2011, p. 163). Next, the student identifies or creates other types of cases, borderline, related, contrary, invented, and illegitimate cases, which are then examined to "help you make better judgments about which defining attributes or characteristics have the best 'fit'" and "help you decide what 'counts' and what 'doesn't count'" (p. 164). The final step is to identify the antecedents and the consequences of the concept.

The most important aspect that differentiates Walker and Avant's method from others is that it is not interpretative, but descriptive; unfortunately, this results in little insight or development of new understandings. Using created cases as "data" is a limitation also previously noted (Hupcey, Morse, Lenz, & Tasón, 1996).

Walker and Avant (2011, pp. 169–170) have identified a number of studies they consider to be excellent examples of studies using their method and covering a variety of topics serving as examples of concept analysis. For instance, see Ellis-Stoll and Popkess-Vawter (1998), Mulder (2006), and Trendall (2000).

Rodgers (1993), Rogders and Knafl (2000): The Evolutionary Method

Concepts develop, and maturation is through malleable processes of application, significance, and use which, over time, change its meaning. Rodgers's method of concept analysis, the *evolutionary view,* closely resembles Walker and Avant's method, with several important differences. First, data used for analysis is the professional literature, within a particular context. The second important difference is that exemplars are selected from the literature. The interactive tasks are similar, but are developed to the level of hypothesis testing:

1. Identify the concept of interest and associated expressions (including surrogate terms);
2. Identify and select and appropriate realm (setting and sample) or data collection;
3. Collect data relevant to identify:
   a. the attributes of the concept,
   b. the contextual basis of the concept, including interdisciplinary sociocultural, and temporal (antecedent and consequential occurrences) variations;
4. Analyze data regarding the above characteristics of the concept;
5. Identify an exemplar of the concept, if appropriate;
6. Identify implications, hypotheses, and implications for further development of the concept. (Rodgers & Knaft, 2000, p. 85)

Examples of concept analysis conducted using the Evolutionary Method are those by Johnson (2007); Rodgers (1989); Schilling, Grey, and Knafl (2002); and Suh (2004).

META-ANALYTIC METHODS

Meta-analytic methods are methods of analyzing the concept as it is used in the literature. "The literature" is usually the scientific literature, but occasionally fiction has been used, or the popular press, such as news releases and newspapers. Analytic methods have been used in nursing for both scientific concepts and lay concepts, have been used to develop the concepts and to develop models (see Chapter 32) and even mid-range theory (see Chapter 21).

Finfgeld-Connett (2008a,b): Concept Synthesis

Once the concept has been identified, professional literature of all types (editorials, anecdotes, case studies, interviews, commentary/letters, biography, and brief items) is retrieved, and forms data. A content analysis is conducted to extract the relevant text, using strategies from qualitative data analysis. Text is coded, categorized, and memos written. The conceptual structure is then identified, and antecedents and outcomes are identified.

Examples are the work by Finfgeld-Connett (2005, 2006 [Chapters 30 and 31, this volume], 2008a, 2008b).

Morse (2000): Pragmatic Utility

Pragmatic utility is described in detail in Chapters 17 and 18. Briefly, it is a method of concept analysis to be used for concepts that are at least partially mature[1] and have a reasonable amount of literature available for analysis. Briefly, when using pragmatic utility, first review the professional (research) literature about the concept of interest, then identify perspectives, or "schools of thought," and sort the literature accordingly. Next, identify "analytical questions"—key questions that provide some variation and will sort data further according to the responses. This provides significant information about the attributes, perspectives, and use of the concept of interest. Pragmatic utility is an interpretive method, so that the results both reveal and provide new insights into the concept.

Examples of studies using pragmatic utility are Hupcey, Penrod, Morse, and Mitcham (2001); McCormick (2002); Olson and Morse (2005); Weaver, Morse, and Mitcham (2008); and Weaver and Olson (2006).

COMBINED METHODS: METHODS USING THE LITERATURE AND QUALITATIVE DATA

Schwartz-Barcott and Kim (2000): The Hybrid Model of Concept Development

The Hybrid Model of Concept Development consists of three phases: *a theoretical phase* (drawing directly from clinical practice); *a fieldwork phase* (qualitative data are collected to further enrich the description of the concept—an important validity check); and *a final analytic phase*, of weighing, working, and writing up the findings (Schwartz-Barcott & Kim, 2000, pp. 131–132).

---

[1] For a discussion on concept maturity, see Chapter 11.

However, even the fieldwork phase follows Walker and Avant's pattern of seeking cases to illustrate the emerging concept.

The final analytic phase brings the concept directly back to nursing, asking:

1. How much is the concept applicable and important to nursing?
2. Does the initial selection of the concept seem justified?
3. To what extent do the review of the literature, theoretical analysis and empirical findings support the presence and frequency of this concept within the population selected for the empirical study? (Schwartz-Barcott & Kim, 2000, p. 147)

Examples of studies that have used the Hybrid Model are Browne (1997); Hagerty, Lynch-Sauer, Patusky, Bouwsema, and Collier (1992); and Madden (1990).

Morse: The Prototypical Method

The Prototypical Method begins with an exemplar that typifies an experience surrounding the concept. The exemplar must be a thick description of the experience (including much detail). It may be a documentary film (as used with hope in Chapter 16), an interview, or an autobiography. From this, the conceptual attributes are identified.

In the second phase, the phase of confirmation, other exemplars in which the researcher also expects to find illustrations of the experience are analyzed deductively, searching for the same attributes. These exemplars may not be in the same context as the first exemplar, but the researcher expects to find the same concept present. These attributes in this second group of experiences are then mapped and compared and contrasted with the first set of attributes.

What happens if the attributes do not match? Two things are possible: either the first exemplar was selected or analyzed poorly, or the second group was a poorly selected sample. In either case, the researcher is wrong, and should begin again.

An example of a study that has used this method is Morse and Doberneck (1995); see Chapter 16.

METHODS USING QUALITATIVE INQUIRY

Qualitative inquiry is the major method used to develop concepts that are immature. Standard techniques in qualitative inquiry to systematically observe, target interviews, and apply analytic techniques to segment data, to identify characteristics, and to abstract and decontextualize, all contribute to the identification and development of new concepts, or the delineation and expansion of concepts moving from the lay to the scientific arena. In this book, Chapter 14 addresses qualitative inquiry as a tool for identifying concepts and Chapter 15 addresses qualitative structured techniques for building concepts.

SUMMARY

There are many choices of *method* for conducting your concept analysis. Which do you choose?

When selecting a method, consider the following:

- What is the level of maturity of the concept I want to study? If I choose to use a meta-analytic technique, is there adequate literature available for the analysis?
- Will the method selected "move the concept along" by providing new insights, or will I only discover the obvious, that which is already known?
- Do the methods (and the examples of those who used the method) provide adequate instructions for me to follow?

And finally, remember Bob's mother's advice. Do it *properly*.

REFERENCES

Browne, A. J. (1997). A concept analysis of respect applying the hybrid model in cross-cultural settings. *Western Journal of Nursing Research, 19*(6), 762–780.

Ellis-Stoll, C. C., & Popkess-Vawter, S. A. (1998). A concept analysis on the concept of empowerment. *Advances in Nursing Science, 21*(2), 62–68.

Finfgeld-Connett, D. (2005). Clarification of social support. *Journal of Nursing Scholarship, 37*(1), 4–9.

Finfgeld-Connett, D. (2006). Meta-synthesis of presence in nursing. *Journal of Advanced Nursing, 55*(6), 708–714.

Finfgeld-Connet, D. (2008a). Concept synthesis art of nursing. *Journal of Advanced Nursing 62*(3), 381–388. doi:10.1111/j.1365-2648.2008.04601.x

Finfgeld-Connett, D. (2008b). Meta-synthesis of caring in of the nursing. *Journal of Clinical Nursing, 17*(2), 196–204.

Hagerty, B. M., Lynch-Sauer, J., Patusky, K. L., Bouwsema, M., & Collier, P. (1992). Sense of belonging: A vital mental health concept. *Archives of Psychiatric Nursing, 6*(3), 172–177.

Hupcey, J. E., Morse, J. M., Lenz, E., & Tasón, M. (1996). Wilsonian methods of concept analysis: A critique. *Scholarly Inquiry for Nursing Practice, 10*(3), 185–210.

Hupcey, J. E., Penrod, J., Morse, J. M., & Mitcham, C. (2001). An exploration and advancement of the concept of trust. *Journal of Advanced Nursing, 36*(2), 282–293.

Johnson, S. (2007). Hope in terminal illness: An evolutionary concept analysis. *International Journal of Palliative Nursing, 13*(9), 451–461.

Madden, B. P. (1990). The hybrid model for concept development: Its value for the study of therapeutic alliance. *Advances in Nursing Science, 12*(3), 75–87.

McCormick, K. M. (2002). A concept analysis of uncertainty in illness. *Journal of Nursing Scholarship, 34*(2), 127–131.

Morse, J. M. (2000). Exploring pragmatic utility: Concept analysis by critically appraising the Literature. In B. Rodgers & K. Knafl (Eds.), *Concept development in nursing* (pp. 333–352). Philadelphia, PA: Saunders.

Morse, J. M., & Doberneck, B. M. (1995). Delineating the concept of hope. *Image: Journal of Nursing Scholarship, 27*(4), 277–285.

Mulder, P. I. (2006). A concept analysis of effective breastfeeding. *Journal of Gynecological and Neonatal Nursing, 3593*, 332–339.

Olson, K., & Morse, J. M. (2005). Delineating the concept of fatigue using a pragmatic utility approach. In J. Cutcliffe & H. McKenna (Eds.), *The essential concepts of nursing: Building blocks for practice* (pp. 141–160). Edinburgh: Elsevier.

Rodgers, B. L. (1989). Exploring health policy as a concept. *Western Journal of Nursing Research, 11*, 694–702.

Rodgers, B. L. (1993). Concept analysis: An evolutionary view. In B. L. Rodgers & K. A. Knafl (Eds.), *Concept development in nursing: Foundations, techniques and applications* (pp. 73–106). Philadelphia, PA: W. B. Saunders.

Rodgers, B. L., & Knafl, K. A. (2000). Concept analysis: An evolutionary view. In B. L. Rodgers & K. A. Knafl (Eds.), *Concept development in nursing* (2nd ed., pp. 77–117). Philadelphia, PA: Saunders.

Schilling, L. S., Grey, M., & Knafl, K. A. (2002). The concept of self-management of type 1 diabetes in children and adolescents: An evolutionary concept analysis. *Journal of Advanced Nursing, 37*(1), 87–99.

Schwartz-Barcott, D., & Kim, S. (2000). An expansion and elaboration of the hybrid model of concept development. In B. L. Rodgers & K. A. Knafl (Eds.), *Concept development in nursing: Foundation, techniques and applications* (2nd ed., pp. 107–133). Philadelphia, PA: Sanders.

Suh, E. E. (2004). The model of cultural competence through an evolutionary concept analysis. *Journal of Transcultural Nursing, 15*(2), 93–102.

Trendall, J. (2000). Concept analysis: Chronic fatigue. *Journal of Advanced Nursing, 32*(5), 1126–1131.

Walker, L. O., & Avant, K. C. (1983). *Strategies for theory construction in nursing* (1st ed.). Norwalk, CT: Appleton-Century-Crofts.

Walker, L. O., & Avant, K. C. (2011). *Strategies for theory construction in nursing* (5th ed.). Upper Saddle River, NJ: Pearson.

Weaver, K., & Olson, J. K. (2006). Understanding paradigms used for nursing research. *Journal of Advanced Nursing, 53*(4), 459–469.

Weaver, K., Morse, J., & Mitcham, C. (2008). Ethical sensitivity in professional practice: Concept analysis. *Journal of Advanced Nursing, 62*(5), 607–618.

Wilson, J. (1969). *Thinking with concepts*. New York, NY: Cambridge University Press. (Original work published 1963)

9

INDUCTIVE–DEDUCTIVE PITFALLS IN CONCEPT DEVELOPMENT[1]

> *[A] concept is not an isolated, ossified changeless formation, but an active part of an intellectual process, constantly engaged in serving communication, understanding and problem solving.*
>
> —Lev Vygotsky (1962)

The challenge of qualitative inquiry is essentially one of validity. Although much literature exists on methods of controlling or countering threats to validity when the goal of research is description, these problems are compounded when one begins working abstractly. Not only is the research most at risk with this research approach, but also these problems have been poorly addressed in the methodological literature.

Recall the goal of qualitative science twofold: first, to develop concepts in order to get a better grasp on the phenomena represented by the concepts themselves, and second, to develop generalizable and valid theories from this. We believe it is these tasks, essentially those involving interpretation, conceptualization, and abstraction, that will eventually provide qualitative inquiry with a legitimate place in the social sciences and ultimately earn its respect and contribution to knowledge.

Presently, ways of controlling threats to inductive validity with descriptive research are only partially successful. Briefly, strategies used prior to commencement of data analysis such as bracketing (Janesick, 2000; van Manen, 1990), rejection of preconceived theoretical frameworks (Miles & Huberman, 1994), or techniques of verification used during the conduct of inquiry (Meadows & Morse, 2001) demand that inquiry begins from the data with each new project, and do not facilitate the incremental

---

[1] An earlier version of this chapter was published as "Exploring qualitatively-derived concepts: inductive-deductive pitfalls" (Morse et al., 2002).

compounding of research projects. Post hoc methods to ensure validity, such as testing results by implementation and subsequent inquiry (Morse, Swanson, & Kuzel, 2001), although important, occur too late in the process of inquiry to expedite the process of inquiry itself. Although these checks and balances guide inquiry toward validity, there is a need to explore the problem of conducting qualitative inquiry using concepts as a starting point within the analytic processes of induction/deduction, and to bring to the fore ways that more advanced inquiry implicitly proceeds. In particular, there is a need to explore the problem in instances in which inquiry begins with a concept itself, rather than commencing with a basic description. Here, we have attempted to identify and to formalize techniques by which inductive processes may be *sustained* (and deductive tendencies avoided) when commencing inquiry at the conceptual level.

Induction is a sacred tenet of qualitative inquiry. Therefore, when one begins a project with a concept of interest (rather than allowing the concepts to emerge from the data per se), how does one *maintain a valid approach?* We previously discussed this problem: Even obtaining consent from a participant may violate the principle of induction and "lead" the participant, thereby invalidating data (Morse, 2008). Therefore, when commencing inquiry with a chosen concept or phenomenon of interest, rather than with a question from the data about what is going on, how does one control deductive tendencies that threaten validity?

Difficulties stem from the *nature of induction itself*—is induction an impossible operation in qualitative research, as Popper (1963/1965) suggests? In this section, we first discuss Popper's concern, followed by a discussion of two major threats that may prevent an inductive approach in qualitative research. The first threat is the *pink elephant paradox;* the second is the avoidance of *conceptual tunnel vision* or, specifically, *how* does the researcher decontextualize the concept of interest from the surrounding context and thereby avoid the tendency to consider *all* data to be pertinent to the concept of interest? How do we maintain both the integrity of the concept and the integrity of the research?

THE MYTH OF INDUCTION

Popper (1963/1965) identified the most well-known threat to inductive soundness, which has become the Achilles's heel of qualitative inquiry. He summed up his challenge to the notion of induction with an example of a group of physics students in Vienna in the 1940s:

> Take a pencil and paper; carefully observe, and write down what you have observed! They asked, of course, what I wanted them to observe. Clearly the instruction, "Observe!" is absurd. (p. 46)

With this example, Popper is implying that just as observation is "always selective," induction is not presuppositionless. From this criticism, fear of violating inductive processes has resulted in researchers' reluctance to focus on a concept until it "emerges," and some researchers even avoid the literature before commencing fieldwork (Glaser, 1992).[2]

But because Popper has removed the process of induction from the context of research itself, we suggest that Popper's concern is unwarranted. Let us explain, and at the same time consider the history of the development of this problem, which we call the *myth of induction*.

The problem of induction is already hinted at in the 4th century BCE by Aristotle, although his approach is not so much to reject what will not fit into a tight logical box as to explain how something like induction, which obviously takes place, must in fact be able to do so. In an important passage from *On Interpretation* (Aristotle, 2000), he suggests that the formation of concepts is a little like what goes on as an army retreats under attack, constantly falling back here and then there looking for a place to make a firm stand. The passage easily reminds one of Piaget's (1959) notion of equilibration, of how concepts are developed through trial and error engagement with phenomena. In both cases, induction is accepted as a real process, and one that is not subject to deductive logical formulation. This is not to deny that some skill-based rules of thumb might help guide induction, although it has been left to later phenomenologists and qualitative researchers to attempt to formulate such rules or guidelines.

When Hume (1960) formulated the classic riddle of induction, the upshot was simply to note that thinking involves two different kinds of concepts: those that can be linked or connected by necessity and those that cannot. But there is no need to deny the reality of concepts that cannot be connected by necessity. The fact that the concept of a triangle necessitates that the sum of the interior angles be 180 degrees, whereas the concept of a *dog* does not with the same necessity mean that it is a mammal, in no way requires that dog and mammal be rejected as being unsound or illegitimate concepts.

Thus, when Popper goes so far as to reject induction as a myth and to replace it with capricious conjecture, which we simply accept as long as we cannot empirically refute it by finding some phenomenon that falsifies it, he reveals his own inherently rationalist biases. It may well be true that this is how some sciences, especially the highly mathematized ones, tend to work. But it is certainly not how all science has to work, or in fact does work. Biology, for instance, clearly proceeds in its classification of organisms more like a well-organized army faced with ever-new experiences.

In this way, Popper's argument is itself unsound precisely because he has removed the process of induction from its real-world context in different

---

[2] Popper also defines research narrowly, as refutation rather than discovery. This perspective also challenges qualitative inquiry, which, of course, does not proceed by using hypotheses and the classical scientific method.

kinds of research. Consider another example: A *race* is defined by certain characteristics or parameters (i.e., there must be a start and a finish, something to race against such as more than one competitor or time, there must be a system of measuring whatever is being challenged, and so forth), and without these characteristics one cannot have a race. Similarly, *research* has defining characteristics, one of which is a *focus of inquiry*. You cannot have research without something to be inquiring about. Thus taken in the *context* of research, Popper's classic criticism of induction in qualitative inquiry ("What shall I observe?") is in itself invalid.

The issue is not *if* the inductive process can be used in qualitative research, but *how* induction should be used.

Nevertheless, our concerns regarding the *pink elephant paradox* remain, and are concerns that the concept of *bracketing* does not resolve. Bracketing works very well for formal knowledge, but less well in instances when the threat to induction is less conscious, as may occur with conceptual tunnel vision. The alternative offered, a priori theoretical frameworks that *prescribe* coding schemes, has been rightly discarded as a source of invalidity for qualitative inquiry.

The Pink Elephant Paradox

"Don't think of a pink elephant!" is an impossible instruction, for once the idea of a pink elephant is mentioned, it cannot be erased from one's consciousness. The *pink elephant paradox* raises the possibility that one could think of an idea or concept that one was trying to avoid, and indeed confirm the existence of the phenomenon to which the concept refers, since once a person starts to think of pink elephants, the person also easily starts not just to think of them. It is possible, for instance, that the mere adoption of some particular coding (or theoretical) framework might lead one to "prove anything," as Popper and others have noted.

We argue that pink elephants are less of a risk in sound qualitative inquiry because they are controlled, to some extent, by processes of saturation, replication, and verification. At the same time, by accruing multiple examples of the same event/relationship/phenomenon in the data, from different times or different circumstances, by asking critical questions of these data, and by constantly looking for alternative explanations, the risk of misattribution or miscategorization is reduced. Thus, the risk of pink elephants is greatest in thin data sets (see Chapter 10).

However, to some extent, the risk always remains and we admit vast pink elephant problems have occurred in social science research, both qualitative and quantitative. One historical example is the theory that masturbation causes madness, which was "experimentally" supported at that time (Engelhardt, 1974).

Conceptual Tunnel Vision

Conceptual tunnel vision exemplifies the researcher's problem in deciding which data do and which do not pertain to a concept, or are and are not examples of the concept. *Conceptual tunnel vision* is the overcategorization of data, assigning more data to one category than actually belongs, or seeing or justifying most things as being related to, or considered examples of, the concept being investigated. This problem is inflated with the value in qualitative inquiry on holism, so that the process of encompassing all data—and the fear of missing something—is embedded in this problem. The questions that the researcher must struggle with are: What is and what is not pertinent to inquiry? And how can I be certain?

When conducting research into a concept, tunnel vision becomes the analytic anathema and overattribution inflates both the contents and the role of a concept in the results.

How can this problem be controlled? One method is to bring critical inquiry out into the open and demand that categories earn their way into the analytic scheme. For instance, in Morse's research program on comfort, we ask: Is thus and so an example of caring or comforting? What is the relationship between caring and comforting? Is caring a part of comfort, or comfort a part of caring? Do they share attributes, or are their attributes distinct? In this way, by constantly being alert to hidden and underlying assumptions, and by only allowing legitimate facts and relationships to be used, we control the use of poorly linked or irrelevant contextual characteristics into the developing theory.

EXPLORING QUALITATIVELY DERIVED CONCEPTS: INDUCTIVE TECHNIQUES

The intermediate solutions or approaches to controlling validity are strategies that are probably already used in qualitative inquiry, but have not been yet formalized and described.

Deconstruction: Techniques of Concept Analysis

The first step is using the literature to conduct a concept analysis of the concept. While we disagree with Glaser (1978, 1992) that one enters qualitative inquiry without using the knowledge of others, either conceptual or substantive, we also disagree with the process of simplistic bracketing. Rather, the researcher should act as an informed consumer when using this literature, assume that it is correct, and critically analyze it all as a whole, deconstructing the concept to identify the attributes or characteristics, assumptions, gaps, limitations, differing perspectives (including the way the concept has been developed in different contexts or disciplines), and different forms of the concept for different functions. Then, once this analysis is completed, the researcher is working wisely, perhaps selectively bracketing, perhaps using this information to refine one's proposal, perhaps using this information as a comparative template in the process of data collection. Regardless of how the information is used, knowledge makes one's questioning of data smarter as data collection proceeds. The researcher is not blinded by ignorance or by the present "partly line" of theories, models, and myths that seem pervasive in the literature. We concede that Popper was correct when he stated that inquiry does not begin from nothing, but by using concept analysis as described elsewhere (Morse, 2000), qualitative inquiry begins its inductive processes by deconstructing all the implicit assumptions, building from a carefully inspected base, by an informed researcher.

Focusing: Development of a Skeletal Framework

Inquiry then proceeds depending on the "maturity" of the concept (Morse, Mitcham, Hupcey, & Tasón, 1996). When concepts are immature or little is known about the concept, the next step in inquiry is to identify and develop a *skeletal framework*.

How then do you proceed? Normally with ethnographic research, data collection begins as a comprehensive and complete "fishing trip"—the holistic approach, or "scoping" (Morse & Richards, 2002). Indeed, broad "maps" are available to ensure such comprehensive data collection, such as Leininger's (1988) Sunrise Model or Spradley's (1980) Descriptive Question Matrix. Basically, these schemata ensure that inquiry is broad, so that necessary data are available when, later in the study, the researcher focuses on a particular topic of inquiry. It is a way to ensure validity—by ensuring a complete data set is available, by ensuring that the concept developed is comprehensive and complete, and by ensuring that "premature closure" has not occurred. For instance, Leininger's Sunrise Model includes categories such as technological factors, religious and philosophical factors, kinship and social factors, and so forth, and how these broad categories influence care patterns and health. Spradley's model is more particular and action-oriented, and includes categories such as space, object, act, activity, event, actor, goal, and feelings (1980, p. 82). Each topic is linked in a matrix to every other topic but, again, these data must be placed within the context of the question asked. In our case, the careful conceptual analysis work preceding the stage of data collection reduces this fumbling, and enables the researcher to move more quickly through the fieldwork. This background work allows the researcher to focus more quickly, thus expediting the research process.

Note that the researcher is only partially rescued from the invalidity dilemma. We discussed what to call the "level of theory" developed from this type of semifocused observations and interview, and decided that the analogy of the skeleton best summed up what we were trying to convey. From the concept analysis, we have some information about the essential characteristics or attributes of the concept, so we know where to direct our attentions but much still remains unknown. As an archaeologist does when discovering a skeleton, we knew roughly the shape of the original dinosaur—and perhaps even how it moved and worked—but we only had a general idea of its actual appearance. As the concept boundaries remain unclear, the risk of omission in data collection remains. To compensate for this risk of missing, ignoring, or omitting essential data, the scope of data collection needs to remain somewhat broader than the actual concept. Thus, researchers should initially sample more data than is required, and refine focus as the study proceeds. However, we avoid the mistake of assuming that all data are relevant—to conduct such a fishing trip is not using inductive principles for inquiry. Only by collecting rich and relevant data around the bare bones of what is known, using principles of saturation and verification, can we recognize the pertinent data from other data.

In summary, a skeletal framework serves to sensitize the researcher and facilitate focusing the inquiry at an early stage. It provides internal structure to study, thus enabling observations, interviews, and analysis to proceed. As an archaeologist tries to piece bones together, the inductive puzzle of inquiry is maintained, and, as inquiry proceeds, falls into place, the skeletal framework is padded, and provides the emerging model with indices of purpose and function.

Toward Verification: Using a Scaffold

When using a scaffold, one is reasonably confident of the type of concept, either from the literature or from previous inquiry, and the concept may be considered at least partially mature. In this way, the investigator may recognize that a particular setting will provide the researcher with a good example of exploring a particular concept. The investigator is reasonably confident about the domain of the concepts—of what is and what is not an example of the concept. Boundaries have been established, so that the scope of the concept is known (Morse & Richards, 2002). However, the researcher may still have questions about the attributes or characteristics that comprise the concept. Thus, a scaffold delineates a concept, but still enables inductive exploration of the internal compositions of the concept to take shape.

When using a scaffold, the boundaries of the concept may be known, thereby focusing on sampling and data collection. However, the internal structures require further investigation. Compared to the previous skeletal framework, sampling is more focused, data are collected in increasing depth, and event sampling may be used. Internally, the researcher maintains loosely held assumptions about the attributes. These are inductively explored, with what is already known drawn as a comparative template over the emerging scheme. Thus, previous work, while focusing inquiry, still enables the internal structure of the concept to be malleable and to "emerge." Data collection proceeds inductively, with the investigator seeking new insights, verification, and saturation. Once the work is completed, the scaffold is dismantled and the theory stands on its own.

From our previous work, developed from interviews, we had an understanding of reports of enduring and manifestation of emotional suffering behaviors, but we did not know if we could differentiate these states observationally. We also had little information about the interaction between family members who are also enduring or emotionally suffering. In this case, we recognized the pink elephant, but explored it closely to collect rich and detailed behavioral descriptions.

Theoretical Frameworks?

Once a concept has been explored and described in depth, inquiry has proceeded to the level that quantitative inquiry and a theoretical framework may, at this stage, be used. A theoretical framework organizes a coding scheme, and it is this structure that deductively prescribes the form of data collection instruments, measurements, and even types of analysis. Note, however, that inquiry has now moved to the deductive quantitative stages, and it should therefore be used cautiously in qualitative inquiry. The use of theoretical frameworks in quantitative inquiry is discussed in Chapter 27.

SUMMARY

To summarize, the systematic exploration of concepts, using interview or observational methods, progresses sequentially from deconstruction of *concept analysis of the literature* to the use of these *data as a skeleton*, or to *using prior knowledge as a scaffold*. All of these stages continue to use induction, but in different ways and in varying degrees. Awareness of the stage of development of the concept, and of how you are using previous inquiry, will expedite inquiry and enhance, rather than threaten, validity.

REFERENCES

Aristotle. (2000). *On interpretation.* London, UK: Duckworth.

Engelhardt, H. T., Jr. (1974). The disease of masturbation: Values and the concept of disease. *Bulletin of the History of Medicine, 48*, 234–248.

Glaser, B. G. (1978). *Theoretical sensitivity.* Mill Valley, CA: Sociology Press.

Glaser, B. G. (1992). *Basis of grounded theory analysis.* Mill Valley, CA: Sociology Press.

Hume, D. (1960). *A treatise on human nature.* In L. A. Selby-Bigge (Ed.), Reprinted from the original in three volumes. Oxford, UK: Oxford University Press.

Janesick, V. J. (2000). The choreography of qualitative research design: Minuets, improvisations, and crystallization. In N. K. Denzin & Y. S. Lincoln (Eds.), *Handbook of qualitative research* (2nd ed., pp. 379–399). Thousand Oaks, CA: Sage.

Leininger, M. M. (1988). Leininger's theory of nursing: Culture care diversity and universality. *Nursing Science Quarterly, 1*(4), 151–160.

Meadows, L., & Morse, J. M. (2001). Constructing evidence within the qualitative project. In J. M. Morse, J. Swanson, & A. Kuzel (Eds.), *The nature of evidence in qualitative inquiry* (pp. 187–200). Newbury Park, CA: Sage.

Miles, M. B., & Huberman, A. M. (1994). *Qualitative data analysis* (2nd ed.). Thousand Oaks, CA: Sage.

Morse J. M., Mitcham C., Hupcey J. E., & Tasón, M. C. (1996). Criteria for concept evaluation. *Journal of Advanced Nursing, 24*, 385–390.

Morse, J. M. (2000). Exploring pragmatic utility: Concept analysis by critically appraising the Literature. In B. Rodgers & K. Knafl (Eds.), *Concept development in nursing* (pp. 333–352). Philadelphia, PA: Saunders.

Morse, J. M. (2008). Does informed consent interfere with induction? [Editorial]. *Qualitative Health Research, 18*(4), 439–440. doi:10.1177/1049732307313614

Morse, J. M., & Richards, L. (2002). *Readme first for a researcher's guide to qualitative methods.* Thousand Oaks, CA: Sage.

Morse, J. M., Hupcey, J. E., Penrod, J., Spiers, J. A., Pooler, C., & Mitcham, C. (2002). Issues in validity: Behavioral concepts, their derivation and interpretation. *International Journal of Qualitative Methods, 1*(4). Symposium introduction. Article 3. Conclusion. Article 9. Retrieved from http://www.ualberta.ca/~ijqm

Morse, J. M., Swanson, J., & Kuzel, A. (Eds.). (2001). *The nature of qualitative evidence.* Thousand Oaks, CA: Sage.

Piaget, J. (1959). *The language and thought of the child* (3rd ed.). London, UK: Routledge & Kegan Paul.

Popper, K. R. (1963/1965). *Conjectures and refutations: The growth of scientific knowledge.* New York, NY: Harper Torchbooks.

Spradley, J. P. (1980). *Participant observation.* New York, NY: Holt, Rinehart, Winston.

Van Manen, M. (1990). *Researching lived experiences.* Albany, NY: State University of New York.

Vygotsky, L. (1962). *Thought and language* (E. Hanfmann & G. Walker, Trans.). Cambridge, MA: MIT Press.

Judith A. Spiers   **10**

THE PINK ELEPHANT PARADOX (OR, AVOIDING THE MISATTRIBUTION OF DATA)[1]

> *One day Alice came to a fork in the road and saw a Cheshire cat in a*
> *tree. "Which road do I take?" she asked.*
> *"Where do you want to go?" was his response.*
> *"I don't know," Alice answered.*
> *"Then," said the cat, "it doesn't matter."*
>
> —Lewis Carroll (1865)

The pink elephant paradox refers to the threat to inductive thinking caused by the difficulty of inadvertently proving the existence of a concept or phenomenon just because it overtly or surreptitiously exists in one's thoughts, leading to misattribution, or miscategorization of data, and thus subverting inductive processes. As Morse and Mitcham (2002) discuss, this is reduced through inductive strategies, including processes of saturation, replication, and verification. Here, I present a story of how the phenomenon of interest in nurse–patient interaction evolved and emerged through a number of qualitative projects. At each stage, concepts were identified, explored, and developed in order to more elucidate the central phenomenon. I will show how, while at times I could identify and avoid the pink elephant, at other times there were one or a herd lurking in the shadows or rampaging through my work. I think that discussing both the successes and pitfalls is one way to acknowledge and address the fact that, although we accept the evolution in ideas and thought processes in qualitative research, we still may not be comfortable in articulating the far more complex and insidious threats to inductive processes.

---

[1] Spiers (2002b). Reprinted with permission of the author.

Some schools of qualitative inquiry consider analysis of the literature a hindrance—in fact, an invalidity—before commencing fieldwork. To the contrary, when a researcher is studying a concept rather than letting a concept emerge from a setting, it is essential to undertake a thorough theoretical and conceptual analysis of the literature (Morse, 2000; Morse, Hupcey, Mitcham, & Lenz, 1996). In my own program of research, the concept analysis was a study in and of itself, with the purpose of examining the maturity of concepts and the explicit and implicit theoretical and research models. The literature constituted data that could be analyzed and formed the basis for a reconceptualization of the original concept by contrasting it with the theory derived from the fieldwork studies.

THE IMPORTANCE OF NURSE–PATIENT COMMUNICATION

My area of interest is interpersonal communication in nurse–patient interaction. Specifically, I am interested in understanding how nurses and patients with uniquely different paradigms of understanding illness experience can, within very short spaces of times, make profound interpersonal connections, perceive and avoid unnecessary interpersonal conflict, and, at times, address issues of significant personal vulnerability.

This dimension of nurse–patient interaction was conceptualized by Christensen (1990) as a paradoxical determinant of the context of nursing partnerships. She called it *anonymous intimacy*, or the significant degree of immediate socially sanctioned closeness between strangers. She described this as the ability for nurses and patients, who are strangers, to forge a high degree of intimacy as the patient surrenders privacy for nursing care. The essence of anonymous intimacy is that patients identify with nursing and nurses rather than individuals.

Although the concept was described well in her data set of 87 nurses and 21 patients in a hospital setting, it was not developed theoretically—the meaning, definitions, assumptions of intimacy and anonymity, and the means through which anonymity and intimacy were combined or resolved in interaction were unclear. Nevertheless, it was a very interesting concept and one that immediately attracted a sense of recognition from nurses. In my conceptual exploration of *anonymous intimacy* in the literature, it quickly became clear that although Christensen's (1990) conceptualization was unique, it in fact represented a way of co-orientating to desired ways of relating to each other. It was a style of interacting, not a contextual feature of interactions. It was about using common social knowledge of nursing and patient roles, along with individual ability and desire to enhance a more personal relationship in order to increase or decrease social distance (Spiers, 1998). Of critical importance was the notion of being able to change the degree of interpersonal space in an interaction according to the flow of events in the encounter.

The ability to manipulate the degree of familiarity is important because many of the activities nurses do on a daily basis create social and personal discomfort and vulnerability for the patient. We know this well; that is why we have different ways of communicating the same information in different contexts. Each approach recognizes the need for diplomacy, politeness, directness, or indirectness. But it is not just the patient's sense of vulnerability at issue—nurses, too, deal with needs for privacy, boundaries, and formality and also can be vulnerable in their interactions. From the standpoint of a theoretical understanding of *anonymous intimacy*, it became evident that the ways nurses and patients interact have something to do with trying to *save face* in interaction, to prevent or minimize interpersonal discomfort and embarrassment. Thus, in order to comprehend the essence of *anonymous intimacy*, the concept of face became important.

Saving Face

The idea of face as personal vulnerability in interaction is an interesting one. *Saving face* is a well-recognized phenomenon in many cultural groups, in which *face* refers to preserving or losing one's social standing by deferring to social norms of behavior. As an ethnolinguistic concept, it has been developed by Brown and Levinson (1987) in a model of the work involved in social interaction to protect and address threats to face, or the threats to an individual's sense of public image in social interaction. Interestingly, face is defined more by its loss and threats, than, in fact, what it is.

Face would seem to be a highly pertinent concept for nursing interactions. Think of the number of situations that threaten not only patients' face, but that have implications for our own as well—patients becoming embarrassed at the loss of bodily or emotional control, the difficulty of conveying distressing news, and how one approaches a procedure never attempted before. Yet, the concept is absent in the nursing literature. The concepts that come closest—such as quality of relatedness, trust, and cocreation of meaning—work at a level of abstraction often developed from nurses' and patients' reflection of their interpersonal relationships (Spiers, 1998). This means that the behaviors, the social actions involved in enacting this dimension of interaction, were still largely obscured because they do not occur at a conscious level of behavior (Byrd, 1995).

Face is related to our sense of personal vulnerability, to our sense of social image, or presentation in social interaction (Brown & Levinson, 1987). Moving away from a macroview of *anonymous intimacy* as a way of relating that minimizes embarrassment and discomfort in interaction by creating a sense of anonymity, it became evident that communicative processes of *saving face* were the key to understanding nursing interactions. However, it is problematic to just borrow a concept from another discipline without thoroughly investigating it. Thus, my attention turned to the concept of face. I needed to explore the philosophical, theoretical, and methodological assumptions underlying the concept of face in order to move forward in my investigations. An article, "The Use of Face Work and Politeness Theory," was published in *Qualitative Health Research* (Spiers, 1998).

I had moved from *anonymous* intimacy to the concept of *face* in order to draw closer to comprehending that elusive dimension of nurse–patient interaction. Face represents personal vulnerability in interaction. The work involved in saving face—face work—referred to the continual process of identifying, constructing, and enhancing one's own and the other person's sense of face and avoiding or mitigating situations that threatened face (Holtgraves & Yang, 1990). Face, an interpersonal social phenomenon rather than an intrapersonal psychological construct, is mutually constructed in the interaction and is something that is strategically manipulated in response to the flow of events in the encounter (Holtgraves, 1992). In other words, the context of the encounter and the events within that encounter change the nature of the face one wishes to claim for oneself and that one is willing to recognize for the other person. That is why talking about a highly intimate and private topic feels different—and is handled differently—when talking with a best friend, an employer, or a health professional. It seemed to revolve around the idea of vulnerability. To understand that part of the nursing experience Christensen (1990) called *anonymous intimacy*, it was necessary to establish an interpersonal context of face. In order to understand the nature of face, the concept of vulnerability emerged in my theoretical analysis. So far, there was little sign of the pink elephant.

THE CONCEPT OF VULNERABILITY

There are literally thousands of references to vulnerability in the literature as it is a fundamental aspect of the experience of health and illness. Yet, when I started to explore how the concept was used in the clinical and research literature, it was evident that there were two primary approaches, neither of which was of much use in looking at the experience of nursing or the behaviors related to influencing social distance in interpersonal interaction (Spiers, 2000). Vulnerability can be used to identify individuals and groups at risk of harm (Aday, 1993). This is based on epidemiological characteristics that assign people or groups to higher than normal standards of risk. This risk is objectively derived, most frequently by some source external to the person being assessed. Thus, vulnerability is located intrapersonally as a personal attribute of some kind of deficiency in comparison to the normative standard, which requires intervention in order to protect the subject from harm or endangerment (Ferguson, 1978). Alternatively, vulnerability can be a more experiential and qualitative phenomenon, a sense of challenge to one's sense of personal integrity (Morse, 1997b; Stevens, Hall, & Meleis, 1992). Being able to distinguish between emic and etic views allows us to differentiate between being at risk and feeling vulnerable (Spiers, 2002a). However, the problem that the concept of face in interaction posed remained—the idea of mutual vulnerability as a social construct, rather than an intrapersonal state in interaction. The definitions used in the literature were still intrapersonal, whether the view was *emically* or *etically* derived.[2]

Moving to Fieldwork

This, then, was the theoretical background for my research on the nature of vulnerability in the interactions between home care nurses and their patients (Spiers, 2002a). It seemed that none of the frameworks I had explored—from anonymous intimacy, to quality of relatedness, to face—were adequate conceptualizations of that elusive dimension of nursing: the ability to move a sense of intimacy and distance in order to deal with the interpersonal implications of the event in the moment. The concept of *face*, although useful and interesting, was defined more by what it was not, and the categories within the model were largely fixed. If I had used this, I would have run the risk of approaching my interpretation deductively, with a priori definitions, and with categories of behavior that were largely decontextualized because face, in Brown and Levinson's (1987) approach, specifically addressed only one distinct dimension of social interaction. The various conceptualizations of vulnerability in the nursing and health literature were likewise problematic, limiting my ability to combine both etic and emic views.

It is important to emphasize that in going to the literature, I was not developing a conceptual framework but trying to clarify assumptions and perspectives to put together the beginning of the skeleton that would give my study shape and direction. To make the fieldwork viable, I needed to have some clarity and a theoretical understanding of the kinds of concepts and phenomena at work in constructing the topic that piqued my interest. Creating this skeleton through systematic concept analysis processes allowed me to articulate my assumptions and perspectives. This would provide direction in sampling and data collection. It had started to build the internal structure for my study. Sometimes, these assumptions were more questions than beliefs—could vulnerability be an interpersonal phenomenon? As a mutual experience related to the events in the interaction, could it be observable in the behaviors of the nurse and patient. These are the ideas that sparked the phase of inductive clinical fieldwork. If I had not done this, but had just leapt into fieldwork, I would have been at extreme risk of floundering—of seeing everything as related to my phenomenon of interest—which, at the beginning, was extremely poorly delineated. Without this theoretical work, not only would the pink elephant have entered the picture, it would have picked me up, set me on its back, and we would have merrily ridden away.

---

[2] "Emic" means "self-focused"; "etic" means focused on the other (or a world view).

EXPLORING VULNERABILITY IN HOME CARE
NURSE–PATIENT INTERACTIONS

As is common in qualitative work, researchers seek the context in which we can best see the phenomenon of interest. I was looking for nursing situations in which the nature and characteristics of vulnerability would be highly apparent. To do this, I videotaped home care nurses' visits to patients. The unit of analysis was the speech or communication act within the interaction, captured in 31 videotaped visits providing more than 19 hours of video data. Now, it is important to remember that I was not seeking representativeness and generalizability, but an in-depth understanding of common social experiences in home care nursing situations. This is where the issue of pink elephants, or issues of inductive/deductive traps, truly began to raise its head—or trunk.

On the Trail of Pink Elephants

The importance of scoping to locate a concept and focusing is discussed in Chapter 8. It is important to find the balance between entering the research with such a wide view that the researcher is left to fumble in the dark and walking in knowing what to look for and where to find it. Issues of bracketing, as they noted, were difficult to resolve, especially when one has invested so much time and energy in theoretical concept exploration. I had tried to avoid the pink elephant through my evolving concept explorations and analyses. The problem was that now I was trying to explore vulnerability, and I had an idea of what it could look like. It was clear that nurses and patients experienced episodes of difficulty in their interactions—both very minor and quite major difficulties. Yet, I could not make sense of my data. Despite an excruciating level of description of my data, and extensive challenges from my colleagues, it did not make sense; the idea of vulnerability simply did not match what I thought I saw in the data. It seemed that *everything* could be related to vulnerability.

As I continued to look at different interactions and nurse–patient dyads, it became clear that until I could understand *what it was* the nurse and patient were trying to achieve, the notion of vulnerability was meaningless. As my study evolved, the research questions became not *what is vulnerability*, but how the patients' and nurses' paradigms of understanding or worldviews were coconstructed through their interaction. I had to explore the kinds of goals in terms of cocreated meaning that both the nurse and patient were working toward in order to understand the interpersonal conditions in which vulnerability could be manifested Spiers (2002a).

To return to the idea of a conceptual skeleton, it turned out that I had the "bones" the wrong way up. It was only through attention to preserving and ensuring principles of inductive reasoning that I came to realize this problem. It was only by suspending ideas from face work theory and models of vulnerability that I could see this, and then more productively use the concepts of face and emic–etic vulnerability later in my inquiry to explore the communicative means by which the interpersonal contexts of mutual interpersonal vulnerability were created and resolved. The following sections are some very concrete and pragmatic examples of the pink elephant threats in this phase of my research.

Overwhelming Amounts of Data

A necessary design feature in my research, dictated by the need to understand the vulnerability as part of cocreation of meaning, meant that my sampling and data collection were extremely broad. Remember that my unit of analysis was not the nurse–patient dyad, but the speech act—the smallest unit of meaning, verbal or nonverbal, which could be indicative of successful or unsuccessful cocreation of meaning, and thus vulnerability. In each interaction, there could be anywhere from 500 to 2,500 speech turns. This was a huge amount of data. However, this breadth was necessary to describe the context of what I was interested in—cocreation of meaning across the nursing and patient paradigms of understanding, and situations in which this did not occur and which was evident in only some data.

I needed to look at multiple levels of the interaction and from different perspectives. For example, I needed to move between very macroperspectives of identifying the activities and tasks they engaged in, from wound care, to pain management, to coordination of services, to types of interaction, from very rote and apparently superficial, to highly attentive interactions, to ones in which each person juggled the degree of involvement. All of this was layered with the immediate and longer terms goals of interaction that were part of every action. By doing this, I could work out what nurses and patients were trying to do, and the nature of the interaction and consequences when this was not successful, or when one person's attempts or goals were not recognized or matched by the other. At this point, my skeletal framework enabled me to more successfully sensitize me to instances of vulnerability as both a process and outcome, or, even more likely, instances of *near misses.*

The *near-miss* instances were very important to avoiding the pink elephant. Essentially, vulnerability emerged as a result of the nurses' and patients' inability to cocreate common meaning and understanding of the situation or the intentions of the other. Vulnerability was more often a potential manifestation rather than an actual one. Why? This was because of the communicative skill of nurses and patients in averting problems in the interaction that could result in overt vulnerability and, often, communication breakdown. The following example illustrates this.

A major type of work in the interactions was creating and sustaining an amicable working relationship. This involved negotiating the level of formality as nurse and patient, and familiarity and liking, as individuals. It was deciding how, and to what extent, to get to know each other. Both nurses and patients volunteered information about themselves and showed interest in finding out about the other. This could range from finding an acceptable level of social talk to inviting or offering self-disclosure. For example, one patient deflected all personal probes from the nurse but would happily engage in detailed conversation about their mutual tastes and habits in their community of shops and restaurants. Mutual vulnerability occurred when someone was trying to establish personal boundaries without appearing rude, dismissive, or offended. If a question was declined in a way that was respectful, it identified the boundaries of the relationship. If it was not performed tactfully, then it had the effect of rejecting the other person. In one dyad, the patient was always interested in flattering her nurse and validating the importance of the exclusivity of their relationship. This created difficulties, because sometimes the nurse could not visit, and a substitute was sent. In trying to offer a compliment to the usual nurse, this could be construed as criticism of the other nurse, creating a situation of mutual vulnerability.

N: Well, I was away last week.
P: I missed you too!
N: I know. [both laugh]
P: Don't get me wrong!
N: No!
P: Nothing wrong with the other nurse.
N: Yeah.
P: She's nice—
N: I know!
P: —She's just not as friendly. She doesn't laugh like you or I do.
N: Yeah. Yeah, yeah, she's more—she's different.
P: She's mostly (XX) on her work and THAT'S IT. Nothing else.
N: Yeah …, you know (yeah). [both laugh]

Intra- or Interpersonal Characteristics of Vulnerability

One of the most apparent deductive–inductive threats in this research was working out the extent to which vulnerability represented an idiosyncratic characteristic or a phenomenon related to the interpersonal context. In dealing with this, my main strategy was pursuing comparative cases. In order to ascertain the extent to which the vulnerability was related to the flow of events in the encounter, rather than to the people, I needed to change the context to see if the nature and characteristics of the vulnerabilities I had identified held across different nurse–patient dyads. It was very interesting to explore how, for example, the kind of vulnerability that was demonstrated in a very well-established dyad had significant commonalties and dimensions, as well as differences, with dyads that were the opposite—a new dyad, a first encounter. I was fortunate in being able to observe different nurses with the same patient, which was another way of determining the extent to which the kinds of vulnerabilities or interactive events were intrapersonally situated or, as I was discovering, idiosyncratically influenced, but located as mutual interpersonal concern.

Attaching Meaning to Behaviors

Another very interesting conundrum I faced was my ability to attribute meaning to particular behaviors. I noted earlier that I was working on the premise that vulnerability was observable, indicated in not only the content of the interaction but also in the flow of the interaction. In other words, vulnerability or otherwise was not only evident in *what* was said, but *how* it was said. This placed me in an interesting position when, from my observer's stance, my interpretation of what happened, and how, differed markedly from the patient, the nurse, or both. I had tried to minimize this problem by incorporating interviews in my data collection. I would talk to the patient and nurse each after every visit, asking them about what happened, what they each were trying to do, why and how, and their perceptions of the other person. And of course, I asked if there had been any difficulties. As I expected, they were very rarely able to give me the kind of information that would help me in my interpretation. Why? This was for two primary reasons, the first being that the kinds of interactive behaviors I was interested in were simply not at a conscious level of awareness or recall. We are so accustomed to dealing with the hiccups and transient communication difficulties that can occur that we simply do not notice them. So, although major communication problems, such as becoming angry or making accusations, were available to my participants for conscious recall, much of what I ultimately found interesting did not exist at a conscious level.

Second, there are interpersonal implications for vulnerability in the researcher–participant relationship and interaction, not just the interaction I was trying to examine. It is bad enough having a researcher observing a nurse's or patient's faults or stupid acts, misunderstanding, being inappropriate or coercive during the actual interaction, let alone having to talk about it afterwards. In this example, the patient's challenge to the nurse's claim to be able to anticipate the physician's actions, her subsequent attempts to explain her assumptions, and the patient's realization that he had embarrassed her by disputing her right—and competence—to do this created acute embarrassment for both:

[Nurse is engaged in changing the dressing of the patient's abdominal wound.]

N: I wonder if he'll take the rest of those staples out. I know. Are they kind of pulling—can you feel them?

P: No, no, that's one thing I don't do—tell him how to do his job. No-no-no-no-no. [fast sing song voice]

N: No-No! I'm just curious!

P: No, I'm just—I'm not even curious!

N: I know—whenever he's ready to take them out, that's (yeah) ok by you!

P: Yes, that's fine. I tell you it doesn't bother me one way or the other.

N: Yeah, yeah. Sometimes people—they irritate, you know, they kind of pull and—but he'll take—he might take—I wouldn't be surprised—

P: Oh, whatever. That's what he gets paid big bucks for.

N: Yeah, that's right.

Reactions to this kind of interaction would be discounting, denying, and laughing it off. Ideally, it could have been useful to take the actual video back to the participants, although I do not think it would have overcome the difficulties inherent in seeing one's own behavior as an observer (Lomax & Casey, 1998). Thus, there was always the risk of misjudging the intent and meaning of the actions. I addressed this in my analysis by being extremely detailed in my description of behaviors and then in my writing, by a textual rendering that tried to draw the reader into the participant's world I was observing.

SUMMARY

Let us reiterate that the process I engaged in to pursue a clinical phenomenon of interest was an exciting voyage of discovery that has demanded flexibility and willingness to pursue a number of productive and less productive routes. All of the processes and stages of these projects were directed toward developing a skeletal framework to guide and refine my research, to provide purposeful seeking and sensitivity to know what is relevant to build up flesh around the skeleton. The result, to date, of vulnerability as an interpersonal phenomenon in nursing relationships is still excessively broad and there are many areas where the boundaries and attributes are less clear than is desirable. The value of this research focusing on vulnerability within the home care nursing context, however, is that it is generating far more specific directions for even more focused research that, cumulatively, will develop the idea of mutual vulnerability in nursing interactions further.

REFERENCES

Aday, L. A. (1993). *At risk in America: The health and health care needs of vulnerable populations in the United States*. San Francisco, CA: Jossey-Bass.

Brown, P., & Levinson, S. C. (1987). *Politeness: Some universals in language*. Cambridge, UK: Cambridge University.

Byrd, M. E. (1995). The home visiting process in the contexts of the voluntary vs. required visit: Examples from fieldwork. *Public Health Nursing, 12*(3), 196–202.

Carroll, L. (1865). *Alice in wonderland*. New York, NY: Macmillan

Christensen, J. (1990). *Nursing partnership; A model for nursing practice, Hauora Takirua: He tauira nga kaupapa hauora*. Wellington, New Zealand: Daphne Brasell.

Ferguson, E. J. (1978). *Protecting the vulnerable adult: A perspectives on policy and program issues in adult protective services*. Ann Arbor, MI: The University of Michigan/Wayne State University.

Holtgraves, T. (1992). The linguistic realization of face management: Implications for language production and comprehension, person perception, and cross-cultural communication. Special Issue: Theoretical advances in social psychology. *Social Psychology Quarterly, 55*(2), 141–159.

Holtgraves, T., & Yang, J. N. (1990). Politeness as universal: Cross-cultural perceptions of request strategies and inferences based on their use. *Journal of Personality and Social Psychology, 59*, 719–729.

Lomax, H., & Casey, N. (1998). Recording social life: Reflexivity and video methodology. *Sociological Research Online, 3*(2). Retrieved from http://www.socresonline.org.uk/3/lomax/lomax_doc.html

Morse, J. M. (1997b). "Perfectly healthy, but dead": The myth of inter-rater reliability. *Qualitative Health Research, 7*(4), 445–447.

Morse, J. M. (2000). Exploring pragmatic utility: Concept analysis by critically appraising the Literature. In B. Rodgers & K. Knafl (Eds.), *Concept development in nursing* (pp. 333–352). Philadelphia, PA: Saunders.

Morse, J. M., & Mitcham, C. (2002). Exploring qualitatively-derived concepts: Inductive—deductive pitfalls. *International Journal of Qualitative Methods, 1*(4), 28–35. Retrieved from http://ijq.sagepub.com/content/1/4/28.short

Morse, J. M., Hupcey, J. E., Penrod, J., Spiers, J. A., Pooler, C., & Mitcham, C. (2002). Issues in validity: Behavioral concepts, their derivation and interpretation. *International Journal of Qualitative Methods, 1*(4), Article 3. Retrieved from http://ijq.sagepub.com/content/1/4/28.full.pdf+html

Morse, J. M., Hupcey, J., Mitcham, C., & Lenz, E. (1996). Concept analysis in nursing research: A critical appraisal. *Scholarly Inquiry for Nursing Practice, 10*(3), 253–277.

Spiers, J. A. (1998). The use of face work and politeness theory. *Qualitative Health Research, 8*(1), 25–47.

Spiers, J. A. (2000). New perspectives on vulnerability using emic and etic approaches. *Journal of Advanced Nursing, 31*, 715–721.

Spiers, J. A. (2002a). The interpersonal contexts of negotiating care in home care nurse–patient interactions. *Qualitative Health Research, 12*(8), 1033–1057. doi:10.1177/104973202129120430

Spiers, J. A. (2002b). The pink elephant paradox (or, avoiding the misattribution of data). *International Journal of Qualitative Methods, 1*(4), 36–44. Retrieved from http://ijq.sagepub.com/content/1/4/36.full.pdf+html

Stevens, P. E., Hall, J. M., & Meleis, A. I. (1992). Examining vulnerability of women clerical workers from five ethnic/racial groups. *Western Journal of Nursing Research, 14,* 754–774.

11

CONCEPT EVALUATION: DETERMINING APPROPRIATE STRATEGIES FOR CONCEPT DEVELOPMENT[1]

Trust, but verify.
—Ronald Reagan

Concepts do not dichotomously simply exist or not exist. Rather, scientific concepts are created and are tentatively introduced to the scientific community, and often undergo significant transformations in the process of development (Thagard, 1992), that is, of reaching consensus. Over time, with continued use and acceptance, concepts are refined, modified, and eventually reach maturity. Lay concepts emerge to accommodate new perspectives, new phenomena, new ideas, and even changing fads. As the context changes, the concepts also change and are modified. Thus, as they mature, so do the things they refer to—the class, or category to which they belong, as well as the scope to which they refer.

Similarly, concepts vary in level of maturity, ranging from immature, poorly defined, poorly understood, and ambiguous concepts, to clear, unambiguous, well-developed concepts.

When concepts are immature, two or more concepts may compete to explain the same phenomenon, or may even be the same concept but with different labels, or else be similar concepts, sharing some attributes and competing for acceptance (i.e., allied concepts). A good example of competing allied concepts in nursing is the five concepts that compete to explain receptivity and insight in the nursing assessment process: intuition, insight,

---

[1] Sections of this chapter were previously published as: Morse, Mitcham, Hupcey, and Tasón (1996) and Morse, Hupcey, Mitcham, and Lenz (1996); reprinted with permission.

inference, empathy, and compathy (see Morse, Miles, Clark, & Doberneck, 1994). Another example is in Chapter 20, in which self-transcendence and self-reformulation compete. As concepts mature and their meanings are clarified, concepts become distinct, their attributes are identified, and the boundaries become well delineated.

Think about this. Students often e-mail me to ask, "How can I validate a concept?" If concepts are neither true nor false, how can they be "validated?" Truth as a criterion has no place in determining the adequacy of concepts. The closest we get to such a criterion would be determining *adequate and appropriate for the purposes you wish to use it for*, and that is the criterion we will use in this book. If we try to validate using "truth," we must have an external criterion with which to compare it—that which is true—and many concepts do not have such criteria—and this lack does not make them less of a concept. Recall that if an external criterion is available, the concept is, by definition, a *perception*, a mental construction, an image, soft and malleable, of that particular external criterion. And, of course the *meaning* (the "external criterion") that a concept represents may be constantly changing: Concepts are malleable. They must be malleable: They emerge, develop, change, and disappear. If concepts were "true," then they would have to be static, and knowledge could no longer develop. This is a very important fact to understand, and will be on your final exam. Therefore, I prefer the Wizard of Oz's definition: "The truth is not fact or reason. The truth is just what ev'ryone agrees on" (Côté, 2005, p. 167; see also Chapter 29). Also, if the external criterion is available to "verify" the concept, researchers would then study the actual object, and not bother studying peoples' perceptions of the object; therefore, using any criterion to determine the truth or falsity of a concept is absurd, and an exercise in futility. Nevertheless, the fact that concepts are neither true nor false is contested by some authors: in fact, "truth" is considered the goal of principle-based concept analysis, named by Penrod and Hupcey (2005a).

However, concept analysis and the evaluation of concepts is not an open field in which anything goes. And for researchers interested in concepts, for nursing in general and for our students, it would be useful to examine the concept of interest, in order to determine if further work needs to be conducted in delineating or clarifying a particular concept (and if so, perhaps at the same time, identifying a topic for a dissertation). Concepts, therefore, may be assessed on an immature–mature continuum, according to their description of the thing(s) to which they refer and represent. *Concept assessment* is determined by considering adequacy of the descriptive criteria, that is, the quality of the description and its referents. We consider the richness of the descriptions of the concept and the formal or informal theory in which it is used. We consider its adequacy for the purposes for which we intend to use it. We consider its level of maturity.

DETERMINING LEVEL OF MATURITY

What is conceptual maturity? Concepts exist in various degrees of "maturity": from simply a named phenomenon, to one that is mature. Mature concepts are those that are well defined, have clear and concise attributes, delineated boundaries, and documented preconditions and outcomes. That is, we know a considerable amount about them, the contexts in which they occur have been well described, and they are ready to be used in research and applied to practice. There is consistency, agreement, and acceptance in their presentation. The consistency should (but not necessarily always) extend beyond a discipline to include other disciplines, such as theology or philosophy. This consistency is important, because concepts "maximize the coherence of theories" (van der Steen, 1993, p. 23).

Concepts must be mature before they can be presented to the scientific community and used in quantitative research. To be included in quantitative inquiry, a concept must be definable in measurable units, in a form that may be converted to measurement, or minimally, have adequate information to be able to recognize its equivalence in another study, so that an instrument or measure, already available, may be used—or if not available, be developed as demanded according to the needs of the theory.

Further, recognizing the preconditions, the outcomes, and the boundaries of the concepts permits the application of the concepts for practice. The attributes must be clearly presented and the concept defined and *in use* (Morse, Mitcham, Hupcey, & Tasón, 1996). Prior to therapeutic application to change practice outcomes, the concept must be understood—and developed—as much as possible. Once a concept is so defined, examples may easily and reliably be identified in the clinical setting. Phenomena that are, and are not, related to the concept are evident.

Although many scientific concepts refer to a less abstract phenomenon than do behavioral concepts, they also must be adequately developed before they can be tested and used in other contexts. Using the attributes, concept analysis may ultimately enable the identification of those variables relevant for measurement. Scientific concepts are usually tested within theory, using scientific methods of testing to determine proof. They are used consistently, and there is consensus for use between theoreticians, researchers, and practitioners.

Considering this progression of science, concept development is a task that must be placed early in the agenda of all research programs and is foundational, integral, and essential to all research programs. In quantitative inquiry, concept clarification must precede the development of project research design, for if a concept is not delineated and if its attributes are unknown, then it cannot be a candidate for measurement. In this case, the researcher must turn to qualitative inquiry to achieve the task of description and identification of the attributes.

If the concept of interest is assessed as mature, then the researcher can with confidence proceed directly to measurement (quantitative inquiry), the manipulation of the concept, or even directly to clinical application.

A concept developed to an intermediate state will reveal a lot of literature, some contradictory, some competing, and some with the same label, but once examined, interpretation may reveal different attributes (and therefore an allied or different concept) using the same concept label. In this case *pragmatic utility* (Morse, 2000a; Chapters 17 & 18) could be used to reveal the different dimensions of the concept.

THE PROCESS OF ASSESSING CONCEPTS

The process of assessing the maturity of concepts is a systematic process, one of first assessing the adequacy of the concept in the literature. According to that preliminary decision, the researcher can then evaluate the adequacy of the concept for the next step: If it is immature, then the research must investigate the concept in context and use qualitative inquiry to create the necessary description to develop the concept; if there is literature available, this must be analyzed for conceptual coherence, to determine if there are competing attributes and concepts within the concept label, or if the concept is ready for quantitative inquiry or theory development. Note that the goal of such inquiry is always theory development, recontextualization of the theory, and application. Concepts themselves are useful clinically, to enable communication and class or category recognition; that is, the recognition of future instances of the concept.

Selecting a Concept

When selecting a concept for assessment of its level of maturity, select one that is important to your discipline and program of research. The concept should be theoretically significant and key—that is, selected because it maximizes the coherence of theory (van der Steen, 1993, p. 23). This means that the researcher must be familiar with the literature and unable to proceed to quantitative inquiry because there is not a measure for the concept of interest. While reviewing the literature, look in other disciplines, to see if the meaning remains the same across disciplinary boundaries and how the concept is used in other contexts. Also, explore the historical development of the concept, tracing its major citations over time.

The assessment of the concepts should begin with a comprehensive review of the literature, including tracing the concept back using a citation trail, as far as possible. This broad review will enable you to see the concept in all of its usage contexts and meanings remembering, of course, that some of the very early meanings may have been since discarded.

Surveying the Literature

Surveying the literature at this point is essential. Although it is not necessary (or possible) to pull *all* the literature at this point, it is necessary to locate the major sources. This includes the publications of researchers who are presently actively researching the concept, as well as the researchers who introduced the concept. If the concept is old, more than approximately 30 years old, then it will be necessary to follow citation trails back by "hand searching" for the publications that introduced the concept. Because you may now be reaching beyond available digital copies and databases, this must be done by searching the citations listed at the end of important articles and locating those, again searching the citations listed at the end of those articles and requesting those, and so forth.

By obtaining the "classical" articles, you will be able to see how the concept originated and, if the meaning has changed over time, where and when it changed. It is also necessary to see how the concept is operationalized when it is used in research, so that any discrepancies between the original definitions and current practice will be evident.

For the current literature (i.e., within the past 30 years), locate all rich descriptions of the concept—that is, qualitative descriptive studies, and any instruments developed to measure the concept quantitatively. Both of these sources will provide important information about the nature of the attributes.

Consider the amount of literature available, both from nursing and other disciplines. If it is voluminous, look to see if the literature contains citations to one or to several definitions. Is it a cohesive field, with consistent definitions used in most studies? If so, and there is agreement—at least in the definition used—that may be one indicator of maturity.

If the definitions used are divergent and scattered into several areas or "schools of thought," this is one indicator of competing concepts and that the concept is less mature. Search the literature according to these various perceptions of the concept, and this will help you later in your investigation.

Assessing the Concept for Appropriateness

Selecting a concept may be simple or straightforward, or else rather difficult, depending on how many concept labels are competing to describe the same concept and have been used by researchers. Often, scientific concepts are rather straightforward, and these authors do tend to use the same label as the researchers who first introduced the concept. However, as noted previously, in qualitative inquiry, researchers unfortunately tend to keep the emic label for the concepts, and this may result in "theoretical congestion" (Morse, 2000b), in difficulty locating articles, and of those identified, in deciding if the concept is relevant, allied, or the same concept as the one you are interested in.

If the concept has been published under a plethora of labels, you have no choice but initially to go through the stack, carefully examining the articles for their relevance. Examine the way the author has defined the concept, and the fit of the concept to your definition of the concept. At this point, do not discard allied concepts. These concepts may share some, but not all of the attributes in your concept, for you may decide to include them in your analysis: either now, or later, when you begin model building.

Assessing the Concept for Adequacy

Next, the researcher must assess the literature by reviewing and summarizing the descriptions of the concept, using concepts of epistemological, logical, and linguistic philosophy, as well as the pragmatic principle, to identify the adequacy and appropriateness of the concept and to determine how to proceed.[1] This following set of criteria proposed in Morse, Mitcham, et al. (1996) will assist in assessing the level of maturity, and determining the subsequent steps in the course of developing the concepts.

Epistemological Principle
Concepts should be clear and distinct, that is, clearly defined, internally consistent, and well differentiated from other concepts.

Ask:

"Is the concept clearly defined and well differentiated from other concepts?"

The epistemological principle refers to assessing both the *internal structure* of the concept (the development of the definitions, attributes, boundary, preconditions, and outcomes) as well as its *external position* in relation to applied concepts and the extent to which it is independently separated from other concepts.

---

[1] Principles to evaluate the pragmatic, epistemological, linguistic, and logical dimensions of concepts were developed in 1996 (Morse, Hupcey, et al., 1996), so that researchers may then proceed with appropriate methods of concept development. Penrod and Hupcey later used these criteria, as "principle-based concept analysis" (Hupcey & Penrod, 2003; Penrod & Hupcey, 2005b) to advance concepts. However, until these strategies for advancement are developed, these principles remain as originally intended by Morse, Hupcey, et al., (1996), as criteria for *assessment of the level of maturity.*

Internal assessment

Is there a clear and commonly used definition? If a concept is poorly developed, definitions are difficult to locate, are skimpy, or inadequately describe the phenomenon. Note that development of the definitions of concepts has little to do with the age of the concept per se. Some concepts that are commonly used in everyday life (such as *privacy*), are relatively poorly defined, whereas newer scientific concepts that have been extensively used in research, such as *bonding*, are well described and researched (Morse, Mitcham, et al., 1996), and are now used in everyday life.

A concept definition obtained from the dictionary is not very useful from the perspective of concept analysis, except to ensure that everyone is talking, more or less, about the same concept. Dictionary definitions, while they may help to superficially describe the concept, are inadequate and too skimpy to be used for concept assessment (Morse, Mitcham, et al., 1996). For instance, look up lemon ("A yellow or green citrus fruit"). It does not tell you about its shape, taste, purpose, or even that it grows on the tree and costs 50 cents in the store. It tells you nothing about the nature of the lemon—indeed, without attributes the definition is not very much useful at all, and certainly not the basis to form nursing knowledge. Dictionaries do not usually list scientific definitions, and therefore should not be used as a source in concept analysis. Rather the definitions, usually obtained from qualitative inquiry, in the discipline concerned should be used.

Furthermore, dictionaries list *all* meanings of the term as it has been used or is currently used in everyday discourse, and these meanings include, from the perspective of a researcher's program of research, irrelevant usages and ambiguous usages. Including ambiguous and irrelevant definitions of the concept does not assist the researcher with the analysis of the concept for the present project, and distracts, or leads the researcher away from the task at hand. As definitions do not list the attributes of the concept, they do not facilitate identifying the conceptual attributes.

Do dictionary definitions clarify the preliminary boundaries of a concept so that it is distinct from other concepts? No, often not—and to delineate concepts is not the purpose of a dictionary definition. As noted earlier, the task of the dictionary definition is to show current use, and therefore it tolerates the ambiguities, dual meanings, and makes cross-references to other words with similar meanings.

Definitions of scientific concepts are not listed in the dictionary (unless they have been identified into the lay lexicon) but are defined in research articles or encyclopedias. For instance, scientific concepts that are well established, such as *gravity*, may be defined in the dictionary, but the definition is written in a form that is comprehensible for the lay reader; in the scientific literature, one would find a more technical definition.

Van der Steen (1993) presents five definitional rules for evaluating definitions: Definitions must be clear, not circular, and neither too broad nor too narrow; they should not include accompanying features (only the attributes), and should refer to the features that are present (rather than referring to features that are absent).

Are the attributes well described? Internally the attributes as a whole must form a strong and coherent concept, independent from allied concepts. Through the attributes, the concept must be understandable to others, that is, recognizable in the present context, in other contexts, as well as in future instances of the concept. The attributes are derived both from the rich description of the concept and from the combined cumulative meaning of the attributes.

The attributes must be clearly stated in a form that does not particularize the concept to a certain context, but rather enables generalization of many instances and forms of the concept to other contexts. Each attribute should be relatively independent of the other attributes (i.e., there is little overlap or crossover), and the attributes should be parsimoniously presented.

If it is a new concept being introduced to the scientific community, then the concept should emerge from the rich description of the context, be logically derived from the description, and be recognizable to the reader. It is the responsibility of the researcher presenting the concept to justify the selection of attributes, and to separate out the "noise," or the inconsistently present and serendipitous features inherent in the context. In qualitative inquiry, this is achieved using various techniques such as template comparison, card sorts, and constructing taxonomies. When using the literature, it is achieved by constant comparison, using large matrixes.

External assessment

Are the boundaries identified? Where the attributes are weak and coexist with the attributes of allied and competing concepts, there comes a point at which the example is no longer an instance of the concept; this is the boundary. Boundaries are not always sharply delineated—often they are "fuzzy" and messy, with weak examples of the concept present. Occasionally, two concepts will merge or intercept, changing the nature of one or both concepts, and this may be the boundary point.

It is the boundaries that make the concept an entity that is recognizable. Although we hope that the boundaries make it self-contained, concepts always coexist with other concepts in the context.

Antecedents and outcomes

Again, concepts do not occur in isolation. They occur because of patterned events within the context that "set the stage," and are linked to predictable and specified outcomes. These should be specified, demonstrated, and described in theoretical and research articles. Set conditions that lead to the concept and to predictable outcomes, suggest process and theory: indeed the most mature concepts may have reached this level.

Pragmatic Principle

Concepts should be applicable to the world or be operationalized.
 Ask:

> **"Does the concept fit with the phenomenon commonly found in your discipline? Is it useful to the discipline?"**

Pragmatists purport that if it works, we should use it. Their methods are defined by their usefulness in research and application in the research setting, and they often use approaches that combine characteristics. Therefore, the pragmatic criterion evaluates the concept's application and its usefulness to its discipline. If it is a scientific concept, has it been operationalized? Is it used in research? Is there much literature available describing or using the concept?

If the concept is a poor fit with the phenomenon it purports to describe or if it has not been well described or operationalized, then it is rated as immature. If it is considered to be a good fit with the phenomenon and is well described and operationalized, then it is considered mature.

Linguistic Principle

Concepts should be appropriate to their use in context.
 Ask:

> **"Is the concept used consistently and appropriately within the context? Is it contextualized or decontextualized?"**

This is an external criterion, in which the concept is evaluated as it performs with context and as it adequately represents the external criterion. Linguists work with a theory of grammar in which the rules and specified constraints of grammar are clear, and with a theory of "natural language" (anything represented by the grammar; Katz, 1999). It is the latter, natural language and the concepts they represent and are developed, that is of interest here. For instance, psychologists specializing in cognition and semantics explore linguistic uses of concepts, developmentally—that is, how infants learn, and how others perceive the world, classify it and is represented conceptually.

Linguists interested in concepts usually work with spoken text, in context (Osswald & Peterson, 2002; Priss, 2004). Linguistics involves the identification and inductive analysis of semantic components, phonemes, syntactical and grammatical markers that reveal classification systems, hierarchies, and taxonomies, with the verbs serving as conceptual attributes. They remove ambiguities from words, attempting to sort into which class they belong. Note—"to which *class* they belong" (not context). Stripping the concept of all features that are not common to multiple settings is the process of *decontextualization*. This process of abstraction—of removing the noise from particular contexts—is a means of obtaining generalization.

In our assessment of the adequacy of the linguistic component, we look to see if there is confusion in the use of the concept, or if it is used consistently in lay or scientific practice. If the concept is immature, it may not be included in nursing's scientific literature; if the concept is immature and if it is a lay concept, it may not appear there at all. If it is partially mature, it may be addressed in the qualitative literature, but not the quantitative, in its process of development; if it is mature, there is no confusion in meaning, and it will be integrated into nursing research and texts.

Logical Principle
Concepts should be coherently and systematically related to other concepts.
 Ask:
"Is the concept coherently and systematically related to other concepts?"
Philosophers are interested in the logical relationship between concepts, as well as the logical relationships between attributes. Philosophers rely on rules. For instance, by seeking commonalities within examples of a particular concept, they may identify that which is common to all examples, called "family resemblances" (Wittgenstein, 1999), and by comparing various forms of the concept, or concepts in which it appears, they seek "what is common," and common relationships, called "disjunction of all their common properties" (Wittgenstein, 1999, pp. 171–174). When used as an assessment criterion, we assess the concept with its external criterion, for what it represents in various situations, and how it competes with allied concepts.

 Concepts that do not meet the logical criteria do not hold their boundaries—this means that you cannot tell exactly to what the concept is referring. When theoretically integrated into other concepts they "bundle" and overlap. They compete to describe the same phenomenon. With partially mature concepts, there is confusion and ambiguity.

THE LEVEL OF MATURITY

These criteria are summarized in Table 11.1. In making a decision about the level of maturity of a concept, one should not restrict consideration of the use of the concept entirely to one's own discipline, for a mature concept should "hold" over disciplinary boundaries. Deciding on the level of maturity is an overall decision, involving all criteria.

 When we examine the structure of the concept, and compare immature or emerging concepts with mature concepts, we find that immature concepts do not have the adequate anatomy (structure) to move forward with inquiry.

Developing the Theoretical Basis of Nursing

Assessing the level of maturity of a concept is only the first step in your research program, but one that is essential. Most importantly, it tells you what the next step should be:

TABLE 11.1
Summary of Criteria for Concept Evaluation

PRINCIPLE	IMMATURE	PARTIALLY MATURE	MATURE
Epistemological Definitions differentiated?	No definitions or inadequate definitions, Competing concepts	Multiple competing definitions	Well defined No competing concepts
Pragmatical Application and usefulness to the discipline. Operationalized?	Dubious fit with phenomenon Not operationalized	Partial fit with phenomenon Partially operationalized	Fit with phenomenon Operationalized
Linguistical Used consistently and appropriately in context	Confusion Not included in social science context	Partially linked to context	No confusion Integrated into social science context
Logical Coherently and systematically related to other concepts	Does not hold its boundaries when theoretically integrated with other concepts	Beginning linkages to other concepts established	Used in theory

Source: Morse, Hupcey, Penrod, and Mitcham (2002). Reprinted with permission.

- If the concept is mature, you may move into quantitative inquiry, measurement, and modeling.
- If the concept is immature and the literature is scant, there is no description and few publications, the concept should be developed using qualitative inquiry.
- If there is considerable literature but the concept appears confusing, or competing with allied concepts, methods of meta-analysis, such as pragmatic utility, will enable concept clarification, delineation, and how the concepts should be developed.
- Once the literature is copious, clear, and consistent you may move onto quantitative inquiry and to modeling and theory development.

Students often ask me if the literature is scant—perhaps only one book or a solid article—is that adequate to move toward quantitative inquiry? Of course, it depends on the quality of the book—the depth of the description. For instance Goffman's *Stigma* (1963) is only one book, but with adequate description to conduct quantitative inquiry or modeling.

Immature Concepts: Concept Identification

When the literature about a concept is scant, the concept is probably immature. Sometimes the term appears in the literature but with little description.
Privacy is such a term, about which much policy has been developed, but
there is very little literature describing privacy, explaining the attributes,
boundaries, and so forth. Immature concepts arise from two sources:

1. Concepts may appear in the literature to be without
   description or development. This necessitates a search in the
   library or in a context using qualitative methods to identify
   and develop the concept. When one finds such a concept, it is
   important to recognize that the concept may exist, but
   perhaps you are using the wrong search term. Continue
   searching using all equivalent terms or approximations of the
   label until you are certain that the concept is unique and does
   not appear in the library.
2. *Those that emerge from data during analysis:* The concept may
   appear as a part of qualitative inquiry, as a category (or
   several related categories) that does not fit the descriptions of
   any known concepts, or be adequately encompassed in any
   known concept or concept cluster. This occurred with data
   for the trauma room that did not fit the concept of empathy,
   as it referred to the vicarious sharing of pain—a *somatic*
   empathy, or *compathy*. (We developed this concept, and it is
   discussed in Chapter 13.)

Partially Mature Concepts: Concept Delineation

Partially mature concepts have some articles that describe their use and anatomy, but are in need of delineation or further development. Perhaps authors
disagree about their context, and this leads to disagreement about their attributes and how they are presented. For instance, the concept of "insight" as
used in nursing is accounted for with terms for the ability to "sense" patient
needs: intuition, inference, emotional empathy, knowing, countertransference, compathy, and embodiment (Morse, et al., 1994). Further inquiry, first
using the literature, is essential to find out if these various concept labels are
competing for the same concept, or if there are allied concepts involved.

Partially Mature Concepts: Concept Comparison

In the case that a single concept has apparently several meanings, it is essential that the concept be compared at all levels: the definitions, the attributes,

the antecedents, and the consequences and the outcomes, to determine if more than one concept is involved. Occasionally, the differences come about in the use of the term—as in Hupcey's (1998a, 1998b) analysis of social support. In this case the scientific concept was defined correctly, but the *application* of the concept—how it was used in research—had changed from the original meaning.

Occasionally, a concept changes its meaning as it is applied in different disciplines. The difference in application molds the way the concept is used and consequently, its meaning. Thus, comparison of a concept between disciplines is sometimes helpful (see Hupcey, Penrod, Morse, & Mitcham's [2001] analysis of trust; Chapter 19).

The most important use of concept comparison is with internal comparison of a concept that appears to be cohesive, but interpretive comparison of the internal conceptual components and the assumptions surrounding the use of the concepts reveals distinct differences in the concept, for instance, a comparison of the conceptualizations of caring, conducted in 1991 (Morse, Bottorff, Neander, & Solberg, 1991; Morse, Bottorff, Anderson, O'Brien, & Solberg, 1992). Most of these studies comparing concepts were conducted using pragmatic utility (Morse, 2000a), a meta-analytic technique that was developed between 1990 and 2000, and asking interpretative questions and comparing each perspective of the concept (Pragmatic utility is discussed in Chapters 17 and 18).

Emerging Concepts: Quantitative Inquiry

Quantitative researchers are primarily interested in mature concepts: those that have established definitions, with attributes described, and the preconditions and outcomes known. Given this, they are interested in confirming the factors of concepts, concept measurement for therapeutic purposes, or in modeling two or more concepts within a theory for the purpose of testing.

The concepts used by quantitative researchers must be approaching maturity, or be already mature, for purposes of measurement. Most frequently, they find an instrument already available to measure their main concepts, or one that approximates the concept of interest, with which they may compare results of the instrument that they are developing.

Qualitatively Derived Mid-Range Theory

Qualitatively derived mid-range theory usually is the product of a single qualitative research project, or the product of a research program, or several studies on a single concept, conducted sequentially by a single researcher. Less often, they are the combined product of several investigators, working separately, but it is possible that the techniques of qualitative meta-analysis will eventually replace such methods.

Depending on the qualitative method used, there will be differences in the level of theory, the complexity of the theory, and the theoretical structure. The most frequently used method for the development of mid-range theory is grounded theory, although ethnography or even mixed-method designs may also be used.

Mature Concepts: Theory and Application

How mature must a concept be before it is used in quantitative inquiry? This is an important question that those who are struggling to understand concept analysis are often asked. But the answer depends on the researcher's intended use, the design of the study, the type of measure intended to be developed, and so forth. A researcher can see if the selected concepts are mature enough to be applied in the clinical setting, to be measured and manipulated quantitatively, and if they can identify measurement instruments or will need to construct their own. If clinicians are intending to use a qualitatively derived theory, they will be concerned about the adequacy and level of description, the "match" between the theory and their perceived clinical problem, and whether or not the form of the theory fits their patient population and their intended use (This is further addressed in Chapter 23).

REFERENCES

Côté, D. (2005). *Wicked the grimmerie*. New York, NY: Hyperion.

Goffman, E. (1963). *Stigma: Notes on a spoiled identity*. New York, NY: Simon & Schuster.

Hupcey, J. E. (1998a). Social support: Assessing conceptual coherence. *Qualitative Health Research, 8*, 304–318.

Hupcey, J. E. (1998b). Clarifying the social support theory-research linkage. *Journal of Advanced Nursing, 27*, 1231–1241.

Hupcey, J. E., & Penrod, J. (2003). Concept advancement: Enhancing inductive validity. *Research and Theory for Nursing Practice, 17*(1), 19–30.

Hupcey, J., Penrod, J., Morse, J. M., & Mitcham, C. (2001). An exploration of the advancement of the concept of trust. *Journal of Advanced Nursing, 36*(2), 282–293.

Katz, J. (1999). On the general character of semantic theory. In E. Margolis & S. Laurence (Eds.), *Concepts: Core readings* (pp. 126–149). Cambridge, MA: MIT.

Morse, J. M. (2000a). Theoretical congestion [Editorial]. *Qualitative Health Research, 10*(6), 715–716.

Morse, J. M. (2000b). Exploring pragmatic utility: Concept analysis by critically appraising the Literature. In B. Rodgers & K. Knafl (Eds.), *Concept development in nursing* (pp. 333–352). Philadelphia, PA: Saunders.

Morse, J. M., Anderson, G., Bottorff, J., Yonge, O., O'Brien, B., Solberg, S., & McIlveen, K. (1992). Exploring empathy: A conceptual fit for nursing practice? *Image: Journal of Nursing Scholarship, 24*(4), 274–280.

Morse, J. M., Bottorff, J., Anderson, G., O'Brien, B., & Solberg, S. (1992/2006). Beyond empathy. Expanding expressions of caring. *Journal of Advanced Nursing, 17,* 809–821. (Reprinted, *53*(1), 75–87)

Morse, J. M., Bottorff, J., Neander, W., & Solberg, S. (1991). Comparative analysis of the conceptualizations and theories of caring. *Image: Journal of Nursing Scholarship, 23*(2), 119–126.

Morse, J. M., Hupcey, J., Mitcham, C., & Lenz, E. (1996). Concept analysis in nursing research: A critical appraisal. *Scholarly Inquiry for Nursing Practice, 10*(3), 253–277.

Morse, J. M., Hupcey, J., Penrod, J., & Mitcham, C. (2002). Integrating concepts for the development of qualitatively-derived theory. *Research and Theory for Nursing Practice: An International Journal, 16*(1), 5–18.

Morse, J. M., Miles, M. W., Clark, D. A., & Doberneck, B. M. (1994). "Sensing" patient needs exploring concepts of nursing insight and receptivity used in nursing assessment. *Scholarly Inquiry for Nursing Practice, 8*(3), 233–254.

Morse, J. M., Mitcham, C., Hupcey, J. E., & Tasón, M. C. (1996). Criteria for concept evaluation. *Journal of Advanced Nursing, 24,* 385–390.

Osswald, R., & Petersen, W. (2002, July). Induction of classifications from linguistic data. In *Proceedings of the 15th European Conferernce, ECAI* (Vol. 2, pp. 75–84). Amsterdam, Netherlands: ISO Press.

Penrod, J., & Hupcey, J. E. (2005a). Concept advancement: Extending science through concept-driven research. *Research and Theory in Nursing Practice, 19*(3), 231–241.

Penrod, J., & Hupcey, J. E. (2005b). Enhancing methodological clarity: Principle-based concept analysis. *Journal of Advanced Nursing, 50,* 403–409.

Priss, U. (2004). *Linguistic approaches to formal concept analysis.* The first international conference on formal concept analysis. Retrieved from http://goo.gl/eMb3M5

Thagard, P. (1992). *Conceptual revolutions.* Princeton, NJ: Princeton University Press.

van der Steen, W. J. (1993). *A practical philosophy for the life sciences.* State Albany, New York: University of New York.

Wittgenstein, L. (1999). Philosophical investigation. In E. Margolis & S. Laurence (Eds.), *Concepts: Core readings* (pp. 171–174). Cambridge, MA: MIT Press.

SECTION III

EMERGING CONCEPTS

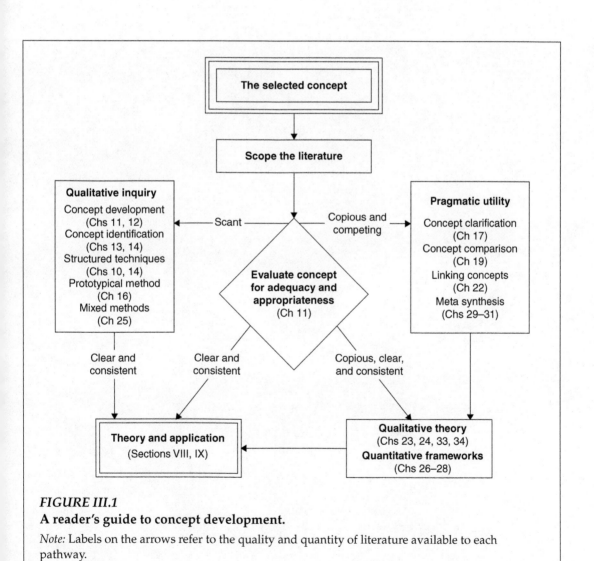

FIGURE III.1
A reader's guide to concept development.

Note: Labels on the arrows refer to the quality and quantity of literature available to each pathway.

QUALITATIVE STRATEGIES FOR CONCEPT DEVELOPMENT

> *Concepts shape how we think about the patients, families, and
> communities with whom we work. They direct our observations and
> our actions based on those observations. Important in their own
> right . . . , they merit our careful attention and nurturance.*
> —Knafl and Deatrick (2000, p. 365)

Qualitative inquiry does not take place in a vacuum, with the investigator blindly using inductive strategies and hoping that a concept or theory will eventually emerge from the data. Neither do qualitative findings emerge from a base of ignorance. Social scientists usually have a fair idea of "what is going on" in a context or with participant behavior, and that is why they ask certain questions about a topic area when developing a proposal. These researchers have developed research programs and conducted previous studies in their program of research; they are familiar with the literature, the state of the art, and in which direction the work of other investigators is moving. Researchers never start from scratch, with a "blank slate." Indeed, to obtain funding for their research, they must review their previous work, situate it in the publications of others, and make a case for the significance of the proposed study within this context.

Some qualitative researchers argue that it is important to go into a setting naive, without preconceptions, to prevent bias—a view now largely discarded (Hegelund, 2005). But there are different kinds of bias, and all of these should be considered. *Value-laden bias* is problematic in qualitative inquiry: One does not do qualitative research to prove a point, in particular, a sensitive point, such as the worth (or lack of worth) of some behavior, opinion, and so forth. And, in this light, I always advise students that doing qualitative research is not a way to resolve their own problems. You cannot be both immersed in grief for the death of your father, or upset about the injustices of your divorce, and at the same time explore the responses of participants to the death of their parents or their divorces. Having experienced the experience you are studying increases the pain, gives you reason to continue with your own suffering or indignation or whatever—but it does not necessarily add insight. In fact, your own experience is a bias that may overwhelm your data and the experiences of your participants, introducing a source of invalidity.

On the other hand, *bias*, for the purpose of *maximizing the behavior of interest*, is essential for good qualitative inquiry, and it is this bias that undergirds the principles of qualitative sampling. If we are interested in pain behaviors, we must sample from a context in which we would see participants responding to maximal pain—not slight pain or average pain; if we are interested in uncertainty, then we sample from a setting in which uncertainty is going to be evident and frequent—otherwise we will be a long time collecting data, waiting for instances of uncertainty to occur so it can be observed, or for participants to think of uncertain situations to tell us about in an interview.

TARGETING CONCEPTS USING QUALITATIVE INQUIRY

When asking questions, qualitative researchers usually are interested, and frame their questions about a lay concept. Look at any issue of the qualitative journal on your desk and read the titles. The issue of *Qualitative Health Research* (December 2015) on my desk has the following concepts addressed in the titles:

- Hemispatial neglect (after a stroke; Klinke, Zahavi, Hjaltason, Thorsteinsson, & B Jónsdóttir, 2015)
- Cultural safety (Hole et al., 2105)
- Embodiment, disclosure, and vulnerability (Harris, 2015)
- Countertransference (Thompson et al., 2015)
- Existential absence (Day & Higgins, 2015)
- Cultural sensitivity (in lifestyle behavior change; Schwingel et al., 2015)

In short, we cannot do qualitative inquiry without some level of understanding of concepts (what they are) and concept analysis (how to recognize them and their components) or concept development (how to build them). The trick is to know what type of concept you are working with, and its level of development, what will be the most appropriate methods and strategies to delineate and to develop the concept. Because concepts do not exist in a vacuum, you must also consider how to link the concept you are working with other established concepts. From there you can move to theory development.

To begin, you must be able to recognize if the concept is a lay concept or a scientific concept—or something in between. If the concept is a scientific concept, it has been developed, defined and the attributes assigned in the process of development. There is little use in using concept analysis techniques or qualitative inquiry to try to determine the meaning of a scientific concept. This information—the definition, the attributes, the boundaries, and so forth—was developed by the originator of the concept when the concept was first introduced. Usually there is no confusion about the meaning of such concepts: think of such scientific concepts as health promotion, public health, nursing, health, and so forth.

But remember that I said something about concepts that were "in between" lay and scientific—you can use the *analytic* strategies or techniques presented in this chapter or the structured techniques presented in Chapter 15, if you have some idea that concept drift has occurred, and if the concept is no longer being used as originally intended or as defined. Alternatively, you may use analytic techniques presented in this chapter if you find published descriptive studies of lay concepts that are partially developed. But once more: These qualitative techniques for concept analysis are useful only for lay concepts, and are not helpful for scientific concepts—concepts that have been initially defined and operationalized when they were created.

In this chapter, I examine the ways in which qualitative inquiry contributes to the development of established lay concepts, and qualitative strategies—analytic techniques—that may be used in defining the attributes or delineating the boundaries of developing data-derived concepts.

BUILDING LAY CONCEPTS EPISTEMOLOGICALLY

Lay concepts are not entities floating without referents. Because of their abstractness and lack of direct connection to reality, they require rich descriptions and theory to "locate" them. If this is not available for the concept, the concept is considered immature, and the first task is to create rich descriptions of the concept in its context. Nevertheless, inspecting your concept as described in Chapter 11, and by searching for a reasonable amount of literature, you will be able to make a decision about how the concept that you are focused on meets the adequacy criteria and how you should proceed with developing the concept. *If* the concept definition lacks clarity in the articles you have pulled, *if* you have to hunt for the definition, or use implied meanings, then the concept is probably immature. On the other hand, if the concept definition is clear, consistent, and consensual, it is probably mature. I use the

TABLE 12.1
Criteria for Concept Assessment

	INDICES OF CONCEPT MATURITY		
CRITERIA	IMMATURE	EMERGING	MATURE
1. Concept definition	Not defined beyond dictionary definition	Lacks clarity Competing definitions	Clear Consensual
2. Attributes	Not identified	Described, but unclear	Clearly described
3. Preconditions and outcomes	Not identified	Evident, but not examined	Described fully and demonstrated
4. Boundaries	Not identified	Murky	Delineated

Adapted from Morse, Mitcham, Hupcey, and Tasón (1996).

word "probably," because the decision for the level of concept maturity is not made on the basis of one criterion, but by assessing all four criteria discussed in Chapter 11, and again summarized in Table 12.1.

Next, check the presence and quality of the attributes and ensure they are clearly described. If they are easily located and appear adequate, the concept is mature; if they are not identified, the concept is listed as immature.

Again, this is on a continuum, and one may locate some attributes (but not all), ranking the concepts as "partially mature" or emerging.

For a mature concept, the antecedents and outcomes must be clearly identified, fully described, and demonstrated. If they are not listed and described, then the concept is considered to be immature. Finally, the boundaries should be delineated, and it should be clear to the reader what cases are examples of the concepts, which are not, and why. Remember that qualitative methods, as shown in Figure 12.1, are used for identifying concepts or for developing immature lay concepts.

QUALITATIVE METHODS FOR *DEVELOPING* CONCEPTS

Qualitative methods provide researchers with different methods for describing and interpreting reality. These methods are designed to best answer particular research questions, for identifying concepts, developing the anatomy and the physiology of concepts, and in theory building. Each method offers a different perspective, and the methods should be chosen according to what the researcher wants to accomplish. In this light, an excellent methodologist is one with a large repertoire of available methods and research strategies, so that what he or she wants or needs to know from the data, or what he or she wants to accomplish as a research goal, is possible given the methods and strategies accessible to him or her.

The various methods that may be available for concept development in qualitative inquiry are listed on Table 12.2. At a broad level, some methods are more appropriate than others for certain tasks. For instance, phenomenology is appropriate for concept identification, and I will demonstrate this in Chapter 13. However, knowledge of the structure of concepts and of other

TABLE 12.2
Qualitative Strategies to Delineate and Develop Concepts

QUALITATIVE METHOD	QUALITATIVE STRATEGIES	APPLICATION FOR CONCEPT DEVELOPMENT
Phenomenology	Phenomenological conversations	Concept identification (epistemological)
	Bracketing	Enables inductive development of concept (epistemological)
	Thematic development	Identification of conceptual attributes (linguistic and epistemological)
Ethnography	Unstructured interviews	Description of concepts from experience (linguistic and epistemological)
	Participant observation	Detailed description of behaviors (epistemological)
Ethnoscience	*Card sorts *Template comparison *Concept comparison	Identification of attributes of the concept Identification of the boundaries (logical and epistemological)
	*Construction of a taxonomy	Discerning relationship between attributes (logical)
Grounded theory	Unstructured interviews	Identification of antecedents and consequences Rich description of the concept over time (epistemological and linguistic) Identification of conceptual boundaries (logical)
	Constant comparison	Identification of attributes (epistemological) Comparison of two apparently allied concepts
	Concept comparison	(ontological) Relationship between concepts (logical)
	2x2s	

Adapted from Morse, Hupcey, Mitcham, and Lenz (1996).

research strategies is necessary if the researcher desires to continue with the development of the concept.

Ethnography and grounded theory are well suited for the development of concepts and subsequently, for the development of theory (see Table 12.2). In nursing, qualitative researchers are mainly using methods that develop concepts and theories from unstructured interviews, in particular, using ethnography and grounded theory. Less commonly, there are structured techniques for concept development, primarily from ethnoscience (a method of cognitive ethnography), which has many strategies for the delineation of attributes and identification of conceptual boundaries. These structured methods are denoted by an asterisk in Table 12.2, and will be described in Chapter 15.

Note that the *strategies* for concept development do not include the entire research method, but rather are techniques to clarify concepts or themes in the process of doing a grounded theory or ethnography. This is because these methods embody creating concepts as a part of the process when using the complete method. In fact, becoming adept in qualitative concept development will greatly assist you in the most difficult parts of qualitative analysis—theory development—when you are doing qualitative research in general.

A MAPPING METHOD TO LOCATE A CONCEPT[1]

Kristy K. Martyn

> *Getting lost is just another way of saying 'going exploring'.*
> —Chen (2009, p.156)

Concept location is a process of identifying a concept in the context in which the behavior or phenomenon of interest actually occurs. A mapping process can help locate a concept using your own experiences and qualitative research findings, and serve as a descriptive analytic tool that facilitates the communication of your ideas.

Mapping processes involve using a diagrammatic tool for a variety of purposes, including idea formation (mind mapping) and facilitating critical thinking about concepts, seeing relationships between concepts, and visually representing complex information (concept mapping; Davies, 2010). Mapping processes are limited primarily by structure (e.g., hierarchy designation) and selection of appropriate concepts and linking words. A mapping method used for concept location could also be used to address these limitations.

---

[1] Reprinted with permission of the author.

Mapping can be done individually or collaboratively (e.g., in student groups). Software programs for mapping such as *Cmap* Tools are available free from the Institute of Human and Machine Cognition (www.ihmc.us). Compendium software is available at the Compendium Institute at http://compendium.open.ac.uk/institute/download/download.htm (Davies, 2010).

The concept mapping method described by Novak and Gowin (1984) is modified to outline a mapping method for identifying concepts in context:

1. Select a behavior or phenomenon of interest. Place it at the center of the page to start a map.
2. Use personal experience and qualitatively derived concepts to develop your map of concepts in context.
   a. First, reflect on personal experiences related to the phenomenon to identify aspects relevant to nursing.
   b. Then identify behaviors, characteristics, environment/setting, and circumstances/action associated with the phenomenon and select representative one- to two-word labels for the aspects you decide are most important.
   c. Next conduct a search of qualitative research using search terms identified from your experience to identify the most important or general concepts.
   d. Then identify behaviors, characteristics, environment/setting, and circumstances/action associated with the concepts/phenomenon. Select representative one- to two-word labels for the most important concepts and related aspects.
3. Identify the environment/setting and circumstances/action that are common to the concepts derived from experience and qualitative research (in steps 2. a–d). Label context clusters.
4. Record these context cluster labels on your map.
5. For the map as a whole and within each cluster order concepts from top to bottom from most general and inclusive to the most specific; this facilitates representation of hierarchical arrangements.
6. Once the clusters of concepts have been identified and ordered on the map, links can be added to show characteristics that link concepts and clusters of concepts. Cross-links help to elaborate how concepts are interrelated.
7. Linking phrases can be added to describe the relationships among concepts.

8. The map can then be evaluated (e.g., inductively, with colleagues and mentors, and deductively using scientific concepts and the literature).
9. Finally, the map is reviewed and the concept is located in context. An example is given in Figure 12.1.

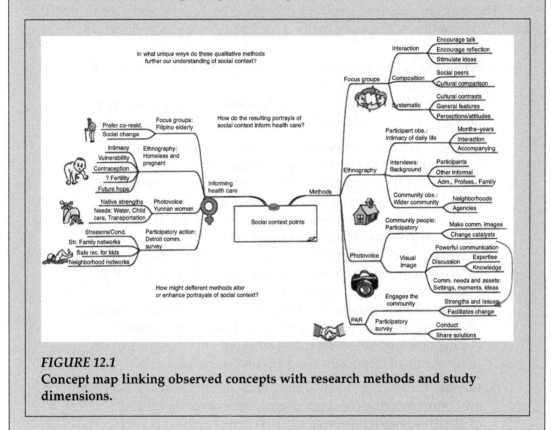

FIGURE 12.1
Concept map linking observed concepts with research methods and study dimensions.

QUALITATIVE STRATEGIES FOR *IDENTIFYING* CONCEPTS

This section consists of a compendium of qualitative strategies for delineating data to support concept development or analysis using qualitative data. As mentioned earlier, these strategies are a part of major qualitative methods, extracted from the methods to facilitate concept development, when you do not need to conduct an entire study.

Nevertheless, the principles of qualitative inquiry still hold.[2] If you are using qualitative inquiry for identifying a concept or developing an immature

---

[2] It is beyond the scope of this text to fully describe all aspects of qualitative inquiry. For further details, see Richards and Morse (2012).

concept, data adequacy and appropriateness are essential. You must attend to your sampling techniques for saturation, scoping, and must attend to obtaining variation in data. Principles of induction and abduction remain important.

Unstructured (Narrative) Interviews

Although the *form* of interviews may vary according to method, qualitative interviews share the common characteristic of inductively allowing participants the freedom to tell their stories without interruption. Participants talk about the general topic of the research project, each telling their story as they wish, and taking as long as they wish.

Rich Description

Interview data or unstructured interviews must be in the form of narrative description, preferably without prompts, guidance, corrections, or queries by the interviewer. The participants must be permitted to tell their story their own way, with the interviewer listening intently. These interviews, when transcribed, produce *rich description*—descriptions that are in-depth, detailed, and use words arising from the interviewee's own experiences. The researcher can check that the interview is indeed unadulterated by the interviewer's interruptions—simply look at the transcribed interview. One should find that the text appears in large blocks on the page, without showing lines of interjection from the interviewer. In fact, Corbin and Morse (2003) note that when the participant is immersed in interview, the interviewer no longer exists for the interviewee. The interviewee becomes totally immersed in his or her own story including the time and circumstances in which it happened. The emotions experienced at that time are reflected in their present emotion as *emotional reenactment* (Morse, 2002).

Qualitative Strategies That Facilitate Concept Development

Because the researcher is learning about the topic incrementally (as the study proceeds), the inductive approach to data collection is most unstructured during the first interviews, but it may become more targeted as the researcher begins to understand the area, to focus the study, and to strategically (or theoretically) sample for particular information.

Interpretative Coding

The nature of this particular information may come from the initial coding of categories (and sometimes themes). The category is given an *emic label*, that is, a label derived from the interviews themselves, and it may be a slang term, an already accepted and used concept label, or even simply a descriptive phrase used by some of the participants.

Building categories requires that interviewing continue until the category of interest has adequate data—a lot of data. There must be enough data to provide the researcher with many instances of all aspects of the category. Use techniques of content analysis to select the relevant blocks of text according to topic, and sort them by placing them into categories, which are initially broadly titled. Warning: Do not have many categories—at this time, up to 12 categories is ample for a data set. If you have too many categories, sorting becomes too difficult and you find yourself splitting hairs trying to decide into which category a piece of text belongs. Your analysis is slowed, and you tend to forget your category labels.

This art, the researcher's skill of analyzing and developing concepts, lies in the ability to sensitively and critically appraise data and ask analytic questions of these data. Using your library knowledge of the concept, compare the library descriptions of the concepts with those from your data. Look at your data for what it is, look at it for what it implies and implicates, and look at it for what it represents. Ask analytic questions—the why, what, and how— questions that will enable variation in responses across author perspectives, between studies, and within different contexts and topics.

Interview techniques assist in processes of sifting and sorting; comparing and contrasting. Look for things that are the same, as well as those that are different. Look for differences in use, differences in form, differences in function, and similarities in use, form, and function. And many things that you need to see are hidden behind the lines of the transcript, and behind the text, concealed in metaphor, silence, contradictions, and riddles. The trick is to ask analytic question to obtain the answers, often by inference rather than expecting the answers to be directly in the body of the text. Working in a seminar is helpful. We look for what *is there* (is said), as well as what is *not there* (is not said). We look for reported behaviors that signify the presence of the concept. We look for metaphors and other linguistic indicators.

EXAMPLE OF INTERPRETATIVE CODING: GETTING BEHIND THE DATA

Janice M. Morse, Kim Martz, and Terrie Vann-Ward

I am sitting with dissertation students, Kim and Terrie in a dissertation seminar. Kim is conducting a study exploring the experiences of families during their elderly loved ones' transition from assisted living to a nursing home; Terrie is attending to provide reflective questions and insights; and I am listening/questioning/ providing poor jokes. A digital recorder is recording, in case we need to listen again to a particularly brilliant comment.

Kim has conducted about 15 interviews and is conceptually "stuck." In this situation, Kim is asked to "tell her participants' story" as a synthesized, single storyline (without notes); others listen and ask analytic questions. This process is different from coding, as the purpose is to open Kim's data, give her study theoretical direction, and facilitate the building of concepts. The process also builds theoretical sensitivity, so the style of interviewing changes with the new insights, and theory building commences.

Let us look at the coding session. The dialogue is on the left, and the theoretical/ methodological comments are on the right.

Example 1: Initial Interpretative Coding Seminar

DIALOGUE	RATIONALE
Kim: I am really stuck with the coding. I thought about *uncertainty*, I thought about *grief*; and I thought about *powerlessness* . . .	Jan realizes that Kim is thinking theoretically about relevant concepts—a good start when moving toward abstraction.
Jan: Tell me what is going on . . .	
Kim: I see *guilt*. Lots of *guilt*. The women I interviewed yesterday—she cried the whole time . . .	Kim has chosen this concept to focus on. This is what emergence is all about.
Jan: Tell me about the guilt.	
Kim: Lots of *dysfunctional grieving*.	Kim has immediately linked guilt with grieving—but Jan does not immediately explore *dysfunctional grieving*, rather builds on the relationship between the two concepts. For the time being, *dysfunctional* (a value) is sidelined.
Jan: Oh. Let's think about that: Does guilt lead to grief? Or do they co-occur? That is, does the guilt remain, and the grief overlay it? Or, do you have to resolve the guilt in order to grieve?	First, slowly and carefully the two concepts are separated and their relationship explored.
How does one transition from guilt to grief?	These data should be in the story interviews, but may have to be teased out.
How do you distinguish between guilt and grief?	
Are there different types of guilt?	
Kim: Oh. [Mulling these thoughts over.]	Leave time in the discussion for "conceptual whirling"—a cognitive state, common in analysts.

Jan: How is guilt resolved? Don't look in the literature; look in your data.

A common mistake is to be led by the literature, not one's data. Your analysis is about analyzing the data—at this point stay there. This is the only way your study can eventually add to the literature.

Kim: (They say) talking about it is cathartic. They say, *"I am sad, but I can move on."*

Yes—this response to unstructured interviewing is well documented BUT here we are analyzing the interviews—take the student to that space.

But others say:

"My parents had me and took care of me. But who says I have to take care of them when they are older? They had me by choice—I don't have the choice."

Jan: Great. Now name that kind of argument/justification.

Name the content—do not label the person.

Terrie: "Failed" or "rejected reciprocity?"

Keep all suggestions on the table, but do not close the discussion.

Jan: Mmmm. Close.

Kim: "Unspoken," "unfulfilled reciprocity?"

Critique all suggestions.

Jan: The problem is, it *can't be met.* That is important. It is an "unspoken reciprocity that *is not met.*" It is the "not met" part that causes guilt.
Think of a better label—then we will be doing real science.

Keep looking at all of the characteristics. The label MUST be inclusive.

Kim: The literature uses "family obligation." How about "unfulfilled family obligation?"

This is exactly why qualitative researchers must be theoretically literature smart.

Jan: That still does not capture it head on—so our label is better.

Use data comparatively.

Go back and see what they all say, and use your conceptual scalpel.

You need a rich, dense data set.

Remember: you are analyzing the guilt; the feelings that underlie guilt; the causes of guilt.

Keep focused.

Look at their expectations of themselves; of their mother, their husband, their kids. Expectations of their friends; from work, church, community, and society at large.

Use different contexts.
Different roles.
Consider antecedents.
Scope data.

Look in your data for different forms or types of guilt that accompany different situations. Look at the families reported behaviors and see if those provide clues about managing guilt. Make a lot of notes.

Sort data.

Identify the types.

Kim: Remember the son who was in a different city, yet he micromanaged his mother's care over the phone?

Discuss variation.

Terrie: Oh yes—too guilty to step away.

Identify characteristics that differentiate types

Kim: Jan, by "go back" do you want me to reinterview the ones I have done?

Yes—as new questions arise. You already have relations ships with those participants—do not close at the end of the first interview.

Jan: Look first in your data with these new eyes. When you do a new interview, continue the interview—do not interrupt in the middle. At the end of the interview, take the participant back to that point, and ask direct questions: Say: *"I am really trying to get handle on how it feels to leave your mother in nursing home. You told me you felt terrible—tell me. . ."*

Loop the interview back to the "rich points" to obtain additional data.

Ask: *"You said you felt guilty. Tell me. . ."*

Ask: *"You talked with other families in the nursing home—was it like this for them also?"* Use shadowed data (Morse, 2001). Sort. List the characteristics. At this point, try and get stories from all of the families. If you do not have the information in your interviews, call them back.

Shadowed data is asking your participant to report on others who felt or did not feel this way.

Compare/contrast.

Look at your nurses' data and incorporate those perspectives.

Once you have started to identify the characteristics of guilt and its interaction with grief, the types of grief, and answered the questions listed earlier, then look in the literature, and see if you have something new. But at this point, build the concepts and analyze as much as possible, before you go back to the literature.

Once you have developed your concepts THEN go back to the literature.

Link to the literature.

The concept of guilt you develop may or may not be the central theme in your emerging theory—you are in the driver's seat, so you decide on the direction our study takes. But today, guilt and its relation to the families' behavior, and to grieving, seems to be an important piece of the puzzle.

Remember the AIM of your study—do not get lost, unless you have to—really MUST—reconceptualize your entire study.

Jan: Super. Build me a table that will enlighten us next week. And write! Write this piece now. And diagram. This will be a very important study, Kim.

Always write as you go. Tables clarify. Diagrams illustrate.

Of course, at this preliminary phase when abstraction and interpretation are starting, the analysis is not "written in stone." It can, and should be, modified and developed further.

Issues With Data Adequacy

How do you know when you have enough data? You must have enough data to be *certain*. During the process of analysis, as questions arise and as you ask analytic questions of your data, you must be able to answer questions adequately and confidently, recognizing the variation within the answers: "Some people do this, and some do that," and the content for each behavior. Qualitative researchers talk of saturation, a concept that is often operationalized, as you are "not hearing anything new in your interviews." But it is one of the most misunderstood concepts (Morse, 1995), with many researchers thinking it means that the data are replicating. A better indicator of saturation was used by Margret Mead: that of *boredom*. Keep interviewing until you have heard it all, in all of its forms, and contexts.

Can a single piece of text be placed into two categories? This is possible, but make a note on the piece of text with the name of the two categories into which it has been sorted. Make certain that these two categories are quite different, and that you do not have two categories representing the same topic.

Once data have been sorted into broad, first-level categories, you will notice that the categories contain lots of examples, perhaps about more than one topic. Then sort the category again, into subcategories. This second-level sort is an internal analysis of the category, and as coding continues, these subcategories may become categories in their own right. Alternatively, they may become attributes, they may be a part of another category and combined with those data, or they may be "dross"—contextual data that is not a part of the category or the concepts, but particular to the context. In the last case, these data are set aside in case, in the future, they gain relevance and are brought back into the analysis.

Digging Deeper Into Data

Digging deeper into the data is not searching for commonalities in the entire data set, again looking for commonalities, variation, and differences. Look at each incident in context and look at groups of incidents. Most important is the attitude of the investigator—which should be one of skepticism. Convince yourself first, build the evidence, and then convince others. This is the most important strategy for maintaining validity, accuracy, and a good night's sleep.

Example 2: Digging Deeper

Back to Kim and her discovery of "guilt" in her interviews. Now she begins looking at her category guilt in the context to the entire data set. From Jan's e-mail to Kim, you can see it is a process of asking analytic questions of the entire data set:

1. Was anyone not guilty? Why? What were those circumstances?
2. *Feeling guilty* is an admission of something not very nice about themselves. At what part of the interview did they tell you (e.g., was it when trust was established)?
3. Are they telling you they felt guilty without using the g-word?
4. What are the behavioral indicators of guilt? Were those reported?
5. Again, if they were not guilty—why not? And how do you know?

Question for you:

Are you on a "witch hunt?" Where is the inductive balance when looking at guilt, and what would (Carl) Popper say about this?

This *witch-hunt* question is for you—to make certain you are SURE about your conclusions and not just cognitively agreeing because it is an easy or obvious category. You can be sure that someone on the (examining) committee will ask you this question, and you have to have your answer ready.

Answer the question with evidence:

1. Line up the characteristics of guilt that you see. List the quotes. List the behaviors. Answer all of the analytic questions.
2. Identify its absence. The reason for its absence.

In other words: Work on guilt

Hold out against guilt until you convince yourself. By this I mean do not accept guilt easily as a category. Work to *not* convince yourself.

BTW: I think you have found the core variable, and conjectures may be: the more disruptive the move, the greater the guilt; the more unexpected the move, the greater the guilt; the more unsettled the resident, the greater the guilt; and look at where the resident's move is from (is it from the daughter's home?) and how that affects the guilt.

Now don't forget the *call back* interviews for additional data.

Think about:

- Are there different types and manifestations of guilt?
- How does feeling guilty affect the interactions/relationships with staff?

Note to Kim: Get busy . . . the great secret is you saturate by asking analytic questions of the data, not by word search for "guilt"; not by coding, and categorizing also has its limitations.

Is a category a concept? The answer is, "maybe." A category is a concept if data are so consistent that you cannot sort the category into subcategories, and move directly into identifying its attributes. However, there is a warning: when following other qualitative texts, look carefully to see how the author is using the term. For instance, Glaser (1978) uses the terms *category* and *concept* interchangeably, and uses the term "concept" very loosely: He does not concern himself with the internal structure of concepts, as we do.

If data within the category is copious, these data may be sorted into *types*. In Kim's case this would be types of guilt, according to the causes (antecedents) and manifestations (reported behaviors) of guilt.

Positioning the Category

At this point your initial category must be "inspected" for its completeness as a concept. As you continue with your analysis and sort the data in your categories, you may find that:

1. The category is adequate to serve as a concept. The category contains adequate appropriate data for thick description of the concept, content recurs as several similar examples, (although not exactly the same), replicates, and is saturated. In this case, further content analysis reveals the attributes. These attributes are then also succinctly labeled.
2. If some of the data in the category appear to be a part of another category, those data should be combined with the second category before analysis continues; or
3. If the category is too broad in scope, it should be further subdivided into two or more subcategories, and data collection continues in order to saturate each component. These data eventually become two or more concepts. Each of these categories should be saturated before further internal analysis to identify the attributes of each is continued.

Analysis continues to identify the concept boundaries by asking: "Is this case a member of this category?" Look for the presence or absence of the attributes in the new case. All must be present for the new case to be a member of the class. Finding many examples that have only some of the attributes, or which are not a member of the class, provides understanding about the position of the boundaries.

Transforming Categories to Concepts

Next, check the emic (descriptive) label you have given each category, and because your category is about to be transformed into a concept, label it with an appropriate noun, and give it a very tight definition.

The next step is most important: Check social science indexes and bibliographies for closely resembling concepts. Is your concept identical, similar, or different? How is it the same and how is it different? Do you really have something unique, or is it a different *type* of the other concept?

If you decide that you have developed something new, by comparing the literature and by continuing to explore your data, tidy your concept. Ensure the boundaries are clear, definitions are tight; attributes are will described and labeled. Can you identify antecedents and outcomes?

Determining the Relationship Between Categories

Our concepts, which are supposed to be relatively static, have precursors and outcomes. And our concepts themselves do not occur all at once, but are ordered. Some concepts occur before others; some things are results of previous actions; some co-occur. Once solid concepts have been developed, list your concepts and the attributes of each on sticky labels. Place these onto a table in order—by relationship, temporal, or hierarchal. Ask yourself:

- Which concepts are closely associated?
- Can they be ordered? Which come before another?
- Do any encompass lower level ones?
- Do some cluster?
- Are some precursors? Outcomes?
- Do some contain processes that go right though the data?
- Do some parallel others? Transect? Split? Or merge?
- Do some link by sharing attributes?

This process requires much thought, discussion, and, often, returning to the data to find exemplars and exceptions. You are looking at your data now, from a distance, thinking of groups, sets, and types of participants and identifying patterns. And it is this—the view-from-afar-while-considering-exceptions—that makes for fine mid-range theory.

Concepts Built From Themes?

Themes differ structurally from categories, in that rather than being segmented as topics in blocks of text, they run right through the data. When analyzing themes, researchers are working much more interpretatively than when working with content analysis to develop categories. Relevant data are often obscured by inferences, metaphors, by oblique references, and even by omission. Therefore, to use thematic analysis for concept development, data may be incomplete and unclear, so that, although not impossible, identifying and defining attributes is a much more difficult task than using content analysis. Why hit a nail with the heel of your shoe when a hammer is available?

Other Techniques

Can you build a concept from data other than rich description? Perhaps.

Observation

Recall that we have defined a concept as a collection of *behaviors*—which means that concepts may often be seen. Furthermore, while we are observing, particularly if we are using videotape, participants may accompany or supplement the behaviors by conversing, and these ongoing conversations may provide additional data for concept development.

One such example is the concept of *talking through*. When a patient is in severe pain and is distraught, as in during resuscitation in the emergency room (ER), the nurse may lean over the patient, hold his or her gaze, en face, use palmer touch, and speak to the patient to help them "hold on." The nurse's speech is a particular style and intonation: it is immediately responsive to the patient's cries; it is soothing ("there, there"), using a special register documented as the *Comfort Talk Register* (Morse & Proctor, 1998; Proctor, Morse, & Khonsari, 1996).

Semi-structured Interviews

Semi-structured interviews do not provide as in-depth, rich data as unstructured interviews (McIntosh & Morse, 2015). The semi-structured (open-ended) questions provide a frame that guides the conversation and encapsulates the topic so that the data obtained are confined to what the researcher wants to know—thus also restricting induction. Categories are usually developed from single items in the questionnaire, and because data are restricted to an open-ended item response, data are thinner than with unstructured interview data, so that a larger sample is essential. Recognizing these limitations, the semi-structured interview data may be used for concept development, but cautiously, and it is not usually recognized as a stand-alone data source.

ANALYTIC STRATEGIES FOR IDENTIFYING ATTRIBUTES

Identifying attributes is a process of sorting the interview data in the category into "dimensions" that, as a set, reveal the nature of the concept. After they are initially developed, they are then decontextualized, defined, and the attribute label written in a clear and succinct form. This strategy allows for the detailed descriptions to be parsimoniously transformed into a decontextualized and abstract statement, which may be applied to other contexts (Table 12.3). In this way, generalization is achieved.

TABLE 12.3
From Description to Identifying Attributes: The Example of Enduring

DESCRIPTION FROM CATEGORY	DEFINITION	ATTRIBUTE
When learning their diagnosis, fear may "grip at the heart." These people instinctively suppress their emotions so that they may remain in control, until the diagnosis becomes real, and they may think what to do and who to tell, when and where and how. Enduring requires deliberate effort and focus to keep going, to do what is required to get through each day, and to bear whatever must be endured.	Deliberately suppress the emotions of despair, grief, or terror or panic.	1. Maintain control of self
They hope to get through the next hour—or sometimes only the next minute—unable to comprehend what must be done in a whole day. For instance, trauma victims narrow their perception by focusing on breathing in and breathing out in an attempt to maintain control; burn victims in the intensive care unit by watching the hands of the clock move or counting the tiles of the roof or the number of treatments. Those bereaving take "one step at a time." All state that they cannot see the big picture, focusing on getting through the minute, the next hour, or the day.	Individuals are present-focused, concentrating on what is happening now and unable to think of their past or contemplate their future. They feel overwhelmed and are unable to consider several tasks at once, focusing on one small thing at a time. Cognitively, individuals put whatever is being endured deliberately to the "back of their mind." They may refuse to let thoughts that may cause the suffering enter their consciousness. They work hard, focusing intensely and concentrating on work, or special tasks they have set themselves.	2. Live in the present moment
Afraid they "will not be able to stop," they resist sympathetic or empathetic interactions, avoiding those who may offer condolences, as such responses "break through" the stoicism of enduring.	Those who are enduring resist crying, and report they are afraid to cry. They avoid and resist acknowledgments from others of the event they are suffering.	3. Remove oneself from the situation

(continued)

TABLE 12.3
From Description to Identifying Attributes: The Example of Enduring (*continued*)

DESCRIPTION FROM CATEGORY	DEFINITION	ATTRIBUTE
Afraid if they are emotionally suffering, that they will not be there to do what needs to be done, and metaphorically afraid they will "break down" and they would not be there for others.	They remove themselves from situations where they must be in contact with others.	4. Aware of the danger or consequences of emotional disintegration
The effort to suppress emotion gives their faces a blank appearance. Facial muscles lack tone and shape. Their lips and mouths move only slightly during speech, their eyes are unfocused and rarely blink, and their gaze is centered in the distance, away from the interviewer.	They "shut down" emotionally and behaviorally, and assume an enduring facial expression, stance, and gait, assuming the enduring appearance.	5. Shut down emotionally and behaviorally

Adapted from Morse (2011).

Sorting: Categorization of Attributes

The first step is sorting the data into categories. These data provide in-depth descriptions of numerous examples of similar events and circumstances, and the emotional and behavioral responses of many participants. Initially, in this example, the category name is "enduring," and all data pertaining to enduring responses are placed in this category. Once these data become dense, the researcher may develop a definition for the category, and decide if the label—in this case "enduring"—remains or is changed to fit with concept labels used in previously published studies.

Eventually, as the study progresses, the researcher begins to recognize that there are different parts or components to the enduring response. Data are now copious and appear to contain several incidences of each emerging subcategory, and the category is then opened to divide into subcategories.

The process of sorting into subcategories is the same as sorting data into the initial categories: Place data that are alike into separate categories. This is usually obvious, but on occasions, it may be necessary to work interpretatively and tentatively ("I think the person means . . ."). Each of these subcategories is then placed into a different file, and the subcategories named and defined. Considering that some of the subcategories may be "misplaced" within the concept, check your total database to ensure that the subcategories are actually a part of the main emerging concept and are not a part of another category, and therefore should not be placed within another concept and set of subconcepts or be treated as a category in its own right. Also, keep in the back of your mind that concepts may link, and that this linkage occurs through the attributes. Ask yourself: Does this subconcept resemble any other subconcepts in other groupings?

It is these "subcategories" or "subconcepts" that form the attributes of the concept. From these data, each subconcept is then described, definitions developed, and the attribute labeled.

This process is illustrated in Table 12.3.

Locating the Boundaries
Not all of your data will be a part of the concept that you have identified. Some of these data will have been sorted into different categories; others will have been considered to be irrelevant when you were coding (and this we call *dross*—do not discard these supposedly unwanted pieces of data, for you may find that you need them later, when you have gained more insight).

The key to locating the concept boundary is to ask what is *not* an example of the case that you are interested. Clearly, the further removed the example that is not a case of your concept, the easier it to see. In reality recall, concepts overlap and the borders are not always clear. When they overlap and share attributes, and have wide fuzzy boundaries, it is that point that decision must be made if this is or is not an example of your concept. At the boundaries the attributes become weak and there are other attributes from allied concepts muddying the waters, so that analysis of these borderline cases should not be attempted until you have the attributes of the concept clearly identified, so that you, at least, know what you are looking for.

Attribute Labels
The *form* of the attribute labels is so important that they deserve a special section in this chapter.

The attribute labels must be:

- Highly pertinent: They must encapsulate the essence of the described category
- Succinct: They must be short, tight
- Descriptive: As a set, represent the meaning of the concept
- As a set, complete: Together the attributes must comprehensively describe the concept, differentiating it from allied concepts

Processes of Decontextualizing
This process of moving from data to description to attribute, is one of deliberately decontextualizing. The researcher is systematically removing

features pertaining to the context, and leaving the primary structure of the concept intact. This process of abstraction is important, for the features pertaining to the context do not belong to the concept per se, but may be considered "noise," or dross—extraneous data. If we maintain these contextual data, then we have difficulty seeing the actual concept in itself—it cloaks or hides the concept. More importantly, we will not see those local features in other instances of the concepts (remember they are attached to the immediate situation). Thus, maintaining that "noise" (i.e., conceptual data) inhibits the application of the concept to other situations; that is, it prevents abstraction and generalization. Maintaining only the essential features of the attributes is a critical step toward tightening the concepts and eventually to theory construction.

QUALITATIVE RESEARCH STRATEGIES FOR EXPANDING CONCEPTS

Qualitative research methods are rarely implemented without a concept focus. The exceptions are a researcher who wants to find out "what is going on" in a particular setting and a researcher who is interested in a particular phenomenon (not a concept). The majority of researchers are interested in "something"—that is, a concept at some level of development. Of course, concepts in the research setting do not occur in isolation—but rather occur with other concepts that influence the target concept's "performance." No matter how hard we try, the second concept continues to interfere whenever we speak of our first concept. Therefore, to understand the target concept, we have to also document, or at least discuss, the second concept. It may not be an allied concept in the sense that it is closely associated with the attributes, and competing with the target concept, but that it co-occurs, and by including both concepts in our findings, we add to our understanding of the target concept in which we have primary interest.

The Dependence of Privacy on Types of Interpersonal Relations

The study discussed here is an example of the study of privacy (Applegate & Morse, 1994). Mary Applegate was extraordinarily interested in *privacy*, particularly privacy maintenance for clients residing in nursing homes. At that time, there was little research on the concept of privacy, and most of the literature in nursing consisted of educational articles on why it was important to respect privacy and strategies for doing so. Some articles existed in the philosophy literature, but not many. Thus, privacy was lay concept, immature, and ideally suited for development using qualitative methods.

But how should the student approach the problem? Applegate could easily make a checklist of all instances of privacy violations, but if she then went and used this list as an observational tool, at the end of her fieldwork she would have nothing more than a frequency count of all of the instances of privacy violation that she had observed. It would not even be a complete list, for many would occur when she was not there, or not looking.

So Applegate's study was designed as an ethnography, and it was agreed that every day she would observe in the nursing home and return to the office at the end of the day to report her findings. She reported many things that were typical of nursing homes. She said, "Many residents do not even know other's names, even though they eat together every day."

"Go and find out who knows whose names," she was told. And so she did.

"Often," she said, "the men treat one another as friends, but other times it seems they don't care about each other. For instance, today one man dashed down the hallway with his walker and sent everyone flying. Yet yesterday a man fell and his room and his roommate spent the day with him to make certain he was all right."

She said: "The men don't talk to one another—but Thursday night is pub night. They gather for a beer and the room sounds like a pub!"

She noted: "Nurses would ignore some residents. Even when residents were waiting at the nursing stations, they refused to make eye contact with them." The discounted residents' reports: One resident reported a blocked toilet; so to confirm his report, the nurse went and flushed the toilet, and it flowed onto the floor. "Doesn't she think I can tell when a toilet is flushed!" said the angry resident. At other times nurses were caring and gave special privileges—one resident was give lemon juice in his water glass at night. Once, they went on a bus trip, and two residents who normally shared a room, had a wonderful time. But on return, the noncommunications returned. One resident even sent a note to his roommate, thanking him for the nice holiday.

And, of course, there were data on privacy violations: of men having wet trousers changed in the residents' lounge in full view of others; of staff sharing personal stories of residents during reports that had little to do with care; of some residents receiving special privileges and others being ignored. And patients occasionally treated staff poorly, as one would order a servant about.

As the field notes accumulated, it seemed that Mary was recording how the residents were being treated, and how they treated each other. Reflecting on these data, the content of these data involved interpersonal relationships between residents, between residents and staff, between staff and residents, and from staff member to staff member. It was clear that we could not separate, or decontextualize privacy from interpersonal relationships. We created a chart of the direction of the interaction by type of relationship: friend, stranger, and as an object, and sorted all of the privacy violations, according to the type of relationship between the persons when the violations occurred.

TABLE 12.4

Patterns of Interaction in a Long-Term Care Setting: Relationship to Privacy

	PATTERNS OF INTERACTION		
COMMUNICATION ROUTE	**AS A FRIEND**	**AS A STRANGER**	**AS AN OBJECT**
Resident to resident	*Caring behaviors* • Anticipated needs of others • Offered assistance or advocacy *Relationship* • Friendship warmth, sharing humor, reciprocal	• Lacked involvement • Formal superficial, cordial conversations trite	• Ignored each other • No relationship courtesies ignored no acknowledgment of frailties
Resident to staff	*Appreciation of the person* • Acknowledged in the total social context • Mutual respect • Sharing of personal information	• Acknowledged in caregiving role • Care rewarded or punished • Employee–employer relationship	• Acknowledged in task context • Manipulation • Master/servant relationship
Staff to resident	*Appreciation of the social context of the resident* • "Care of the person" • Bends rules/ routines to allow for individual preferences • Care is past, present, and future-oriented.	*Interaction context is role-based* • "Care of the resident" • Bends rules/routines to accomplish care activities • Care is present and future-oriented • Distant, professional	*Interaction context is task-based* • "Completion of the task" • Unit routine is enforced • Care is present-oriented • Invisible
Staff to staff	*Interactions about residents aimed at a personalized plan of care* • Mutual goal setting between resident and staff • Residents' confidences are respected • Shared stories reveal the personhood of the resident	*Interactions about residents aimed at staff control over the plan of care* • Resident input into the plan of care controlled • Residents' confidences are shared by the staff • Stories told for interest	*Interactions aimed at organizing and completing tasks efficiently/expediently* • Shared stories criticize, demean, or ridicule the resident

(continued)

TABLE 12.4
Patterns of Interaction in a Long-Term Care Setting: Relationship to Privacy (continued)

COMMUNICATION ROUTE	PATTERNS OF INTERACTION		
	AS A FRIEND	AS A STRANGER	AS AN OBJECT
Relationship to privacy	*Privacy is respected*	*Social norms of privacy are acknowledged*	*Privacy is violated*
	• Personal respect is conveyed naturally (inherent in relationship) • Function of relationship	• Compliance with ascribed rules of privacy	• Privacy not considered necessary or important

Source: Applegate and Morse (1994). Reprinted with permission.

To our excitement, these data were surprisingly consistent: All of the privacy violations occurred when the persons were being treated *as if* they were an object. These data are presented in Table 12.4.

Once into data collection and analysis it becomes clear that one cannot focus on the single concept as originally intended: The first concept is intractably intertwined with another allied concept, and only by exploring *both* concepts will the study make sense. This is because there is an astonishingly clear relationship between interaction pattern and privacy maintenance or violation. When people treated one another as friends or as strangers, privacy norms were respected; all of the violations, either staff to staff, staff to resident, resident to staff, or resident to resident, occurred when they were treating one another as an object.

This is amazingly important for us. First, you will notice that Applegate commenced her study with a definition, but not with an analysis of the concept of privacy. Yet it seems, from the analysis, that type of relationship is an attribute or privacy. In order for privacy to be respected, the relationship must be *as a person* (a friend or a stranger), and for privacy violations to occur, the individual must be perceived *as an object* and *must be treated as an object*. Are there one concept or two? If two, are they codependent?

My second point is just as important: *Relationship* is an attribute of privacy? But, you may argue, relationship is a concept. How can it possibly be an attribute? Can we flip it around the other way: Is respect for privacy an attribute if we consider relationship as a concept?

This is a very significant point. Lay theories and concepts are not concrete; are not fixed. You are in the driver's seat. You may manipulate, organize, display attributes, concept theories, as *demanded by your data, by reality* and *by your common sense.* And yes your work is sometime constrained by others, and must somehow fit in with what has been published before. At the same time you must be true to your data and how you have conceptualized it. Relationship may be a concept in some studies, or it may be an attribute in your study on privacy. How we conceptualize a concept depends on how it will be used in your theory. It is not fixed: Its positions and use may change from study to study.

Is this true for scientific concepts? No—recall scientific concepts are fixed, defined concretely, and must be used the way the developer intended. Any modification must be done carefully, for solid reasons, and preferably with consultation with the original developer.

Abstraction and Generalization

In Table 12.4, notice how the categories have been removed from the context of the nursing home. The process of decontextualization removes the concept from the setting to a level of abstraction, so it can be reapplied to other settings, provided these setting have the same major main characteristics.

What are these characteristics in this case? The nursing home could be considered a total institution, in which the residents are in a somewhat ambiguous situation. There is a status differential between the carers and the cared for. The residents are being cared *for*; they *need* this care; independence is *limited*. The privacy violations are one way—usually from the caregiver to the one being cared for. Sometimes the privacy violations are essential—the caregivers need to access a purse for the patient's identification, or need to attend to intimate parts of the body. But whether the violation is physical, property-related, or informational, it could possibly be justified as a part of the caregiving role.

We can think of other situations in which these are a total institution, status differential, and one group dependent on the other: a prison, a boarding school, and a hospital unit. In each of these situations, the framework of the concept of privacy and the differing relationship and privacy violation, holds. We do not look for, as in quantitative inquiry, similarities between demographic characteristics in the two populations. Yet our findings are generalizable.

TO DO 12.1. IDENTIFYING CO-OCCURRING CONCEPTS

Read the article: Personal privacy and interaction patterns in a nursing home (Applegate & Morse, 1994).

Now, explore the data as it is presented. What other concepts are described? Are those concepts "restricted" to certain interaction types? Are they significant to privacy, or are they just coincidental in the study?

SUMMARY

This chapter examined the process of developing concepts from transcribed interviews, following the process of categorizing, forming subcategories, defining and naming concepts, and forming and naming attributes was examined. The next chapter provides two working examples: identifying a concept from a phenomenological study, and the development of a concept over time, using multiple studies to develop the concept of "preserving self."

TO DO 12.2. IDENTIFYING CONCEPTS FROM TEXTUAL DATA

Examine the following data, which have been formed into a category: "Responding to biopsy for possible breast cancer."

1. Code, using highlighters and making notes in the margin.
2. Identify a category.
3. Sort all relevant data into the category.
4. Develop a definition and label the category.
5. Inspect your category—are they subcategories? If so, sort again, and label the subcategories.
6. Identify and name the attributes of your concept.
7. Have you developed a concept? Is it a new category or does it resemble one "in use?"

DATA

PARTICIPANT #1

I: What was that waiting like for you?
S: I didn't really, I didn't, it, it didn't sit on my mind because the, the first one was, they considered it, it was just a precaution. And um . . . I probably just put it out of mind. I didn't dwell on it. But I guess that's what I'm saying. Now who knows, if, if they had said well it looks like it, I can't say what, what would have happened to me. Uh . . . I think it would have been except, I think I would have had my cry. And then after that, you have, you know, you have, you know, you have to . . . I guess that my opinion is you, that you're, you've got it. There's not much you're going to do about it. You know uh . . . screaming and yelling or, or whatever is not going to do anything. My husband's of the same attitude too.

And um . . . it's like when I became diabetic. What can I do? There's, there's worse than being a diabetic. But you just have to go on and, and do it. If I was dying, I don't know how I would handle that. I could probably sit and cry all of, you know, I don't know.

It's, it's, it's so hard to say. I don't know. But I did not. And maybe, maybe that's not good on my part either not to dwell on it.

PARTICIPANT #2

I found out that I had cancer. And I mean, from, from that time on, I'm sure between the diagnosis and the first stage of my surgery, that is a biopsy um, I um . . . I had like a knot in my stomach I am sure for a good month and that was a daily thing for me. And uh, but I um, I just took one step at a time because that's the way it had to be. And I went to the motions of different surgeries and um . . . it was interesting. Um . . . I had surgery. I had my diagnosis confirmed as pre-cancerous at the time.

PARTICIPANT #3

It weighs on you somewhere in the back of my mind. And, and then when uh . . . when she phoned and said it was just a confirmation of what she'd previously said and that for now, I was okay.

PARTICIPANT #4

S: Well, it's not a, a good thought. I, I wasn't, I don't think—I didn't get upset. I've got upset on probably minor, more minor things than that. I think my feeling came home is there's not much I can do about it. It's there uh . . . you know, I was more upset with the doctor in his attitude for some—we've never had any real major problems that we had to have you know, a doctor really worry about something. And my opinion with some doctors is sometimes they panic. And then when you panic, then they come out with well why did you worry about it? You know, they, they, they kind of create the panic. But um . . . I didn't, I guess maybe, back in my mind, I thought there is no history. And, and based on my mom having cysts out oh you know like, probably 40 years ago. And she's had a number of them out. And um, I don't think I overly panicked. But mind you, when I went back this last time and she felt the lump, it was a little scary thinking that well maybe it was um . . . but I didn't, I wasn't, when I went there, I wasn't upset or anything like that.

My main worry, in some cases, is if it was cancer is my husband has MS. And he um . . . he's not really bad. He, he can walk not a great distance. He can drive. But you know, we don't go out. So he would be, he could manage but not totally on his own. So that was more my fear of, you know, what would happen to him.

I: So you were just . . .
S: If something happened like that.
I: Okay. There was, fear was entering into it.

PARTICIPANT #5

But anyway, it was just once, uh, I, when it comes to something like this, I just always say I have to deal with this one step at a time. I can't sort of look at the whole picture. I, I seem to function better when I do things in small increments

PARTICIPANT #6

S: I wouldn't have this, maybe some of the support that I needed if, if something happens. Like I don't have a husband to take me to the doctor or, or you know, what things like that. Uh . . . but uh . . . no, I have to say I really, that's why I felt I wasn't really good for this thing because I did not panic. And, and uh, and I did not discuss it with anybody. The only other person that knows other than my husband is my daughter. I did not tell my son until, unless we had decided we would just not say anything.
If there was something there, we would, we would say. And then in that case, I would have to inform my sisters and my mother. But to this day, they know nothing.

PARTICIPANT #7

It's that waiting and waiting and waiting and waiting and wondering and wondering and wondering if I have cancer. Um, what happened to me. So. That was kinda tough. . . . You just go day to day to day. And, it's not, it's not that I was, I wasn't crying, I wasn't emotional, I wasn't depressed . . . I kept telling myself, "okay, one more day." And that's tough. Not knowing.

PARTICIPANT #8

What helped me was the fact that he was so upset I knew I had to have that strength, even at night when you know you could cry, I didn't. I thought I've gotta be strong I have to keep that strength cause I thought of it in the future—in the future, if I do have cancer I have to be the strong one and we have to do it a step at a time and it's going to be harder for them but if I could be strong and if they could see I could handle it.

    I mean, at night you know, when you're lying there, of course, bad thoughts get into your head but you've got to push them out and say you know, even if this is cancer, we can deal with it . . . I was lucky. It wasn't, it wasn't bad so uh, but you do find, you do find strength within you. Especially I think with the kids, you know. You've got to find that strength cause you can't, you can't break down and you know, you have to, you have to be strong.

PARTICIPANT #9

I kept busy. That's important so that I didn't have too much time to dwell on it. My family was going through other crisis at the time. So I couldn't just think of me. That was important. Um . . . important not to; not to stop working. I also go to the gym. And uh . . . I found that if I went each day rather than the three times a week that I had been going, that it really helped me . . . .to have exercise, more exercise than a normal working mother has.

PARTICIPANT #10

It was a real uh struggle for me to keep the, the tears back. I was just very frightened, you know, that what if something isn't quite right . . . I did talk to, to a couple of people and cried a little bit.

REFERENCES

Applegate, M., & Morse, J. M. (1994). Personal privacy and interaction patterns in a nursing home. *Journal of Aging Studies, 8*(4), 413–434. doi:10.1016/0890-4065(94)90012-4

Chen, J. (2009). *North of Beautiful.* New York, NY: Little, Brown.

Corbin, J., & Morse, J. M. (2003). The unstructured interactive interview: Issues of reciprocity and risks. *Qualitative Inquiry, 9*(3), 335–354.

Davies, M. (2010). Concept mapping, mind mapping and argument mapping: What are the differences and do they matter? *Higher Education, 62,* 279–301. doi:10.1007/s10734-010-9387-6

Day, J., & Higgins, I. (2015). Existential absence: The lived experience of family members during their older loved one's delirium. *Qualitative Health Research, 25,* 1700–1718. doi:10.1177/1049732314568321

Glaser, B. G. (1978). *Theoretical sensitivity.* Mill Creek, CA: Sociology Press.

Harris, M. (2015). "Three in the room": Embodiment, disclosure, and vulnerability in qualitative research. *Qualitative Health Research, 25,* 1689–1699. doi:10.1177/1049732314566324

Hegelund, A. S. (2005). Objectivity and subjectivity in the ethnographic method. *Qualitative Health Research, 15,* 647–668. doi:10.1177/1049732304273933

Hole, R. D., Evans, M., Berg, L. D., Bottorff, J. L., Dingwall, C., Alexis, C., . . . Smith, M. L. (2015). Visibility and voice Aboriginal people experience culturally safe and unsafe health care. *Qualitative Health Research, 25,* 1662–1674. doi:10.1177/1049732314566325

Klinke, M. E., Zahavi, D., Hjaltason, H., Thorsteinsson, B., & Jónsdóttir, H. (2015). "Getting the left right": The experience of hemispatial neglect after stroke. *Qualitative Health Research, 25,* 1623–1632. doi:10.1177/1049732314566328

Knafl, K., & Deatrick, J. (2000). Research careers and concept development: The case of normalization. In B. L. Rodgers & K. A. Knafl (Eds.), *Concept development in nursing: Foundations, techniques, and applications* (2nd ed., pp. 353–368). Philadelphia, PA: W. B. Saunders.

McIntosh, M., & Morse, J. M. (2015). Situating and constructing diversity in semi-structured interviews. *Global Qualitative Nursing Research,* 1–12. doi:10.1177/2333393615597674

Morse, J. M. (1995). The significance of saturation [Editorial]. *Qualitative Health Research, 5*(2), 147–148.

Morse, J. M. (2001). Using shadowed data [Editorial]. *Qualitative Health Research, 11*(3), 291.

Morse, J. M. (2002). Emotional re-enactment [Editorial]. *Qualitative Health Research, 12*(2), 147.

Morse, J. M. (2011). The Praxis Theory of Suffering. In J. B. Butts & K. L. Rich (Eds.), *Philosophies and theories in advanced nursing practice* (pp. 569–602). Burlington, MA: Jones & Bartlett.

Morse, J. M., & Proctor, A. (1998). Maintaining patient endurance: The comfort work of trauma nurses. *Clinical Nursing Research, 7*(3), 250–274.

Morse, J. M., Hupcey, J., Mitcham, C., & Lenz, E. (1996). Concept analysis in nursing research: A critical appraisal. *Scholarly Inquiry for Nursing Practice, 10*(3), 263.

Morse, J. M., Mitcham, C., Hupcey, J. E., & Tasón, M. C. (1996). Criteria for concept evaluation. *Journal of Advanced Nursing, 24,* 385–390.

Novak, J. D., & Gowin, D. B. (1984). *Learning how to learn.* Cambridge, UK: Cambridge University.

Proctor, A., Morse, J. M., & Khonsari, E. S. (1996). Sounds of comfort in the trauma center: How nurses talk to patients in pain. *Social Science & Medicine, 42*(12), 1669–1680. doi:10.1016/0277-9536(95)00298-7

Richards, L., & Morse, J. M. (2012). *Readme first for a user's guide to qualitative inquiry.* Thousand Oaks, CA: Sage.

Schwingel, A., Linares, D. E., Gálvez, P., Adamson, B., Aguayo, L., Bobbit, J., . . . Marquez, D. X. (2015). Developing a culturally sensitive lifestyle behavior change program for older Latinas. *Qualitative Health Research, 25,* 1733–1746. doi:10.1177/1049732314568323

Thompson, M. N., Nitzarim, R. S., Cole, O. D., Frost, N. D., Stege, A. R., & Vue, P. T. (2015). Clinical experiences with clients who are low-income mental health practitioners perspectives. *Qualitative Health Research, 25,* 1675–1688. doi:10.1177/1049732314566327

CONCEPT IDENTIFICATION USING QUALITATIVE INQUIRY

> *What is wrong with health care are its concepts and words, rather than its picayune—but rather costly—procedures.*
>
> —Ivan Illich (1994)

Concept identification is a crucial process within all qualitative methods, and the goal of most. As described in Chapter 12, qualitative methods inductively use the description necessary for identifying and constructing attributes and defining boundaries, and use techniques of categorization and comparison for delineating concepts. This chapter consists of examples of concept identification and development using data. It is divided into three sections. In the first section, *data-derived concepts*, the concept is identified and developed directly from data, using the example of *compathy*. In this chapter, *concept-supporting data* in which data (or indices) seeking a concept are applied directly from data to develop concepts, uses the example of disembodiment for the self-management of excruciating pain.

DEVELOPING A CONCEPT FROM DATA: THE EXAMPLE OF COMPATHY

In the 1990s, with funding from the National Center for Nursing Research (NCNR; now the National Institute of Nursing Research [NINR]) to critically assess the meaning and role of comfort in nursing, we initiated phenomenological research into enhancing endurance in acutely distressed patients. We began to investigate how burned and traumatized patients themselves attained comfort (i.e., self-comfort) and how nurses sought to nonpharma-ceutically provide it. In this research, experiential descriptions of responses to the distress of others began to surface. These descriptions did not fit the standard conceptions of empathy in the literature. Initially, inquiry focused on the suppression of such responses—of steeling or bracing oneself, and controlling one's expressions of dismay, distress, or disgust, in order to continue providing care. Eventually, however, we realized that we had data that did not fit descriptions of empathy, and recognized that they were in the presence of an experience of singular importance—one (with the exception of Hoffman [1990]) that had not been discussed in the literature.

We were using phenomenology, the goal of which is to understand, to elicit the meaning or the essence (van Manen, 1990) of the concept. But those interested in concepts take this one step further: Phenomenology enables the development of adequate description to *identify* behavioral concepts, and to explore the context and produce rich descriptions that will enable the *development of attributes*.

Examples From Data: Nurses' Descriptions of Compathy and the Compathetic Response

Interviews with nurses about aspects in patient care that evoked a compa-thetic response were:

- Providing emergency care, such as doing mouth to mouth if a mouthpiece is not available—especially if the patient vomits
- Having to inflict pain, especially when the person does not really understand what you are doing, such as having to take blood from a small child
- Shaving around a wound that has to be sutured, such as a scalp lacerations "makes me feel weak and sweaty, especially if there is dried blood that I have to wash away."

Many nurses reported that the smell of burned flesh, fecal vomiting, blood, melena, and amniotic fluid all evoked a physical response. These noxious odors were different from the compathetic response, because patients' distress was not the trigger for the nurses' response. Similarly, sounds were also offensive, such as: someone blowing his or her nose and about to spit; bones grating, scraping, but removed from a distressed person, but again, removed from signals of distress, they were not the same as a compathetic response. Interestingly, although the sound of vomiting has been reported in an international Internet survey and was ranked as the "most horrible sound" (Cox, 2008), nurses reported that "it was not so bad" and "you got used to it."

Nurses reposted that the sight of trauma was not so distressing if the person was not behaviorally and emotionally distressed:

> One sight sticks in my mind. I remember a gentleman who had been riding a motorcycle and took out a metal guardrail along the side of a road—no one felt sick—it was kind of intriguing for the anatomy, because he came in ventilated and the whole of his chest was open. So every time you bagged him and gave him a breath, you could see his lungs inflate and deflate. It was interesting, but you didn't have time to feel sick.

Describing Compathy

In the next section, I will use these data to illustrate the process of developing a concept from phenomenological data. In this case the concept was identified from the phenomenological study, but I will continue beyond identification to develop the concept anatomically to the level of model building.

Data Summary

When an individual is injured or experiences a painful condition, the injury or pain may be immediately manifested in various ways. Persons may posture to guard or to protect the painful part, may grimace and become pale, sweat, and display other indices of physical distress. They may also express pain by crying out or describing it to others. The posturing, physiological signs, sounds, and verbal descriptions all communicate to others (and to some degree to oneself) the level of distress or nature and intensity of the pain being experienced. Furthermore, in the case of injury, disfiguring disease, or illness, such signs as damaged tissue, bleeding, the sounds of grating bones or labored breathing, the odor of blood or decaying tissue, and the cold, clammy sensation of the skin of a person in shock all indicate aspects of the severity of a condition and the character of its experience. Someone may thus perceive not only the extent and possible ramifications of the injury, which may cause shock and horror, fear, anxiety, sympathy, and compassion, and would amount to emotional empathy; but in addition to this, someone may have a sense of what the experience of such injury must feel like to the sufferer.

Through experience and training, especially among professional caregivers, it is possible for persons to learn to control for the compathetic response. Caregivers are motivated and guided by compathy to give better care, but they also have to learn to shield or otherwise protect themselves from some aspects of the compathetic response, at least in its stronger forms. Physicians and nurses must learn not only to limit empathetic identification with their patients but also to control for compathetic identification.[1] When a patient reminds the caregiver of a relative or a friend—or in fact is a relative or friend—the compathetic response is not so easily controlled, and shielding mechanisms readily break down. In one instance a nurse reported having to leave the room to maintain control: "And when I looked at him, I thought it was my dad. And I just lost it . . . I just had to leave the room. I could not nurse in that room. I could not work on this guy."

Triggers for Compathy

The notion of *contagion of physiological response* is not new, but has been relatively ignored in the literature. What is the result of this "contagion?"

The triggers for the compathetic response (i.e., the antecedents) usually arise from directly viewing the person suffering. The response is particularly strong if the observer has a close relationship, that is, is embodied with the sufferer. It can be conceptualized as a *contagion of physiological response*. The various responses that occurred in the individual as a result of the compathetic arousal, identified from observations, personal knowledge, and the literature, may be sorted into four levels, and evident in various degrees:

- By *seeing* the illness/suffering
- By *hearing* descriptions of illness/suffering
- By *reading* descriptions of illness/suffering, or
- When the phenomena is dissociated from a known person, even by *thinking* about it

Level 1. Mimicking of Physical Behaviors

The first level is evident in infant development as the modeling of nurturing/comforting behaviors that form the basis of socialization of infants and children. In the first year of life, infants are taught to respect others and not to cause pain; that others feel as they themselves feel; that when they are hurt, others "make them feel better"; and that they too may comfort others. These behaviors are taught by modeling and by imitating others (Davis, 1985; Hoffman, 1981) and by the repetitive instruction that occurs in the parent–child relationship. Infants are taught not to bite, push, or to hit others, and mothers may even give their own infant a small hit "to see how it feels." Small children are constantly reminded to "be gentle with others" and not hurt others. This learning continues as parents try to monitor playground and keep older children from observing violence on TV.

An example of modeling is shown on Figure 13.1, a newspaper photograph of a grandson imitating his grandmother while she receives a flu shot.

---

[1] A scientific concept developed from qualitative data.

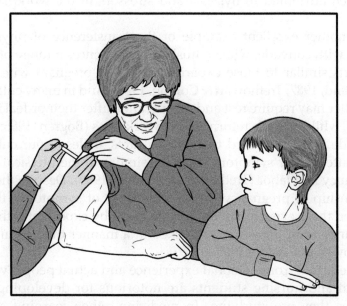

FIGURE 13.1
Learning by modeling: grandson vicariously experiences his grandmother's flu shot.

Level 2. Contagion of Physiological Responses

The contagion of involuntary responses to pain is evident in this level, with some of these responses based on shared emotions. For example, uncontrolled giggling (especially in adolescents) is classic, and serves a function of reducing social stress (Glenn, 1989). Other emotional responses that are manifest physiologically, such as, crying, sadness, and group hysteria are also common. These behaviors are stimulated by triggers, which occur in groups and are involuntary.

Not all of these contagious physiological responses are based on pain. Yawning is of particular interest for a contagious physiological response that can be easily triggered by observing a yawn in another (i.e., a yawn-evoked yawn [Provine, 1986]), and one that has even been well described by Dr. Seuss (Geisel 1962, p. 2). A yawn may be triggered, or the desire to yawn stimulated, even by thinking or reading about yawning; because once initiated the response must go to completion, it is known as a *released fixed action pattern* (Provine, 1986).

Level 3. The Contagion of Physiological Conditions; Often Pathophysiological

These syndromes, or set of physiological symptoms, are more complex. For example, psychogenic epidemics in the workplace have been documented, with symptoms including dizziness, vomiting, fainting, hyperventilation, skin disorders, and epileptic-type seizures. Such mass psychogenic illness has been attributed to hysteria and stressors in the workplace (Olkinuora, 1984).

Another excellent example of the transference of physical responses occurs with couvade; when a husband experiences a range of pains and discomforts similar to those experienced by his pregnant wife (Bogren, 1986; Strickland, 1987; Trethowan & Conlon, 1965). And in many cultures an expectant father may require rest and recuperation after their ordeal in the postnatal period, while his wife returns to her work roles (Bogren, 1986; Clinton, 1985). Couvade is not restricted to exotic cultures; males in our culture are sometimes affected by symptoms that are similar to the physical discomforts of pregnancy and labor (Trethowan & Conlon, 1965). Despite the chronological relationship of pregnancy to the occurrence of symptoms, the relationship between these events may not be perceived by expectant fathers. Yet certain pregnancy symptoms are "mimicked in a manner that is quite remarkable" (Trethowan & Conlon, 1965, p. 59).

Detached from personal experience and actual people with the illness, medical and nursing students are notorious for developing symptoms of diseases they are studying. In medicine, when learning about diseases, hearing descriptions of symptoms, they compared their own body and any symptoms they might have been experiencing, with those diseases. They self-diagnose the same symptoms in themselves, or recognize them in their own healthy bodies—usually with a grim prognosis. Medical students in their first course of anatomy, when dissecting cadavers (Gustavson, 1988), particularly had somatic symptoms when dissecting the hands, genitals, and face.

Finally, the contagion of pain is evident in some at the scene of accidents. Children in a school yard may gather around a friend with a scraped knee, feeling the pain in their own knee, even holding their own knee, and experiencing the stinging with a voiced implosive ("Oooh!" or with a vocalized sucking sound in the throat).

TO DO 13.1. ANALYZING BYSTANDER BEHAVIORS AT ACCIDENT SCENES

Look for newspaper photos of accident scenes, and study the expressions and physical posturing of bystanders. Often the shared pain experience injured victims of pedestrian or a motor vehicle accident is reflected on the faces of the bystanders.

The contagion of nausea and vomiting, although not well documented, is a phenomenon with which we may all identify. In interviews, nurses report struggling against the urge to "throw up" as they assist the vomiting patient. Other nurses refuse this task and leave the room, send in another nurse, or ignore the patient's distress until the episode passes. Several movies have recently exploited this phenomena—most notably the story of Lard Butt and barf-o-rama in *The Pie-Eating Contest* (Evans, Scheinman, & Reiner, 1986) and Mr. Creosote and the French restaurant vomiting scene from Monty Python's *Meaning of Life* (Goldstone & Jones, 1983).

Level 4. Suppression of the Response

In the fourth level, the response becomes disabling, intolerable and is suppressed. We are taught to treat other humans (and some animals) respectfully as living, feeling entities. When this principle must be violated, we must deliberately then relearn to detach ourselves from the reality and depersonalize the *person* to the status of an object. This is a learned process, one that allows us to inflict pain. By treating the person as an object, we convince ourselves that the person does not feel; and as an object without feeling, the compathetic response is inhibited or blocked. Alternatively, we justify our actions as essential for the other's health and recovery, as being "for their own good" and "will be better (for the person) in the long run."

Examples of this behavior are taught to us as adolescents when learning to dissect frogs in the biology lab (Shapiro, 1990). Similarly, surgeons must depersonalize patients—and make patients into cases, concealing their faces and all areas but the sterile, operative area with drapes, before being able to cut the skin. Even then the learning process is slow, and medical students fainting in their first exposure to surgery is classical.

Suppression of compathetic responses is also important for medical students learning in the anatomy lab. The stress responses that develop while learning dissection are well documented (Finkelstein & Mathers, 1990). Students report "strong negative arousal (that is, feelings of anxiety, disgust and dislike) with first incisions" and with dissection of the genitals, female breast, face, and hands (Gustavson, 1988, p. 62). Symptoms include a close identification with the cadaver and describing the cadaver "as an image of the self in a morbid condition" (p. 63). In extreme cases, students have recurring "death images" and become "preoccupied with their own health" with "persistent thoughts of their own death" and "the increasing fragility of their tissues as they age" (Finkelstein & Mathers, 1990, p. 223). Students must learn detachment and to distance themselves, or leave medicine.

Shielding or Blocking the Compathetic Response

When physicians order nurses to conduct particularly painful procedures, nurses often rationalize or justify these actions to themselves as "for the patient's own good." On occasion, such a rationalization can become so pervasive as to preclude seeing what is obvious. This narrow focus is a structural feature of medicine regarding attitudes toward patients. The social distance between physician and patient is culturally prescribed. Posture, formality of address, and strict norms regarding acceptable types of touch are professionally prescribed. In medicine, a person is first cognitively perceived as a patient, and then as a case. In the operating room, a person is further distanced by the covering of drapes, concealing all but the operative area. Medical dialogue focuses on disease rather than the afflicted person.

When the patient is first brought into the trauma room, prior to the administration of any analgesic, and in pain and distress, we noted that any observers postured, holding one arm around their chest and the other hand over their mouth, to contain their own distress, and in a posture that we now recognize as enduring, almost at transition (Morse, Beres, Spiers, Mayan, & Olson, 2003).

Suppression of the compathetic response is seen daily. Persons learn to block the response and "hold themselves together." They put their arms around their chest and hold themselves, and place a hand over their mouths, as if to block the news. A recent example of this posturing is the file photos of the National Security staff observing the attack on Bin Laden (Sept 28, 2011). Secretary of State Hillary Clinton portrays a compathetic response while the others passively observe, perhaps blocking this response.[2]

The extreme of this level is the detachment manifest in psychotic behavior with murderers and rapists treating their victims as objects, rather than human. This phenomenon is also documented with advice given to protect victims as to make themselves human to their attackers, as this will reverse this process of depersonalization, and hence stop the attack.

Developing Types of Compathetic Response

From the previous discussion, we can schematically represent the types of compathetic response and their relationship to compathy, as we further delineate it from empathy (see Figure 13.2).

Formally Developing the Concept Structure

Once we are convinced that we have a new and unique concept, the next task is to develop its definition: its attributes, boundaries, antecedent, and consequences.

Defining Compathy

Our definition, derived from data, is as follows:

> A *compathetic response* is the response/arousal that is evoked in an individual observing the suffering. The suffering and symptoms experienced by the observer mimic those experienced by

---

[2] See: http://goo.gl/tofyrN (Photo 1, White House: Intense: President Obama watches . . .).

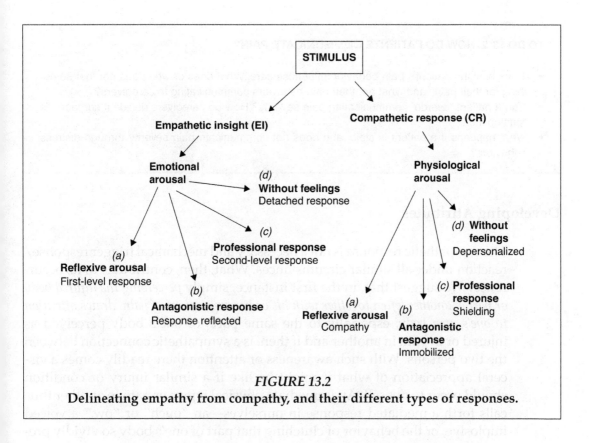

FIGURE 13.2
Delineating empathy from compathy, and their different types of responses.

the individual with the affliction. Although the distress is precipitated by the experiences of the other, it is something that is reflexively simultaneously occurring in the observer. Compathetic response may therefore be considered a psychogenic contagion. (Morse & Mitcham, 1997; Morse, Mitcham, & van der Steen, 1998)

We selected compathy as a neoclassical hybrid term from the Latin prefix cum (meaning "together with") and the Greek word pathos (meaning "experience" or "suffering"). We also considered the more appropriate terms of "compassion" and "sympathy," but both of these terms were already defined differently, and we wanted to emphasize the sharing of the physical states. Compathy did not have a formal label, albeit the concept is now appearing in the literature as "vicarious pain" (see, e.g., Vachon-Preseau et al., 2011).

All of us may envision scenes that involve a compathetic response. They usually involve painful procedures, such as of dentists drilling, fingernails being pulled off, teeth extracted, or broken bones grating. Interestingly, envisioning a scene that results in a compathetic response requires previous experience with a painful experience and the memory of a sound. Less frequently, these responses involve the previous witnessing of an incident or the sense of smell.

TO DO 13.2. HOW DO PATIENTS COMMUNICATE PAIN?

- Think how the patient's pain behavior influences care. What does or who does not "get something for their pain," and what are their pain behaviors communicating to caregivers?
- Can a patient "overdo" communicating pain severity? How do caregivers decide if someone is "putting it on?"
- What happens if a patient is stoic, and does not communicate pain severity through distress behaviors?

Developing Attributes

The compathetic response is not a necessary and mechanical trigger response/ reaction under all similar circumstances. What, then, contributes to its occurrence? We suggest that, in the first instance, simply *perceiving the injured body or part of another, often together with his or her expressions of pain, draws attention to one's own body*, especially to the same parts of one's body perceived as injured or in pain in another and if there is a sympathetic connection between the two persons. With such awareness or attention there readily comes a visceral appreciation of what it might be like if a similar injury or condition should occur to oneself. An immediate physical injury or pain in another thus calls forth a mediated response in ourselves—an "ouch" or "ow," a voiced implosive, or the behavior of clutching that part of one's body so vividly presented in the pain of another.

1. *Attribute 1*: The compathetic responder embodies the pain experience of the other. *Perceiving the injured body part of another, together with the person's pain response, draws attention to one's own body with immediate* visceral appreciation of what it might be like if a similar injury or condition should occur to oneself.
2. *Attribute 2*: The person immediately responds by experiencing:
   a. A compathetic response (identical, initiated, transferred, or converted), or
   b. By blocking the compathetic response (shielding/ steeling). Blocking may be postulated to originate in deliberate and conscious efforts *not* to experience. Nurses talk about "taking a deep breath" and pausing to collect themselves before unwrapping a wound or entering a trauma room. If the compathetic response surfaces, they may have to struggle to control facial expressions by focusing intently on the task at hand rather than on the

patient as a person who is suffering. Eventually nurses speak of "getting their comfort level up" by blocking the impact of sights, sounds, and odors that would otherwise trigger a compathetic response.

Generalizing: Moving Beyond the Emergency Department Caregiving Context

Once we understood the concept and learned to recognize compathy, examples of compathy were everywhere: in everyday usage, in poetry, in lay (trade) literature and even as evidence of injury severity in court. The examples are interesting.

To Modify Behavior

Those who review too many citations for exceeding the speed limit are required to attend sessions offered by the police. These sessions include slides of accidents—car smashes with passenger or pedestrian injury, using the compathetic response to recognize the injury ramification of speeding, and hence to change driving habits and slow down.

Another example is on cigarette packets in Canada. The "warnings" of the dangers of smoking include actual photographs of dental disease, chest x-rays showing cancerous lesions, and cancer of the tongue and lips. The not so implicit message is, "This could happen to you."

Safety programs often use the compathetic response as an incentive for workers to avoid certain behaviors and to comply with safety standards. Stephen Pile (1979) in his *Official Handbook of the Not Terribly Good Club of Great Britain* reported on the least successful safety film, merging this category with the next, to entertainment:

> In 1976, the British Aircraft Corporation showed a film on the dangers of not wearing protective goggles to employees at its Preston Factory. It was so horrific that 13 employees had to be helped out by work mates and State Registered Nurses.
>
> One scene was so realistic that a welder fell off his chair in fright and had to have seven stitches. During the same scene another worker fainted and had to be carried out. In one full-color close-up, a group of machine minders had to be led out feeling sick and faint.
>
> The divisional safety officer, Mr. Ron Hesketh, said the film was being withdrawn because it was not safe . . . (Pile, 1979, p. 33)

Entertainment

Think about horror movies, war movies, and other violent actions on the screen that involve pain and injury. Does the viewing of such injuries make you cringe? Feel discomfort? Even feel nauseated?

Consider fair grounds: What use is "commercial" use of the compathetic response? Bert Almon's poem is interesting, because the compathetic response is conveyed to the audience without signs of distress by the person who should be feeling and should be suffering:

> The tattooed man, a neural freak
> who drove a nail up one nostril,
>
> smiles, then inserted a screwdriver
> into the other, dark ichor running
>
> in the heavy light, and as finale
> (your eyes were shut now, unbearable
>
> for you the pain he couldn't feel)
> offered to pass a safety pin through
>
> the bunched flesh of his arm, and snap it shut
> Almon (1984, p. 40. Reprinted with permission of the author).

Legal

In the courtroom, the compathetic response has been used as evidence of injury severity. Below is an account of the trial of a barroom bouncer who roughly ejected a woman who died with a fractured skull late the same day:

> Other bar patrons testified that they saw [the victim] Cardinal's
> head hit the doorframe as [the bouncer] Pirie took her out of the
> bar, before heading up the steps. 'It was loud enough that we
> heard. The people I was with, we all said, "Oooooo, ouch"',
> testified Delores Delver. (Coldlter, 1991, p. B16)

TO DO 13.3. COMPATHY EVERY DAY?

Find everyday examples of compathy. Have you found an example of compathy—or a category—that is not listed in this chapter?

Toward Modeling: The Physiology of Compathy

There is a paradoxical relationship between compathy and the provision of care (Morse, Mitcham, & van der Steen, 1998). On one hand, compathy may serve to motivate the caregiver to provide care; on the other it may overwhelm the caregiver and inhibit care or drastically alter the type of care provided. Experienced caregivers learn to block the compathetic response, but this may also inhibit a useful caregiving motivator. The process is modeled in Figure 13.3.

Compathy is manifest (Figure 13.3, pathway a), and may be reflected in the individual as *manifest* in as similar or dissimilar form (see Table 13.1). If the caregiver has a similar response and the patient is vomiting, the caregiver's response may be to vomit or feel nauseated. If the caregiver's response is dissimilar and a *converted* response, the caregiver may develop a backache.

When the response is suppressed (pathway b), then the caregiver alters his or her perceptions of the *patient* or the experience. The caregiver may degrade or minimalize the patient's experience ("the pain is not that bad"), depersonalize the patient ("acting out"), or justify the treatments as being "for her own good."

In the third pathway, experienced caregivers have learned to block the compathetic response entirely. Caregivers are able to provide care while shielding, maintaining control. Shielding, the deliberate and conscious efforts not to experience, involves self control: physical "deep breathing",

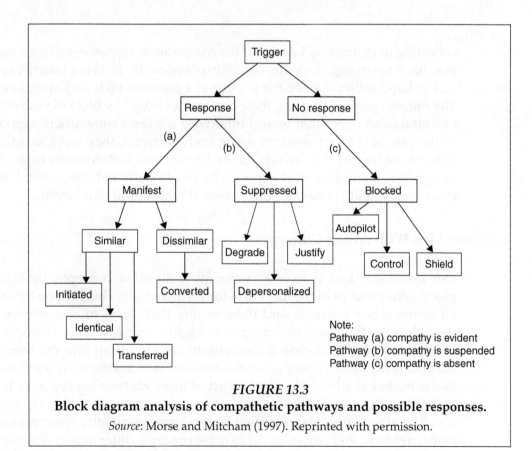

Note:
Pathway (a) compathy is evident
Pathway (b) compathy is suspended
Pathway (c) compathy is absent

FIGURE 13.3

Block diagram analysis of compathetic pathways and possible responses.

Source: Morse and Mitcham (1997). Reprinted with permission.

TABLE 13.1
Types of Compathetic Responses

RESPONSE	DESCRIPTION	EXAMPLE
Identical	Mediated symptoms mimic those of the immediate response	Mother reports her child's injection "as if" the needle were going into her own arm
Initiated	Mediated symptoms are of the same type but not of the same extent or intensity as the immediate response	Vomiting in a sufferer provokes nausea in a witness
Transferred	Mediated symptoms are worse or more exaggerated than an immediate response	Couvade: Husband experiences the wife's pain during childbirth
Converted	Mediated symptoms are quite differing from an immediate response	A sufferer's limb trauma experienced as nausea, fainting, or abdominal pain in a witness

Source: Morse, Mitcham, and van der Steen (1998). Reprinted with permission.

collecting or distracting oneself. If the compathetic response surfaces, nurses may have to struggle to control facial expressions by focusing intently on the task at hand rather than on the patient as a person who is suffering. Eventually nurses speak of "getting their comfort level up" by blocking the impact of sounds and odors that would otherwise trigger a compathetic response. In the case of disaster workers doing body retrieval, they work in an emotionless manner by rote, which can be labeled *autopilot*. Another example of autopilot is a surgeon working with an emotionally flat affect, resulting in emotionally "flat" behavior and patterned mechanical movements.

Relationships With Allied Concepts

Our remaining task is to link compathy with other concepts, by *logically* placing the concept in the literature for further study. This is done by listing all of the allied concepts and determining their level of abstraction: Are they close to the data, mid-range, or highly abstract? This is important because we need to decide if the concept we are fitting into the literature fits beside the other concepts (on the same level of abstraction), sits beneath and is nested at a lower level as a part of more abstract concepts, or is at a higher level.

The allied concepts identified as bordering compathy were psychosomatic, neurotic, and empathy. All of these concepts differ in two dimensions:

whether the caregiver's focus is on him or herself or the patient and whether the response is physical is psychological (see Figure 13.4).

When the response in the caregiver is on the sufferer (the other) and the response is somatic, the reflexive, sufferer-focused response is that of compathy, of sharing the pain with the other (see Figure 13.4, cell *b*). When the caregiver focuses on him or herself and the manifestation is somatic, the result is the development of symptoms as psychosomatic disorder (cell *a*). The caregivers focus on the other, and the sharing of the emotion is empathy (cell *d*). Finally, if the focus is on self and is psychological, the response is neurotic (cell *c*). With neurotic behavior, the focus may be so internalized that the person becomes preoccupied with self, constantly dwelling on symptoms.

Assessment of the Concept

Using the four principles for assessment—epistemological, logical, linguistic, and pragmatic—we find that:

- The epistemological principle has been met: The concept was developed from qualitative data, labeled, and defined. Adequacy was demonstrated by seeking numerous examples from disparate sources, confirming that the concept was not an artifact of a particular setting.
- The linguistic principle, demanding consistency in use of the concept by others, has yet to be demonstrated. As a new

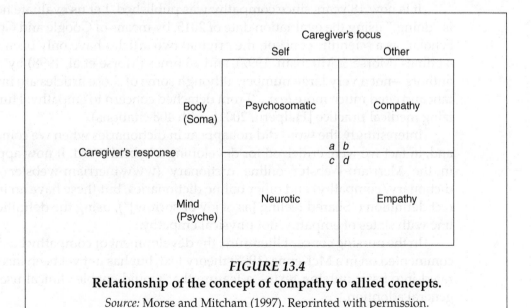

FIGURE 13.4
Relationship of the concept of compathy to allied concepts.
Source: Morse and Mitcham (1997). Reprinted with permission.

concept it remains to be seen how the concept will be adopted into everyday usage in the clinical setting and become part of the professional vocabulary.
- The logical principle has been met. The components are well described: the precondition is a trigger experience; the outcome a physical response. The physical response may closely resemble the condition of the sufferer; may be similar, but less severe (e.g., nausea, rather than vomiting); may be an unrelated response (such as a stress symptom in another part of the body); or the response may be blocked by deliberate learned disembodiment/detachment of the observer from the sufferer.
- The conceptual boundaries include the condition that the compathetic response must be a physical response. These boundaries may be less clear if the response is both physical and emotional. While it is presumed that compathy may co-occur with empathy, if this is the case, it must be recognized as a dual response, each distinct. (see, Morse and Mitcham, 1997, p. 656)

ROLE OF COMPATHY IN KNOWLEDGE DEVELOPMENT

Before we examine its utilization and adoption, let us first consider what type of concept *compathy* is. Because it was deliberately developed from science and is not used in the lay lexicon, it is a scientific concept.

It is now 18 years since compathy was published. Let us evaluate how it is "doing," using the evaluation date of 2015, by means of Google and Google Scholar: as a scientific concept, the original two articles have only been cited 44 times (Morse & Mitcham, 1997), and 35 times (Morse et al, 1998) by other authors—not a very large number, although some of those articles are important and cited much more (e.g., "From detached concern to empathy: Humanizing medical practice [Halpern, 2001], with 408 citations).

Interestingly, the word did not appear in dictionaries when we coined it, and, in fact we were criticized for developing a hybrid word. It now appears in the Merriam-Webster online dictionary (www.merriam-webster.com/dictionary/compathy) and other online dictionaries, but these have an incorrect definition ("Shared feeling [as of joy or sorrow]"), using the definition in line with states of empathy, not physical empathy.

In the nursing concept literature, the development of compathy has been commented on in a McKenna (1997) theory text, but has not yet been incorporated into basic nursing texts—a feature that would enable clinical use and general adoption.

Vicarious empathy appears to have emerged as the primarily competing concept, with the top citations numbering 323, or 10 times the citation of compathy. However, several articles loosely link "vicarious" and "emotions" or "empathy" (e.g., discuss the phenomenon as "vicariously instigated emotions"), as if these authors have not seen the development of the scientific concept.

The bottom line is that the concept must still be considered "new," despite the length of time since it was first introduced into the literature. It remains to be seen if this work will "take off" or die a natural death. This topic, the introduction and utilization of new knowledge, is further discussed in Chapter 39.

REFERENCES

Almon, B. (1984). Palace of illusion. In *Deep north* (p. 40). Saskatoon, Canada: Thistledown Press.

Bogren, L. Y. (1986). The couvade syndrome. *International Journal of Family Psychiatry, 7*(2), 123–136.

Clinton, J. (1985). Couvade: patterns, predictors, and nursing management: A research proposal submitted to the division of nursing. *Western Journal of Nursing Research, 7,* 221–243.

Coldter, D. (1991). Head made dull "thump," bouncer tells inquiry. *Edmonton Journal, 19,* B16.

Cox, T. (2008). Scraping sounds and disgusting noises. *Applied Acoustics, 69,* 1195–1204. doi:10.1016/j.apacoust.2007.11.004

Davis, M. R. (1985). Perceptual and effective reverberation components. In A. P. Goldstein & G. Y. Michaels (Eds.), *Empathy: Development, training, consequences* (pp. 62–108). Hillsdale, NJ: Erlbaum.

Evans, B.A., & Scheinman, A. (Producers), & Reiner, R. (Director), (1986). *Stand by Me* [Motion picture]. United States: Columbia Pictures.

Finkelstein, P., & Mathers L. (1990). Post-traumatic stress among medical students in the anatomy dissection laboratory. *Clinical Anatomy, 3,* 219–226.

Geisel, T. S. (1962). *Dr. Seuss's sleep book.* New York, NY: Random House.

Glenn P. J. (1989). Initiating shared laughter in multi-party conversations. *Western Journal of Speech Communication, 53,* 127–149.

Goldstone, J. (Producer). & Jones, T. (Director). (1983). *Monty Python's the meaning of life* [Motion picture]. United Kingdom: Universal Pictures.

Gustavson, N. (1988). The effect of human dissection on first-year students and implications for the doctor-patient relationship. *Journal of Medical Education, 63,* 62–64.

Halpern, J. (2001). *From detached concern to empathy: Humanizing medical practice* (p. 17). New York, NY: Oxford University.

Hoffman, M. (1981). The development of empathy. In J. Rushton & R. Sorrentino (Ed.), *Altruism and helping behavior: Social personality and developmental perspectives* (pp. 41–63). Hillsdale, New Jersey: Erlbaum.

Hoffman, M. L. (1990). Empathy and justice motivation. *Motivation Emotion, 14,* 151–172.

Illich, I. (1994, June 11). *Against coping.* Presented at Qualitative Health Research conference. Hershey, PA. (Tape #SON 94-2, Berkeley, CA: Conference Recording Service).

McKenna, H. P. (1997). *Nursing theories and models.* New York, NY: Psychology Press.

Morse, J. M., & Mitcham, C. (1997). Compathy: The contagion of physical distress. *Journal of Advanced Nursing, 26,* 649–657.

Morse, J. M., Beres, M., Spiers, J., Mayan, M., & Olson, K. (2003). Identifying signals of suffering by linking verbal and facial cues. *Qualitative Health Research, 13*(8), 1063–1077.

Morse, J. M., Mitcham, C., & van der Steen, V. (1998). Compathy or physical empathy: Implications for the caregiver relationship. *Journal of Medical Humanities, 19*(1), 51–65.

Olkinuora, M. (1984). Psychogenic epidemics and work. *Scandinavian Journal of Work Environmental Health, 10,* 501–504.

Pile S. (1979). *The book of heroic failures: The official handbook of the not terribly good club of Great Britain.* London, UK: Futura.

Provine, R. R. (1986). Yawning as a stereotyped action pattern and releasing stimulus. *Ecology, 72,* 109–122.

Shapiro, K. J. (1990). The pedagogy of learning and unlearning empathy. *Phenomenology and Pedagogy, 8,* 43–48.

Strickland, O. L. (1987). The occurrence of symptoms in expectant fathers: The couvade syndrome. *Nursing Research, 36,* 184–189.

Trethowan, W. H., & Conlon, M. F. (1965) The couvade syndrome. *British Journal of Psychiatry, 111,* 57–66.

Vachon-Preseau, E., Martel, M. O., Roy, M., Caron, E., Jackson, P. L., & Rainville. P. (2011). The multilevel organization of various pain responses: Effects of pain cues and empathy traits on spinal nociception and acute pain. *Pain, 152,* 1525–1531.

van Manen, M. (1990). *Researching the lived experience: Human science for an action sensitive pedagogy.* London, ONT: University of Western Ontario Press.

Janice M. Morse

14

BUILDING CONCEPTS

> *A concept . . . refers to the properties of a phenomenon, not the phenomenon itself. It gives meaning to what can be seen, heard, tasted, smelled and touched. Thus, a concept enables us to categorize, interpret, and structure the phenomenon.*
> —Fawcett & Downs (1992, p. 19)

Concepts do not always emerge directly from data. Often a phenomenon emerges in the data, and it is richly described in an article but not developed (at least initially) to the level of a concept. But as these observations and descriptions accrue, eventually these studies will provide data for the development of a concept. Often these descriptions emerge slowly in articles in which they are at first tentatively addressed, perhaps not even as the main focus of inquiry. In this chapter the first example of the phenomenon of depersonalization during agonizing pain illustrates such a data source. The second example, the emergence of a concept called "preserving self," suggested by diverse sources and disciplines, is the same process, but further along the continuum than our pain example. In both cases these data may be subsequently used to support the development of an emerging concept.

CONCEPT-SUPPORTING DATA

A major strategy for using qualitative data is the use of data to support the development of a concept. This may occur in two situations: The first is when you find interesting data in an interview and seek to "attach" or label it to an established concept. Here we discuss linking data with *disembodiment*. The second situation may occur when your research program is *developing* an immature or partially mature concept, and we discuss the case of *preserving self*.

THE DATA–CONCEPT LINK

Induction is the sacred cow of qualitative inquiry. We teach students that cognitive leaps, moving from data to a concept in one bound, are very risky; for the concept label, no matter how tempting a shortcut to expedite one's analysis, one must take such leaps in baby steps: Develop and saturate your categories and move carefully developing attributes. Once you are certain about your data and the concepts, move it across the developed concept as if a template, to compare the fit, similarities, and comparisons of the two concepts.

But is this process always necessary? Our data are full of others' concepts. Every sentence we utter has at least one established concept—that is how we communicate, for goodness sake. But in the example below, I describe how I found some very interesting data that could have been explained and better understood if I had placed it immediately within the context of a developed concept. Let us have a look.

The Experience of Agonizing Pain

At this point in my research program I was investigating how patients controlled agonizing pain, how they managed to maintain control of self. I had observed pain behavior in emergency and seen vocalizations and behaviors of the severely injured, and identified various states of discomfort from scared to out of control. I had conducted interviews, yet continued to feel that I had not reached the core of "what was going on." One day while analyzing an interview from a lineman who had received a serious electrical burn, I walked away from my computer and came back to look at this text on the screen with new eyes:

> . . . both hands and wrists were burnt, which were the [electrical] entry sites. And . . . both feet were burnt . . . the right side being the worst . . . right side of both hands and feet because— my right hand was up high—so naturally it entered the right the most . . . whatever was left over came down and went into the left . . . it still sustained some damage . . . the right hand had to be removed. . . . And the right leg was burnt quite badly, and the whole outside of the leg was burnt down to the bone—you could see bones and sinews in there, and at the very bottom—it also exited—not on the bottom of the foot—but . . . on the bottom of the leg, like right at the side of the foot was really burnt bad, too.

This person was talking about himself! Yet he was using depersonalized language. He was talking about himself as if his body were not his own. Let us code this piece of text using italics, so we can see the instances of depersonalization:

> . . . *both hands and wrists were burnt*, which were the [electrical] entry sites. And . . . *both feet* were burnt . . . *the right side* being the worst . . . *right side* of *both hands and feet* because—my right hand was up high—so naturally it entered the right the most . . . whatever was left over came down and went into *the left* . . . *it* still sustained some damage . . . *the right hand* had to be removed. . . . And *the right leg* was burnt quite badly, and the whole outside of *the leg* was burnt down to *the bone*—you could see *bones and sinews* in there, and at the very bottom—it also exited—not on the bottom of *the foot*—but . . . on the bottom of *the leg*, like right at the side of *the foot* was really burnt bad, too. (Morse & Mitcham, 1998, p. 670)

The next step was to further analyze the text to see when the definitive article was used and not used. He said, "my right hand was up high—so naturally it entered the right the most" giving an instance of reverting to the possessive pronoun, perhaps indicting that before the burn, his body was still his.

An obvious conjecture could be: The way that persons with excruciating pain cognitively "manage" the pain, is to remove the pain from themselves (using "self" in the sociological sense), which is reflected in their language. In other words, when experiencing excruciating pain, processes of embodiment break down and painful body parts are disembodied. This disembodiment is reflected in their speech.

Therefore, are we seeing *disembodiment*? Can we immediately tag these data as disembodiment? Possibly.

Confirming the Phenomenon

At this moment in your analysis, the limitation is that we have only one case, and from that case made a cognitive leap from data to a concept. But with this new insight let us examine other cases from the data set for these "signals of disembodiment."

First, we examined the descriptions of the pain experience of six other burn patients. All described the pain as "engulfing" and "overwhelming." Four patients experienced amputations of digits, hands or feet or legs, and two had at least one prosthetic limb.

Therefore the next step was to conduct a secondary analysis of participants' narratives to understand their experiences of illness, using data that were collected for previous studies but were not collected specifically to understand the pain experience. This point is important, as it removes any bias that may be with the interaction between the interviewer and the interviewee. If the interviews are already collected, the interviewee can't possibly be responding to cues received from the interviewer. So we examined carefully the selected interviews that we decided to examine. Our rationale for the selection were:

1. *Patients with spinal cord injury:* Does the objectification of the body occur with loss of sensation and loss of control? Do patients who cannot feel parts of their body, treat those parts objectively?
2. *Patients who had transplants (five heart, one heart–lung, one liver transplant, and one kidney transplant):* Personal control and the amount of sensation of the body part remained unchanged before and after the transplant. Postoperative pain was controlled with analgesics.
3. *Patients who had experienced myocardial infarction:* These patients had no alteration in control of their hearts, nor loss of sensation. The patient experienced was less intense than burn patients.

Identification of Alternative Competing Explanatory Conjectures

The next step was to consider what this form of detached speech signifies. Our first two conjectures addressed the objectification of the self related to the transformation of body parts into a separated "object" or "thing" because the injury resulted in loss of sensation in the affected part or in the inability to control or to move the body part. These were:

1. *When individuals lose control of a body part, some disembody that part to maintain control of the self.*
2. *When individuals lose sensation in a body part, disembodiment can be a psychological strategy for "disengaging" the body part from the self.*

These two conjectures were tested by systematically comparing burn patient transcripts with patient groups who have and who have not lost sensation and control. Support for these conjectures is provided if the members of those populations that have lost sensation and/or control also used the definite article in reference to their bodies and if those who have not lost sensation or control do not use this form of speech.

3. *Patients learn disembodying language from physicians.*

Linguistically, modes of detachment are a normal pattern of "doctor talk" as a way of objectifying parts of the body. Patients learn these linguistic patterns of speech by hearing physicians discuss themselves as "cases" on rounds, and so forth.

4. *Disembodiment is used in life-threatening trauma, in an effort to protect the self.*

Here disembodiment would be viewed as a strategy encouraged by a threat to life in which removing the injured part of the self could remove the threat to the self. To support this conjecture, linguistic signals of disembodiment should occur in the transcripts during periods when patients face any life-threatening injury or illness.

5. *Disembodiment is a strategy used to remove the body part, hence to remove the pain, when the agony is overwhelming.*

This conjecture may be tested by comparing the burn patients with comparison groups that experienced varying amounts of pain in the course of their injury or illness.

Testing Conjectures

At this point the presence or absence of each criterion is recorded for each conjecture for each patient group. It is important to note that the use of the criterion that a phenomenon be present in all cases during initial coding introduces an important standard of rigor required in qualitative work, especially considering the small samples used. But this need not mean that the appearance of one single negative case discounts or invalidates an observation. In quantitative inquiry a score of zero on a scale does not indicate that a phenomenon does not exist—only that it was not present in that particular case. One may thus suggest that these same standards could apply to qualitative inquiry. Yet in qualitative work, when the sample is obtained and analyzed case by case, if the negative case is the first case analyzed, there is a risk that this case could inadvertently redirect inquiry. The results are shown in Table 14.1.

From Table 14.1, the only conjecture clearly supported related to extreme pain. This supports the conclusion that *disembodiment "disengages" a body part when a sensation is lost.* Further examination of transcripts showed that burn patients tended to refer to their amputated limbs using the definitive article, "the leg" and to their prosthetic limbs using the possessive "my." For example:

> So [my wife] said, "Come up there with me." And I started
> jumping about a foot, two feet in the air. I was doing fine until
> one leg pulled out and twisted sideways so I had to hang on to
> [my wife], and we had to . . . I sat down on the trampoline, and
> they had to get me off and put my leg back on . . . (laughter). So
> that was pretty hilarious. My brother was there, and he was just
> in tears laughing.

TABLE 14.1
Presence of Characteristics of Disembodiment in Four Patient Groups

CHARACTERISTICS	SAMPLE			
	BURN	SPINAL CORD INJURY	TRANSPLANT	MYOCARDIAL INFARCTION
Loss of control of body part	Some loss of movement	Yes	No	No
Loss of sensation	Some loss of prostheses used	Yes	No	No
Need to protect self	Yes	Yes	Yes	Yes
Opportunity to learn language from physicians	Yes	Yes	Yes	Yes
Extreme pain	Yes	No	No	No
Evidence of linguistic signals of disembodiment	Yes	No	No	No

Source: Morse and Mitcham (1998). Reprinted with permission.

DEVELOPING CONCEPTS TO USING STUDIES TO SUPPORT AN EMERGING CONCEPT

The third way that we use qualitative inquiry is collectively, to develop a concept. The concept first peeks into the literature and is barely noticed. Then it occurs again, and then described in another study, yet again. In each study, the name used is the same or similar. Gradually, the concept is recognized, becomes searchable, is described, and researchers then move to the stage of intentionally exploring and developing the concept. Over time, the concept will be developed enough to be quantified, and then eventually developed into a theory.

In the early stages of development, the greatest threat to validity is the "pink elephant phenomenon," which carries the risk of violating the qualitative principle of induction. The pink elephant illustrates how difficult it is to remain objective while looking for subjective phenomena, and how easy it is to see something you want to see in the data. If we say "don't think of a pink elephant!" everyone immediately thinks of a pink elephant—and could see one in their data. Therefore, the essence of qualitative work at this stage is verification. The researcher must move cautiously, *abductively* verifying each new finding, checking with other participants, other data sets, other literature, and constantly verify, verify, verify, within and outside the dataset.

Later, as there is agreement between studies and among investigators about the concept, the definition, the attributes, and the boundaries, the research changes, with the approach of the researcher not quite so inductive. The researcher does not wait for the concept to emerge, but uses the concept as the central focus of the research and holds the objective of refining the attributes. These phases of the process of accruing qualitative knowledge have been described elsewhere (Morse, 2012, pp. 124–125), but pertinent to the developing of concepts, we are only interested in the first three stages: Stage I: description, Stage II: toward conceptualization, and Stage III: abstraction. This process of developing new concepts with multiple studies and investigators will be illustrated using the example of *preserving self*.

EMERGING CONCEPTS

Concepts are normally identified in qualitative inquiry inductively. The investigator, in the process of analysis, finds a category and gives it a name selected from the data itself (i.e., from words used by the participants that seem the best descriptor). At this stage, it is not usually considered a concept, but a category label. Study #2 deals with the same phenomenon and the same outcome, hopefully with the researcher selecting a label that is similar to or the same as the first study. This second investigator may or may not be associated with the first, and may or may not have even read the first article. Most importantly, the article may or may not be situated in the same context.

The process continues until there are several articles identifying and describing the new category/concept. This is shown in Figure 14.1 as the inductive phase. Researchers do not set out to explore the concept—it is something that emerges in the process of inquiry, and is labeled. In the discussion, later articles may or may not acknowledge the earlier finding of the category or concept.

Eventually, enough articles appear to pique the interest of researchers, and articles start to appear using the concept name as targeting topics of the research. These researchers may be working in different areas or context, but work to build the concept: they make an effort to define the concepts, to identify the attributes, the boundaries, the preconditions, and the outcomes. The concept is used as a key word.

This is called the *abductive phase* as the researcher enters the phase deductively, using what is known about the concept as a skeleton (in which case the data are placed using the skeletal outline and inductively built, padding the frame) or a scaffold (framing the outline and filling in the interior; Morse & Mitcham, 2002). It is called abduction, following Charles Sanders Peirce (in Josephson & Josephson, 1996), with the researcher making a deductive

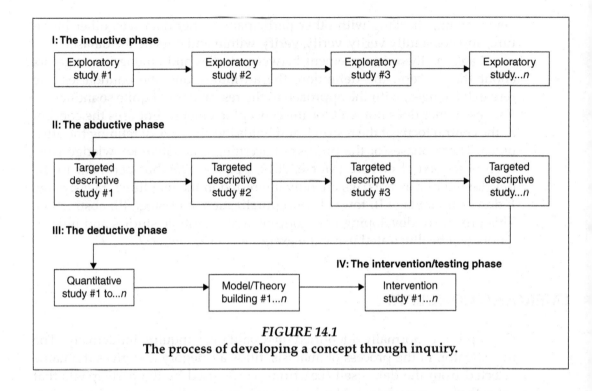

FIGURE 14.1
The process of developing a concept through inquiry.

inference, followed by an inductive verification from data; and the process is repeated. It is in this phase that the anatomy of the concept is developed, the concept is separated from overlapping allied concepts, and the concept eventually reaches maturity.

Phase III is the deductive phase, in which the concept is used in quantitative methods, measurement of the concept is developed; models and theories are designed and used in inquiry. Shortly after, *Phase IV* is the intervention phase: interventions are used, and the efficacy measured.

THE CASE OF "PRESERVING SELF"

As an example, we will examine a concept that is now entering the abductive phase, Phase II in the model (Figure 14.1). The concept is *preserving self* (sometimes called preserving *the* self; Howard, Balneaves, Bottorff, & Rodney, 2011) and preserving the *integrity* of self (Irurita & Williams, 2001).

Definitions for *preserving self* are listed in Table 14.2 and are defined variably as they relate to the context in which they are studied:

- A process for managing role transitions, thereby allowing women to maintain their "sense of self" (Johnson & Morse, 1991, p. 130)

- Strategies that enable the persons to "confront and regroup, meeting the old and new realities (after major trauma) to redefine the self" (Morse & O'Brien, 1995, p. 859)
- Developing personal measures aimed at preventing or reducing harm inflicted by others as a result of one's infertility (Mogobe, 2005)
- The overarching decision-making process evident in the participants' descriptions. This process was shaped by contextual conditions including the characteristics of health services, the nature of hereditary breast and ovarian cancer risk-reduction decisions, gendered roles, and the women's perceived proximity to cancer (Howard, Balneaves, Bottorff, & Rodney, 2011, p. 502).

Despite the differences in the definitions, there are clear commonalities, which will, as the concept moves to Phase II, be identified and the attributes clarified.

The concept was first identified by Johnson (Johnson & Morse, 1991, pp. 130–131) as a component of the process of recovery of women from a myocardial infarction for "managing role transitions." The heart attack undermined the woman's "confidence and self-worth, threatened independence, and consequently jeopardizes a person's sense of self." This resulted in a role transition, from a healthy person to a patient, to an invalid, to a "heart attack victim," and the belief that the dramatic shift in her life as a less robust person, living with restrictions, could never be the same. Women found it difficult to sit and watch others do "their work" in the home, and reframed the daily tasks as "not real work." They "bent the rules" to "engage in prohibited activities, rather than feel dependent and watch others do their work." All publications have described *preserving self* as having a large cognitive component with behavioral manifestations that enable the acceptance of a changed state, which has occurred in the case of a serious physical threat (Table 14.2).

At this time, *preserving self* remains a "contextualized concept." Although it has been used in a number of studies, it is still in Phase I, concept description, and is explored within contexts where there is a threat to the physical or psychological self. Is this concept ready for meta-analysis? Not quite—more studies are needed.

Tracing the Development of Concepts

Should the concept be more developed (or have a larger number of citations), an interesting exercise is to trace the emergence and development of the concept. It is advisable to use multiple data bases initially, as by looking at *preserving self*, you will note that the citations are not all from PubMed, but also from social science sources. Do not rely entirely on databases when you are

TABLE 14.2
Development of the Concept of **Preserving Self** *Using Multiple Studies*

DATE	AUTHOR(S)	TITLE	DEFINITION OF "PRESERVING SELF"
1990	Johnson & Morse	Regaining control: Women having cardiac surgery	A process for managing role transitions, thereby allowing women to maintain their "sense of self" and regain control (p. 130).
1991	Morse & Johnson	Towards a theory of illness: The Illness-Constellation Model	Preserving self was resituated from Johnson & Morse (1991, pp. 329–331) and generalized from Johnson's (1991) study of women with MI, to a strategy of the Illness-Constellation Model, *Striving to regain self*. In order to preserve self, the individual asserts him- or herself and works to regaining control.
1993	King & Jensen	Preserving the self: Women having cardiac surgery	Getting through the surgical experience (waiting, getting there, surviving, being there and moving on) was achieved using the following strategies: relating, making sense, managing and normalizing what was happening to them. These behaviors were directed toward preserving self (p. 99).
1995	Morse & O'Brien	Preserving self: From victim, to patient, to disabled person	The strategies used to preserve self required deliberate action, focused energy and tremendous effort, and changed at each stage of the model. At the beginning, when physical survival was in jeopardy, the strategies were primarily physical. Protecting self was a process of "taking time out" and of shutting down in the stage of disruption. During the stage of enduring the self, the strategy was passively learning to "take it" and to bear the treatments. Finally, in the stage of striving to regain and preserve the self, the work was in redefining the self as a disabled person (p. 886).
2001	Irurita & Williams	Balancing and compromising: Nurses and patients preserving integrity of self and each other	"This reciprocal process used by nurses and patients to preserve their own and each other's integrity involved: contributing to care—cooperating; prioritizing and rational sacrificing; justifying compromised care and lowering expectations; and protecting self by attracting or repelling" (p. 597).

(continued)

TABLE 14.2
Development of the Concept of **Preserving Self** *Using Multiple Studies (continued)*

DATE	AUTHOR(S)	TITLE	DEFINITION OF "PRESERVING SELF"
2007	Mackintosh	Protecting the self: A descriptive qualitative exploration of how registered nurses cope with working in surgical areas	"The need to switch off in order to protect the individual self, a process which is facilitated by the adoption of a working or role specific persona that is discrete from their own personal persona and is enhanced by their length of experience" (pp. 988–989).
2011	Bagarozzi	A closer look at couple collusion: Protecting the self and preserving the system	A "group of defenses that some spouses use to protect their respective selves and to preserve dyadic equilibrium" (p. 390).
2011	Howard, Balneaves, Bottorff, & Rodney	Preserving the self: the process of decision making about hereditary breast cancer and ovarian cancer risk reduction.	Preserving the self was the process of "conceptualized engaging in decision making as a way for women to attend to their physical health and protect themselves from cancer, as well as protect their self-identity as a woman, their emotional well-being, and their relationships" (p. 512).

Republished with permission of Taylor & Francis, Group LLC Books, from Morse (2012). Permission conveyed through Copyright Clearance Center, Inc.

searching early citations: Supplement this with check of the citations in the reference lists of the major articles. Sometime when searching "way back" you will find that concepts are not always referred to consistently with the same names.

TO DO 14.1. THE DEVELOPMENT OF A CONCEPT OVER TIME

Select a concept and trace its development from the point that it was first introduced into the litera-ture to the present time. What is the concept's level of development? Can you identify the periods of transition from Phase I to Phase II, and to Phase III?

SUMMARY

In this chapter, we examined the ways that qualitative research develops from data to a concept. Three methods were identified. The first is identifying the concept within the data, and the concept of *compathy* was used to illustrate how a concept may be developed from a single project. Second, data were used to develop a concept. Interesting data were "matched" with the concept of disembodiment. To prevent the risk of a "cognitive leap" and the misapplication of these data, other data sorts were used to strengthen and support the application and subsequent identification of the use of *disembodiment* as a strategy to control the management of agonizing pain.

The third method was the development of the concept of *preserving self*, as the concept emerged from many descriptive studies over a period of two decades. The level of development of this concept is still in the descriptive stage—but watch it as it emerges—it will not be long before the anatomy of the concept is delineated and it moves into Stage II, the *abductive phase*.

Now it is your turn to develop a concept. The first assignment may serve as your term paper: to develop a concept by using the literature as data. The second assignment is more fun, and uses observational data and an Opus cartoon.

TO DO 14.2. DEVELOPMENT OF A SCIENTIFIC CONCEPT

QUESTION:
How has an important concept developed in nursing?
To what level has it developed conceptually?
What use is it to nursing?

Conduct a literature search using a lay concept (such as hope). Use your selected concept and *concept* as key words. Look at the development of the concept from 1990—or an appropriate date—to the present time. Consider citation streams—who cites whom—and the development refinement of the concept, both as a concept and perhaps as a theory, to the present time.

Has the concept been primarily developed within nursing, was it "adopted" into nursing, or is it used differently in nursing than other disciplines?

Present your findings as a narrative, supplemented with a table.

Be certain to include a conclusion/summary statement

To Read: Greene, J. A. (2004). 2002 Roy porter memorial prize essay: Therapeutic infidelities: "Noncompliance" enters the medical literature, 1955–1975. *Social History of Medicine, 17*(3), 327–343.

REFERENCES

Bagarozzi, D. A. (2011). A closer look at couple collusion: Protecting the self and preserving the system. *The American Journals of Family Therapy, 39*, 390–403. doi:10.1080/01926187.2011.575633

Fawcett, J., & Downs, F. (1992). *The relationship of theory and research* (2nd ed.). Philadelphia, PA: F. A. Davis.

Howard, A. F., Balneaves, L. G., Bottorff, J. L., & Rodney, P. (2011). Preserving the self: The process of decision-making about heredity breast cancer and ovarian cancer risk reduction. *Qualitative Health Research, 21,* 502–519. doi:10.1177/1049732310387798

Irurita, V. F., & Williams, A. M. (2001). Balancing and compromising: Nurses and patients preserving integrity of self and each other. *International Journal of Nursing Studies, 38,* 579–589.

Johnson, J. (1991). Learning to live again: The process of adjustment following a heart attack, In J. M. Morse and J. L. Johnson (Eds.), *The illness experience: Dimensions of suffering.* Newbury Park, CA: Sage.

Johnson, J. J., & Morse J. M. (1990). Regaining control: The process of adjustment following myocardial infarction. *Heart and Lung, 19*(2), 126–135.

Josephson, R., & Josephson, G. (1996). *Abductive inference: Computation, philosophy, technology.* New York, NY: Cambridge University Press.

King, K. M., & Jensen, L. (1993). Preserving the self: Women having cardiac surgery. *Heart & Lung: The Journal of Critical Care, 23*(2), 99–105.

Mackintosh, C. (2007). Protecting the self: A descriptive qualitative exploration of how registered nurses cope with working in surgical areas. *International Journal of Nursing Studies, 44*(6), 982–990.

Mogobe, D. K. (2005). Denying and preserving self: Batswana women's experiences of infertility. *African Journal of Reproductive Health, 9*(2), 26.

Morse, J. M. (2012). *Qualitative health research: Creating a new discipline.* Walnut Creek, CA: Left Coast Press.

Morse, J. M., & Johnson, J. (1991). *The illness experience: Dimensions of suffering.* Newbury Park, CA: Sage. Retrieved from http://goo.gl/6va9Ql

Morse, J. M., & Mitcham, C. (1998). The experience of agonizing pain and signals of disembodiment. *Journal of Psychosomatic Research, 44*(6) 667–680.

Morse, J. M., & Mitcham, C. (2002). Exploring qualitatively-derived concepts: Inductive-deductive pitfalls. *International Journal of Qualitative Methods, 1*(4), Article 3.

Morse, J. M., & O'Brien, B. (1995). Preserving self: From victim, to patient, to disabled person. *Journal of Advanced Nursing, 21,* 886–896. doi:10.1046/j.1365-2648.1995.21050886.x

Janice M. Morse

15

QUALITATIVE STRUCTURED TECHNIQUES

> *Analysis of any kind involves a way of thinking. It refers to the*
> *systematic examination of something to determine its parts, the*
> *relationship among parts and their relationship to the whole.*
> —Spradley (1979, p. 92)

Since the 1960s, as a part of ethnographic fieldwork, cognitive anthropologists have used structured methods of ethnoscience for eliciting lay concepts from participants. Their goal has been to try and find a way to access and describe their participants' worldviews using culturally embedded implicit knowledge. But for our purposes of identifying lay concepts, these techniques provide an excellent way to access concepts used by participants in their everyday discourse and to explicate those lay concepts. These techniques also help us to determine the various forms of a particular lay concept, to identify and delineate reporting of lay concepts (such as symptom reporting), and to move and develop these lay concepts toward scientific use.

Anthropologists use methods of *structured interviewing* to elicit what they call cognitive domains of cultural groups, using linguistic techniques and logical relations between and within classes. These techniques allow for the emic identification of concepts—that is, to identify concepts from the person's perspective, and not from the perspective of the researcher. These strategies form an important set of techniques for the use of researchers who are interested in concept development.

TARGETED STRATEGIES FOR CONCEPT AND ATTRIBUTE DEVELOPMENT

The key, when eliciting the meaning of terms, is not to ask for meaning per se, but to ask for *use* (Spradley, 1979, p. 97). Although we do need to develop definitions as labels in concept development, the definition in itself is inadequate for understanding and is of very limited use in research.

Each concept belongs to a *meaning system,* or a collection of allied concepts. The meaning of any concept is derived from its relationship to these other concepts. Further, we must differentiate between what a concept denotes (i.e., things the concept defines) and what it connotes (refers to over and above their immediate referential meaning). For example, a *lemon* denotes a fruit of a certain color and flavor: That is, the characteristics of the thing in itself. But in the connotative sense, it may refer to something else—that is, a referent that shares a particular characteristic of the lemon, but not all. For instance, it could refer to something sour, bitter; to a color; to something faulty (as, "that car is a lemon"); to the shape of the fruit; and so forth. The referent (the thing that the concept refers to or represents) may be anything, either concrete or symbolic, but what is important is the relationship between the referent and the concept, and the fact that the referent may be using only one or more of the attributes, so it is not an exact replica.

The final way we infer meaning is to examine the parts of the concept or the parts of the whole. Recall that a concept refers to something—and a behavioral concept refers to a collection of behaviors. Techniques of eliciting what the concept refers to, its components, and the relationships between them may be obtained from the use of particular types of structured interviewing techniques. These techniques, such as, "free listing," "semantic relations," "sentence frames," and "20 questions," enable the associations between the concept and its referents, between the parts of the whole, or by identifying and examining its components.

Fieldwork: Identifying a Lay Concept

The process invariably begins with fieldwork. By observing the group, the researcher becomes familiar with the local forms of speech, the participant's "world," and the things that are mutually important to the researcher and to the participants. During the course of these observations, the researcher may stumble across an unfamiliar term, one with which the researcher is unfamiliar, and that warrants further inquiry as the concept of interest. For instance, Spradley (1970), when studying tramps in the Pacific Northwest, became interested in the term "flop" or "making a flop." He was told that "the most important thing to a tramp is something to eat and a place to flop" (pp. 98–99), so that a *flop* was a term that tramps used to refer to the place where they slept. But what exactly is a flop? And how do tramps rate or rank the quality of their flops? This became a significant part of Spradley's (1979) ethnography, describing the lives of urban nomads.

Another example: While doing fieldwork in emergency rooms, Morse noticed that nurses reported patient's condition when asked: "What's his comfort level?" The responses to *comfort level* appeared to be concerning the patient's emotional and behavioral states: Patients were reported to be: "resting comfortably," "really scared," "tolerating it well," and so forth. Yet, although *comfort level* was clearly an important concept used widely for rapid assessment and reporting of stages of relative comfort and discomfort, and was almost universally understood in clinical practice, it was not a concept that was found in nursing texts. That is, comfort level assessments were not formally taught or even acknowledged in the classroom.

Free Lists: Identifying the Domain

At this point, if the concept appears obvious, meaning that it is a term used frequently by the group and is not a one-time specialist word, the researcher may move directly to *free listing*. Free listing is a technique in which the researcher asks participants to list as many examples as possible of a particular term (or concept). These examples provide the researchers with the domain (scope) and variation. For example, you may ask the participant to list freely the words used to describe types of pain; the researcher would record the words, attending to both the accrual word used and the order is which the participants listed it. Using free lists ensures that your domain is developed inductively. Thus, it provides "an extremely useful and powerful tool" (Bernard, 2012, p. 233) for concept identification.

The conceptual domain (or the scope) may be elicited from participants' words, lay concepts, and sentences used in everyday language, that are all in the same level of contrast, using free lists and pile sorts (Bernard, 2012, pp. 233–235). By asking participants to quickly and out loud to list terms enables the concept to be explicated by the participants, and from these lists, examples of the concept, what it is not, and where the boundary lies, may be developed.

The terms selected by the participant are usually at the same level (i.e., they are not components of parts; Weller & Romney, 1988). In other words, asking this question of 10, 20, 30, or more people will give you lists of equivalent terms. Some terms will be offered by many of the participants. Count them and sort them according to the frequency that they are used. Those that occur most frequently are the more common terms, and may be more important, or salient. Some may be mentioned by only one participant, and therefore occur only once. As your sample size increases, so will your list become more stable, and new terms will be less likely to appear (Weller & Romney, 1988).

When compiling a *free list*, the researcher asks the participants: "Name all of the types of_____ that you know?" or "What types of_____ are there?" For instance, Spradley (1970), used free lists, supplemented with interviews, and found that drunks listed almost 100 types of *flops* or places to sleep (pp. 99–104). If we continue our example of comfort levels, we would ask: "Name all of the types of comfort levels that you can think of_____?" and "What types of comfort levels are there?"

These terms, representing examples of your comfort level, provide you with your concept, or what anthropologists call your conceptual domain. The descriptors of terms for types of *comfort level* as listed by 15 nurses as examples of emergency department patients' comfort level are listed by frequency in Table 15.1. Note there are no restrictions on the number of terms a

---

TABLE 15.1
Types of Comfort Levels of Patients in the Emergency Department (Hypothetical Data)

WORD SORTED	n (TIMES LISTED)	WORD SORTED	n (TIMES LISTED)	WORD SORTED	n (TIMES LISTED)
Scared	15	Resting quietly	6	Frightened	1
Anxious	15	In a lot of pain	6	Terrified	1
Frightened	11	Sleeping	5	Jumping off the table	1
Really scared	8	Pain is in control	5	Screaming	1
Holding on	8	More comfortable now	5	Easily roused	1
Relaxed	8	Pretty jumpy	4	Quieted down	1
Crying	7	Scared stiff	4	Not trusting	1
Watching our every move	7	Sobbing his heart out	3	Taking it	1
Hollering	7	Pretty sad	3	Semiconscious	1
Restless	7	Comfortable	3	Not complaining of pain	1
Broken up	7	Complaining	2	Fighting restraints	1
Irritable	7	Asking repetitively about _____	2	No complaints	1
Dozing quietly	7	Out of control	1		

n = 15 participants.

participants may provide—in this hypothetical study, the most terms listed by any one participant were 20.

All of the nurse participants thought that patients' comfort level may be scared, anxious; most thought of frightened patients. The states that are listed less frequently may be patients who are not seen so often, or lesser known terms.

What sorts of concepts are best suited to free listing techniques? Bernard (2012) suggests rich domains, subjects that are not concrete, not taught, not structured. Questions must be carefully considered: For instance, if you were asking about ingredients used to bake a cake, most would respond with flour, sugar, baking powder, eggs, salt, and flavoring (chocolate, lemon, vanilla), and there would be little variation in the responses; but if you were asking flavors of cakes or types of cakes, the variation would increase. We would, for instance, ask for types of cakes and get answers such as Christmas cakes, birthday cakes, sponge cakes, chocolate cakes, pavlova, cream cakes, fruit cakes, and so forth. As most researchers use the technique in areas or topics with which they are not familiar, the answers are always interesting. Hopefully your topic, obtained from 20 or 30 participants, will produce at least 30 items from which you will be able to produce a frequency list.

Guided Interviews

The format of the interviews for identifying folk concepts are somewhat structured, with the researcher planning to ask a few questions, to which the participant may respond freely. For instance, to get more contextual information about comfort levels, the interviewer may ask:

"Tell me about _____" (a particular type of patient).

Then ask, "What is his comfort level?"

"What are the signs that a patient has a _____ comfort level?"

"Describe other patients who have had a _____ comfort level?"

And you may ask: "Is 'comfort level' a term used by nurses, or do you use it when reporting to non-nurses, such as physicians or physical therapists?"

The goal of these guided interviews is to get as much contextual information as possible that will later help you understand, define, and describe the term (in this case, comfort level), to determine appropriate usage, where, when and why it is used, and to what it refers. These interviews are transcribed and analyzed. Categories are developed showing the use of the term, the scope, and the possible attributes. Once this information is obtained, the investigator then moves onto conducting structured interviews, such as semantic relations.

Semantic Relations

Semantic relations are the identification of terms within a language, and the terms with which they are related or linked (Spradley, 1979, pp. 100–101). Research is conducted as follows:

- They are identified by listening carefully when participants talk and when reading the interview text. They may be related to the names of things and occur in a set of two or more in relationship to each other. The concept may be of one of three types of relationships:
  Inclusion: An X is a kind of Y.
  Attribution: An X has Y.
  Sequence: From X comes Y.
- Prepare to interview about the particular concept. Prepare question prompts from an extended list of relationships. The types of semantic relationships and type of questions to be asked to elicit this are as follows:

1. Strict inclusion is asked as: X is a kind of Y?
2. Spatial is asked as: X is a place of Y, Y is a part of X?
3. Cause and effect is asked as: X is a result of Y, X is a cause of Y?
4. Rationale is asked as: X is a reason for doing Y?
5. Location for action is asked as: X is a place for doing Y?
6. Function is asked as: X is used for Y?
7. Means-end is asked as: X is a way to do Y?
8. Sequence is asked as: X is a step (stage) in Y?
9. Attribution is asked as: X is an attribute (characteristic) of Y?

(Spradley, 1979, p. 111)

- Integrate the semantic relations questions into interviews that are in process, rather than asking them as a separate list. For instance, when the term is introduced into the interview, ask the appropriate semantic relation question.
- List the examples of the terms provided, order the parts of the whole, and examine relations between them.

Word Associations

Word associations are primarily fill-in-the-blank questions, used to find out new terms, to seek relationships, and to find what Werner and Schoepfle (1987) call a "response chain." In their example, they use the following: "*A sincere person is a good person. It is only good persons that are capable of sincerity. I would imagine that sincerity is a form of honesty*" (p. 83). From this, the characteristics of the stimulus word "sincerity" are *good person* and *honest*. It may be considered:

Sincerity: is a characteristic of a good person. It is a kind of honesty.

OR

Sincerity: . . . is a kind of honesty.
. . . is an attribute of a good person.

(Werner and Schoepfle, 1987, p. 83)

Such analyses enable the researcher to obtain all possible meanings of a term for consideration, rather than using one meaning too quickly in the analysis.

Think of an Animal

This "game" systematically delineates a domain by comparing two objects within the class. The researcher thinks of a bird (or whatever topic is)—for instance, a kiwi. The participant then thinks of an animal, perhaps a duck, and is asked for a question that separates a kiwi from a duck. For instance, this may be: "Does it fly?" And the answer for the duck is "Yes."

The participant then thinks of another bird—for instance, an emu. The researcher then asks, "Can it fly?" The participant says, "no." "Is it a kiwi? The participant says, "no." Ask: "Then give me a question that separates the kiwi from an emu," and the participant says, "Can it run 30 mph?" and the answer for kiwi is "no."

This game therefore sequentially separates the types of birds (think of them as concepts) by distinguishing features. An online version of the game may be found at: http://rogerfrost.com/animaltree/index.htm.

We could do this with our behavioral states of patients in the emergency department.

Researcher: "I am thinking of a patient who is frightened.
Think of another patient's behavioral state."
Participant: "Scared."
Researcher: "Give me a question that distinguishes a frightened patient from a scared patient."
Participant: "Is the patient jumpy?"
Researcher: "And the answer for scared patient is_____."
Participant: "No."

Card Sorts

The next step is conducting card sorts, that is, asking the participants to categorize the lists, so that relationships between the items may be determined. Make the cards to be sorted by writing each item from the free list on a single index card.[1]

---

[1] Actually, make three sets of cards so that as you move from the dyadic to the triadic, to the free sort, the cards will be ready.

Card Sorts/Q-Sorts

Ask each participant to "sort the cards into piles, putting things that are similar in the same pile." Participants may make as many piles as they wish, but each card may only be put into one pile once (i.e., it cannot be duplicated and placed into two piles). Ask participants to think "out loud" while they are soring the cards, so you can record and elicit information about how they make decisions for card placement. The result is that no two participants will make identical piles; some participants will make a few piles; others will make many. If participants find an item that they do not know or recognize, ask them to put that card aside.

The next step is to interview participants about their selected piles, while audio recording their responses. Ask them: "What do the cards in this pile have in common?" "If you could name this pile, what would it be? And, "How does this pile differ from that pile?"

Finally, record the contents of each pile. Place rubber bands around each pile, so that the contents of each pile maybe recorded later—or read the names of each pile into the recorder. Items are analyzed by listing the cards in order of frequency, combining the responses of all participants.

Triadic Card Sorts

The next step is to give the participant another set of the same cards, and ask him or her to sort them into three piles. This forces the classification of some of the smaller piles, and may break up some of the larger piles. Again, while audio recording, ask the participants what each pile has in common; ask them to compare the piles and tell you why they are different, and to name each pile. Place a rubber band around each pile for later analysis of the piles.

Dyadic Card Sorts

We continue with each participant, with a fresh batch of the same cards, asking the participant to sort them again, this time into two piles. It is important not to give the participants three piles from the last round, and ask them to sort them into two, should they simply combine two piles. Again, record their "thinking aloud" while audio recording, ask the participants what each pile has in common, ask them to compare the piles and tell you why they are different, and to name each pile. Again, place a rubber band around each pile for later recording and analysis of the piles.

Analysis of Piles

List the content of each pile for each participant for each type of card sort. Order the contents by name and frequency (i.e., the number of times sorted in a pile by participants). Create a table of your results.

Next, examine the labels given by participants to each pile. These names provide important thematic clues to the overall content. Some labels will be helpful, and others, obvious and unhelpful (for instance, simply reiteration of a name used on a card in the pile is not helpful). Listen to the recordings of the participants' rationale as they sort the piles, as these recordings provide information about the essential characteristics of the piles. However, the final choice of labels selected for the piles is the prerogative of the researcher.

Contrasting From Card Sorts

The insights obtained from the ways that participants sort cards, and the labels for each pile, are then organized by the researchers into contrasting sets. The relationships between the sets are then explored. Ask yourself: "What are the characteristics of each pile?" "What do they have in common?" And most importantly: "What are their differences?"

Example: Delineation of the Characteristics of Fatigue

An important research program by Karin Olson on the somatic experience of fatigue, delineated the lay concepts of tiredness, fatigue, and exhaustion (Olson, Krawchuk, & Quddusi, 2007), cross-culturally (Graffigna, Vegni, Barello, Olson, & Basio, 2011), in extreme experiences of daily life, such as persons who were shift workers, depressed, athletes, and with chronic fatigue syndrome (CFS; Olson & Morse, 2005); in depression (Porr, Olson, & Hegadoren, 2010), melanoma (Booker, Olson, Pilarski, Noon, & Bahlis, 2009); multiple sclerosis (Smith, Hale, Olson, & Schneiders, 2009), lung and colorectal cancer (Olson et al., 2002), and advanced cancer (Graffigna et al., 2011; Olson et al., 2008). At the same time, Olson investigated the relationship between fatigue and: exercise (Booker et al., 2009; Smith et al., 2009), the quality of life (Booker et al., 2009), and the behavioral and physiological indices of fatigue (Olson et al., 2008). She also developed a model of adaptation/nonadaptation to fatigue (Olson, 2007, 2013).

Olson's initial work identified the characteristics and differences in intensity of tiredness, fatigue, and exhaustion, definitions for each, and the signs of each, using card sorts (Table 15.2). All of the symptoms delineating tiredness and exhaustion from fatigue are symptoms recognized and reported by participants themselves, thereby illustrating the importance of developing lay concepts for linking lay and scientific knowledge—in this case, medical and nursing management of fatigue.

Next, Olson further developed her categories, in a preliminary model, to show the linkages to the individuals' ability to adapt or their inability to adapt (Figure 15.1), so that medical intervention became essential.

Construction of a Taxonomy by Classes

The straightforward example is given below of a taxonomy that sorts classes of "beings" by a few simple and obvious characteristics. But it is an excellent example of the way that categories are delineated using primary characteristics, and these primary characteristics identified and sorted.

TABLE 15.2
Key Domains of Fatigue Developed From Card Sorts

TYPE OF FATIGUE	SLEEP QUALITY	COGNITION	STAMINA	EMOTIONAL REACTIVITY	CONTROL OVER BODILY PROCESSES	SOCIAL INTERACTION
Tiredness	Normal sleep pattern, feels rested	Forgetful	Gradual loss of energy in proportion to energy expended	Impatient	Body and mind work together	Engages in normal social activities
Fatigue	Chronic disrupted sleep pattern, does not feel rested	Inability to concentrate	Gradual loss of energy out of proportion to energy expended	Anxious	Mind over body	Saves energy for participation in enjoyable activities
Exhaustion	Erratic sleep pattern, including periods of insomnia and periods of hypersomnolence	Confusion	Sudden loss of energy out of proportion to energy expended	Emotionally numb	Body over mind	Withdraws from all social activities

Source: Olson (2007). Reprinted with permission.

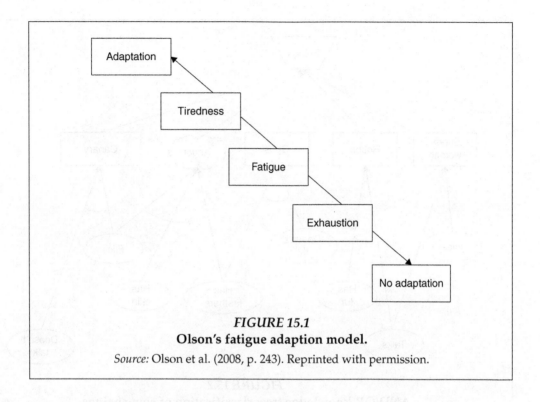

FIGURE 15.1
Olson's fatigue adaption model.
Source: Olson et al. (2008, p. 243). Reprinted with permission.

First, a "rule set" is established, based on inclusion/exclusion criteria (AND/OR) and knowledge developed from the rule set. In this case, the following characteristics were identified as characteristics that delineated one from another. These were: the ability to fly, to talk, the presence of fur, feathers, or skin. The rule set is as follows:

Rule 1: If it flies AND talks, THEN Superwoman
Rule 2: If it talks AND has fur, THEN Hobbs
Rule 3: If doesn't fly AND has feathers, THEN Opus
Rule 4: If has feathers AND has skin AND flies THEN angel
Rule 5: If it Flies AND does not talk THEN canary
                        (Furbee & Benfer, 1994, p. 4)

This classification system may be further diagrammed as a simple taxonomy (Figure 15.2).

Data may also be presented as a decision matrix (Table 15.3), by asking the same questions used on the rule set, and used to produce Figure 15.2.

Example: Sorting by Two Primary Characteristics
It is possible to present data by sorting according to the presence or absence of two primary characteristics, and then identifying the characteristics of those that fill each of the four cells. This technique was described by Glaser (1978) for use in grounded theory. Chassé (1991) provides us with an excellent

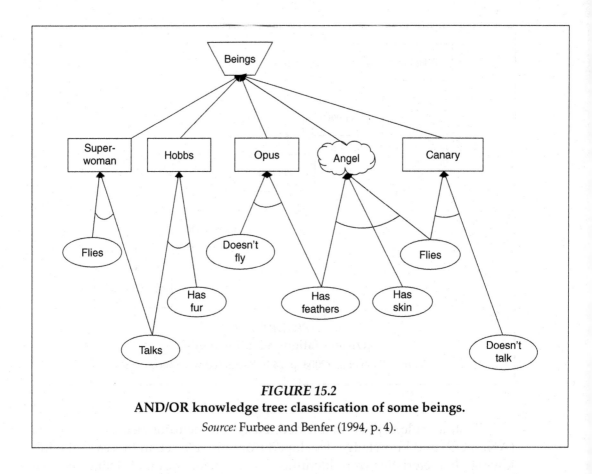

FIGURE 15.2
AND/OR knowledge tree: classification of some beings.
Source: Furbee and Benfer (1994, p. 4).

example in Figure 15.3, when she compares the support for women participants (women who have had a hysterectomy). She considered the accessibility of supportive women (+ = accessible and – = not accessible) with their
husband's recognition of their illness (+ = recognized and – = not recognized).

TABLE 15.3
Decision Matrix of AND/OR Knowledge Tree

	SUPERWOMAN	OPUS	HOBBS	CAT	ANGEL	CANARY
SKIN	Yes	——	——	——	Yes	——
FLIES	Yes	No	——	——	Yes	Yes
FEATHERS	——	Yes	——	——	Yes	Yes
FUR	——	——	Yes	Yes	——	——
TALKS	——	——	Yes	No	——	No

Source: Furbee and Benfer (1994).

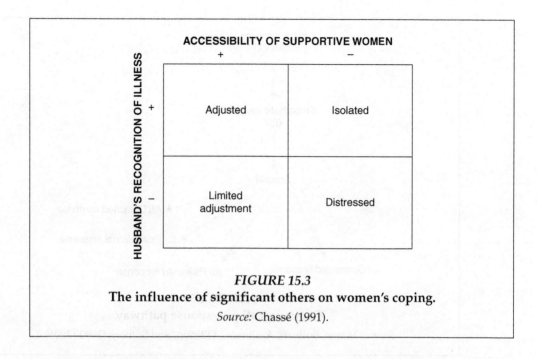

FIGURE 15.3
The influence of significant others on women's coping.
Source: Chassé (1991).

When the husband recognizes his wife's illness, and wife also has accessible, supportive women friends, her participants were adjusted to the surgery; without accessible women, her participants felt isolated. On the other hand if the husband did not recognize the illness, and women participants did have access to supportive women, they had "limited adjustment"; without husband's recognition and supportive women, the participants were distressed.

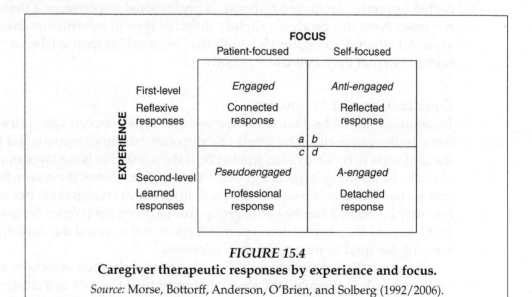

FIGURE 15.4
Caregiver therapeutic responses by experience and focus.
Source: Morse, Bottorff, Anderson, O'Brien, and Solberg (1992/2006).

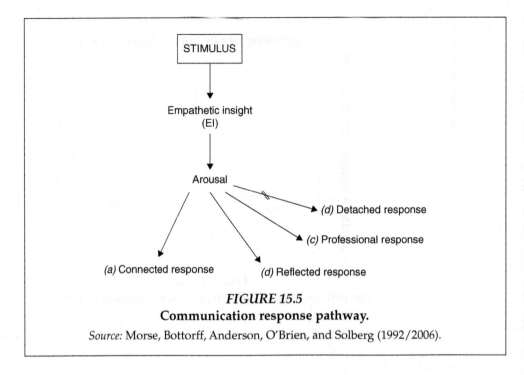

FIGURE 15.5
Communication response pathway.
Source: Morse, Bottorff, Anderson, O'Brien, and Solberg (1992/2006).

The last is another 2 × 2 format, but it allows much more data to be displayed (see Figure 15.4). We are basically using the same data, and this time *examples* of each response are listed in each cell.

Another form of illustrating data is to produce a type of flow diagram (Figure 15.5). This flow chart illustrates the sequence and direction of the response. A stimulus produces empathetic insight into the nurse, who is "aroused" and motivated to respond. The nurse may respond with a connected response, a reflected response, a professional response, or a detached response. Note this produces slightly different type of information from the same data than does Figure 15.3, with the "engaged" response labeled "connected," so that the labels differ slightly.

Construction of a Taxonomy

Taxonomies are tables that show the relationships between categories and items in the categories. The levels of categories are either constructed from the card sorts (free/Q, dyadic, triadic) or, if the researcher has a large number of cards, by splitting large categories into two. This allows the researcher to create a tree structure for each individual, from which an aggregate tree structure may be created for the entire group from a given cut (Weller & Romney, 1988). Record the cards at each split, and again audio record the participants thinking out loud as they make their decisions.

Because all participants will display variation in their selection, rationale, and cards in the piles, the researcher must treat the data as a cluster and

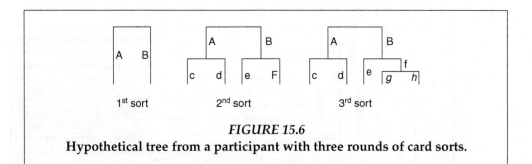

FIGURE 15.6
Hypothetical tree from a participant with three rounds of card sorts.

the relative similarity of data within a cluster, rather than focusing on the relative similarity between clusters. The labels for the piles and the data recorded from the participants thinking while making their selections provide clues to the differences between clusters.

To form a single taxonomic tree, the first cut (i.e., sort) for a single individual may be piles as follows (see Figure 15.6).

First cut: A and B.

Second cut: Sort A into c and d, and B into e and f.

Third cut: Sort cards into *g* and *h*.

Whether or not the researcher decides to continue sorting depends on the size of the pile and the number of apparent variants in the pile. Always record the participants thinking aloud as they sort the cards.

The levels of data sorts are then labeled and placed on the taxonomic grid showing these relationships. The overall label is for the segregate, that is, the category; the next level, subsegregates (or subcategories). The labels chosen for each group are placed the taxonomy, and a full description is provided in the text.

An example of a taxonomy from a study of gifts given to nurses by patients (Morse, 1991a) is in Figure 15.7. Interestingly, gift giving to caregivers is universal, including from patients to nurses, despite hospital administrations' efforts to prohibit such gifts or to redirect the gifts to the hospital foundation. Interviews produced unexpected results: nurses considered gifts not only as presents (a positive), but also considered complaints and even a lawsuit to be a "gift" as in to "give back" as an act or retaliation to equalizing incompetent care or errors. In fact, nurses saw all gifts as equalizing and evaluative of the caregiving relationship. Even the quality of the chocolates given was considered as a message from the patients by nurses—and one that the nurses understood. They considered drugstore chocolates to be ordinary, and given for "usual" care, whereas handmade chocolates were for acknowledging extraordinary care. From these interviews, lists of gifts were developed, and items for the card sorts were derived from these lists.

A taxonomy does not stand on its own, but provides clarity into the meaning of terms and the relationship between the components and

Gifts in the patient–nurse relationship					Item
As beneficiary					Donations to the hospital foundation
As beneficiary					Equipment for the hospital
Serendipitous	Rewards				Spirituality – 'Doing good'
Serendipitous	Rewards				Clinical outcomes (patients condition improves)
Serendipitous	Rewards				Personal growth (insight about self)
Serendipitous	Rewards				Social ('click' with patient)
Serendipitous	Perks				Flowers – left behind by patient
As a perceived obligation	As presents				Seasonal – Christmas, Easter, Valentines Day
As a perceived obligation	As presents	To personally acknowledge nurse			Marriage, birthday, birth of a child
As a perceived obligation	As presents	To personally acknowledge nurse			Career, exams, promotion, graduation
As a perceived obligation	As custom				Ward norm
As a perceived obligation	As custom				Patients cultural norm
To manipulate	To coerce	To change patient-nurse relationship			Invitation to dinner, proposals
To manipulate	To coerce	To change patient-nurse relationship			Overtures to become 'part of the family'
To manipulate	To coerce	To change patient-nurse relationship			Suggestive gifts – lingerie, perfume
To manipulate	To coerce	To obtain privilege			Gift given, later followed by request
To manipulate	To coerce	As advocate			Beg, complain, explain, reiterate, moan
To manipulate	To ensure care				Bribes-$$
To manipulate	To ensure care				Chocolates (individual – on locker)
To manipulate	To ensure care	To reinforce continuance of care	Direct		Chocolates/sweets (individual – on locker)
To manipulate	To ensure care	To reinforce continuance of care	Direct		Tips, gifts of cash
To manipulate	To ensure care	To reinforce continuance of care	Direct		Cajole, false compliments
To manipulate	To ensure care	To reinforce continuance of care	Indirect		Thanks, smiles, praise and waives
To manipulate	To ensure care	To reinforce continuance of care	Indirect		For unit (all staff share)
To manipulate	To ensure care	To reinforce continuance of care	Indirect		For nurse's kids
To reciprocate	As atonement	From family			Food – donuts, cakes, cookies and chocolates
To reciprocate	As atonement	From patient			Gifts from hospital canteen
To reciprocate	As atonement	From patient			Verbal apology, note, card
To reciprocate	As atonement	From patient			Gifts made in occupational therapy
To reciprocate	Of gratitude	At the end of the relationship	Connected nurse–patient relationship		Complete trust
To reciprocate	Of gratitude	At the end of the relationship	Connected nurse–patient relationship		Significant, personal gifts
To reciprocate	Of gratitude	At the end of the relationship	Normal nurse–patient relationship		Flowers, chocolates
To reciprocate	Of gratitude	At the end of the relationship	Normal nurse–patient relationship		Thanks, cards, letters
To reciprocate	Of gratitude	In the midst of the relationship	Celebrate milestones		Party food – cake, pizza
To reciprocate	Of gratitude	In the midst of the relationship	Appreciation		Something admired by nurse
To reciprocate	Of gratitude	In the midst of the relationship	Appreciation		Something made by patient
To reciprocate	Of gratitude	In the midst of the relationship	Nurturance		Give sympathy, withhold requests
To reciprocate	Of gratitude	In the midst of the relationship	Nurturance		Chocolates
To reciprocate	Retaliation	Nurse controlled clinical relationship			Withhold gifts, thanks
To reciprocate	Retaliation	Nurse controlled clinical relationship			Letters of complaint, sabotage
To reciprocate	Retaliation	Incompetence			Sue

FIGURE 15.7

Types of gifts in the patient–nurse relationship.

Source: Morse (1991a).

subcomponents when analyzing lay concepts or anthropological domains. Along with the description accompanying the taxonomy, it makes the study exceedingly rich, providing conceptual clarity and contextual information.

SUMMARY

Structural techniques of interviewing allow the researchers access to *lay* concepts—especially to those that are relatively uncommon and arise in the course of fieldwork or interviews. They enable the delineation of the concept and the identification of the boundaries and provide techniques to identify the components by eliciting examples. These may then be used to facilitate the construction of the attributes and to become actually all it means and understand its use.

TO DO 15.1. PRACTICING CLASSIFICATION

1. Create a decision matrix for the following types of balls:

Basketball	Golf ball
Football	Baseball
Tennis ball	Ice hockey puck

2. Redraw your classification as a knowledge tree diagram.

3. Find a friend who is interested in a sport or a musical instrument that you know little about. In an unstructured interview, ask them to explain the sport to you. Identify some concepts that you have not heard before.
    Develop sematic relation questions to develop the concept as much as you can.

4. To develop an understanding of the construction of taxonomies, play "think of an animal" (http://rogerfrost.com/animaltree/index.htm).

REFERENCES

Bernard, H. R. (2012). *Research methods in anthropology: Qualitative and quantaitive approaches.* Lanham, MD: Altamira.

Booker, R., Olson, K., Pilarski, L. M., Noon, J. P., & Bahlis, N. J. (2009). The relationships among physiologic variables, quality of life, and fatigue in patients with multiple myeloma. *Oncology Nursing Forum, 36*(2), 209–216. doi:10.1188/09.ONF.209-216

Chassé, M. A. (1991). The experience of women having a hysterectomy. In J. Morse & J. Johnson (Ed.), *The illness experience: Dimensions of suffering* (pp. 89–139). Newbury Park, CA: Sage.

Furbee, L., & Benfer, R. A. (1994). A beginning guide to expert systems: 2. Implicit knowledge. *CAM: Field Methods, 6*(3), 3–4.

Glaser, B. G. (1978). *Theoretical sensitivity.* Mill Creek, CA: Sociology Press.

Graffigna, G., Vegni, E., Barello, S., Olson, K., & Basio, C. A. (2011). Studying the social construction of cancer-related fatigue experience: The heuristic value of ethnoscience. *Patient Education and Counseling, 82,* 402–409. doi:10.1016/j.pec.2010.12.017

Morse, J. M. (1991a). The structure and function of gift-giving in the patient–nurse relationship. *Western Journal of Nursing Research, 13,* 597–615.

Morse, J. M., Bottorff, J., Anderson, G., O'Brien, B., & Solberg, S. (1992/2006). Beyond empathy. Expanding expressions of caring. *Journal of Advanced Nursing, 17,* 809–821. (Reprinted, *53*(1), 75–87)

Olson, K. (2007). A new way of thinking about fatigue: A reconceptualization. *Oncology Nursing Forum, 34*(1), 93–99. doi:10.1188/07.ONF.93-99

Olson, K. (2013). Learning about the nature of fatigue. In C. T. Beck (Ed.), *Routledge international handbook of qualitative research* (pp. 64–74). New York, NY: Routledge.

Olson, K., Krawchuk, A., & Quddusi, T. (2007). Fatigue in individuals with advanced cancer in active treatment and palliative settings. *Cancer Nursing, 30*(4), E1–E10.

Olson, K., & Morse, J. M. (2005). Delineating the concept of fatigue using a pragmatic utility approach. In J. R. Cutcliffe & H. P. McKenna (Eds.), *The essential concepts of nursing* (pp. 1141–1160). London, UK: Churchill Livingston.

Olson, K., Tom, B., Hewitt, J., Whittingham, J., Buchanan, L., & Canton, G. (2002). Evolving routines: Preventing fatigue associated with lung and colorectal cancer. *Qualitative Health Research, 12*(5), 655–670. doi:10.1177/104973202129120160

Olson, K., Turner, A. R., Courneya, K. S., Field, C., Man, G., Cree, M., & Hanson, J. (2008). Possible links between behavioral and physiological indices of tiredness, fatigue, and exhaustion in advanced cancer. *Support Care Cancer, 16,* 241–249.

Porr, C., Olson, K., & Hegadoren, K. (2010). Tiredness, fatigue and exhaustion in the context of a major depressive disorder. *Qualitative Health Research, 20*(10), 1315–1326.

Smith, C., Hale, L., Olson, K., Schneiders, A. G. (2009). How does exercise influence fatigue in people with multiple sclerosis? *Disability and Rehabilitation, 31*(9), 685–692. doi:10.1080/09638280802273473

Spradley, J. P. (1979). *The ethnographic interview.* New York, NY: Holt, Rinehart, Winston.

Spradley, J. P. (1970). *You owe yourself a drunk: An ethnography of urban nomads.* Boston, MA: Little, Brown.

Think of an animal. Retrieved from http://www.learninggamesforkids.com/animal_and_nature_games/randomals/animal-twenty-questions.html

Weller, S. C., & Romney, A. K. (1988). *Systematic data collection (qualitative research methods, Volume 10).* Newbury Park, CA: Sage.

Werner, O., & Schoepfle, G. M. (1987). *Systematic Fieldwork: Ethnographic analysis and data management, Vol 2.* Newbury Park, CA: Sage.

THE PROTOTYPICAL METHOD

Q: How many people of a certain classification
does it take to screw in a lightbulb?
A: More than one.

Recall the definition of a *behavioral* concept: It is a representation of a collection of behaviors that have been given a name.

It is the shared agreement of these labels and what they represent that enables communication. However, reality is messy, and we often find that behavioral concepts are a poor fit, and sometimes there is no concept label for what we are interested in. In these instances, we communicate using description, analogies, metaphors, and so forth. On the other hand, we may find several concepts fitting, or competing for, the same phenomena, or, alternatively, a range of phenomena or examples fitting the same concept label (Figure 16.1a and 16.1b). In these cases it is important to determine the actual differences between the concepts or the phenomena. (These techniques are discussed when we need to compare concepts in Chapter 19.) Importantly, sometimes we find a situation or phenomenon that fits the concept label exactly—a perfect exemplar (Figure 16.1c). It is this last type of exemplar that we analyze in the first part of the prototypical method for concept development.

THE PROTOTYPICAL METHOD

What level of concept is most suited for analysis or development using the prototypical method? The best are lay concepts that are well established in the lexicon but have not been well developed. Their definition in the literature may be clear, but the attributes have not been identified. In the literature,

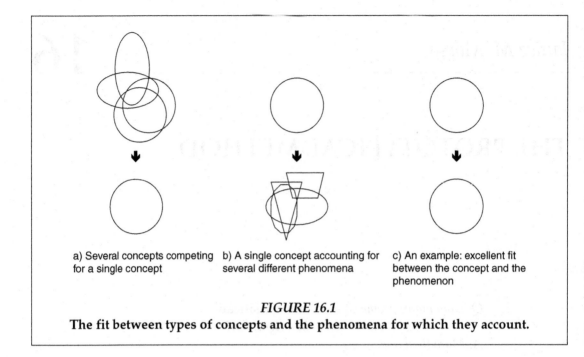

a) Several concepts competing for a single concept

b) A single concept accounting for several different phenomena

c) An example: excellent fit between the concept and the phenomenon

FIGURE 16.1
The fit between types of concepts and the phenomena for which they account.

there may be some descriptive qualitative studies available, and even some quantitative, but these studies are not explanatory—they do not help us understand the nature of the concept. Thus, the concept that you are interested in may be classified as being in the upper level of immature, bordering on partially mature. It may be commonly used, and even considered important in nursing care.

As we learned from our analysis of compathy, once a concept is identified, it is easy to see it everywhere. The concept suddenly appears obvious or commonplace.

Using the Prototypical Method

The prototypical method of concept identification and development consists of two stages: (a) an inductive phase, the identification and analysis of the exemplar and the concept, and (b) a deductive phase, exploring the presence of the concept in other situations, of confirmation of the concept as a concept.

Phase 1: The Identification and Analysis of the Exemplar

The prototypical analysis usually starts with the investigator's analysis in a particular concept, followed by a rather frustrating and unfruitful literature review. Then, in desperation, the investigator may find a documentary movie or a short biographical story that seems to be an excellent example of the phenomenon of interest. If it is a story presented as an oral history, one should be certain to audiotape it, as the story must be in a form suitable for analysis. Remember, this is your primary data for developing the concept.

Next, listen carefully to the story or watch the video several times. Make notes on the course of events and the nature of the phenomena. You must be able to sort out the dross—the irrelevant incidents or events—from those events associated with the concept. Some early important features will be those that set up the concept, that is, the preconditions. Strong characteristics are probably attributes; weaker characteristics may also be attributes, but are those that are not dominant in this form of the concept. Alternatively, they may be attributes that are shared with allied concepts. Or, they may even be just noise, coincidental events that may be disregarded.[1]

If your story is complete (i.e., not an ongoing episode), events that occur at the end of the story are probably outcomes. Spend time examining these outcomes, and the transition or boundary that just precedes the outcome.

Now develop the attributes. These events/incidents or descriptive features should be described as cleanly as possible. Preferably, give them a name that is not too colloquial—that is, select a label that is general and descriptive, and is possibly a concept name that is already used in the literature. Do not choose an emic label; that is, one that uses the words of the participants, for these are too local. Remember you are developing a concept and contributing to the literature. These labels will, hopefully, be used by others.

Delineating the Concept

Next, work on the attributes. Write a description of each and select a reasonable name for each. Each must be distinct from the names from other concepts. Usually, the attributes all may co-occur and are not ordered—that is, one occurring before another. If an attribute does precede another (i.e., is sequenced), you will find that you are developing a model, albeit primitive.

Phase 2: Exploring the Presence of the Concept in Other Situations

At this point you have developed a concept from a single case. It is possible that your concept is *right*, but we must ensure that is it correct and generalizable, and not some local phenomenon.

The first step is to find other sources of data that may be used to confirm the attributes. In the example of hope (that follows in this chapter), it used other data sets—data collected for other purposes, but in which hope was likely to be present. Examine these sets of data using your knowledge about the concepts deductively. Look for the attributes—are they all present? Does the description hold?

---

[1] How long does it take a nurse to change a light bulb?

One should note that concepts appear in different forms in different contexts—later in the chapter we discuss different types of hope. Each type of hope has all of the attributes, but in some forms of hope some attributes are stronger, more dominant, than others, and others are weaker. They are still present, but have been backgrounded. And this pattern varies with the type of hope. Therefore, in your data, some of the variations that you see may be from different forms of the concept, but it is still the same concept. In the hope example, we have diagrammed the different forms of hope.

Near the boundaries, the concept becomes weaker, as it interfaces with allied concepts. Look to see where the boundaries are: When the concept no longer becomes an example of the phenomenon, that is the point where the boundary lies.[2]

Finally, check the antecedents and the consequences. Do the conditions to setting up the concept and the outcomes still hold?

And one final step: Visit the library and check that the concept you have just delineated has not been developed by someone else. If it has, check for similarities and dissimilarities. Look at their context; check their definitions. If their conceptualization is very close to yours, adopt their terms. They identified it first; so acknowledge that. As it is highly unlikely that their concept description will be exactly the same as yours, yes, you have done original work, and will be acknowledged for it. But do make it simple for the rest of the world, and link your findings with theirs.

THE CASE OF HOPE[3]

In the early 1990s much had been written about hope, but the literature was not clear: hope, as a concept, had not yet been delineated. Although hope was defined in the dictionary, the attributes were not explicated. We needed to identify the antecedents and we needed to identify the outcomes. Neither had the boundaries been identified. Importantly, we wanted to know if the many forms of hope were pertaining to one malleable concept as the strengths of attributes changed, or to many allied concepts that appeared as the patient's condition changed or as the prognosis was confirmed.

Research Context

Some years earlier, I worked with a student, Sharon Laskiwski, to conduct an ethnography in a spinal cord unit exploring the role of hope in the early stages of a spinal cord injury. From those data, we documented the changing nature of hope—this was the first study that viewed hope as a dynamic concept, capable of changing form as the phenomenon changes—in this case, the

---

[2] ANS: 15 seconds to change it; 30 seconds to chart it.

[3] *Source:* Morse and Doberneck (1995), reprinted with permission.

prognosis of the spinal cord patient changed as the injury was assessed and realized in the days following injury (Laskiwski & Morse, 1993).

At this time, why was hope to be considered a phenomenon and not a concept? As noted, hope was defined in the dictionary, but was poorly developed, and had not reached the developmental stage of a concept. Hope was considered an *emotion,* a collection of behaviors that roughly occurred together, but these emotions or behaviors had not been described in detail and had not been delineated. In the research presented in this section, we first described hope in detail (Laskiwski & Morse, 1993) and then developed the attributes of the concept of hope (Morse & Doberneck, 1995) using the *prototypical method of concept development.* Once completed, and recognizing that the types of hope were a single concept, we used these attributes to develop an assessment guide, so that clinicians could support or modify the development of hope (Penrod & Morse, 1997). This is described later in Chapter 23. Later in the research program, we linked hope to emotional suffering (Morse & Penrod, 1999) in the process of developing the mid-range theory, the *Praxis Theory of Suffering* (Morse, 2001, 2011), described in Chapter 35. Such was the usefulness of the concept to the progression of the research program.

But we are getting ahead of ourselves.

The first descriptive study of hope showed that hope was a malleable concept, changing over time. All parties involved with the patient who had a spinal cord injury—the patient, the family members, and the staff—changed what they were hoping for, very quickly, as they received and were able to accept new information (Laskiwski & Morse, 1993, p. 152).

But such a descriptive study is only the beginning. To develop *hope* as a concept, we need to identify a context and a phenomenon that will lead to hope (the precursors or antecedents of hope), conditions of which we may be reasonably certain.

TO DO 16.1. TAKE A BREAK/STOP AND THINK

Look at the different types of hope (Table 16.1). Each has a different form, yet they all have the same attributes.

Now think of other types of hope: I will get you started: how about "High hopes." Does the concept definition hold? Are all the attributes present?

Can you diagram "high hopes?"

TO DO 16.2. WATCH A MOVIE

How about *My Left Foot?* (Brown, 1989). Christy Brown's mother is listening to her son practicing his speech lessons. She worries: "There is too much hope in his voice."

What does she mean by "too much hope?" Why is an excess of hope a cause for concern?

Now, this is important: Hope apparently may be valued as good or desirable, or bad or harmful. Therefore, as it depends on context, the value that is placed on hope as good or bad is *not* an attribute.

TO DO 16.3. THE STRENGTH OF CONCEPTS

Is "hopeless" or "without hope" a form of the concept hope? If you answer *yes*, discuss the attributes. Are they present and weak? Or not present? Alternatively, if you think "without hope" is not a type of hope, what is it? And why is it called hope?

The strength of the concepts is important. Building on to the hope example, we can put some types of hope on a continuum from absent/weak to excessive.

Finish this series for me: *Hopeless; a glimmer of hope; . . .*

TO DO 16.4. BUILDING A CONCEPT BY SEQUENTIAL CITATIONS

Conduct a literature search using *hope* and *concept* as key words. Look at the development of the concept from 1997—or 1990—to the present time. Consider citation streams (who cites whom?) and the development refinement of the concept of hope both as a concept and as a theory to the present time.

Phase 1: The Identification and Analysis of the Exemplar on Hope

One night I watched a 2-hour documentary, *Snowbound: The Jim and Jennifer Stolpa Story* (Rintels, 1994). This was a made-for-television movie about the plight of a young couple and their infant, who were lost in the Rocky Mountains in a blizzard; it portrayed their story of survival. This documentary become the exemplar of hope—the prototypical example—an example that made one think: "Well, if this is not about hope, then nothing is!"

So, we have a context and phenomenon in which our concept of interest would be highly likely to occur: the context was a blizzard in the Rocky Mountains; the focus was a family travelling across the Rockies; the phenomenon was becoming snowbound and lost, and our concept of interest was hope.

When commencing concept development with a single exemplar, it *must* be an excellent exemplar: the attributes of hope must be so clear that they are easily identified. Now, some may accuse you of using a biased sample, and they would be right. Your example *must be biased*, so that you can easily see the components (attributes) of hope. Later in the process, we will verify our findings in other data sets, but right now our task is to carefully watch the documentary—and watch it again and again, if necessary—to document the components of hope behaviors used in such a desperate situation: being lost in a blizzard.

Essential in the development of hope as a concept is the fact that in order to hope, you must have something to hope *for*. If you have something to hope for, you must also have something to *hope against*. You must be able to develop a plan to reach your hoped-for goal (Morse & Doberneck, 1995, p. 278).

Now let us see how Jim and Jennifer are faring with their hope. First, they realized their predicament—and this predicament is the antecedent of hope.

Next they developed a plan for walking out of the mountains, determined the route (cutting over the mountain versus walking 18 miles down the road), and prepared their clothing to prevent frostbite and a sleeping bag to carry and keep their child warm. Therefore the first attribute is:

> *The envisioning of alternatives and the setting of goals.* In this
> phase, the individual "scans" to determine all possible solu-
> tions **or** ways out of the predicament. (Morse & Doberneck,
> 1995, p. 278)

Notice that the attribute is not cluttered with details of Jim and Jennifer, or being lost in the snow, but could be applied to any situation involving hope.

The second attribute pertains to what is being hoped against, and building in the possibility that they would not succeed. Jim and Jennifer also prepared for the worst: they left a note in their car to their families, in case they did not make it out. They wrote what happened to them, telling family how much they loved them, and where their ashes should be spread. Therefore:

> *A bracing for negative outcomes* is the next attribute. Because the
> assessment of the negative outcome is realistic, negative out-
> comes are not ignored. Rather, the individual may consider a
> negative outcome a real possibility but one that is *hoped* will not
> occur. It is the fear of a negative outcome that provides a moti-
> vating force for individual action and makes hope powerful.
> (Morse & Doberneck, 1995, p. 278)

Third, Jim and Jennifer evaluated their odds. They were fit and well, had army survival training, had sleeping bags and warm clothing. At the same time, they realized that frostbite was a real possibility, that their infant was particularly vulnerable, and that although Jennifer's breastfeeding was a plus, they did not know how far they had to go, or how long her lactation would last:

> *A realistic assessment of personal resources and of external conditions
> and resources.* The individual(s) recognizes that a negative out-
> come is a real possibility, and because of this does not "play
> games" or set oneself up for failure by being overly optimistic.
> Thus, the assessment of one's resources for solving the problem
> is reality-based and fair. (Morse & Doberneck, 1995, p. 278)

People who are hoping surround themselves with those who support what they are hoping for and avoid those who are negative. Jennifer supported Jim's decision to walk out. Notice that when one of them had doubts about the decision to walk out, the other bolstered and supported the one with doubts, hence alleviating those concerns.

> *The solicitation of mutually supportive relationships.* Hoping is an
> *active process*, and the family actively seeks out supportive rela-
> tionships. The selected plans devised to achieve the goal are
> discussed and mutually agreed upon. One's relationship with
> one's family, or persons providing support, is "balanced."
> When one member is down, the others bolster and reinforce
> that person's hopes. Rarely are all members of the family
> "down" and experiencing doubts about the feasibility of the
> goal at the same time. (Morse & Doberneck, 1995, p. 278)

Jennifer and Jim continuously looked for signs—any signs—that they had made the right decision to leave their vehicle. They looked to the mountain ridge and thought they saw lights of a town on the other side, and decided to cut over the mountain. They even used a shooting star as a good omen: encouraged them and helped them fight fatigue.

> *The continuous evaluation for signs that reinforce the selected*
> *goals.* The seeking of signs that will indicate these individuals
> have made the correct choice is an ongoing procedure,
> and often the signs sought are superstitious signs. However,
> the continual process of evaluation and modification of
> strategies used to reach the goal may result in the modification
> of the means selected to reach the goal or the modification
> and compromise of the goal itself. (Morse & Doberneck, 1995,
> p. 278)

Did they compromise their goals? Yes: when Jenifer was too tired to go further, Jim found a cave for Jennifer and the baby to shelter. He marked with a "flag" (using his shirt on a stick) and walked back down the mountain, then miles down the road until he met a ranger.

Most evident throughout was Jim and Jennifer's determination to endure—for themselves, their infant, their families, and future life. Even when rescued, Jim recognized that he could not let go—he had to assist in telling the rangers where Jennifer and the baby were.

> *A determination to endure.* The maintenance of hope requires
> focused energy to get through the situation and to reach
> the goal (Morse & Doberneck, 1995, p. 278).

TO DO 16.5. THE PROS AND CONS OF USING DOCUMENTARIES AS DATA

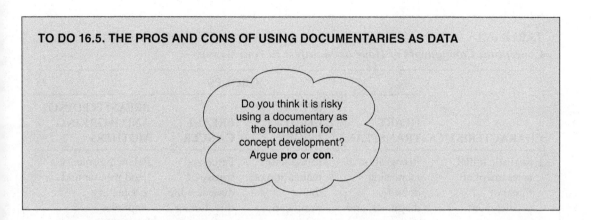

Do you think it is risky using a documentary as the foundation for concept development? Argue **pro** or **con**.

Phase 2: Exploring the Presence of the Concept in Other Situations

Next, because the attributes were identified from a case study of one exemplar, we needed to verify that the attributes were correct. We needed to be certain that we had not missed anything. We needed to be certain that we had not seen something that did not fit and listed it as an attribute only to find that it was associated with Jennifer and Jim's particular experience rather than the concept of hope. This step, identifying and examining the attributes, also lets us determine if the attributes are different (hope is many concepts) or the same (types of hope are one concept).

From previous studies we have many data sets. We selected four of these in which the process of hope was likely, and obtained institutional review board (IRB) approval to reanalyze these data. Importantly, we had not collected these data to examine hope, so we felt that these data were valid: with the exception of one, they were not collected with the participants having been set up to talk about hope. These data were:

- Interviews with seven patients waiting for heart transplantation, interviews with post-transplant patients, and with two nurses and 11 physician's assistants from the transplant team
- Interviews with eight spinal cord injured patients from a previous study on hope (Laskiwski & Morse, 1993)
- Interviews with five women who were breast cancer survivors (18 months–20 years)
- Breastfeeding mothers ($n = 15$) who were maintaining lactation and returning to work

Examine these data for each group by attribute. Do you think all attributes are present for all types of hope? How do they, within their particular context, meet the criteria for each attribute? Examine Table 16.1 carefully.

TABLE 16.1

Conceptual Components of Hope as Manifest in Four Groups

CHARACTERISTICS	GROUPS			
	HEART TRANSPLANT	SPINAL CORD INJURY	BREAST CANCER	BREASTFEEDING AND WORKING MOTHERS
1. Realistic initial assessment of threat or predicament.	Recognition of increasing debility, diagnosis, and prognosis— transplant or death.	Immediate realization of the ramifications of injury = permanent paralysis.	Perceived course of disease = life-threatening and "treatment" involving incapacitating side effects.	Balancing roles of a good mother and satisfactory employee = impossible dilemmas.
2. The envisioning of alternatives and setting of goals.	Envisioning death was unacceptable. Transplant viewed as the key to a "normal life."	Alternatives were to work for small gains and life skills or become completely dependent.	Alternatives were to choose physical deformity for long-term survival or a shortened life.	Envisioned all possible problems and made contingency plans and backup plans for the contingency plans.
3. Bracing for negative outcomes.	Prepared by focusing on the positive as a means to "beat the odds."	Prepared for the increasing probability that mobility would not improve.	Prepared for coping with the onslaught of treatment side effects, and bad news about spread of the disease.	Prepared to wean infant if it refused the breast but not because of lactation problems.
4. A realistic assessment of personal resources and external conditions/ resources.	Sought competent "state-of-the-art" medical care. Recognized need for psychological support.	Recognized dependence on others and constant need for assistance. Planned modifications to home.	Explored options and solicited support and commitment from family.	Used past experience and experience of others. Developed complex schedules involving partner, sitters, and work schedules.
5. The solicitation of mutually supportive relationships.	Primarily obtained from former transplant patients, hospital staff, and family.	Other spinal cord injury patients and often spouses or boy/ girlfriends.	Support groups, spouses, friends, or other family members.	Sought support from other breastfeeding mothers, spouses, or La Leche League.

(continued)

TABLE 16.1
Conceptual Components of Hope as Manifest in Four Groups (continued)

		GROUPS		
CHARACTERISTICS	HEART TRANSPLANT	SPINAL CORD INJURY	BREAST CANCER	BREASTFEEDING AND WORKING MOTHERS
6. The continuous evaluation for signs that reinforce the selected goals.	Solicited positive survival stories. Watchfully waited for the heart.	Focused on tiny physical gains.	Constantly assessed for signs of recurrence.	Constantly evaluated how baby thrived and level of contentment.
7. A determination to endure.	Desperate. Transplant considered the *only* way to achieving a normal life.	The greater the determination, the greater the progress.	Endured in smaller frames by setting attainable events as milestones.	Determined to do what is best for baby.

Source: Morse and Doberneck (1995). Reprinted with permission.

Although the value of looking for similarities is important, so is looking for differences, and these are also presented in Table 16.1. From the differences, that is, from the different strengths of the attributes in each context or situation, we can then identify the emic labels for the types of hope in each situation. The different patterns (types) of hope are diagrammed in Figure 16.2(a–d).

Hoping for a chance (Figure 16.2a), heart transplant patients realize that they had only "one shot" for what they hoped for. The alternative, dying, was not an option. They focused on their goal and tried to maximize their chances for the hoped-for goal.

Mothers who were breastfeeding and hoping to maintain their lactation when they returned to work used hope to formulate plans and backup plans and backup plans for the backup plans. That enabled them to identify a variety of caregivers that they may use if necessary, so they could go to work if the baby was ill. This we called *provisional hope*. For instance, they planned, *if* baby was sick and it was Monday, then maybe dad could stay home, or the baby could go to her mother's. If it was Tuesday, her neighbor can watch the baby and so forth. We have indicated these various alternate decision points with an asterisk in Figure 16.2b.

An example of *hoping against hope* is long-term survivors of breast cancer (Figure 16.2c). These women would go for a checkup hoping everything would be clear, and perhaps the doctor would find a new node. They

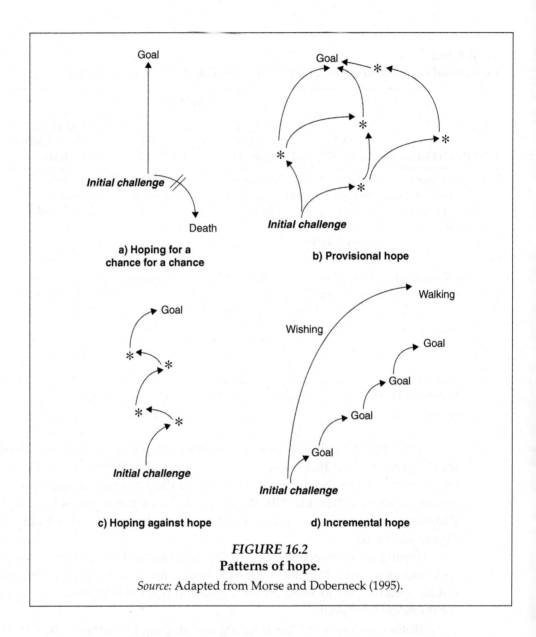

FIGURE 16.2
Patterns of hope.
Source: Adapted from Morse and Doberneck (1995).

would then hope that the node was negative, that it was localized, and so forth, so that their hope changed constantly with the new diagnostic procedures.[4]

An example of *incremental hope* was the rehabilitation of spinal cord injured patients (Figure 16.2d). These patients would hope for a small advance, perhaps to move one finger, then hope to move several fingers, then hope to be able to hold a spoon, and so forth. In this figure, we have illustrated the difference between hoping and wishing: Hope is something that is always worked toward; wishing is not. Consider the case of walking: the

---

[4] Is there a difference between wishing for an A and hoping for an A?

spinal cord patient may work toward walking in incremental steps as he or she progressed. But if he or she wishes to walk, it would be a distant goal—or even a dream.

Variation in the form of a concept occurs with variation in the strength of some of the concepts. All of the attributes of hope are present in every example of hope, but these attributes occur in different strengths, are paced differently, and this gives rise to the various patterns or types of hope. Can you extend this list?

TO DO 16.6. IDENTIFY TYPES OF HOPE

High hopes
False Hopes
A glimmer of hope
Hopeless
No-Hoper
Hoping against hope
Daring to hope

SUMMARY

Concept identification using the prototypical method is for relatively undeveloped concepts for which the literature does not provide an adequate example of the concept per se. But, on the other hand, the lay concept is used frequently enough to find an exemplar that fits one's conceptualization of the concept exactly. This exemplar is used to identify the components of the concept, and then, in the second stage to explore these components in other data sets or exemplars to verify the concept and its components.

REFERENCES

Laskiwski, S., & Morse, J. M. (1993). The spinal cord injured patient: The modification of hope and expressions of despair. *Canadian Journal of Rehabilitation, 6*(3), 143–153.

Morse, J. M. (2001). Toward a Praxis Theory of Suffering. *Advances in Nursing Science, 24*(1), 47–59.

Morse, J. M. (2011). The Praxis Theory of Suffering. In J. B. Butts & K. L. Rich (Eds.), *Philosophies and theories in advanced nursing practice* (pp. 569–602). Sudbury, MA: Jones & Bartlett.

Morse, J. M., & Doberneck, B. M. (1995). Delineating the concept of hope. *Image: Journal of Nursing Scholarship, 27*(4), 277–285.

Morse, J. M., & Penrod, J. (1999). Linking concepts of enduring, suffering, and hope. *Image: Journal of Nursing Scholarship, 31*(2), 145–150.

Pearson, N. (Producer), & Sheridan, J. (Director), (1989). *My left foot* [Motion picture]. United States: Mirimax.

Penrod, J., & Morse, J. M. (1997). Strategies for assessing and fostering hope: The hope assessment guide. *Oncology Nurses Forum, 24*(6), 1055–1063.

Rintels, J. (1994) *Snowbound: The Jim and Jennifer Stolpa Story.* Los Angeles, CA: Jaffe/Bronstein Films.

SECTION IV

PARTIALLY DEVELOPED CONCEPTS

*I'm sure we all agree that we ought to love one another, and I know
there are people in the world who do not love their fellow human
beings—and I hate people like that!*
                    Tom Lehrer (1965), for National Brotherhood Week

*Thank you, Tom Lehrer! Your song is a perfect example of conceptual confusion, of the
inconsistencies we find in everyday language. In this section, I demonstrate techniques to
finding the more subtle discrepancies, incongruities, confusions, divergences, and even holes
in everyday concepts. And we address the topic of confusions about scientific concepts,
including concept drift.*

CONCEPT CLARIFICATION: THE USE OF PRAGMATIC UTILITY[1]

> *Words . . . should be discarded as soon as they begin to conceal what they ought to illuminate. Our terminology should be flexible in order to bring more and more human experience into the range of our theory.*
> —Goldenburg (1990, p. 215)

Concepts are dynamic. As our world changes and develops, so do concepts emerge, change, and develop. Consider how many concepts have developed with the coming of the digital age—with cell phones, computers, and online music, books, movies, and information.

In order to understand concepts pertinent to nursing practice and research, it is helpful to examine how they have been used and developed in nursing research. At least it seems to be an approach that would please the Wizard (Coté, 2005, p. 167), for concepts are by their very nature subjective, created perspectives of reality, which are shared and that allow us to communicate. If we can determine what everyone agrees on, what they *are*, and *what they represent*, then we are one step closer to developing the theoretical basis of nursing. In Chapter 12, we discussed how to elicit lay concepts that are implicit and undeveloped, but nevertheless a part of our reality. Here, we start one level above this, examining concepts that are partially developed, and that have been used in research and discussed in our literature. Using the concept of caring as an example, we explore *how* various authors have used this lay concept, how they defined it, and considered its scope and its attributes. If there is some variation in its presentation and use, we examine the agreements and disagreements about the concept, and the different assumptions and perspectives as presented in the literature.

[1] Portions of this chapter have been previously published in Morse, J. M. (2000). Exploring pragmatic utility: Concept analysis by critically appraising the literature. In. B. Rodgers & K. Knafl (Eds.), *Concept development in nursing.* (pp. 333–352). Philadelphia, PA: W.B. Saunders Co. Reprinted with permission.

Recall this method of analysis is for *lay* concepts, not scientific concepts: there should be agreement about scientific concepts, and their components clearly presented when they were introduced. As they have, by definition, been introduced into research as mature concepts, there is no reason to conduct a concept analysis or be concerned with concept development.

However, the fact that a concept may not be developed to the state of maturity does not deter researchers from using the concept in research. In fact, in qualitative inquiry, where the goal is to develop theory and concepts, concept maturity is not often reached, even as an outcome of the study. In quantitative inquiry, where the majority of the major concepts used are scientific concepts, lay concepts, with all their limitations, are also used. Rarely however, are immature lay concepts used in quantitative research, although we do find them in qualitative inquiry.

Therefore, the goal of pragmatic utility is the development of *partially mature* concepts by using the literature as data. Pragmatic utility is a meta-analytic technique that, rather than synthesizing the literature, moves inquiry forward by examining or appraising the way the lay concept has been *used* by other researchers and authors in their publications. When conducting pragmatic utility, the researcher systematically examines the definitions, attributes, and uses of partially mature concepts as described by each author, and *asks analytic questions* about the components of authors' conceptualizations of the concept, then comparing, contrasting, and synthesizing that data. In this way, the researcher may identify the implied and the explicit assumptions, overt and inferred meanings, and implicit and explicit conceptual components. Thus, the commonalities and the differences of the use of the lay concept may be identified, the different perspectives or usages of the lay concept described, and the degree to which the lay concept has been operationalized can be determined.

Note that pragmatic utility is mainly used for lay concepts, for eliciting hidden meanings. The technique may not be very useful for scientific concepts, as scientific concepts have been purposefully developed, and should in the process of development be published as a mature concept, so that there is nothing "hidden" to reveal. But there is an exception: sometimes scientific concepts, as they are used in research by various researchers, are subtly, consciously, or unconsciously changed, and these changes become significant, yet remain covert. In Chapter 19, we discuss one such example, social support, and Hupcey's (1998a, 1998b) analysis of the changes that occurred over time.

Pragmatic utility is not a literature review, in which all of the research pertaining to a particular topic is summarized. It differs from a critical analysis, in which the researcher criticizes or challenges the ideas of other authors. It differs from a research review or critique, in which the researcher synthesizes the major contributions to research in a particular area and attempts to identify what is known and where the gaps in the research are or to identify the next logical step, hypotheses, or research questions to be tackled in order to continue inquiry. And it is more than a meta-analysis, in which the perspectives of various authors are synthesized and compared, and even a new model created.

Using procedures that differ from other types of literature summaries and syntheses, pragmatic utility is a method that explores concepts as determined by critically appraising the literature and the role they play in inquiry. Pragmatic utility provides a method to compare attributes of a concept suggested by various authors, to elicit the underlying assumptions of their perspectives, to identify the attributes of the concept, and its application or use in practice. Pragmatic utility may be used to compare, to clarify, or to develop lay concepts (Morse, 2000). It may be used to explore various forms of a particular concept or the relationship of a concept to its allied or competing concepts. It is an important method that moves knowledge forward.

PROCEDURES: DOING PRAGMATIC UTILITY

Pragmatic utility represents serious scholarship, with lots of hard thinking. It has been criticized for the amount of work it entails, for the lack of clear guidelines, for the open-ended nature of the literature search, and for the lack of a clear end goal (Weaver & Mitcham, 2008). I address these criticisms as I describe the process and procedures. Certainly, pragmatic utility is not a trivial technique, but with concentrated effort, it can be accomplished in a semester, and the results sometimes result in seminal contributions (Paley, 2002).

Why does the method not include fieldwork (or a combination of analyzing the literature and fieldwork) as does the hybrid model of concept development (Schwartz-Barcott & Kim, 2000) and recommended by Fawcett (2008a)? Because pragmatic utility is used for partially mature concepts, some published research about the concept of interest is available, and this research contains descriptive data from qualitative fieldwork—interviews and observations. Therefore, some knowledge that may be gained from conducting fieldwork should be available in the literature, so let us use it, reflect on it, synthesize it, and analyze it. Fieldwork is appropriate for the identification and analysis of immature concepts, when the literature is not available or scarce, as we discussed in Chapter 13.

Be Clear About the Purpose of the Inquiry

Doing concept analysis as a class exercise is not an adequate reason for using pragmatic utility. Rather, the purpose of your inquiry will direct your approach, determine the way the literature is segregated, and guide the types of analytic questions you will be asking. While it appears simple, doing concept analysis

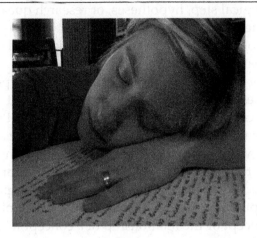

FIGURE 17.1
The essence of analysis is actively asking analytic questions.

is actually hard work! (see Figure 17.1). Granted, at the very beginning, before you have delved into the literature, you may not be very clear exactly *why* you are doing it. But some good reasons for using pragmatic utility are:

- *Concept development:* To develop the conceptual structure, identify and clarify the attributes
- *Concept clarification:* To identify types of concepts, according to the strength of the attributes present in each type; to clarify the concept as it is used by various authors or schools
- *Concept delineation:* To delineate a concept from allied or competing concepts
- *Concept comparison:* To compare two or more allied concepts that account for a particular phenomenon
- *Concept correction:* To explore and to "correct" concept drift in scientific concepts

Each of these goals may be attained using pragmatic utility and be reflected in your research question. As with all research, it begins with a research question. This question arises from your open inquiring attitude as you read about the concept:

- Think—Is there consensus within the literature about the definition of the concept? Do definitions vary from article to article?
- Are definitions missing or not stated? How are they implied?

- Is the concept used in the same way in each study and is it used consistently from study to study, and from situation to situation?
- Is the concept used consistently among different disciplines?

Note that while your question about a concept arises from a curiosity present at the beginning of the study, it may be reconceptualized in the process of reading the copious literature available on the topic. Indeed, you may not have been aware of the specifics or the problems or strengths in the concept before delving into the literature.

Be careful not to combine too many questions or purposes in one study. Each time data are "split," the amount of data in each category is further reduced, and introduces a problem of *thin data* or an inadequate number of articles (data) available for analysis in each category. Moreover, your analysis may become confusing if you try to do too much at once.

The Research Question Dictates The Organization of Data

Researchers must always be aware of their rationale for asking a research question, and they should be able to see the project through to the expected completion (results) and be aware of the type of results that they intend to obtain. This is essential—research is not an exercise of fumbling in the dark, but there is a fine line between knowing what you are looking for, and violating the principles of induction. Always keep your research questions and your goal in mind, so that you do not become completely lost in your data.

The rationale for conducting the study remains a constant reminder of the overall desired goals. For instance, you may be interested in different *disciplinary perspectives* on the concept. Whereas the conceptual attributes remain the same, the various disciplinary contexts emphasize different attributes and de-emphasize others, resulting in different forms of the concept. Similarly, as authors or major schools of inquiry tend to cluster in disciplines (or even within disciplines, institutions, or geographic areas), the analysis may cluster by major contributors or researchers who tend to use the same conceptual definitions. Occasionally, one or two authors will have made significant contributions, and therefore, it may be pertinent to the research goals to sort the concept by definition: for example, to sort *stress* by articles using Selye's (1976) definition versus "others." Often such an excellent definition becomes influential, is cited (and used) frequently, and developed into a "school" of thought.

Another question that may be of interest to researchers, and influence design, is by method. By *method*, I do not mean research method (as in *qualitative method*), but rather how the concept is researched and described, for exploring this provides insight into how the concept or phenomenon has been perceived. For example, the phenomenon of nurses' ability to assess the patient's condition without the patient verbalizing complaints has been accounted for by the concepts of intuition, inference, sublimation, empathy, and insight (Morse, Miles, Clark, & Doberneck, 1994). Consider *how* the phenomena were researched: With each concept, did the researcher obtain information about the concepts by *interviewing* nurses or *observing* nurses assessing patients to describe the concepts used? Did the researcher interview nurses about unsuccessful as well as successful incidents when exploring nurses' insights? As discussed later, these five concepts all have distinct attributes, and using different methods to examine the same phenomenon sheds light on how such concepts are perceived.

Identifying a Partially Mature Lay Concept

In order to achieve the interpretative and descriptive goals of pragmatic utility, you must have:

- Identified a *partially* mature lay concept
- Adequate pertinent literature

Identifying a *concept of interest* is the easy part. Because concepts are all around us in our personal and professional lives, students often come up with a concept that they are passionate about. Or they come with a list of scientific concepts, thinking that lay concepts are not relevant to our profession.

As previously mentioned, because scientific concepts are created in the course of science and the operational definitions and attributes are described in the course of development, all of the components are published at the time. The concept is introduced. Therefore it would be a waste of our time to "analyze" these concepts to identify the attributes, because we should simply be able to look them up. Yet many students make that mistake: we find concept analyses of scientific concepts, such as *health promotion*, *public health*, and so forth. Therefore, if you are unsure about the status of your concept, the first task is to determine whether your concept is a scientific or a lay concept.

Usually the type of concept you have is obvious—lay concepts are derived from everyday terms. But occasionally this may be difficult: Recall that some scientific concepts are adopted into the lay lexicon and vice versa. Therefore, if you are uncertain, follow the concept back in the literature to see when it was introduced. This is often done by *citation tracking*, by tracing citations back from article to article, to the first citation and then its original source. (For instance, *compliance* was introduced into the medical literature in 1955 [Greene, 2004].) If you suspect that the scientific concept has drifted from its original description, you may be able to conduct an interesting analysis of that drift (e.g., see Hupcey's analysis of social support [Hupcey, 1998a, 1998b; Chapter 19]). If you find that a lay concept has subsequently been adopted and described as a scientific concept, then consider it a scientific concept, clear and concise—and select another concept, a lay concept.

Identifying Concept Maturity

Assessment for concept maturity has been explained in Chapter 11, so this section is just a reminder. To determine the concept's level of maturity, first ask: *Is the concept used consistently across the discipline?* Then, examine its origin and the pragmatic, linguistic, logical, and epistemological principles. If lay concepts are "undeveloped," and used in nursing practice but have not been used in research, they may appear only in the clinical, descriptive literature. If this is the case, use qualitative methods to develop the concept, rather than pragmatic utility, for you need rich description to understand what the concept represents. If there is a lot of literature, clear and concise, then the concept is probably mature. In this case, select another concept, using pragmatic utility. If it is a scientific concept, select another lay concept.

Examine your concept to consider the level of development and the anatomy of the concept:

- To identify the boundaries, ask: *What are the preconditions and the outcomes of the concept?*
- To identify boundaries and allied concepts, ask: *What other concepts occur with the concept?*
- To identify the attributes, ask: *Are the characteristics of the concept clearly and succinctly described?*
- To identify the context, ask: *When, where, with whom, and how is the concept used?*

Do you have a partially mature concept? Great! Move to identifying the literature, which will be used as your data.

Identifying Adequate and Pertinent Literature

Having adequate and appropriate literature is essential to ensure that your analysis is probably right. Adequate and appropriate literature, with enough variation to enable comprehensiveness, ensures that the scope of the lay concept is complete. But this is only the beginning. Identifying the literature is not enough—you have to read the literature carefully and in a particular way, and attend to sorting and coding these data, asking critical questions, and developing a summary chart.

Having adequate and appropriate literature means having enough studies—a large pile of articles to analyze: Remember that this is your data source. Also remember that you are analyzing the concept *per se*, so do not select studies from one specific area, and that the final results must be decontextualized. If, for example, your concept is *vigilance*, but you are actually interested in nurse vigilance for the prevention of patient falls, at this stage of the inquiry, *do not* restrict your search to vigilance as it is only associated with "falls." Rather, your first task is to learn about the concept of vigilance and select all reports on vigilance in nursing, regardless of the topic in which vigilance was applied.

How much literature is adequate? You would like me to give you a number? Guessing, I could recommend that you need at least 30 studies, preferably 60 studies but of course, I have no idea. The number of articles needed depends on the quality of description about the concept, the level of development, the scope and level of abstractness, the variation within the concept, and what is known about the concept.

The basic principle is that you must have enough literature to provide an in-depth description. These studies may have been conducted in one context, yet, if your goal is to develop the concept for *nursing* beyond the limitations of one specialty, then you will have to look further. To ensure that your concept will be *well scoped*, you will need adequate literature from all areas. You do not restrict your search to research articles—you should also include clinical descriptions and philosophical essays, if available. Include classical research even if they are not from nursing. For instance if you have selected *stigma*, be certain that you include Goffman's (1963) seminal work, for the basic structure of the concept may not have changed, and the 5- or 10-year expiration embargo that we place on literature searches for clinical topics does not apply. One can usually identify the major sources by looking at citation rates for articles, or by hand searching the bibliographies to see which articles are generally cited. If you have identified only a few articles, unless those few articles are rich and theoretically comprehensive, your sample will be inadequate.

Develop and Use a System for Classifying and Maintaining Bibliographic Records

The amount of literature identified—as a simple count of the number of articles—should be large, and it needs to be large if you are using this method of concept analysis. But it is easy to lose track of citations with this method. An automatic bibliographic referencing system will be useful, but tag all pieces of data, so you know where they came from and so that they may be correctly cited.

Getting Inside the Literature

Copy the whole of each article, not just the abstract. As you are reading each article, pay particular attention to (and highlight) any definitions of the term (and any attribution for the term), the study's research question, and any assumptions listed. Consider exploration of the concept within a "school of thought," and if possible, organize the articles according to underlying assumptions or how similar concept definitions are used or who cites whom. If working in teams, at this point, each member may be responsible for analyzing the literature from a particular perspective.

In examining conceptual components in the literature, Weaver developed a tracking system (see Figure 17.2) for each major citation (Weaver & Morse, 2006). This system expedited the examination of the concept, the identification of incomplete and competing definitions, overlapping boundaries, and allied concepts. Of course, it does not shortcut the process of detailed reading of the articles and recognizing important phrases and components, but it makes your research process transparent.

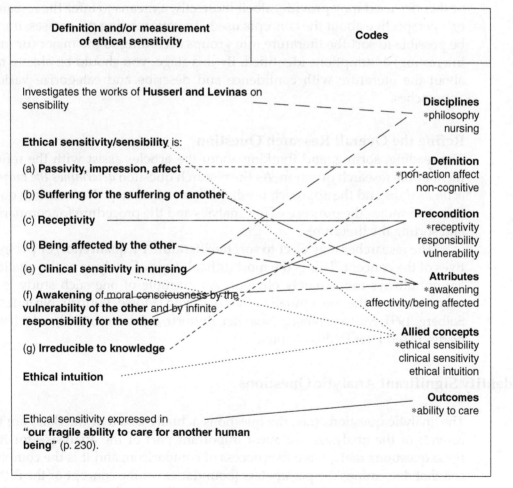

FIGURE 17.2

Coding showing linkages between articles and categories.

Reprinted with permission from Weaver and Morse (2006).

Read Interpretatively Behind the Text

If the attributes are not presented clearly in an article, it may be necessary for you to seek out, identify, and record assumptions used in the articles. The assumptions or author's perspectives may be "hidden" as assumptions, and may be inferred from: (a) the research question(s) asked in the study, (b) identifying the researcher's focus or "bias," or (c) from the general content of the article, such as, analyzing the variables used in the article or examining the items listed in the instruments used. When examining the items used in questionnaires, ask:

Why did the authors ask this particular question?

What perspective does this question represent? (Warning, beware of miscoding reversed items!)

Recall that research is not value-free, and the author's bias, perspective, or theories used may provide, albeit indirectly, a means to infer the researcher's perspective about the concepts used. As your reading progresses, it may be possible to sort the literature into groups according to the major (or most interesting) assumptions identified. By this stage, you should be able to talk about the literature with confidence and describe and categorize various approaches.

Refine the Overall Research Question

The reading, sorting, and thinking about the articles assist with the refinement of the research question. As the research question *determines the purpose of the analysis* and the approach used, this is a critical step. The research question determines the purpose of the analysis and the procedure for comparing and sorting the literature.

The researcher may elect to sort the literature by quality(ies) or perspectives of the concept. This is the most difficult type of analysis as the qualities are not always immediately obvious. An example of one such study is an examination of the conceptualizations of caring (Morse, Bottorff, Neander, & Solberg, 1991; Morse, Solberg, Neander, Bottorff, & Johnson, 1990), which will be discussed later in this chapter.

Identify Significant Analytic Questions

The analytic questions (i.e., the questions actually asked of the data) are the essence of the analysis—the most important part of the analysis—for it is these questions that enable the process of comparison; and it is the comparison that determines the parameters (boundaries) of the concept or the differences between perceptions of the concept or differences in the attributes when comparing concepts. I cannot emphasize enough that these questions, which come from a deep understanding of the literature, are the most significant contribution to the analysis and the strength of your study.

Analytic questions are developed from the interpretative reading of the data (i.e., the literature) and placed on the data summary charts. The strength of the analysis depends on identifying significant questions, and these questions are derived from your interpretative analysis of major articles. They can only be identified once the researcher is familiar with the literature. Until the researcher has an excellent grasp on the concept and its components and has looked at the literature critically, he or she will not be able to identify questions that may be asked of all conceptual dimensions.

Some of the analytic questions used by Weaver to elicit the nature of ethical sensitivity, the ethical requirements for praxis, and to prepare the professional for practice (Weaver & Morse, 2006, p. 203) were:

- Is ethical sensitivity applied in all practice situations or just in particular ones?
- Does ethical sensitivity have an anticipatory function or does it emerge only within ongoing dilemmas?
- Are there variations in types of ethical sensitivity?
- Does the nature of ethical sensitivity change with the level of involvement (e.g., as observer or actor) in the situation?
- Is ethical sensitivity innate or acquired?
- What is the relationship between technical competency and ethical sensitivity?
- Is ethical sensitivity discipline-specific (e.g., could a physician recognize ethical content in an accounting situation)?
- What personal and interpersonal characteristics are required for developing ethical sensitivity in professional and interdisciplinary praxis?
- Do employing organizations foster ethical sensitivity?
- Assuming that ethical sensitivity or at least some aspect of it can be taught or learned, what, if any, strategies best prepare professionals to develop ethical sensitivity?

Asking these questions across major authors, difference in use, in perspective, and in application will provide important insights into the concept.

Record Responses on a Data Collection Sheet

Set the "stage" so you can see the whole: This is the key to developing an adequate means and appreciating the dimensions of difference. Seeing the whole matrix allows the researcher to ask analytic questions across dimensions and identify commonalities and differences.

Prepare a worksheet by taking a roll of art paper and cutting a sheet the size of your tabletop (or by taping large sheets of paper together so that they cover a tabletop). This is large, at least 4 by 8 feet. With a long ruler, construct a matrix, with the analytic questions in the left column and the selected dimensions across the top. Draw in the columns and complete the matrix. Questions answered appropriately may minimally have "Yes," "No," or "Exceptions," the names of the first author, and the bibliographic number of the article written in the cells. Occasionally the best quotation—or most represented summary, or notes—may be written in the cell for comparison of authors and for future reference. Or the analytic question may demand that the description be listed in the cell—again with the citation number of the article.

Because you cannot view the whole matrix at once on the screen, there is a distinct *dis*advantage to using a computer for recording responses to comparative analytic questions. Even if the matrix is relatively complete, it will require much printing and taping of pages together to form the complete sheet. My recommendation for this task is to use a pencil and paper; more specifically, obtain a very large sheet of paper and draw multiple columns and cells.

One word of warning: It is important not to consider the cells or categories as rigid or inflexible, and do not make value judgments about the appropriateness or inappropriateness of the derivations of the conceptualization. Using cells to identify dimensions is merely an analytic tool, and the process of abbreviating and separating necessarily simplifies, perhaps unfairly separating the statements from the context of the article as a whole. But it is a technique that enables the identification of differences and makes the process of analysis exciting, interesting, and possible.

If working as a team, *divide the task into cohesive areas within each topic and allocate tasks accordingly.* Making a team member responsible for distinct areas within the topic enables analytic questions to be asked within the context of team meetings by comparing and contrasting areas. For example, if the analysis of the topic is by comparing disciplines, each member of the team may be responsible for the literature in one or two disciplines; if it is by perspectives within the topic (as with the caring example presented next), each member may be responsible for one of the emerging categories. The adage "many heads are better than one" is true in this context, especially if you are working with a multidisciplinary team. The different theoretical bases, or insights, of each team member stimulate a greater variety of questions, which, in turn, moves the analysis along more quickly and results in a richer, more comprehensive product. Initially, the answers to questions may be abbreviated on the chart, with the chart "fleshed out" and completed at a later time.

Synthesize Results

Once the analysis has been completed, the researchers must then compare cells and perspectives, and synthesize the findings to accurately report the results. Look at each set of responses on your chart, and summarize those findings in a few sentences or paragraphs. You may need to cull them down further when you begin writing, but at this point, keep it comprehensive. In addition, as you write, make comparative notes and paragraphs about the in-between—about the comparison and differences between perspectives. If necessary, make figure(s) to show the relationship between perspectives, or between attributes and the concept as a whole.

Make the important aspect of your large worksheet into a table, for insertion into your manuscript. Publication requirements may limit the size of your table, and this will force further synthesis, so consider your emerging groups—let us call them categories—carefully. Because you primarily write about your tables in your article, make certain that you work with them until they are in final form, before you start writing your text.

Writing

The first step in writing your manuscript, always, is to outline the article and insert the tables or figures into your outline in the proper place. One needs to be creative about the best way to present data from so many authors on a single table or figure, giving consideration to the format of the journal to which the completed article will be submitted. Occasionally, your article will exceed the number of references that a journal editor will permit and will allow space for only the major references. Negotiate for a full bibliographic list to be included with the article, perhaps on a linked website. If this fails, include a footnote inviting readers to e-mail the senior author for the complete bibliographic list. If it is essential for attribution, a coding system may be developed to identify the primary author for each citation.

When writing the article, it is important to maintain a balanced and fair perspective. Be certain to point out *new findings* and points that reinforce the status quo. Above all, be clear; contrast and explain facts in detail so that your reader does not struggle to follow you or to seek out your point.

REFERENCES

Côté, D. (2005). *Wicked the Grimmerie*. New York, NY: Hyperion.

Fawcett, J. (2008a). Advancing development of nursing theory: An innovative approach. *Journal of Advanced Nursing, 63*(5), 429. doi:10.1111/j.1365-2648.2008.04766.x

Goffman, E. (1963). *Stigma: Notes on a spoiled identity*. New York, NY: Simon & Schuster.

Goldenburg, N. R. (1990). *Returning to words of flesh: Feminism, psychoanalysis and the resurrection of the body*. Boston, MA: Beacon.

Greene, J. A. (2004). 2002 Roy Porter memorial prize essay: Therapeutic infidelities: "Noncompliance" enters the medical literature, 1955–1975. *Social History of Medicine, 17*(3), 327–343.

Hupcey, J. E. (1998a). Social support: Assessing conceptual coherence. *Qualitative Heath Research, 8*, 304–318.

Hupcey, J. E. (1998b). Clarifying the social support theory-research linkage. *Journal of Advanced Nursing, 27*, 1231–1241.

Morse, J. M. (2000). Exploring pragmatic utility: Concept analysis by critically appraising the literature. In. B. Rodgers & K. Knafl (Eds.), *Concept development in nursing* (pp. 333–352). Philadelphia, PA: W. B. Saunders.

Morse, J. M., Bottorff, J., Neander, W., & Solberg, S. (1991). Comparative analysis of the conceptualizations and theories of caring. *Image: Journal of Nursing Scholarship, 23*(2), 119–126.

Morse, J. M., Miles, M. W., Clark, D. A., & Doberneck, B. M. (1994). "Sensing" patient needs exploring concepts of nursing insight and receptivity used in nursing assessment. *Scholarly Inquiry for Nursing Practice, 8*(3), 233–254.

Morse, J. M., Solberg, S. M., Neander, W. L., Bottorff, J. L., & Johnson, J. L. (1990). Concepts of caring and caring as a concept. *Advances in Nursing Science, 13*, 1–14.

Paley, J. (2002). Benner's remnants: Culture, tradition and everyday understanding. *Journal of Advanced Nursing, 38*(6), 566–573.

Schwartz-Barcott, D., & Kim, S. (2000). An expansion and elaboration of the hybrid model of concept development. In B. L. Rodgers & K. A. Knafl (Eds.), *Concept development in nursing: Foundation, techniques and applications* (2nd ed., pp. 107–133). Philadelphia, PA: W. B. Sanders.

Selye, H. (1976). *The stress of life*. Boston, MA: Butterworths.

Weaver, K., & Mitcham, C. (2008). Nursing concept analysis in North America: State of the art. *Nursing Philosophy, 9*(3), 180–189.

Weaver, K., & Morse, J. M. (2006). Using Pragmatic Utility to analyze the concept of ethical sensitivity. *Research and Theory in Nursing Practice, 20*(3), 191–214.

Janice M. Morse

18

RESEARCH USING PRAGMATIC UTILITY

> *Researchers who disagree about facts will often use concepts in different ways, rightly so. After all concepts are not designed to "fit" the facts as researchers see them . . . if vagueness and ambiguity cannot be avoided, they must be brought out into the open whenever that is possible, to prevent necessary confusion.*
>
> —Wim J. van der Steen (1993, p. 11)

Pragmatic utility is a meta-analytic and interpretative technique for eliciting the complex meanings within concepts. This means two things. First, because it is a meta-analytic technique, it uses a large amount of data. By this I mean a quantity of good professional theoretical and research articles, and because many people have used the concept that you are studying, it must fit the criteria for partially mature or mature. Second, because it uses interpretative methods of inquiry, it provides new insights, new perspective, and new understanding of the concept(s) being explored. In other words, it is an activity worth doing, as it provides understanding and insights that moves the field along—which is what research is all about.

Other authors say it is hard; they say that when doing pragmatic utility it is difficult to follow from instructions available (Weaver & Mitcham, 2008). I hope the additional information in this book corrects that shortcoming. Others whisper that the process is exhausting, but finishing is exhilarating. And others complain that it gives them a headache. Nothing comes easy. At graduate school you are paying to learn to think.

EXAMPLE I: CONCEPT CLARIFICATION INSIDE A CONCEPT: THE CONCEPTUALIZATIONS OF CARING AND CARING AS A CONCEPT[1]

The problem, in 1990, was that the concept of caring was elusive and confusing. Beyond the obvious dual definitions of caring as an action (to care for) and caring as an affect (a feeling of endearment), there was no consensus in nursing regarding a definition of caring, nor the components of care, nor the process or the outcomes of caring.[2] There was no discussion, debate, or even comment in the literature on the lack of clarity or differences in perspectives between authors. For instance, *care, caring,* and *nursing* care were used interchangeably. Although *care* or *caring* may specify the actions performed, as "to take care of" or to exhibit concern, as in "to care about," these differences in meaning were ignored. Morse and her colleagues argued that if caring was to be retained as the "essence of nursing" and if research was to advance as a caring profession, then caring as a concept must be clarified and the strengths and limitations of the conceptualizations identified (Morse, Bottorff, Neander, & Solberg, 1991; Morse, Solberg, Neander, Bottorff, & Johnson, 1990). The purpose of this research therefore, was in the area of *concept clarification,* using the method of pragmatic utility.

Literature as Data

The major nurse theorists and researchers who had authored articles on caring were identified, and their literature carefully read and coded. Major references included in the analysis are listed in Box 18.1.

BOX 18.1. CITATION OF CARING LITERATURE INCLUDED IN THE CARING ANALYSIS

Benner, P. (1984). *From novice to expert.* Menlo Park: Addison Wesley.

Benner, P., & Wrubel, J. (1989). *The primacy of caring: Stress and coping in health and illness.* Menlo Park, CA: Addison Wesley.

Benaira, Z. (1990). Book review [Review of *The primacy of caring: Stress and coping in health and illness*]. *Social Science and Medicine, 30,* 517–519.

Bevis, E. O. (1981). Caring: A life force. In M. M. Leininger (Ed.), *Caring: An essential human need. Proceedings of Three National Caring Conferences* (pp. 49–59). Thorofare, NJ: Slack.

Brody, J. K. (1988). Virtue ethics, caring and nursing. *Scholarly Inquiry for Nursing Practice: An International Journal, 2,* 87–101.

Brown, L. (1986). The experiences of care: Patient perspectives. *Topics in Clinical Nursing, 8,* 56–62.

Dunlop, M. J. (1986). Is a science of caring possible? *Journal of Advanced Nursing, 11,* 661–670.

---

[1] Acknowledgments. Reprinted with permission from Morse, Solberg, Neander, Bottorff, and Johnson (1990) and Morse, Bottorff, Neander, and Solberg (1991).

[2] Do you think caring is the essence of nursing? Argue!

Fanslow, J. (1987). Compassionate nursing care: Is it a lost art? *Journal of Practical Nursing, 37*(2), 40–43.

Forrest, D. (1989). The experience of caring. *Journal of Advanced Nursing, 14*, 815–823.

Fry, F. T. (1989). Toward a theory of nursing ethics. *Advances in Nursing Science, 11*(4), 422.

Gadow, S. A. (1985). *Nurse and patient: The caring relationships.* In A. H. Bishop & J. R. Scudder (Eds.), *Caring, curing, coping* (pp. 31–43). Birmingham: University of Alabama Press.

Gaut, D. A. (1986). Evaluating caring competencies in nursing. *Topics in Clinical Nursing, 8,* 77–83.

Gendron, D. (1988). *The expressive form of caring.* Toronto: University of Toronto.

Griffin, A. P. (1980). Philosophy and nursing. *Journal of Advanced Nursing, 5*, 261–272.

Griffin, A. P. (1983). A philosophical analysis of caring in nursing. *Journal of Advanced Nursing, 8*, 261–272.

Horner, S. (1988). Intersubjective presence in a caring model. In *Caring and nursing explorations in the feminist perspective.* (pp. 166–180). Denver, Co: Center for Human Caring, University of Colorado Health Sciences Centre.

Kahn, D. L. & Steeves, R. H. (1988). Caring and practice: Construction of the nurse's world. *Scholarly Inquiry for Nursing Practice, 2,* 201–216.

Knowlden, V. (1988). Nurse caring as constructed knowledge. In *Caring and nursing explorations in the feminist perspective.* (pp. 318–339). Denver, Co: Center for Human Caring, University of Colorado Health Sciences Centre.

Larson, P. J. (1984). Important nurse caring behaviors perceived by patients with cancer. *Oncology Nursing Forum, 11*(6), 46–50.

Leininger, M. M. (1981). The phenomenon of caring: Importance, research questions and theoretical considerations. In M. M. Leininger (Ed.), *Caring: An essential human need* (p. 316). Thorofare, NJ: Charles B. Slack.

Leininger, M. M. (1988). Leininger's theory of nursing: Cultural care diversity and universality. *Nursing Science Quarterly, 1*, 152–160.

Lundh, U., Soder, M., & Waerness, K. (1988). Nursing theories: A critical view. *IMAGE: Journal of Nursing Scholarship, 20*, 36–40.

McFarlane, J. (1976). A charter for caring. *Journal of Advanced Nursing, 1,* 187–196.

Orem, D. E. (1985). *Nursing concepts of practice.* Chevy Chase, MD: McGraw-Hill.

Ray, M. A. (1989). The theory of bureaucratic caring for nursing practice in the organizational culture. *Nursing Administration Quarterly, 13*(2), 31–42.

Roach, M. S. (1987). *The human act of caring: A blueprint for health professions.* Toronto: Canadian Hospital Association.

Swanson-Kauffman, K. (1988). Caring needs of women who miscarried. In M. Leininger (Ed.), *Care discovery and uses in clinical and community nursing* (pp. 55–70). Detroit, MI: Wayne State University Press.

Watson, J. (1988a). *Nursing: Human science and human care: A theory of nursing.* New York, NY: National League for Nursing.

Watson, J. (1988b). Response to caring and practice: Construction of the nurse's world. *Scholarly Inquiry for Nursing Practice: An International Journal, 2*, 217–221.

Weiss, C. J. (1988). Model to discover, validate, and use care in nursing. In M. M. Leininger (Ed.), *Care: Discovery and uses in clinical and community nursing* (pp. 139–149). Detroit, MI: Wayne State University Press.

Wolf, Z. R. (1986). The caring concept and nurse identified caring behaviors. *Topics in Clinical Nursing, 8*, 84–93.

Note: Although some of these authors may have updated or revised their stance on caring and therefore not agree with the way they are categorized here, this section is presented to illustrate the methods of pragmatic utility.

Definitions of caring were delineated and analyzed. Content analysis of 25 of these definitions revealed five different perspectives on the nature of caring, not according to the major focus of the theory, but rather according to the basis from which the perspective was derived. When caring was not explicitly defined, theoretic perspectives were identified and classified from examination of research approaches and their underlying assumptions. For example, Stevenson (1990) reviewed the quantitative literature and sampled all nursing articles that used *care* in the title, thus implying that care is inherent in all nursing procedures. On the other hand, Aamodt (1994) explored care from the patient's perspective, implying that care is a concept that is reflected in nursing behaviors and is recognizable by the patient. When the conceptualization of caring was described as a process, the explicit or implied linkages are shown on arrows (see Figure 18.1). For example, Forrest (1989) and Fanslow (1987) view caring as an affect, do not consider outcomes, and therefore their perspective remains within the *affect* category. These categories are not intended as rigid or inflexible sales, nor is any value judgment intended as to the appropriateness or inappropriateness of the derivations of the conceptualizations. They are merely identified to clarify aspects inherent in the complexity of the literature rather than to imply causal relationships.

The five categories of caring identified were caring as a human trait, caring as a moral imperative or ideal, caring as an affect, caring as an interpersonal relationship, and caring as a therapeutic intervention. In addition to these, two outcomes that were identified were: caring as the subject of experience of the patient and caring as a physical response. In each case, the decision to classify a different definition was based on the theorist's epistemological perspective. If the theorist viewed caring as a process and described the means and outcome of caring, or the changing nature of the caring relationship, then pathways linked these categories (as shown in Figure 18.1). For example, Leininger (1978, 1981a, 1981b, 1984a, 1984b, 1988, 1995, 2002) reiterates that humans are caring beings and that caring is a universal trait vital to human survival; therefore, this definition was categorized with those who purported that caring is a human trait. The examples of care constructs identified by Leininger are behavioral attributes representative of caring; consequently her definition of caring extends from the human-trait category to "the direct (or indirect) nutrient and skillful activities related to the assisting people" (1984a, p. 4) or the therapeutic intervention category. (For further illustration of this analysis, see Morse, Bottorff, Neander, & Solberg, 1991, pp. 120–121).

Caring as a Human Trait

From this perspective, caring is an innate human trait, the "human mode of being." Although all humans have the potential to care, this ability is not uniform. Roach (1987) suggests that one's own experience of being cared for and expressing caring influences one's ability to care. The nurse's educational experience professionalizes this caring to the acquisition of knowledge and skills. Despite this assertion that one's ability to care is influenced by life

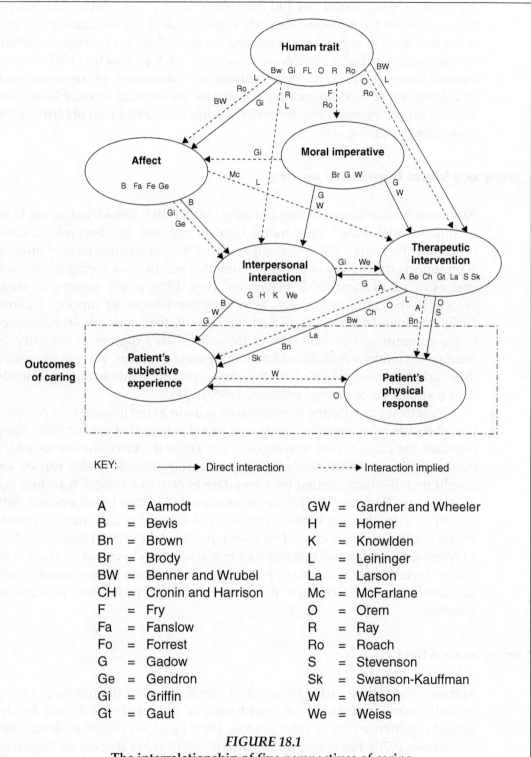

FIGURE 18.1
The interrelationship of five perspectives of caring.
Source: Morse, Solberg, Neander, Bottorff, and Johnson (1990).

experiences, being cared for, and expressing caring, this relationship has yet to be examined by exploring the early experiences of nurses. Leininger (1995) states that diverse expressions, meanings, and modalities of caring are culturally derived. Attributes of professional caring, such as Roach's (1987) dimensions of compassion, competence, confidence, conscience, and commitment, or Leininger's (1984a) 55 curative constructs, are derived from or have their locus in caring. According to these definitions, the human trait of caring is the motivator of nursing actions.

Caring as a Moral Imperative or Ideal

Authors who considered caring as a moral imperative considered caring to be a "fundamental value" or a moral ideal in nursing. For example, Gadow (1985) and Watson (1985, 1988a) suggest that the substantive base of nursing is preserving the dignity of patients. From this perspective, caring is not manifest as a "set of identifiable behaviors" (Fry, 1989, p. 48), images, or traits evident in the caring nurse (e.g., sympathy, tenderness, or support; Gadow, 1985), nor does it encompass all that nurses *do*. Rather, caring is the adherence to the commitment of maintaining the individual's dignity or integrity. In contrast to Gadow's realistic and attainable view or praxis, Watson suggested that caring actions revealed in the nurse–patient relationship are merely "approximations of caring" (Watson, 1985, p. 34).

In agreement with the theorists who adhere to the human-trait perspective, theorists who describe caring as a moral imperative concur that caring provides the basis for all nursing actions. Thus, the environment in which nurses work must facilitate and support caring. Paradoxically, nurses are caught in a dilemma created by a mandate to care in a society that does not value caring (Reverby, 1987). Nurses are expected to care for others as a duty (i.e., to be altruistic), yet without professional autonomy (i.e., they are unable to exercise their right to control their own practice). Fry (1989) notes that if, as a profession, nursing holds caring as a moral ideal, and present working conditions increasingly limit the opportunity to care (for instance, unsafe staffing conditions persist), then the survival of the profession remains in question.

Caring as an Affect

Authors who define caring as an affect emphasize that the nature of caring extends from emotional involvement with or an empathetic feeling for the patient experience (Bevis, 1981; Forrest, 1989; Fanslow, 1987; Gendron, 1988; McFarlane, 1976). For example, McFarlane (1976) states that caring "signifies a feeling of concern, of interest, of oversight with a view to protection." Bevis (1981) considers caring to be a feeling of dedication, a feeling that motivates nursing actions. It is a response that is primarily based on increasing intimacy between the nurse and the patient, and this, in turn, enhances mutual self-actualization. Self-actualization consists of four developmental stages: attachment, assiduity, intimacy, and confirmation. The nurse is moved to act selfishly without immediate gratification or the expectation of material reward.

Caring as It Is Manifest in the Nurse–Patient Relationship

Authors who write from this perspective believe the interaction between the nurse and the patient expresses and defines caring. Caring encompasses both the feeling and behaviors occurring within the relationship (Horner, 1998). For example, the relationship (i.e., the feeling) and the content (i.e., the behavior) of caring include such specific aspects as "showing concern" and "health teaching," touch, being there, and technical competence (Knowlden, 1988). Alternatively, these may be manifest in the supportive relationships nurses have with their patients (Gardner & Wheeler, 1981).

Caring as a Therapeutic Intervention

By defining specific nursing interventions or therapeutics as caring (Stevenson, 1990) or by describing conditions as necessary for caring actions (Gaut, 1986), these theorists have linked caring more directly than others with the work of nurses. Caring actions may be specific, such as attentive listening, patient teaching, patient advocacy, touch, "being there," and technical competence (Brown, 1986; Larson, 1984; Wolf, 1986) or caring may include all nursing actions (e.g., all nursing procedures for interventions; Stevenson, 1990) that enable or assist patients (Mayer, 1986). Emphasis is placed on the necessity for adequate knowledge and skill as a basis for these caring actions as well as on the congruence between nursing actions and the patient's perception of need.

Outcomes of Care and Caring

Rather than studying the concept of care and caring, some researchers have examined the concept of care by exploring patient physiological or psychological outcomes. This perspective is primarily used by those researchers who focus on quality assurance and use physiological outcomes as indicators of care (e.g., injuries from patient falls). For example, these outcomes may be the level of care determined by using selected statistical indices, such as morbidity and mortality statistics, length of stay in hospital, or the number of patient incident reports, thus removing the indicators of care to the

group level. Alternatively, researchers and auditors may use physical examination to observe for the absence of indicators of poor care, such as skin
conditions (pressure ulcers and abrasions), poor muscle tone, or even the
patient's state of hygiene, to ensure that an individual patient has been cared
for. The patient's subjective responses to care are also a part of these quality
assurance programs.

COMPARING THE CONCEPTUALIZATIONS AND THEORIES OF CARE

The next phase was to explore the implications of these diverse conceptualizations of caring for nursing practice and examine the commonalties,
strengths, and weaknesses of each perspective. This is conducted by sorting
all the caring articles into the five definitions of caring (identified in the previous stage), and comparing and contrasting articles in each perspective by
asking analytic questions.

The analytic questions regarding the focus of care are:

- Is caring considered a human trait?
- Is caring considered a moral imperative?
- Is caring considered an affect?
- Is caring considered an interpersonal interaction?
- Is caring considered a therapeutic intervention?
- Is caring unique in nursing?
- Can caring be reduced to behavioral tasks?

Analytic Questions Regarding Authors' Perspective of Care

As stated, the analytic questions that are asked at this stage are crucial for the
validity and significance of the study. But where do these questions come
from?

Analytic questions are created by extensive reading of the literature and
"reading between the lines," and by reading interpretatively behind the text.
In this study, we identified the following:

- Is caring unique to nursing?
- Does the caring intent of nursing vary between patients?
- Can caring be reduced to behavioral tasks?
- Does caring take place in individuals or in groups?
  - Does the outcome of the caring affect:
    - The patient?
    - The nurse?
  - Both the patient and the nurse?

Preparing a Matrix

Next, on a large sheet of paper (4 foot by 6 foot),[3] we made a large grid. The analytic questions related to the different types of care were placed on the top row of the chart. The authors' name and date of the publication were placed on the left hand row. We prepared a matrix by drawing the rows and columns on the paper, and filled in the matrix by answering the analytic questions from the perspective of each author.

As the analysis proceeded, additional characteristics emerged and raised questions that further illustrated the diversity of conceptualization of caring among theorists. These characteristics included the uniqueness of caring in nursing, the constant or varying nature of the caring capacity of nurses, whether caring may be reduced to behavioral tasks, and whether the outcome of caring influences or affects the nurse, the patient, or both. These results are presented in Table 18.1.

Is Caring Unique to Nursing?

This question is critical if caring is to attain and/or retain a central position in the development of nursing theory. Surprisingly, there is disagreement among nurse theorists regarding the uniqueness of caring in nursing. Although some agree that caring is unique in nursing, several theorists (Benner & Wrubel, 1989; Bevis, 1981; Fry, 1989; Horner, 1998) do not consider caring to be unique in nursing. For example, Benner and Wrubel (1989) state, "Caring practices are lived out in this culture primarily in parenting, child care, nursing, education, counseling and various forms of community life" (p. 408). Others, including Bevis (1981), Fry (1989), and Horner (1998), emphasize the universality of caring as opposed to attempting to identify the unique characteristics of caring in nursing.

Does the Caring Intent of Nursing Vary?

This question considers whether caring is a constant and unchanging motivator within the nurse regardless of characteristics of the patient. Again, several theorists agree that the intent to care changes according to the patient's characteristics or other variables. This position has received some support from Kahn and Steeves's (1988) study of the meaning of the caring relationship for nurses. Although the majority of the informants (who were nurses) believed that caring should be an unconditional aspect of nursing, they provided many examples that indicated that caring depended upon "having enough time, getting along with each other and not having too many other demands" (p. 213). Examples in this study showed that nurses found it

---

[3] Use the back of your supervisor's favorite poster.

TABLE 18.1
Caring Theorists' Perceptions of Selected Characteristics of Caring

Is caring unique in nursing?

Yes	No
Brody	Benner and Wrubel
Knowlden	Bevis
Leininger	Fry
McFarlane	Griffin
Roach	Horner
Watson	Ray

Does the caring intent of nursing vary between patients?

Yes	No
Griffin	Brody
Horner	Fanslow
Ray	Fry
	Gendron
	Leininger
	Watson

Can caring be reduced to behavioral tasks?

Yes	No
Brown	Benner and Wrubel
Gaut	Bevis
Larson	Brody
Leininger	Fanslow
McFarlane	Fry
Orem	Forrest
Swanson-Kauffman	Gadow
Weiss	Griffin
Wolf	Horner
	Knowlden
	Roach
	Watson

Does the outcome of the caring affect

The patient?	The nurse?	Both the patient and the nurse?
Brown	Brody	Benner and Wrubel
Gaut	Fanslow	Bevis
Gendron	Forrest	Gadow
Larson	Fry	Griffin
Leininger	Roach	Horner
Orem		Watson
Swanson-Kauffman		
Wolf		

Source: Morse, Bottorff, Neander, and Solberg (1991).

easier to care for patients whom they liked. The authors stated "nurses indi-cated that those patients who made it easier for them to do the caring activi-ties, to engage in praxis, more readily elicited caring" (p. 214). Nurses have also reported that patients use strategies, including giving manipulative gifts and using behaviors, such as making themselves "no trouble," so that nurses will be more willing to care for them during their illness (Morse, 1991b). Watson (1988b) advocates that whereas caring at the "surface level" may vary in relation to situational factors, caring in nursing at the moral and philosophical level "is underpinned by a moral stance that goes beyond the like or dislike of a patient . . . to touch the human center of the person" (p. 218). Thus, from this perspective, caring is held as a moral ideal in nursing; then the forms of caring may vary due to external constraints, such as the amount of time the nurse and patient have together, while the caring intent remains constant.

Can Caring Be Reduced to Behavioral Tasks?

If caring is to be considered measurable and intervention studies and evalua-tion research developed, this question is critical. Theorists who view caring as a moral ideal unanimously agree that caring is not reflected in a set of tech-niques but provide the stance from which one intervenes as a nurse, thereby influencing judgments, decision making, and action. Brody (1988) states, "It is not just the competent performance of technical skills that evokes the image of caring, but the compassionate attitudes and feelings of the nurses toward the patient as they perform their tasks that is the essence of caring" (p. 92). With the exception of McFarlane (1976), theorists who view caring as an affect do not consider the behavioral tasks of nurses as characteristic of caring: "Caring involvement and interaction incorporates on the part of the nurse a preference for 'being with' rather than 'doing to' a patient" (Forrest, 1989, p. 818). Not surprisingly, all the theorists who were included in the therapeu-tic intervention category considered caring as specific nursing actions. These actions were both indicators of caring and evidence that caring had taken place. Some of these theorists were quite specific in the delineation of car-ing tasks (Brown, 1986; Orem, 1985), whereas others used a more global approach (Leininger, 1981a, 1988; Swanson-Kauffman, 1988).[4]

Does the Outcome of the Caring Affect the Patient, the Nurse, or Both?

With the exception of the theorists who view caring as a therapeutic interven-tion, there was no clear pattern in the caring outcomes for either the nurse or the patient. Nurse outcomes that were identified included personal enrich-ment (Benner & Wrubel, 1989), increased understanding, emotional capacity, sense of personal worth (Griffin, 1983), and increased emotional burdens

---

[4] Why is it necessary to "split hairs" like this?

(Forrest, 1989). When mutual outcomes are discussed these theorists indicate that both the nurse and patient experience self-actualization (Bevis, 1981), enhanced subjectivity (Gadow, 1985), or increased spirituality (as reflected by Watson, 1988a). Watson states: "In a transpersonal caring relationship a spiritual union occurs between the two persons where both are capable of transcending self, time, space and the life history of each other" (p. 66). On the other hand, theorists who describe the outcomes of caring in terms of patient responses include enhanced health, well-being, comfort, self-integration, and patient satisfaction. For these theorists, the goal of caring would be to affect a desirable outcome in the patient. That outcome could be in terms of a subjective experience on the part of the patient or some actual physical response that could be measured. For example, Gaut (1986) operationalizes her conceptualization of caring with an example; that is, ensuring a patient recovering from surgery is adequately hydrated. The different qualities of power associated with caring are emphasized by Benner (1984). Some qualities—the transformative, integrative, advocacy, and healing qualities of the power of caring—have a direct bearing on patient outcomes. For instance, nurses who cared for patients with prolonged and permanent disabilities have been instrumental in "assessing the importance of helping the patient to continue with normal activities to minimize the isolation, loss of meaning and inactivity . . . [and nurses have] offered the option of reintegration by providing the patients and families with new possibilities in the midst of deprivation and loss" (p. 211). On the other hand, the power of creative problem solving associated with caring provides effective care and indirectly influences patient outcomes. The power of caring has not been recognized fully by nurses who see their caring role as a source of their powerlessness; yet, as argued by Benner (1984), any definition of power for nursing must include the power that resides in caring.

DISCUSSION ON CARING AS A CONCEPT

If caring is the "essence of nursing," then the issue of which theoretical perspective of caring is most descriptive of this essence is vital. Given the present diversity in the conceptualizations of caring, all of the attempts to delineate caring may have some application to the central paradigm of nursing. Presently, the concept is poorly developed, and as a result it may not be comprehensive enough to encompass all the components of caring that are necessary to guide clinical practice. There remains a loose link between many definitions of caring and patient outcomes. In particular, the previously unspoken controversy concerning whether caring may be reduced to behavioral tasks and the underdeveloped links to specific patient outcomes form the Achilles heel of caring theory. If the relevance of caring to practice and to the patient cannot be clearly explicated, or if it is claimed that caring cannot be reduced to behavioral tasks, nursing will no longer be a practice discipline. Either the central core of nursing will need to be reformulated or the gap between theory and practice will be widened to insurmountable proportions.[5]

This analysis of caring was conducted two decades ago. At this time it is considered still to be significant, and is still cited—even though some of the caring theorists included in this analysis have gone on to develop their theory further, some in new directions, others to clarify or to expand their original perspectives. Others have not written anything further, and still others have appeared on the horizon—a new cadre of nurse theorists. Nevertheless, the purpose here was to illustrate the power of pragmatic utility and to illustrate the backstage cognitive processes used in making decisions regarding the categories developed, so that others may also use the technique.

EXAMPLE II: CONCEPT CLARIFICATION: ACCOUNTING FOR STRATEGIES OF EMPATHETIC COMFORTING[6]

At this point we became interested in empathy as a *strategy* for expressing caring and providing comfort. Of course, empathy is a scientific concept and therapeutic strategy. It has been carefully defined, yet when we examined the major literature using pragmatic utility, we found four components: moral, cognitive, emotive, and behavioral (see Table 18.2). Each component was based on slightly different assumptions, and used slightly differently.

However, we were not content. We felt, as clinicians, this analysis did not provide us with anything very surprising. Although empathy was extremely helpful in the psychiatric settings in nursing (where nurses had the opportunity to counsel patients), in the "regular medical-surgical settings," with the exceptions of emotive empathy, other "empathetic responses" were used on a day-to-day basis. But these other concepts that were linked to empathy as empathetic responses were considered with varying degrees of "therapeutic-ness." For instance, *compassion* is considered therapeutic, but sympathy and pity are not considered therapeutic, and their use is even actively discouraged.

---

[5] There is a *vast* literature on caring in nursing. Some authors have written on caring many times. Consider the importance of the number of publications by one author as an important strategy for dissemination versus progression in their research program.
Think on these things.

[6] Reprinted with permission from Morse, Bottorff, Anderson, O'Brien, and Solberg (1992).

TABLE 18.2
Definition and Components of Perspectives of Empathy

| | EMOTIVE COMPONENT | MORAL COMPONENT | THERAPEUTIC | |
			COGNITIVE COMPONENT	BEHAVIORAL COMPONENT
Definition	The ability to subjectively experience and share in another's psychological state, emotions, or intrinsic feelings.	An internal altruistic force that motivates the practice of empathy.	The therapist's intellectual ability to identify and understand another person's feelings and perspective from an objective stance.	Communicative response to convey understanding of another's perspective.
Other Labels	"raw" "natural empathy" "trait empathy" "instinctual sensitivity" "emotional empathy" "affective empathy" "raw identification" "an emotional tie"	a "moral predisposition" "a flash of intuition" an "empathetic disposition"	"state empathy" "empathetic response" "sophisticated empathy" "clinical empathy" "role taking" "perspective taking"	"mirroring" of nonverbal behaviors "interactional empathy" "behavioral expression of empathy" "expressed empathy"
Social/Counseling Psychology and Philosophy	Burleson, 1984 Hoffman, 1981 Meyer, Boster, and Hecht, 1988 Rogers, 1957	Hogan, 1969 Buber, 1973 Batson and Coke, 1983 Gladstein, 1983 Stewart, 1973	Kalliopuska, 1986 Meyer, Boster, and Hecht, 1988 Rogers, 1957	Gladstein, 1983 Gazda et al, 1982 Trauz and Carkhuff, 1967 Rogers, 1957

(continued)

TABLE 18.2
Definition and Components of Perspectives of Empathy (continued)

	EMOTIVE COMPONENT	MORAL COMPONENT	THERAPEUTIC COGNITIVE COMPONENT	THERAPEUTIC BEHAVIORAL COMPONENT
Assumptions	1) Emotional distress is contagious (i.e., individuals experience the distress of another vicariously when they perceive the other's distress). 2) The ability to be empathetic is a natural, inherited potential that develops with maturity.	1) The empathetic person must enter into and know oneself before extending empathy to others. Thus, becoming empathetic is a conscious and deliberate process. 2) An empathetic desire is dependent upon: a) an unconditional acceptance of the other; b) a commitment to understand the other; and c) a belief in the universality of human needs and a sense of obligation to assist others to meet their basic needs.	1) The therapist can comprehend the client's experience from a more objective stance than the clients themselves. 2) This component of empathy is a teachable and measurable skill, built on natural abilities.	1) Empathetic behavior may be viewed by an independent observer. 2) Observed behavior is indicative of empathy. 3) Empathetic behavior can be demonstrated with higher or lower degrees of empathy and is measurable. 4) There is a readiness on the part of the client to receive help. 5) Empathetic responses will facilitate the personal growth of the client.
Strategies/ Manifestations	1) Emotional arousal empathizer. 2) The empathizer perceives him or herself responding emotionally to the other's emotional cue.	1) Exercise of one's power of will to either attend to, or engage with another, or to avoid and distance oneself from the other. 2) Attitude of receptivity and availability to others.	1) Imaging, comprehending, reasoning, analyzing, critical review. 2) Using the "as if" quality. 3) Deliberate distancing away from the vicarious emotions and movement toward cognitive processing of the whole situation.	1) Body posturing. 2) Mirroring. 3) Active listening. 4) Four levels of empathetic responses (Carkhuff's model). 5) Perception checking, validation. 6) Reflection. 7) Self-disclosure.

Source: Morse et al. (1992).

Patient Engagement

Underlying our analysis was the concept of engagement, or the identification of the caregiver with the sufferer's experience (see Gadow, 1980, 1984, 1989). Removed from the experience of suffering, the caregiver is not usually consciously aware of his or her own body. However, observing a patient suffering causes distress in the nurse and, consequently, awareness of his or her own body. Thus, the nurse was engaged with the patient's experience of suffering so that the patient's suffering is embodied by the nurse and suffering becomes a shared experience.

Nurses cannot physically escape from the patient's experience of suffering, yet they are in the position of being *responsible for alleviating the suffering.* Some methods of alleviating the suffering are not usually in the direct control of the nursing profession (e.g., the prescribing of adequate analgesics), and some are controlled by the profession (e.g., in the skill of nursing arts, such as positioning, the use of touch, the use of appropriate verbal responses, etc.); and in other cases, the nurse is powerless to alleviate the suffering because the pain is so severe and nothing can alleviate the distress. The patient is forced to endure the agony, and the nurse is forced to witness and, therefore, to share in the experience.

Observing such suffering does not leave the nurse unaffected: A patient's suffering is sensed and experienced by the nurse and evokes an emotive insight (EI) that, in turn, evokes expressions of verbal comfort (e.g., sympathy, pity, compassion, commiseration, consolation, or reflexive reassurance). However, the constant exposure to patient suffering emotionally drains the nurse; consequently, the experience of shared suffering must be controlled by the nurse, (a) so the nurse may leave the distressed patient and move on and care for other patients and (b) so the nurse can limit his or her involvement with the patient's suffering and avoid becoming emotionally drained and exhausted.

Human responses that are reflexive, *first-level, sufferer-focused responses* are responses that are triggered by the emotional insight of the caregiver. These responses are culturally conditioned rather than learned, almost reflexive or automatic, and are naturally comforting to the sufferer. We asked: What are these lay "empathetic concepts" that are used clinically, but not taught? Our list was

- Pity
- Sympathy
- Consolation
- Compassion
- Commiseration
- "Reflective reassurance"

Reflective reassurance was considered as the immediate reassurance provided without facts, such as "I am sure it will turn out for the best." Such reassurance is ambiguous (it does not promise recovery), yet to some degree it is comforting.

When the first-level responses were self-focused, we identified:

- Guarding
- Shielding/steeling or bracing
- Dehumanizing
- Withdrawing, distancing
- Labeling, denying

Second-level responses occurred when the first-level responses were consciously and deliberately suppressed, and replaced with a learned "professional" response. Such suppression frequently occurs in the process of professional socialization or is suppressed as a self-protective mechanism due to fatigue ("burnout") or overexposure to distressful stimuli.

Second-level responses result in the nurse being "pseudoengaged" with the sufferer (that is not embodied with the sufferer, but gives attention). These responses are learned, and were identified as:

- The deliberate sharing of self
- Humor
- Reassurance (informing)
- Therapeutic empathy
- Confronting
- Learned comforting

Those that are self-focused, second level, were:

- The rote professional behaviors
- Legitimizing or justifying
- False reassurance, false pity

Method

Because these first-level concepts were primarily *lay* concepts, our first task was to identify definitions and examples of their use, preferably in the context of nursing. Popular literature biographical or autobiographical accounts provided us with adequate examples. These were advantageous, for not only did they provide us with the dialogue and a description of the context, but they also provided us with a description of the emotive responses, usually those of the patients or their relatives. Second-level concepts were also

FOCUS				
	Sufferer-focused (patient)		**Self-focused (professional)**	
	CHARACTERISTIC	RESPONSE	RESPONSE	CHARACTERISTIC
First-level	Engaged (with sufferer's emotion) Genuine Reflexive	Pity, sympathy Consolation Commiseration Compassion Reflexive reassurance	Guarding Shielding/steeling/bracing Dehumanizing Withdrawing Distancing Labeling Denying	Anti-engaging (against embodiment, protective)
		(a)	*(b)*	
EXPERIENCE		*(c)*	*(d)*	
	Pseudo-engaged Learned Professional	Sharing self Humor Reassurance (informing) Therapeutic empathy Confronting Comforting (learned)	Rote behaviors 'professional style' Legitimizing/justifying Pity (false/professional) Stranger Reassurance (false)	A-engaged (embodiment absent or removed)
Second-level				

FIGURE 18.2
Types of responses by focus and experience of the caregiver.
Source: Morse, Bottorff, Anderson, O'Brien, and Solberg (1992). Used with permission.

described in this biographical or autobiographical literature, and used to illustrate these concepts. Next we identified in their use, whether they were sufferer-centered or nurse-centered concepts. We asked:

- Is the nurse focused on the sufferer's response (i.e., engaged and, therefore, embodying the sufferer' experience) or focused on the self, protecting him or herself from experiencing the sufferer's suffering?
- Is response reflexive and spontaneous (first level) or learned (second level) and, therefore, controlled?

First-Level Lay Concepts

Each of the first-level responses (i.e., pity, sympathy, consolation, compassion, commiseration, and reflexive reassurance) has unique characteristics. Each response evokes particular feelings in the caregiver that are targeted toward specific cues in the sufferer and may be recognized by characteristic verbal expressions and intonations. These responses also differ: They are spontaneous, and in duration, focus, and are targeted toward particular stimuli. Yet, in nursing, these responses are devalued, and nurses are taught to respond to patients more "professionally." We contend that this devaluation of first-level responses in nursing seriously limits the efficacy of nursing care. Interestingly, clinical observations illustrate that despite the fact that these responses are not part of formal nursing education they are used by nurses in their day-to-day work.

The critical factor in eliciting a first-level response from an emotional insight is that the caregiver must engage in the sufferer's experience: That is, the caregiver must be emotionally involved or able to identify with the sufferer. The caregiver must be willing and able to experience or share with the other's suffering in order to respond meaningfully and appropriately to the sufferer. It is this process of engagement between the nurse and the patient that allows for the sharing of the experience. Paradoxically, the caregiver's immersion in another's reality also results in experiencing the other's pain and suffering. The sharing of such an experience requires emotional energy and strength on the part of the caregiver. In the clinical area, there are limits to how much shared suffering the caregiver can tolerate or may find desirable. Because nurses are exposed to so much suffering, constantly bombarded with emotional stresses, and frequently required to inflict pain (i.e., to cause additional suffering), they learn to redirect, alter, or quench the spontaneous arousal of first-level emotive responses.

Sufferer-Focused First-Level Responses

Six sufferer-focused first-level responses have been identified and differentiated, but this list is not intended to be exhaustive. Each of these is discussed and illustrated with examples.

Pity

Pity is an expression of regret or sorrow for one who is suffering, distressed, or unhappy, and it confirms the sufferer's state. This confirmation facilitates the sufferer's acceptance of reality, which hastens the adjustment period and allows the patient to attain comfort sooner. Following her mastectomy, Rollins (1976) wrote,

> Pity is delicious. I was crazy about the pity I got. It was the best kind, too. I did not get, not did I want the drooling, mewing kind. I preferred something more restrained but deep-felt. Quality pity. (p. 72)

This type of "quality" pity may only be required for a short time and is especially useful to the patient during episodes of extreme suffering. The caregiver feels a deep sorrow for the situation that the patient or his or her family members are experiencing, and the caregiver's expressions of pity reflect this sorrow. Thus, pity serves an important function for the sufferer. The sorrow expressed by the caregiver has the effect of endorsing the sufferer's experience, and if the sufferer is in a state of shock or disbelief, it has the effect of *confirming* reality, thereby enabling and enhancing the sufferer's ability to accept reality. Although pity may lead to transient/temporary self-pity (Charmaz, 1980, p. 135), this state may be an important part of the overall psychological process of dealing with an illness when the illness first interrupts or begins to create changes in a person's lifestyle.

Sympathy

In contrast to pity, sympathy is an expression of the caregiver's own sorrow at another's plight. It has an "I" focus, expressing "I'm sorry" rather than "poor you." It is the verbal and nonverbal expression of dismay, and although triggered by the sufferer's state, it is a unilateral response from the caregiver. Given appropriately, sympathy legitimizes and justifies feelings of suffering experienced by the patient, making it "all right" for the patient/sufferer to feel that way. Expressions of sympathy demonstrate acceptance of the sufferer's state and thereby provide comfort.

Some authors suggest that sympathy interferes with the caregiver's ability to accurately perceive the patient's experience or offer assistance (Forsyth, 1980; Kalisch, 1973) because caregivers are dominated by their own sorrow for the sufferer. Others suggest sympathy motivates the caregiver to act in an effort to relieve distress (Travelbee, 1971; Wispe, 1986), but few have focused on the patient's need for or response to sympathy.

To be effective, sympathy must be seen as genuine, as closely as possible approximating the patient's true feelings, and offered at a time when the patient needs confirmation of his or her suffering. When this occurs, the patient's experience changes as it did for these parents when the person they consulted about their premature baby was sympathetic:

> This morning's appointment with Maureen Klein at the
> Children's Bureau did not produce a solution. Yet Maureen
> herself seemed so sympathetic that we left feeling glad we had
> come, which was not at all the emotion I had going in.
> (Stinson & Stinson, 1979/1983, p. 220)[7]

The fear that too much sympathy will inhibit independence and encourage sufferers to feel sorry for themselves or malinger may be unfounded. For example, an oncology patient experiencing alopecia for the first time described her feelings thus:

> Nobody has much sympathy for my feelings about my hair,
> which makes me feel misunderstood. "What's more
> important?" the purveyors of optimism try to convince me,
> "your hair or your life."

---

[7] From Stinson and Stinson (1979/1983). Reprinted by permission of the Harold Matson Co., Inc. All rights reserved.

> I don't need convincing: of *course* my life, of course. But they
> have missed the point. (Cook, 1981, pp. 301–302)

The changes Cook was experiencing, although necessary to preserve her life, were, at least in her mind, sufficient reason to grieve. In reality, if sympathetic responses have undesirable outcomes, it may be related to feelings of responsibility sufferers experience when they feel they are becoming a burden, instigating feelings of suffering in the sympathizer. For example, after her mastectomy when friends offered sympathy, Rollins (1976) responded with her "brave act":

> All I needed to hear was a slightly choked, "Betty, my god, I just
> heard, I can't tell you how sorry . . ." and there was a perfect
> cue for "I'm feeling terrific, absolutely terrific, being spoiled to
> death—oops, guess that's not the best way to put it—heh, heh
> . . ." and so on. (p. 73)

Thus, another function of sympathy may be to move the sufferer from a state of misery to a position of "taking it," which, in turn, elicits admiration from others who observe the resilience of the sufferer. Although this brave act is a facade, it is a facade that enables the sufferer to "get through" or to endure painful experiences.

Consolation

Consolation encompasses soothing and encouraging expressions that are used to ease discomfort or pain. It is the "I" in the caregiver expressing concern and working with the sufferer in order to temporarily reduce distress. During expressions of consolation, the caregiver assumes an active role. The sufferer experiences at least temporary relief from discomfort and pain, thereby attaining some degree of comfort. Consolation may be supportive, include an essence of hope, and is used frequently, although not exclusively, by the clergy. An incident of consolation, which she experienced while waiting for her husband's condition to stabilize in the coronary care unit, is described by Lear (1980):

> The nurse Bonnie came and went. Big Mama, so exquisitely
> attuned to countless women like me, whom she had consoled in
> the waiting room, that she seemed to be inside my head, to
> know exactly what images were trapped in there and how best
> to pet and soothe. Draping herself now about Judy and me,
> whispering news bulletins and cautionary notes: ". . . still
> holding his own . . . we just don't know . . . moment to
> moment . . ." I felt that I needed no cautions. (p. 34)

Although consolation that provides unrealistic hope or is otherwise misdirected potentially can increase rather than alleviate suffering, consolation can also alter perspective, without diminishing the meaning of a crisis. For example, following the premature birth of her baby, weighing 1 pound, 12 ounces, Peggy Stinson recalls,

> Mendelssohn [the doctor] came in to say we had held up well. I nodded through a stream of tears. He put out his hand in a consoling gesture. "You have your health," he said.

> It was all he said, but it was the right thing. We mustn't forget to be thankful for the disasters that didn't happen. We still had what we had before we started. And because I had my health, we had the hope for another baby. (Stinson & Stinson, 1979/1983, p. 22)

Commiseration

Although the circumstances surrounding the individual experiences may differ, commiseration is appropriate when the caregiver has shared the sufferer's predicament (at least to an implicitly agreed level). In essence, commiseration involves reflecting on a mutual response to a common experience. Unlike pity, sympathy, or compassion, which arise from a unilateral response of the sufferer or the caregiver, commiseration may be initiated by either the caregiver or the sufferer. While commiserating, the caregiver and the sufferer share a feeling of identity, enabling the caregiver to listen and communicate sincere expressions of agreement and understanding. It is the comfort derived from commiseration that is the basis of support groups and from which developed the adage "misery loves company." Patients often report that their primary source of support is another patient who is undergoing the same experience and who "intuitively" knows and understands what they are feeling. Although commiseration often occurs between nurses and patients in labor rooms and in emergency situations as an outgrowth of common experience, it does not follow that nurses and sufferers (patients) must have undergone identical experiences in order to be able to commiserate. Despite the adage "all nurses should be a patient, at least once," it is interesting that there is a notable absence of reference literature to support the use of commiseration by nurses. The importance of commiseration is reflected in the following quote:

> By coincidence, I met another woman at the party exactly my age, who had the same operation I had, two weeks before me . . . She was one treatment ahead of me and we couldn't stop talking to each other about everything. "How did this happen?" "What was your blood count on that?" "When is your second-look operation?" She had a scarf on, not a wig, and I kept wanting to just kiss her head because she had the same amount of hair I had—none. It was like going to a party when you were

a teenager and meeting someone you had so much in common with that you just couldn't believe it. (Radner, 1989, p. 152)

Compassion

Compassion is a strong emotion or sentiment stimulated by the presence of suffering that evokes recognition and mutual sharing of the despair or pain of the sufferer. It demonstrates acceptance of the sufferer's plight. But rather than being an expression of the caregiver's sorrow (as in sympathy), the compassionate caregiver echoes the sufferer's sentiment and shares in the suffering. By sharing the other's suffering, the caregiver's expression of compassion strengthens and comforts the sufferer. A good example of compassion is found in Cook's (1981) account of her experience with a compassionate nurse:

> She [the nurse] nods as if she understands. "It's so complicated," she offers. "We all identify with you, with what you're going through, your husband, your kids, your being so young. It could be any of us, nobody is immune. Any of us could have . . ." She breaks off and looks hard at me. (p. 233)

At times, it may be difficult to be compassionate. In being open to another's suffering, nurses must be willing to confront their own mortality, or as Copp (1990) writes, nurses must be willing to confront something "even worse than death, [their] own suffering" (p. 2). It is not possible to avoid pain and still be compassionate; therefore, in some situations, feelings of compassion may lead caregivers to withdraw from the suffering patient or shield themselves in order to avoid further pain or emotional involvement.

Reflexive Reassurance

This is a spontaneous reaction that occurs in the caregiver to counteract feelings of anxiety, uncertainty, or worry about the circumstances in which patients find themselves. Labeled as "optimistic assertion" (Teasdale, 1989), this response reflects the caregiver's attempt to "balance" the sufferer's feelings and to calm the sufferer by using verbal assurances in a tone of voice that is not unlike that of a "parent" (Berne, 1961). When these expressions are acceptable, anxiety is alleviated, and the person attains comfort:

> "Could you tell me, do you think, just as a person, would giving up Andrew for adoption be a bizarre thing to do?" He parroted the words all back to me—"No, I don't think it would be a bizarre thing to do"—with one of those smiles of amused reassurance, the way you would respond if your child suddenly asked you, "Mom, do you think I'm ugly?" So that I had to smile too—as if I had just been caught in the silliest of doubts. (Stinson & Stinson, 1979/1983, p. 207)

Reflexive reassurance is also used by patients to allay their relatives' fears about their obviously poor condition. Thus, a loop of "kind" or well-intentioned deceit may occur, with the patient trying to appear "up" for his or her relatives and the relatives trying to appear optimistic, minimizing the seriousness of the illness for the patient's sake. Lear (1980) writes,

> And still I grieved, without knowing quite why or for what or for whom. . . . On the fifth day, when I entered the cubicle, he was sitting up in bed. . . . "This is ridiculous," he said. Big grin. "I feel great. What the hell am I doing with a heart attack? There must be a mistake." (p. 38)

Analyzing the First-Level Sufferer-Focused Responses

The next step in the analysis was to place the six first-level responses on a chart, asking detailed information about the characteristics of each one, to clarify their role in the empathetic interaction. We asked:

1. Duration, or how long did the interaction take?
2. Who was the recipient of the statement (the caregiver as an "I" statement or the patient as a "you" statement)?
3. What was the nature of the feelings evoked on the caregiver?
4. Consider the participation in the interaction:

   Who led the interaction?
   Was the caregiver active or passive?
   Was the patient (i.e., the sufferer) active or passive?

5. Did the methods used involve verbal or nonverbal?
6. Was the response appropriate?

Table 18.3 shows that each of these lay concepts serves a particular purpose, for certain situations, and should be appropriately acknowledged and used in nursing education. Now all therapeutic interactions occur in a formal counseling setting—in fact, most occur outside. Yet the delegation of "nursing interactions" to psychiatric courses has biased the types of interactions taught and acknowledged as therapeutic.

Self-Focused, First-Level Responses

When first-level responses are focused on the caregiver rather than the patient, the caregiver's feelings are actively blocked or ignored, and the caregiver does not engage with the patient and feelings of embodiment disappear. Self-focused responses at this level (Figure 18.2, cell *b*) have the primary purpose of protecting the caregiver from being enjoined with the suffering experience of the patient. This is done by focusing on oneself rather than on the patient and by fighting and rejecting feelings resulting from *the threat of*

TABLE 18.3
The Components of Comfort, Delineating the Strategies of Talking and Listening

CHARACTERISTIC	PITY	SYMPATHY	CONSOLATION	COMPASSION	COMMISERATION	REFLEXIVE REASSURANCE
				STRATEGY		
Definition	An expression of regret expressed as the other's plight, as the other feels	An expression of one's own sorrow at another's plight	Soothing to ease discomfort/pain	Sensitivity to recognition of despair/pain	Sharing of mutual predicaments	Attempt to counter negative emotions
Duration	Instantaneous/Short	Short	Short	Short > sustained	Short	Short
Recipient	"you" focus (caregiver)	"I" focus (sufferer)	"I" am working with you	Acceptance of the other's plight	Mutual-focused on "thing" stressor	"Thing" (external) focused
Feelings evoked in caregiver	Feeling sorry for	Your sorrow for the sufferer	Concern for another	Feeling the sufferer's misery	Feeling the identity with misery	Attempt to "balance the sufferer's feeling"
Participation	Client-led Unilateral	Client-led Unilateral	Client-led Unilateral	Client-initiated Mutual	Caregiver-driven Mutual	Client-initiated Unilateral
Caregiver	Active	Active	Active	Active	Active	Active
Sufferer	Depersonalized	Passive	Passive	Passive	Active	Passive
Method	Verbal and nonverbal	Verbal and nonverbal expressions of dismay	Easing verbal soothing expressions of encouragement	Echoing of sufferer's sentiment Listening	Passive listening Expression of agreement Shared response	Verbal response
Appropriate use	Confirms sufferer's state	Legitimizes/justifies sufferer's response	Temporarily reduces distress	Enjoins sorrow	Support groups "misery loves company"	Alleviates sufferer's immediate anxiety
Outcome	COMFORT	COMFORT	COMFORT	COMFORT	COMFORT	COMFORT

Source: Morse, Bottorff, Anderson, O'Brien, and Solberg (1992). Used with permission.

engagement with the sufferer. The responses are reflexive and create the emotional and/or psychological distance that is sometimes needed if the caregiver is to remain *disengaged* or detached enough from the suffering to provide the needed care.

Three of these responses, *shielding, withdrawing,* and *guarding,* serve to protect the caregiver by reducing the caregiver's sensitivity to the suffering experience, which keeps the caregiver emotionally separated from the sufferer. The remaining four responses, *labeling, dehumanizing, distancing,* and *denying,* protect the caregiver by changing the caregiver's perception of the sufferer: That is, these responses keep the sufferer psychologically distant from the caregiver. All of these strategies are important to reduce vulnerability and to ensure that caregivers have the stamina necessary to continue to give care. The detachment that results from these strategies often occurs when the caregiver is too tired or burned out to continue to be sensitive to the suffering cues of patients, and any attempt by the patient to change the relationship, to be treated as a person, is met with rejection. An example of this is described by Cook (1981), who struggled to control her feelings, which were unacknowledged by her caregivers:

> I find myself apologizing for being a person rather than a case,
> for having feelings and wanting—needing—to understand
> what they are doing to me . . . what is happening to me. Clearly
> any attempt to assert one's basic dignity and the right to have
> some small measure of control are met with exasperated
> tolerance, dismissal, resentment. (pp. 264–265)

The mechanism of detachment is probably a necessary process that enables nurses to overcome the stress caused by the patient's suffering, which is associated with certain procedures and treatments. Some feelings may be so intense that caregiving would be impossible or disabling if the caregiver permitted him or herself to imagine and, therefore, experience the patient's experience. And it is probably the fear of the inability to give care that underlies the rule that caregivers must not nurse friends and relatives:

> [A] couple of months later a young radiologist who was a
> friend of a friend came by to say hello. He happened to see me
> that day and realized he recognized me—without knowing
> me—having been notified of my impending admission by our
> mutual friend. He remembered my red robe and the masses of
> long hair splashed over the pillow of the stubby ambulance
> stretcher, saw my face only obliquely because I had turned it
> toward the wall. He said it made him sick to look at me; he took
> the rest of the day off. (Cook, 1981, p. 254)

Second-Level Responses

Second-level responses are learned, professional responses. They have been taught in the classroom as a part of communication courses or by role-modeling in the clinical area.

When caregivers try to reduce their own emotional responses to the patient or sufferer, thereby decreasing their personal investment in the suffering, they initiate second-level responses such as the learned professional responses of therapeutic empathy, informing reassurance, humor/distraction, and confronting (Figure 18.2, cell *c*). As their emotional involvement with the sufferer is more limited than during first-level responses, caregivers must try to *imagine* what it is like for the patients rather than becoming genuinely involved in their experience. The term *pseudoengagement* is applied to this level of response. The focus of professional helping responses is the sufferer, and although some of these responses may be off target or not helpful, they are generally therapeutic.

These responses keep the caregiver somewhat detached, objective, and therapeutically "at arm's length" from the sufferer. Learning these distancing responses often forms the basis of communication courses in professional programs such as nursing. Frequently, the primary focus is on understanding the patient's suffering and developing a repertoire of cognitive and behavioral communication strategies that can be used in place of emotional, reflexive processes. Thus, the learned response is deliberate and conscious, and the caregiver is not, or is only minimally, emotionally involved with the sufferer.

Sufferer-Focused, Second-Level Responses

In the following example, a nurse uses *humor* to ignore a patient's pleas for orange juice. The patient responds to the teasing rather than becoming difficult; thus, the relationship between the nurse and the patient is not destroyed:

The nurse Lois asks him to take some pills.

"Bring in a quart of orange juice and we'll negotiate it," he says.

Lois tells him, "But I don't like orange juice."

"Bring vodka too. You'll like it." (Lear, 1980, p. 346)

Therapeutic empathy

The use of therapeutic empathy in nursing, arising from a seemingly uncritical adoption of the concept from psychology, has generally been accepted as an important part of the nurse–patient relationship (Holliday, 1961; MacKay, Carver, & Hughes, 1990; Travelbee, 1963; Triplett, 1969; Zderad, 1969). In discussing the therapeutic use of empathy in nursing, the term has taken on more of a cognitive/behavioral meaning, de-emphasizing the emotional involvement that is central to first-level, emotional empathy. The differences between "clinical" or therapeutic empathy and "natural" or emotional empathy as delineated by nurses (Ehmann, 1971; Zderad, 1970) also point to this fact. It is only in clinical empathy that a detachment or dissociation phase is a prerequisite, removing the nurse from the risk of personal involvement and ensuring that the interaction is professional. When this phase is not actually described, nursing authors stress the need for objectivity on the part of the empathizer (Forsyth, 1980).

Despite the inclusion of empathy training in educational programs, it has not been easy for nurses to incorporate empathy into their practice due to the realities of the clinical setting. Although the use of therapeutic empathy may be appropriate in some nurse–patient interactions, there is a need to identify when it should be used in the clinical setting and the patient outcomes that can be expected.

Informative Reassurance
This type of reassurance is a purposeful, conscious, and deliberate attempt to restore confidence (French, 1979; Teasdale, 1989) and reduce uncertainty (Boyd & Munhall, 1990). Although a range of behaviors may be used to produce a state of calmness or assurance, information giving and explanations primarily are used to produce this state. Others have argued that this type of reassurance is a complex interpersonal skill that can be enhanced by education (French, 1979) and that it is prompted by knowledge of the patient's situation and evidence of his or her unmet and projected needs (Boyd & Munhall, 1990):

> Three days ago, on January, 12, I saw Whitmore. He was reassuring. The prostate is smaller, tough and burned out by the radiation implants. Willet said he could feel some of the seeds. There was some pus in the urine which Gantrisin is supposed to clear up. That is about the extent of what I learned. Whitmore asked me to come back in two months. Will the day ever come when he says, "Give me a call in a year or two"? (Ryan & Ryan, 1979, p. 277)

Although informative reassurance is given with the intention of comforting, the reassurance may not convince those who are distressed because it does not address all of their concerns:

> Logically speaking, there is not a great deal of risk to this operation. "It's the appendectomy of heart operations," they tell us. "Of course there is always the risk in any major surgery; but at this hospital we have one of the best surgeons in the field.

Really, there is no need to worry. Besides, the risks of the operation are less than the risks of leaving the child's heart condition untreated." These words of reassurance do not offer much comfort. . . As parents, we are fearful for our child. "Look, don't worry," chides the physician, "he'll be in good hands. We have a very good record in treating this problem." But can our fears be so unfounded? (Smith, 1989, p. 148)

Self-Focused, Second-Level Responses

If the caregiver experiences a prolonged "assault" (i.e., he or she must continue to provide care for patients in distress or must inflict pain), the process of blocking engagement becomes successful, and the caregiver is without feelings for the patient and *completely detached*. Therefore, patients are treated as objects or as cases rather than as people or as individuals. Caregivers who respond in this way may also appear uncaring and mechanical; at best, their responses appear as "absentminded kindness" (Cook, 1981, p. 303) and, at worst, as callousness:

The male figures were with him for ten minutes a day. They were marginal figures, shadowy and cold. They touched him with instruments—stethoscopes, blood-pressure gadgets. They had condescending airs. They asked him curt questions and grunted at him. He did not like them.

"Do you have trouble breathing?"

"No."

"Do you have chest pain?"

"Yes."

"How bad?"

"Slight."

"Oh. Do you have . . ."

How quickly arrogance had been inbred into these kids, these baby-faced interns and residents. (So young! Had he looked this young when he himself had been an intern, feeling so old in his dewy skin and in his nifty white coat?) How early they grew pompous! (Lear, 1980, pp. 40–41)

Despite the possible therapeutic function of *complete detachment*, it is clear that patients are aware that they are not being treated as persons and that they find this disturbing:

I was sure she would rather I were unconscious. She wouldn't
have to talk to a comatose patient, and Gwenn left no doubt in
my mind that she preferred not having to speak to me. She
wasn't unkind. Just aloof, remote. (Baier & Schomaker,
1985/1986, p. 18)

Furthermore, the effects of such treatment frequently have a devastating
effect on patients and their relatives:

Dr. Carvalho has the bedside manner of a robot. Cold,
emotionless, unaffected by anything you say. Moving from
statements like "Your baby is very sick" (the words once used to
make Andrew's condition comprehensible to 5-year-old Jenny)
to "The hospital's policy is to obtain court orders when parents
don't agree with its decisions" to "These children are precious
to most parents" without even changing expression or tone of
voice. Describing Andrew as still "salvageable," providing
substance-less answers to questions about treatment or
prognosis. Looking at you vacantly when you try to protest.
How incredibly disconcerting and disorienting it is trying to
explain your most private, painful, vulnerable thoughts to a
panel of robots. (Stinson & Stinson, 1979/1983, p. 51)

These responses are effective in enabling the caregiver to continue working by reducing the effort of giving care and by eliminating the need to experience any of the sufferer's pain or suffering. However, these responses are
not beneficial to the patient and may be alienating. Caregivers may also protect themselves from attending to the emotional stimulus and respond with
behaviors such as rote responses, legitimizing or justifying actions, false pity,
acting as "stranger," and false reassurance. This is clearly evident in the Stin-
sons' experience with a social worker who used rote behaviors during an
interview with them:

The effect [of the conversation with the social worker] was just
as disorienting because she was programmed to say warm
sensitive things automatically whether they applied or not.
"You must be very tired," she began solicitously. I wasn't, but I
nodded cooperatively, trying to think why I would be tired. "It
must be very hard to have to see your baby amidst so much
unfamiliar equipment," she continued. I tried to explain that
that wasn't why I hadn't gone in to see Andrew. "It must be
very upsetting, having a baby and knowing that it's so sick."
Weakly now, I started to explain that that wasn't why I was so
upset.

It was no use. She had a whole string of "you musts" and "it must bes" that didn't fit me at all. She was trying hard to make me fit into the normal pattern, to put the right thoughts and feelings onto my tongue so that she could respond with the right sympathetic understanding. Only she wasn't listening to what I was saying, to what Bob and I had both been saying in that claustrophobic room.

I backed away in confusion, trying to get away before I began to look even more abnormal than I did already. Trying to avoid more embarrassing crying. (Stinson & Stinson, 1979/1983, pp. 51–52)

One of the unfortunate ramifications of the lack of engagement is that the absence of feeling for the sufferer results in the lack of an advocate for the patient. Elsewhere (Morse, Bottorff, Anderson, O'Brien, & Solberg, 1992/2006), we argued that the *empathetic insight* (EI) motivates the caregiving interaction, and if the EI *is repressed*, then caregiving may be dangerously absent:

He [the infant] cried with alarming intensity, as if his whole being were nothing but a heart-wrenching plea for someone to do something.

I went back down the hall to tell the nurses about him. "Oh, he's all right," one of them told me cheerfully. "He's just been circumcised today." (Stinson & Stinson, 1979/1983, p. 30)

Often, to protect themselves, the caregivers' detachment is complete, with no personal contact between the caregiver and the sufferer, and the sufferer's needs are completely ignored:

Came home to find that a letter had arrived from Pediatric Hospital. Inside the envelope was a letter bearing the signature of Richard T. Farrell, MD. But it was a form letter. A mimeographed form letter! You try and try to communicate with these people, you drive all the way there again and again to explain and re-explain, you stay up all night writing them letters, but they don't listen. They don't try to understand you. They don't even acknowledge your protest. Then they have the nerve to tell you by form letter that all parents have the same feelings and concerns. (Stinson & Stinson, 1979/1983, p. 78)

Because the caregiver loses *emotional insight* and the ability to observe some of the patient's needs, the patient is in jeopardy by not having a caregiver who will serve as an advocate and by the caregiver not providing necessary care. Thus, with *complete detachment,* the goals for humanistic treatment may change. This may become a serious ethical issue:

> Those doctors go on righteously about their business while our lives fall apart. Andrew is "interesting" to them in some detached way—their own private research project, conveniently underage so that they need no consent for whatever it is that they do. "Oh my, his bones are breaking now—whatever could be causing that? What will be the result of trying this?" Of course they don't see it that way; they're saving the life of an unfortunate child, saving him from his immoral parents. And if it begins to look like Andrew can't be saved? Why stop there? They're still learning something, aren't they? These matters are routine to them—it's not *their* pain and suffering. There's always the next baby; the farther they can push this baby, the more they can do for the next. (Stinson & Stinson, 1979/1983, p. 187)

Discussion

From analyzing comforting interactions, the essence of the nurse–patient relationship is the identification of the nurse with the patient, or level of engagement. The instantaneous recognition of another's plight causes reflexive feelings of helping that trigger expressions of first-level responses in the caregiver. The basis of this response is the emotional insight (EI) or the reflexive emotional response in the nurse that extends from identifying with the patient's experience. Gadow (1980, 1989) argues that engagement allows nurses to "attend to the objectiveness of the person" by "abstracting the condition of the person" without reducing the patient to the "level of objectification" while, at the same time, "allowing them to remain at the center of their experience" (Gadow, 1984). Thus, a nurse identifies with the human experience of a patient. For instance, a nurse may observe a patient in pain or distress and be moved to assist that person *because they are suffering*, without necessarily knowing what is causing the pain or underlying the distress (although such information would be sought in the process of helping).

The communication model presented here expands the repertoire of responses for nurses to use with distressed patients and makes use of "natural" emotions that are aroused spontaneously. It suggests that rather than using a professional but less genuine and less effective learned response, nurses are drawn into a process of willful involvement and engagement with the sufferer. Although the use of pity, sympathy, commiseration, compassion, consolation, and reflexive reassurance may require the nurse to use more energy compared with a rote professional response, such relationships are described as being more rewarding for the caregiver. The reciprocal nature of the exchange should reduce rather than increase the nurse's risk of burnout.

Because the first-level responses are evoked reflexively and without premeditation, these responses are always appropriate, on target, relieve distress, and produce comfort. This is not to argue that pity or sympathy cannot be used inappropriately; rather, it is to point out that when they are expressed reflexively as first-level responses, because the caregiver is engaged with the sufferer, the EI ensures the response given is the appropriate response. When the caregiver is not engaged with the sufferer an expression of pity becomes impossible. Pity, if then offered, appears as "false" pity, thus evoking such feelings as anger in the sufferer. It is important to note that as nurses become more experienced in their work they learn to control the level of engagement with patients, to block the EI and to remain detached (i.e., disengaged), to fight against the EI (i.e., anti-engagement), or to imagine the sufferer's experience as when using empathy in a professional relationship (i.e., pseudoengaged). Each of these types of nurse–patient engagement may be identified by the types of responses the nurse presents to the distressed patient. Although engagement with patients in distress is beneficial to the patient, it is neither beneficial nor desirable to be constantly in an engaged relationship and to be consistently using first-level responses. Other types of responses are often appropriate, and these may protect the caregiver or be needed by the patient and ideal for the situation.

SUMMARY: BACK TO PRAGMATIC UTILITY AS A METHOD

To reiterate, the type of approach to the literature will depend on the level of development of the concept and, consequently, the researcher's purpose in conducting the analysis, from which, of course, the research question is derived. Only those concepts that have some development and adequate literature may be analyzed using these methods. Principles of sampling dictate that there must be adequate literature available in order to conduct this type of analysis.

When asking analytic, comparative questions of the data (i.e., the literature), the researcher must have an adequate database available to answer the questions. If there are too few articles, or the articles do not contain adequate information (i.e., the database is inadequate), then the concept is immature and a qualitative study must be conducted. This is a basic principle of sampling.

The main purpose for conducting pragmatic utility is to assess: to clarify concepts, to compare and contrast the use of concepts in particular disciplines, to compare conceptual adequacy with competing concepts, to identify conceptual gaps and boundaries, and to identify conceptual inconsistencies within a concept (see Box 18.2).

BOX 18.2. OTHER EXAMPLES OF PRAGMATIC UTILITY

Hawkins, S. F., & Morse, J. (2014). The praxis of courage as a foundation for care. *Journal of Nursing Scholarship*, *46*(4), 263–270.

Hupcey, J. E. (2008). Maintaining validity: The development of the concept of trust. *International Journal of Qualitative Methods*, *1*(4), 45–53.

Huynh, T., & Alderson, M. (2009, April). Concept analysis of human ecology. In *Nursing Forum* (Vol. 44, No. 2, pp. 115–128). Blackwell Publishing Inc.

Kunyk, D., & Olson, J. K. (2001). Clarification of conceptualizations of empathy. *Journal of Advanced Nursing*, *35*(3), 317–325.

Olson, K. (2007, January). A new way of thinking about fatigue: A reconceptualization. *Oncology Nursing Forum*, *34*(1), 93–99.

TO DO 18.1. PRAGMATIC UTILITY AS A CLASS PROJECT

An interesting task for the class to do as a joint project, would to be to "update" this work, using theorists from 1991 to the present time. Ask the class to locate the literature and sort it into the five perspectives here. Do these categories still hold?

Then divide the class into five teams, each taking one set of literature. Develop large matrices on huge sheets of paper.

Each team must ask the following analytic questions of their stack of articles:

Do the analytic questions still hold?
Do the differences in perspectives of caring theorists continue in nursing?
Has caring theory developed, and if so how?

REFERENCES

Aamodt, A. (1994). *Topics in case-based reasoning*. New York, NY: Springer-Verlag.

Baier, S., Schomaker, M. Z. (1985/1986). *Bed number ten*. Boca Raton, FL: CRC Press.

Batson, C. D., & Coke, J. S. (1981). Empathy: A source of altruistic motivation for helping? In J. Rushton & R. Sorrentino (Eds.), *Altruism and helping behavior: Social personality and developmental perspectives* (pp. 167–187). Mahwah, NJ: Erlbaum.

Benner, P. (1984). *From novice to expert: Excellence and power in clinical nursing practice*. Menlo Park, CA: Addison Wesley.

Benner, P. E., & Wrubel, J. (1989). *The primacy of caring: Stress and coping in health and illness*. Menlo Park, CA: Addison-Wesley.

Berne, E. (1961). *Transactional analysis in psychotherapy: A systematic individual and social psychiatry*. New York, NY: Grove.

Bevis, E. O. (1981). Caring: A life force. In M. Leininger (Ed.), *Caring, an essential human need: Proceedings of the three National Caring Conferences*. Detroit, MI: Wayne State University.

Boyd, C. O., & Munhall, P. L. (1990). A qualitative investigation of reassurance. *Holistic Nursing Practice, 4*(1), 61–69.

Brody, J. K. (1988). Virtue ethics, caring and nursing. *Scholarly Inquiry for Nursing Practice: An International Journal, 2*, 87–101.

Brown, L. (1986). The experience of care: Patient perspectives. *Topics in Clinical Nursing, 8*(2), 56–62.

Buber, M. (1973). Elements of the interhuman. In J. Stewart (Ed.), *Bridges not walls*. Menlo Park, CA: Addison-Wesley.

Burleson, B. (1984). Comforting communication. In H. Snyder & J. Applegate (Eds.), *Communication by Children and Adults: Social Cogniyive and strategic Processes* (pp. 63–84). London, UK: Sage.

Charmaz, K. (1980). The social construction of self-pity in the chronically ill. In N. Denzin (Ed.), *Studies in symbolic interaction: A research manual* (Vol. 3, pp. 123–145). Greenwich, CO: Jai Press.

Cook, S. (1981). *Second life*. New York, NY: Simon & Schuster.

Copp, L. A. (1990). *Treatment, torture, suffering, and compassion* [Editorial]. *Journal of Professional Nursing, 6*, 1–2.

Ehmann, V. E. (1971). Empathy: Its origin, characteristics, and process. *Perspectives in Psychiatric Care, 9*, 72–80.

Fanslow, J. (1987). Compassionate nursing care: Is it a lost art? *Journal of Practical Nursing, 37*(2), 40–43.

Forrest, D. (1989). The experience of caring. *Journal of Advanced Nursing, 14*, 815–823.

Forsyth, G. L. (1980). Analysis of the concept of empathy: Illustration of one approach. *Advances in Nursing Science, 2*, 33–42.

French, H. P. (1979). Reassurance: A nursing skill. *Journal of Advanced Nursing, 4*, 627–634.

Fry, F. T. (1989). Toward a theory of nursing ethics. *Advances in Nursing Science, 11*(4), 422.

Gadow, S. (1980). Existential advocacy. In S. F. Spicker & S. Gadow (Eds.), *Nursing: Images and ideals* (pp. 79–101). New York, NY: Springer.

Gadow, S. (1984). Touch and technology: Two paradigms of patient care. *Journal of Religion and Health, 23*(1), 63–69.

Gadow, S. (1985). Nurse and patient: The caring relationships. In A. H. Bishop & J. R. Scudder (Eds.), *Caring, curing, coping* (pp. 31–43). Birmingham, AL: University of Alabama.

Gadow, S. (1989). Clinical subjectivity. Advocacy with silent patients. *Nursing Clinics of North America, 24*, 535–541.

Gardner, K. G., & Wheeler, E. (1981). The meaning of caring in the context of nursing. In M. Leininger (Ed.), *Caring: An essential human need* (pp. 69–79). Thorofare, NJ: Charles B. Slack.

Gaut, D. A. (1986). Evaluating caring competencies in nursing. *Topics in Clinical Nursing, 8*, 77–83.

Gazda, G. M., Childers, W. C., & Walters, R. P. (1982). *Interpersonal communications*. Rockville, MD: Aspen.

Gendron, D. (1988). *The expressive form of caring.* Toronto, Canada: University of Toronto.

Gladstein, G. A. (1983). Understanding empathy: Integrating counseling developmental and social psychology perspectives. *Journal of Counseling Psychology, 30,* 467–482.

Griffin, A. P. (1983). A philosophical analysis of caring in nursing. *Journal of Advanced Nursing, 8,* 289–295.

Hoffman, M. (1981). The development of empathy. In J. Rushton & R. Sorrentino (Eds.), *Altruism and helping behavior: Social personality and developmental perspectives* (pp. 41–63). Hillsdale, New Jersey: Erlbaum.

Hogan, R. (1969). Development of the empathy scale. *Journal of Consulting and Clinical Psychology, 33,* 307–318.

Holliday, J. (1961). The ideal characteristics of a professional nurse. *Nursing Research, 10,* 201–210.

Horner, S. D. (1998). Catching the asthma: Family care for school-aged children with asthma. *Journal of Pediatric Nursing, 13*(6), 356–366.

Kahn, D. L., & Steeves, R. H. (1988). Caring and practice: Construction of the nurse's world. *Scholarly Inquiry for Nursing Practice, 2,* 201–216.

Kalisch, B. J. (1973). What is empathy? *American Journal of Nursing, 73,* 1548–1552.

Kalliopuska, M. (1986). Empathy, its measurement and application. *British Journal of Projective Psychology, 31,* 10–19.

Knowlden, V. (1988). Nurse caring as constructed knowledge. In R. McNeil & R. Watts (Eds.), *Caring and nursing: Explorations in the feminist perspective* (pp. 318–339). Denver, CO: Center for Human Caring, University of Colorado Health Sciences Centre.

Larson, P. J. (1984). Important nurse caring behaviors perceived by patients with cancer. *Oncology Nursing Forum, 11*(6), 46–50.

Lear, M. W. (1980). *Heartsounds: The story of a love and loss.* New York, NY: Simon and Schuster.

Leininger, M. M. (1978). *Transcultural nursing: Concepts, theories and practices.* New York, NY: John Wiley & Sons.

Leininger, M. M. (1981a). Some philosophical, historical, and taxonomic aspects of nursing and caring in American culture. In M. M. Leininger (Ed.), *Caring, an essential human need: Proceedings of the three National Caring Conferences* (pp. 133–143). Thorofare, NJ: Slack.

Leininger, M. M. (1981b). Cross-cultural hypothetical functions of caring and nursing care. In *Caring: An essential human need* (pp. 133–143). Thorofare, NJ: Slack.

Leininger, M. M. (1984a). Caring in nursing: Understanding the meaning, importance, and issues. In *Caring: A central focus of nursing and health services.* Detroit, IL: Wayne State University.

Leininger, M. M. (Ed.). (1984b). *Care, discovery and uses in clinical and community nursing.* Detroit, MI: Wayne State University.

Leininger, M. M. (1988). Leininger's theory of nursing: Culture care diversity and universality. *Nursing Science Quarterly, 1*(4), 151–160.

Leininger, M. M. (1995). Overview of Leininger's culture care theory. In M. M. Leininger (Ed.), *Transcultural nursing concepts, theories, research & practices* (2nd ed., College Costom Series, pp. 93–112) New York, NY: McGraw-Hill.

Leininger, M. M. (2002). Culture care theory: A major contribution to advance transcultural nursing knowledge and practices. *Journal of Transcultural Nursing, 13*(3), 189–192.

MacKay, R., Carver, E., & Hughes, J. (1990). The professional's use of empathy and client care outcomes. In R. MacKay, J. Hughes, & J. Carver (Eds.), *Empathy in the helping relationship* (pp. 120–132). New York, NY: Springer.

Mayer, D. K. (1986). Cancer patients' and families' perceptions of nurse caring behaviors. *Topics in Clinical Nursing, 8*(2), 63–69.

McFarlane, J. (1976). A charter for caring. *Journal of Advanced Nursing, 1*, 187–196.

Meyer, D. J., Boster, F. J., & Hetch, M. L. (1988). A model of empathetic communication. *Communication Research Reports, 5*, 19–27.

Morse, J. M. (1991a). The structure and function of gift-giving in the patient-nurse relationship. *Western Journal of Nursing Research, 13*, 597–615.

Morse, J. M. (1991b). Negotiating commitment and involvement in the patient-nurse relationship. *Journal of Advanced Nursing, 16*, 455–468.

Morse, J. M., Anderson, G., Bottorff, J. L., Yonge, O., O'Brien, B., Solberg, S. M., & McIlveen, K. H. (1992). Exploring empathy: a conceptual fit for nursing practice. *Journal of Nursing Scholarship, 24*(4), 813. Used with permission.

Morse, J. M., Bottorff, J., Anderson, G., O'Brien, B., & Solberg, S. (1992/2006). Beyond empathy. Expanding expressions of caring. *Journal of Advanced Nursing, 17*, 809–821. (Reprinted, *53*(1), 75–87)

Morse, J. M., Bottorff, J., Anderson, G., O'Brien, B., & Solberg, S. (1992). Beyond empathy. Expanding expressions of caring. *Journal of Advanced Nursing, 17*, 813. Article reprinted for the *Special 30th Anniversary Issue* of *Journal of Advanced Nursing,* (2006) *53*(1), 75–87. p. 813.

Morse, J. M., Bottorff, J., Neander, W., & Solberg, S. (1991). Comparative analysis of the conceptualizations and theories of caring. *Image: Journal of Nursing Scholarship, 23*(2), 119–126.

Morse, J. M., Solberg, S. M., Neander, W. L., Bottorff, J. L., & Johnson, J. L. (1990). Concepts of caring and caring as a concept. *Advances in Nursing Science, 13*, 1–14.

Orem, D. E. (1985). *Nursing: Concepts of practice* (3rd ed.). Chevy Chase, MD: McGraw-Hill.

Radner, G. (1989). *It's always something.* Toronto, Canada: Simon & Schuster.

Reverby, S. (1987). *Ordered to care: The dilemma of American nursing, 1850–1945.* Cambridge, England: Cambridge University Press.

Roach, M. S. (1987). *The human act of caring: A blueprint for health professions.* Toronto, CA: Canadian Hospital Association.

Rogers, C. R. (1957). The necessary and sufficient conditions of therapeutic personality change. *Journal of Counseling Psychology, 21*, 95–103.

Rollins, B. (1976). *First, you cry.* New York, NY: The New American Library.

Ryan, C., & Ryan, K. M. (1979). *A private battle.* New York, NY: Simon & Schuster.

Smith, S. J. (1989). Operating on a child's heart: A pedagogical view of hospitalization. *Phenomenology and Pedagogy, 7*, 145–162.

Stevenson, J. (1990). A review of the quantitative literature on care. In J. Stevenson & T. Tripp-Reimer (Eds.), *Knowledge about care and caring: State of the art and future development.* Kansas City, KS: American Academy of Nursing.

Stewart, J. (1973). *Bridges not walls*. Menlo Park, CA: Addison-Wesley.

Stinson, R., & Stinson, P. (1979/1983). *The long dying of baby Andrew*. Boston, MA: Little, Brown.

Swanson-Kauffman, K. (1988). Caring needs of women who miscarried. In M. Leininger (Ed.), *Care discover and uses in clinical and community nursing* (pp. 55–70). Detroit, MI: Wayne State University.

Teasdale, K. (1989). The concept of reassurance in nursing. *Journal of Advanced Nursing, 14,* 444–450.

Travelbee, J. (1963). What do we mean by rapport? *The American Journal of Nursing, 63,* 70–72.

Travelbee, J. (1971). *Interpersonal aspects of nursing*. Philadelphia, PA: F. A. Davis.

Triplett, J. L. (1969). Empathy is… *Nursing Clinics of North America, 4,* 673–681.

Truax, C. B., & Carkhuff, R. R. (1967). Toward effective counseling and psychotherapy. Chicago, IL: Aldine.

van der Steen, W. J. (1993) *A practical philosophy for the life sciences*. Albany, NY: State University of New York Press.

Watson, J. (1985). *Nursing: Human science and human care*. New York, NY: Appleton-Century-Crofts.

Watson, J. (1988a). *Nursing: Human science and human care: A theory of nursing*. New York, NY: National League for Nursing.

Watson, J. (1988b). Response to caring and practice: Construction of the nurse's world. *Scholarly Inquiry for Nursing Practice: An International Journal, 2,* 217–221.

Weaver, K., & Mitcham, C. (2008). Nursing concept analysis in North America: State of the art. *Nursing Philosophy, 9*(3), 180–189.

Wispe, L. (1986). The distinction between sympathy and empathy: To call forth a concept, a word is needed. *Journal of Personality and Social Psychology, 50,* 314–321.

Wolf, Z. R. (1986). The caring concept and nurse identified caring behaviors. *Topics in Clinical Nursing, 8,* 84–93.

Zderad, L. T. (1969). Empathic nursing; realization of a human capacity. *The Nursing Clinics of North America, 4*(4), 655–662.

Zderad, L. T. (1970). Empathy—from cliché to construct. In C. M. Norris (Ed.), *Proceedings of the Third Nursing Theory Conference, Kansas City* (pp. 46–75). Kansas City: University of Kansas Medical Center Department of Nursing Education.

19

CONCEPT COMPARISON

> *Why is a raven like a writing desk?*
> —Lewis Carroll (1865/2010, p. 82)

Conceptual comparison is a method used to delineate allied concepts. It may be used if you suspect that a single concept label is being applied to several allied (or slightly different) concepts, it may be used when a number of concepts compete to explain or account for a single phenomenon, or it may be used when a researcher suspects that a concept has subtly undergone changes during the process of application—that is, as it has been used over a period of time, or has been used in different contexts, for instance, adopted into different disciplines and these different contexts have given it a different form. Conceptual comparison is therefore a method identifying small but important changes within or between allied concepts; it is a way to develop conceptual precision.

THE PATTERNS AND USES OF CONCEPT COMPARISON

Concept comparison may be used for different patterns of comparison. We discuss the major types here and, with examples, later in this chapter.

Several Concepts Compete for the Same Phenomenon

Concept comparison enables us to explore, compare, and delineate competing concepts: that is, to examine two or more concepts competing for the same phenomenon. Often these concepts have a lay label and a scientific label that both describe the same phenomenon. For instance, we may consider "being there" and "presence" to be overlapping concepts. This is diagrammed in Figure 19.1(a).

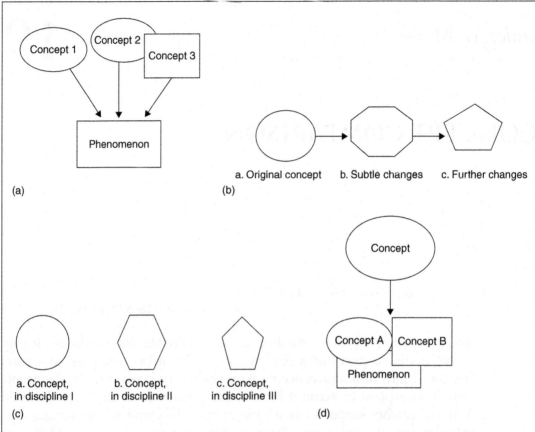

FIGURE 19.1
Patterns of concept comparison: The types of relationships between phenomena and concepts. (a) Several concepts competing for the same phenomenon; (b) the concept has undergone changes as it has been used; (c) the concept is used differently in different contexts; and (d) concept label accounts for several allied concepts (which may actually be the same concept or phenomenon).

The Concept Has Undergone Changes as It Has Been Used

The second reason to use concept comparison is if you suspect that the concept has become *unstable* over time and to determine if the concept has changed or gradually been altered with use (see Figure 19.1b). This method is usually used with scientific concepts, which are supposedly clearly defined in operational definitions. The definitions of scientific concepts remain constant over time. Yet sometimes they may be altered gradually over time, or used in slightly different ways from study to study. Researchers may be unaware that the concept has been altered, yet examination of its use in research may reveal that subtle but important changes have occurred.

The Concept Is Used Differently in Different Contexts

Sometimes the concept acquires different forms in different contexts or may change with different applications. An example of such a change is the different forms acquired when a concept is used in different disciplines. Concept comparison enables us to determine if different *forms* of a concept are indeed a single concept or rather several allied concepts masquerading under a single concept label. (Figure 19.1c).

Several Allied Concepts May Actually Be the Same Concept

Sometimes allied concepts may actually be different concept names for the same concept, so that a broad concept may account for many types or forms. The same attributes are present in the two or more allied concepts, but these attributes are present in different strengths; thus the two concepts are actually different forms of the *same* concept (see Figure 19.1d). An example of this is the concept of hope, which comes in many different forms: In Chapter 16 we discuss hoping against hope, hoping for a chance for a chance, provisional hope, and incremental hope. But there are many other kinds of hope, and we asked you to consider if high hopes, unrealistic hope, and false hope were kinds of hope, allied concepts, or different concepts. Another example would be three terms that are frequently used in nursing: "watching over," "being there," or "presence." Are these the same concept, allied concepts, or different concepts?

ALLIED CONCEPTS

At times, two similar concepts may actually represent slightly different forms of a similar concept—and are "true" allied concepts. These concepts may share one or more attributes and it is this that makes them *similar*, and they may be associated in different ways—within the concept but at a lower level of abstraction, as a component of the larger concept, or nesting. However, as an allied concept represents a different (albeit associated) phenomenon, it is delineating and clarifying these differences that makes an important contribution.

Patterns of Relationships of Allied Concepts

Embedded, More Specialized Concepts

The first pattern of relationship with allied concepts is when a horizontal concept has "lower level" concepts embedded in it. The example given earlier in this text was the horizontal concept of suffering, with "more specialized" and contextualized concepts within it. For instance within suffering we may have the concept of grieving, bereavement, sorrow, and so forth, which may be considered types of suffering.

- *Components, parts of the whole*: These allied concepts may be a part of the larger concept. The example we discuss in Chapter 35 is "enduring," which may be considered the first stage (or part) of suffering. Enduring may be explored as a concept in itself, or we may explore suffering, which consists of two (allied) subconcepts, enduring and emotional suffering.
- *Clustering or neighboring concepts*: These are concepts that account for closely associated concepts. An example may be to differentiate suffering from depression. In this chapter, we illustrate this process by delineating concepts that all account for nursing insight: intuition, emotional empathy, and inference.

When concepts appear similar, the trick is deciding if you are working with the same concept (in different forms) or allied concepts. A student once said, "It is time to get out our conceptual scalpels" (Antasia Wycoff, personal communication). Our task in concept clarification is to sort out (or to clarify) murkiness in our discipline and attack these puzzles. Dictionaries will not help with this task. Dictionaries often use the definition of one concept to define the allied concept.

CONCEPT COMPARISON AS A METHOD

Briefly, conceptual comparison is an active process of comparing the definitions and the significant dimensions (attributes and boundaries) of each concept. These conceptual dimensions are then compared between each allied concept to ensure comprehensive understanding of the differences in the way each allied concept is applied. Alternatively, the attributes of each competing concept are compared and contrasted. Then, from this analysis, comparison continues by asking analytic questions, and identifying significant attributes of a concept, thus enabling the researcher to determine what is unique and what is common between these concepts. (This step is the same as that used in pragmatic utility [Chapter 18], except that you are working with two or more concepts.) The boundaries of each allied concept are compared, to determine if the scope of each concept is similar.

Extending the Strategies of Pragmatic Utility

Constant comparison uses the principles and procedures of pragmatic utility described in Chapter 18. While pragmatic utility has been recommended for use with partially mature concepts, when comparing concepts you may find the following exceptions.

The Inclusion of Scientific Concepts

The concept concerned may be a *scientific concept* rather than a lay concept. Recall that the reason against using pragmatic utility for scientific concepts is that scientific concepts are fully developed when they are introduced: The definition is clear and standardized (as an operational definition), the attributes are clearly articulated, and the boundaries set. Therefore, nothing may be learned from analyzing such a concept.

However, when comparing concepts, we find ourselves looking at subtle and small changes in the same concept. Now, there is nothing wrong with a concept changing: indeed, lay concepts are constantly changing from being introduced to going "out of fashion." A scientific concept also should be changed if it can be improved. (Notice that I said, "should be changed," meaning that the change should be deliberate.) But we may elect to study a particular scientific concept because we *suspect* that the form of the concept has changed subtly over time. These changes may occur from use, acquired by one researcher after another working in different contexts and with different methods, or through debate, confusion, and disagreement between users. Concept comparison allows for the comparison of suspected differences in the form of the same concept, using the techniques of pragmatic utility. By this time, the concepts will have appeared in a large number of articles and be used by many researchers. Concept comparison allows us to compare a scientific concept as it was originally developed, and to look for variation as it has been used over time, comparing the concept as it was developed with the presently used "new version."

Involving Immature Concepts

Occasionally, when comparing several competing concepts, you may find that the concepts involved are not all at the same level of maturity. Some of the concepts involved in the comparison (especially when used to examine competing concepts) may be immature, and there is little literature available describing these concepts. In this case, continue using pragmatic utility, but note the scarcity of literature for one or more of the concepts as a limitation. Excluding them altogether will result in a greater threat to the validity of your analysis. Alternatively, you may introduce the immature concepts after your examination of the analytic questions and compare them broadly at that point.

PATTERNS OF CONCEPT COMPARISON

Comparing Several Concepts Competing for the Same Phenomenon

Often, several concepts compete for the same phenomenon (Figure 19.2). We may call these terms "similes" or allied concepts, but often the terms need to be clarified, and often one is preferred over the other to advance the discipline. For example, we are not certain if nursing "presence" is the same as "being with," and both appear in the literature. These two concepts closely resemble each other; one may be slightly different, and may appear to more closely resemble the phenomenon. Our task would be to determine the differences and the similarities between each of the concepts. At this stage of our research we do not examine the phenomenon itself—that is the task of qualitative inquiry.

Example
Concepts that compete to explicate nursing insight
As an example of the use of concept clarification for competing concepts, we examine the concepts that nurses use to explain nurses' ability to assess a patient condition, or to recognize a patient's state, or an impending crisis, without the patient verbally reporting his or her symptoms, feelings, or need, and before the signs of deterioration are detected on patient monitors. These nurses have the ability to "read" the patient cues, and have the insight to comprehend their meaning (Morse, Miles, Clark, & Doberneck, 1994).

The first step is to identify the concepts in the literature accounting for this phenomenon. Three of the concepts were considered partially mature:

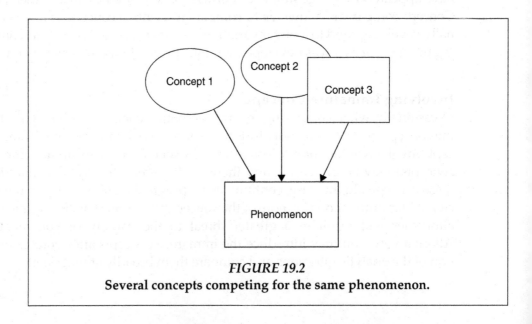

FIGURE 19.2
Several concepts competing for the same phenomenon.

intuition, emotional empathy, and inference. "Knowing" was considered an immature, lay concept. Those that were scientific concepts were: countertransference, compathy, and embodiment. Following the examination of the concepts' definitions, these immature and scientific concepts were placed aside until the partially mature concepts were examined further.

Table 19.1 lists the definitions of each of the concepts. These definitions are derived from a "composite" definition. Displaying the definitions this way enables the researcher (and the reader) to quickly see significant differences in the concepts.

Some of the definitions refer to cognitive processes, others to emotional, and yet others refer to a mixture of both. Countertransference was described as emotional/physical. Which of the concepts occur to one quickly, instantaneously, with conscious thought? Did some concepts imply more certainty to assess the patient's condition/experience than others?

The next step is to identify analytic questions that will enable you to distinguish between concepts. From a close reading of the literature, the following analytic questions associated with preconditions, the process of insight, and the outcomes, were identified.

Preconditions:

- Is the concept a part of human experience?
- Is the concept a gift, talent, or special ability?
- Is the concept influenced by the nurse's personal past?
- Is a previous relationship with the patient necessary for the concept to "work?"
- Can the experience of insight be taught or enhanced in the classroom or in the workplace?

The process of insight:

- Do nurses use emotional, cognitive, or physical responses with the concept?
- At what level of consciousness do nurses use the concept?
- At what level does identification with the patient, occur within the nurse—is it psychological or vicariously physical?

Outcomes:

- Is the concept used to describe a process or a produce?
- Is the experience accurate in terms of predicting patient outcomes?
- Is the concept positive or negative for patient care?

The next step is to take a large (*very* large) sheet of paper and draw a matrix. Place these analytic questions in the first column (one per row). Across the first row, name the major author in the group for each major concept (in this case, authors for intuition, emotional empathy, and inference).

TABLE 19.1
Concepts Used to Describe "Sensing" Patient Needs: Definitions, Mechanisms, and Applications

CONCEPT	DEFINITION	MECHANISM	APPLICATION
Intuition (Agan, 1987; Benner & Tanner, 1987; Correnti, 1992; Rew, 1986, 1988a, 1988b, 1989, 1991; Raw, Agan, Emery, & Harper, 1991)	"Understanding without rationale" (Benner & Tanner, 1987)	Cognitive/emotional	Immediate apprehension, and action on the basis of that conclusion
Inference (Hammond, 1966; Hammond, Kelly, Schneider, & Vancini, 1966; Kelly, 1966; Tanner, Padrick, Westfall, & Putzier, 1987; Westfall, Tanner, Putzier, & Padrick, 1986)	Forming a conclusion based upon premises	Cognitive	Tentative conclusion derived from a process of diagnostic reasoning used by nurses to make judgments about the state of a patient
Emotional Empathy (MacKay, 1990; Morse, Anderson, et al., 1992; Morse, Bottorff, Anderson, O'Brien, & Solberg, 1992; Travelbee, 1972)	"Ability to subjectively experience and to share in another's psychological state, emotions, or intrinsic feelings" (Rogers, 1957, 1962)	Emotional: the distress of the patient is perceived as an emotional insight, which is then followed by an emotional response in the caregiver	Conscious and deliberate role taking to assist the distressed patient
"Knowing" (Tanner, Benner, Chesla, & Gordon, 1993)	Familiarity with patients' responses to therapeutic measures, routines and habits, coping resources, physical capacities and endurance, body typology and characteristics	Cognitive	Involvement with patient permits the use of the optimal intervention
Countertransference (Geach & White, 1974; Miles & Morse, 1995; Schroder, 1985)	A therapist's total response to a client—including conscious and unconscious thoughts and feelings (Hammond, 1966)	Emotional/physical—the reactions of professional caregivers to their clients	A potential therapeutic tool that can enhance a therapist's understanding of a client
Compathy (Morse & Mitchan, 1997)	The response that occurs when a person observes physical distress/suffering in another person, and the observer experiences similar distress or symptoms	Emotional: response reflexively simultaneously occurs in the observer	Motivates the observer (caregiver) to assist to relieve the distress in the patient, in order to relieve the distress in the caregiver
Embodiment (Gadow 1982, 1983, 1989)	Experiencing one's body as lived connection with the self	Emotional: inflicting pain necessitates the nurse to objectify the self—to detach from him or herself	Embodiment results in the nurse acting as an unfeeling instrument. Nurses must "re-embody" in order to serve as patient advocates

Source: Morse et al. (1994).

Working systematically, ask each author the analytic question, recording his or her answer on your matrix. Maintain control by placing direct quotations in quotation marks with the page number, noting the author, year, and page number.

Once this is completed, synthesize each group of responses. The results for this project are presented in Table 19.2. Any difference between concepts—and similarities—should be immediately apparent.

Delineating/Developing the Concepts

In Table 19.3 we show the conceptual attributes of intuition, emotional empathy, and inference. Commonalities are evident: all are for the relief of distress; all provide a nursing intervention. However, the process by which the nurse responds is very different. Intuition and emotional empathy both use the nurses' emotional response and response subconsciously, whereas inference uses clinical knowledge. In addition, the outcomes and the perceived "success" of each, are also different with inference the most tolerant of error. However, difference in reporting were also different. Benner and Tanner (1987), when reporting on nurses' interviews about intuition, had not reported instances in which the intuition was incorrect—on instances in which the nurse, based on intuition, had called a code and the patient had subsequently *not* coded.

Despite the cognitive overlap of these three concepts, there are distinct differences *within* each concept according to their epistemological origin, which impact on the interpretation, translation, and utilization of the concepts. Further, when concepts are borrowed from other disciplines, often their meaning subtly changes, so that two authors discussing the same concept may be using diverse meanings. We noted that:

> . . . there were distinct differences relating to the epistemological origins and/or to the nursing interpretation, translation, adoption, and utilization of the concepts; this divergence of use is a problem for nursing. At times, the fact that these concepts were removed from their theoretical contexts and/or theoretical origins is not discussed. This borrowing has serious ramifications because, in the process of transfer, the meaning subtly changes. Thus, two authors may be apparently discussing the same concept yet applying diverse meanings to the same concept. For example, Benner and Tanner (1987) use the concept "intuition" to describe a model of skill acquisition as developed by Dreyfus and Dreyfus (1980), whereas Gerrity (1987) uses the concept of intuition as a personality trait as described by Jungian psychoanalysts . . . Because these differences have not been made explicit and because the same label is used for both

TABLE 19.2
Comparison on Intuition, Emotional Empathy, and Inference

ANALYTIC QUESTIONS	CONCEPTS		
	INTUITION	EMOTIONAL EMPATHY	INFERENCE
Preconditions			
1. A part of the human experience?	Everyone has the ability, but in differing degrees (Agan, 1987; Rew, 1988a) Only experts (Benner & Tanner, 1987; Schraeder & Fischer, 1987)	Yes—innate human condition (Wheeler, 1988; Zderad, 1969)	Not directly addressed but as a way of reasoning—most people have this capacity
2. Special gift/ability?	Special ability/gift, personality attribute. (Rew, 1988a) Gift that can be enhanced. (Rew, 1989) No—everyone has it. (Agan, 1987; Benner & Tanner, 1987)	No—basic human endowment (Zderad, 1969) Yes—it is an art that is acquired (Hughes, Carver, & MacKay, 1990)	N/A
3. Influenced by the nurses' personal past?	"Lifelong learning experience." (Agan, 1987) Includes personal values and attitudes. (Corcoran-Perry & Bungert, 1992)	Yes (La Monica, 1983; Zderad, 1969)	No—only *clinical* memory—do not discuss
4. A previous relationship with the patient?	No, but it helps (Agan, 1987; Benner & Tanner, 1987; Correnti, 1992; Rew, 1988a; Schraeder & Fischer, 1987)	Yes—"occurs with listening" (Rogers, 1957) A professional relationship; "one shares, but stands apart." (Travelbee, 1972)	No (Kelly, 1966; Tanner, Padrick, Westfall, & Putzier, 1987; Westfall, Tanner, Putzier, & Padrick, 1986)

(continued)

TABLE 19.2
Comparison on Intuition, Emotional Empathy, and Inference (continued)

ANALYTIC QUESTIONS	CONCEPTS		
	INTUITION	EMOTIONAL EMPATHY	INFERENCE
5. Can the experience be taught or enhanced in the classroom or at work?	Yes—mediating/using imagery (Harper, 1991; Rew, Agan, Emery, & Rew, 1986) Yes—with on the job experience (Agan, 1987; Benner & Tanner, 1987; Corcoran-Perry & Bungert, 1992; Rew, 1991; Schraeder & Fischer, 1987) Yes—enhanced in the classroom (Benner & Tanner, 1987) May be taught (Correnti, 1992)	Yes (La Monica, 1983; MacKay, 1990)	May be improved with exposure in classroom and job (Hammond, 1966; Kelly, 1966; Tanner, Padrick, Westfall, & Putzier, 1987) "Memories of knowledge" (Westfall, 1986)
Process			
6. Nurses' response emotional, cognitive, or physical?	Cognitive, emotional, and physical components (Agan, 1987; Benner & Tanner, 1987; Rew, 1988a, 1988b; Rew, Agan, Emery, & Harper, 1991)	Primary emotional "Personality change" (Rogers, 1957) Emotional, cognitive, and physical aspects (Zderad, 1969)	Cognitive "message units," "cues" (Hammond, 1966) "Judgment, intellectual process" process," (Kelly, 1966) "Intelligent, cognitive" (Tanner, Padrick, Westfall, & Putzier, 1987)
7. Level of consciousness	Subconscious knowing (Agan, 1987; Correnti, 1992) Subliminal or unconscious (Rew, 1988a) Not conscious (Schraeder & Fischer, 1987) "Commonsense understanding" (Benner & Tanner, 1987)	Unconscious "Empathic understanding." (Rogers, 1957) "Affective empathy" is both subconscious and unconscious: "cognitive empathy" is intellectual and conscious. (Gladstein, 1983) Conscious and unconscious aspects. (Conscious Travelbee, 1972; Zderad, 1969)	N/A

(continued)

TABLE 19.2
Comparison on Intuition, Emotional Empathy, and Inference (continued)

	CONCEPTS		
ANALYTIC QUESTIONS	INTUITION	EMOTIONAL EMPATHY	INFERENCE
8. Identification occurs with the patient—is it psychological or physical?	N/A	Psychological (Rogers, 1957) Both have "psychological, physiological, and social dimensions." (Zderad, 1969)	N/A
Outcomes			
9. Is the concept used to describe a process or a product?	Process (Agan, 1987; Benner & Tanner 1987; Rew, 1988a, 1988b; Rew et al., 1991) Both process and product (Benner & Tanner, 1987) (used interchangeably) (Correnti, 1992; Young, 1987) Product "intuitive judgment." (Benner & Tanner, 1987) "Something is wrong." (Schraeder & Fischer, 1987)	Process or product—has psychological, physiological, or social dimensions. (MacKay, 1990; Travelbee, 1972; Zderad, 1969)	Process "Making a judgment." (Kelly, 1966) "Information processing." (Hammond, 1966) Product "conclusion itself." (Tanner, Padrick, Westfall, & Putzier, 1987; Westfall, Tanner, Putzier, & Padrick, 1986)
10. Is the experience accurate in terms of predication?	Emphasize accuracy Note that it may be incorrect and recommend using other data. (Agan, 1987; Benner & Tanner, 1987) May be inaccurate. (Gerrity, 1987)	Accurate (by definition)	May be wrong (Hammond, 1966; Kelly, 1966) Either (Westfall, Tanner, Putzier, & Padrick, 1986)
11. Positive or negative for patient care?	Positive is emphasized exclusively (Agan, 1987; Benner & Tanner, 1987; Rew, 1991) Can be negative if not used (Pyles & Stern, 1983)	Positive "If correctly done." (Rogers, 1957)	Because it can be wrong, it may be either.

Source: Morse et al. (1994).

meanings, these two theoretical interpretations of the same concept and the resulting research have been merged and are treated equivalently in the nursing literature. This conceptual sloppiness is a problem that requires urgent attention. (Morse et al., 1994, p. 249)

None of the authors writing about these concepts have suggested that nurses actually use two or even three of the concepts simultaneously—the concepts are distinct, and the competition between them is in the accounting for the phenomenon. Even though the process of instantaneous assessment without patients' verbal complaint or changes in the vital signs on the monitor is still an important part of care, none of the concepts are adequately developed as to be incorporated into nursing theory or clinical teaching, and this problem remains. It is not a problem of monitoring, but in the interpretation of the behaviors of those being monitored. In 1994, we concluded by suggesting that as none of the concepts accurately included nurses' prediction of a patient coding from a "look that patients get" prior to a code (Benner & Tanner, 1987) then perhaps we should transfer our attention to conducting research using subliminal theory. Research could then be conducted by actually coding patient's expressions and looking for signs of this particular expression, rather than continually interviewing nurses (which appears to be a dead-end path to this inquiry). Such research would be clinically useful for assessment, and be suitable for teaching in the classroom, but to my knowledge, this has not been done.

The purpose of listing this 1994 research in this volume was to illustrate the process of conducting concept comparison. However, nurse researchers are still exploring intuition using concept development methods with little progress, or by conducting interview research—which also has serious limitations for understanding this type of question. A systematic review by Rew (2004) concluded that most studies were of descriptive–exploratory design and have remained at that level for "more than 20 years" (p. E24). The microanalytic observational study has not been conducted.

What are we doing about this as a discipline? Research agendas established by federal agencies or foundations do not approach such a basic clinical problem—nor, indeed, do they call for any research problems that are at the core of nursing processes. Tanner (2006) reviewed the research to teaching clinical judgment, but in her article, clinical judgment remains dependent on reflective practice. Without developing a new approach to this research, educators have a difficult time teaching clinical judgment, as do students to learn the skills. Expert nursing remains the purview of mentors, learning by trial and error, and mysterious, unidentified assessment processes (see Paley, 1996, 1997, 2006).

TABLE 19.3
Comparison of the Conceptual Components of Three Major Concepts Accounting for Nurse Insight Permission required

	INTUITION	EMOTIONAL EMPATHY	INFERENCE
Definition	"Understanding without rationale"[1]	Ability to subjectively experience and to share in another's psychological state, emotions, or intrinsic feelings	Forming a conclusion based upon premises
Preconditions	Patient distress	Patient distress	Patient distress
	Particular sensitivity in the nurse, enhanced by learning and experience	The art of psychological and emotional sensitivity in the nurse	Clinical reasoning in the assessment of the patient cues
Attributes	Subconscious	Emotional, subconscious	Cognitive
	Instant recognition of a patient's problem	Emotional sensing of a patient's problem	Recognition, judgment of a patient's problem
	Relationship not necessary, but will aid	Social dimension. Enhanced by relationship	Relationship not necessary
	Nurse: cognitive, emotional, and physical response	Nurse: emotional, psychological, and physical response	Nurse: physical intervention
Boundaries	Physical assessment	Physical/psychological assessment	Physical assessment
Outcomes	Nursing intervention	Nursing intervention	Nursing intervention
	Nurses' responses generally positive, but may be incorrect	Nurse response positive	Nurse response may be correct or incorrect

Source: Morse et al. (1994).

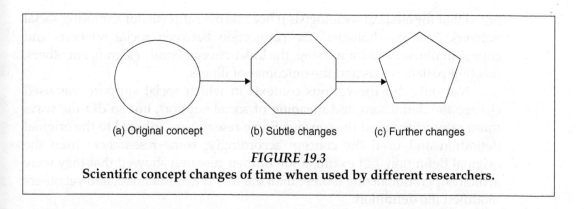

(a) Original concept   (b) Subtle changes   (c) Further changes

FIGURE 19.3
Scientific concept changes of time when used by different researchers.

The Concept Has Undergone Changes as It Has Been Used: Conceptual Drift

Pragmatic utility is a strategy that may be used for comparing a concept as it was developed with the way the concept is currently used. It may be used for scientific concepts, so that it is relatively easy to locate the publications that first introduced the concepts, and later publications that cited the original authors, and use the concept in current research, looking for subtle changes in the meaning or use of the concept (see Figure 19.3).

The problem is that the authors using the concept use the original definition and cite the author who originally introduced the concept, yet may be unaware that they are not using the concept as it was intended.

Do not forget that concepts are dynamic. However, scientific concepts are not supposed to be "informally dynamic." If scientific concepts change (and they may), any modification is supposed to occur purposefully, with supporting theoretical rationale, experimentation, measurement, and debate.

THE EXAMPLE: THE CONCEPTUAL COHESION OF SOCIAL SUPPORT

Judith E. Hupcey

When the concept of social support was introduced by Caplan (1974), Cobb (1976), and Cassel (1976), social support was not suddenly "invented," introducing new types of supportive relationships. Rather, the identification of the concept changed our perception of, and renamed, what was previously—and clumsily—called "caring friendship, community cohesion, or unconditional positive regard" (Tilden, 1985). However, as soon as social support was introduced, the significance of social support was recognized, but it had different research purposes in different disciplines. Hupcey (1998a) noted that for medical sociologists it became the rationale for exploring social networks; for psychologists the connection between social relations and coping in illness; and for nursing, the link between family/significant others, meeting patient needs and the outcomes of illness.

Not only did the various contexts in which social support was used change the definitions and meaning of social support, but so did the ways those researchers used the concept. Some researchers adhered to the original definition and used the concept accordingly; some researchers used the original definition, but examination of their research showed that they were actually operationalizing it other than the way it was intended, and yet others modified the definition.

Suspecting such changes, Hupcey (1998a) proceeded by first examining the original definitions of the concept. When concepts are first introduced, there is often a period of debate and modification to the definition. She then listed the definitions that were presented by each author, and examined them by comparing them with the original definitions, and the components of each definition, and examined their attributes (characteristics) looking for commonalties and differences. From this, analytic questions were developed:

1. Was the relationship between the supporter and the recipient specified?
2. What were the recipients' perceptions of the outcomes of social support?
3. Was the type of support specified?
4. Did the definitions exclude material aid?

Hupcey's (1998a) evaluation of the analytic questions and these enabled her to explore the anatomy of the concept (see Table 19.4). Although all researchers used the term "social support," the theoretical definitions used varied greatly, from the supporter's "act of providing a resource," to the recipient's "having the sense of, or belief, that someone is there for them" (p. 307). As most of the studies do not specify the relationship between the provider and the recipient, "any social relationship (e.g., giving directions to a stranger) would be considered social support" (Hupcey, 1998a, p. 307). However, examining the more recent literature, Hupcey noted that most of the studies are conducted without a theoretical definition (p. 312). Other conceptual issues that are unclear are:

• If an action is given, but not recognized
• If the action provided is not considered positive by the recipient, but really is
• If the action is intended to be positive, but the outcome is negative

- If the action is negative, but considered by the recipient to be positive
- If the action is given by a stranger, organization, the community, or a professional. (Hupcey, 1998a, p. 313)

In the next step in her research, Hupcey was able to determine the anatomy (which she refers to as the "structural features") of the concept of social support (Table 19.5).

Exploring the physiology of the concept, Hupcey (1998a) examined the supporter's intentionality, the congruence between the supporter and the recipient into what was perceived by each as "supportive," and the recipient's awareness of the act. Social support, she concluded, has only occurred when there was "an appropriate need for support," the recipient perceived the need for the support and when the support was given and accepted. Social support had not occurred when the recipient did not appreciate the need to support, when the support was rejected, or when the support was withheld. This analysis is conducted by constructing a 2x2 matrix and asking the analytic questions for each cell by row and column (Figure 19.4).

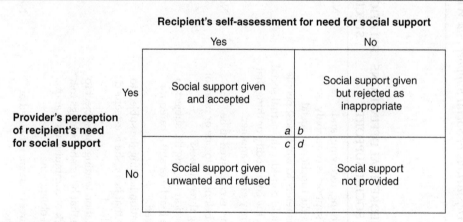

FIGURE 19.4

Matrix explicating the congruency between the provider and the recipient of social support.

Cell *a*: Congruent. The perception of need and action provided is congruent between provider and recipient.

Cell *b*: Incongruency between the provider and recipient. Support is untimely or the wrong type of support; or inappropriate assessment of need by the provider.

Cell *c*: Incongruent. Provider perceives a need and provides support when the recipient does not perceive a need. (Support is stifled—"get off my back." For instance, pushing someone to follow a low fat diet or to stop smoking.)

Cell *d*: Congruent. Provider and recipient perceive no need for support. Support not provided.

Source: Adapted from Hupcey (1998a).

TABLE 19.4
Comparison of Major Theoretical Definitions of Social Support and What is Described

AUTHOR(S)	MAJOR THEORETICAL DEFINITIONS OF SOCIAL SUPPORT	RELATIONSHIP SPECIFIED	INCLUDES RECIPIENTS' PERCEPTIONS OF THE OUTCOMES OF SOCIAL SUPPORT	TYPE OF SUPPORT SPECIFIED	EXCLUDES MATERIAL AID
Antonucci (1985, p. 25)	The actual giving, receiving, and exchange of support is commonly referred to as the function of social support. This refers to what most people probably would consider the actual social support, i.e., the commodity or thing that one person may give to another.	No	No	No	No
Cobb (1976, p. 300)	Social support is conceived to be information belonging to one or more of the following three classes: 1. Information leading the subject to believe that he or she is cared for and loved. 2. Information leading the subject to believe that he or she is esteemed and valued. 3. Information leading the subject to believe that he or she belongs to a network of communication and mutual obligation.	No	Yes	Yes	Yes
Cohen, Mermelstein, Karmarck, and Hoberman (1985, p. 75)	. . . the resources that are provided by other persons	No	No	No	No

(continued)

TABLE 19.4
Comparison of Major Theoretical Definitions of Social Support and What is Described (continued)

AUTHOR(S)	MAJOR THEORETICAL DEFINITIONS OF SOCIAL SUPPORT	RELATIONSHIP SPECIFIED	INCLUDES RECIPIENTS' PERCEPTIONS OF THE OUTCOMES OF SOCIAL SUPPORT	TYPE OF SUPPORT SPECIFIED	EXCLUDES MATERIAL AID
Heller, Swindle, Dusenbury (1986, p. 467)	A social activity is said to involve social support if it is perceived by the recipient of that activity as esteem enhancing or if it involves the provision of stress-related interpersonal aid . . . The term perceived support (Procidano & Heller, 1983) refers to a generalized appraisal that individuals develop in the various role domains of their lives in which they believe that they are cared for and valued, that significant others are available to them in times of need, and that they are satisfied with the relationships they have.	Yes and No	Yes	Yes	Yes
Hilbert (1990, p. 84)	Social support is defined as a diversity of natural helping behaviors of which individuals are recipients in social interactions . . .	No	No	No	No

(continued)

TABLE 19.4
Comparison of Major Theoretical Definitions of Social Support and What is Described (continued)

AUTHOR(S)	MAJOR THEORETICAL DEFINITIONS OF SOCIAL SUPPORT	RELATIONSHIP SPECIFIED	INCLUDES RECIPIENTS' PERCEPTIONS OF THE OUTCOMES OF SOCIAL SUPPORT	TYPE OF SUPPORT SPECIFIED	EXCLUDES MATERIAL AID
Antonucci and Jackson (1990, p. 252)	. . . social support is defined in terms of resources that meet needs . . . Emotional support refers to behavior that fosters feelings of comfort and leads an individual to believe that he or she is admired, respected, and loved, and that others are available to provide caring and security. Cognitive support refers to information, knowledge, and/or advice that helps the individual to understand his or her world and to adjust to changes within it. Material support refers to goods and services that help to solve practical problems.	No	Yes	Yes	No
Kahn and Antonucci (1980)	Social support has been defined as interpersonal transactions that include one or more of the following: affect (expression of liking, love, admiration, respect), affirmation (expressions of agreement or acknowledgment of the appropriateness or rightness of some act, statement, or point of view), and aid (transactions in which direct aid or assistance is given, including things, money, information, advice, time, or entitlement).	No	No	Yes	No

(continued)

TABLE 19.4
Comparison of Major Theoretical Definitions of Social Support and What is Described (continued)

AUTHOR(S)	MAJOR THEORETICAL DEFINITIONS OF SOCIAL SUPPORT	RELATIONSHIP SPECIFIED	INCLUDES RECIPIENTS' PERCEPTIONS OF THE OUTCOMES OF SOCIAL SUPPORT	TYPE OF SUPPORT SPECIFIED	EXCLUDES MATERIAL AID
Lin (1986, p. 18)	Thus, the synthetic definition of social support is the perceived or actual instrumental and/or expressive provisions supplied by the community, social networks, and confiding partners.	Yes—global	No	Yes	No
Pilisuk (1982, p. 20)	Social support refers to those relationships among people that provide not only material help and emotional assurance, but also the sense that one is a continuing object of concern on the part of other people.	No	Yes	Yes	No
Shumaker and Brownell (1984, p. 13)	Social support is an exchange of resources between two individuals perceived by the provider or the recipient to be intended to enhance the well-being of the recipient.	No	Yes + No	No	No
Thoits (1985, p. 53)	Social support most commonly refers to helpful functions performed for an individual by significant others such as family members, friends, coworkers, relatives, and neighbors. These functions typically include socioemotional aid, instrumental aid, and informational aid.	Yes	No	Yes	No

Source: Hupcey (1998a).

TABLE 19.5
Structural Features of Social Support

PRECONDITIONS	CHARACTERISTICS	OUTCOMES	BOUNDARIES
Provider perceives a need in the recipient[†]	Action is toward a particular "person"[†]	There is usually a positive response (or change) in the recipient	It is not social support if the action:
Provider must be motivated to take appropriate action	Action must be well intentioned		is given to or from an organization, the community, or a professional
	Action must be willingly/freely given	This response may be subjective, objective, or delayed.	
			has a negative intent or is known to result in a negative outcome
			is given grudgingly

[†]The recipient and "person" are defined as having a personal (not professional) relationship.
Source: Hupcey (1998a).

Subsequently, from this analysis, the theoretical definition that was developed was:

A well-intentioned action that is given willingly to a person with whom there is a personal relationship and that produces an immediate or delayed positive response in the recipient (Hupcey, 1998a, p. 313).

EVALUATING CONCEPTS FOR APPROPRIATE APPLICATION

The Concept Has Undergone Changes in Application

Concept drift occurs with *use* of the concept over time, by different researchers. If you suspect this has occurred; investigate the phenomenon rigorously, so that your study does not compound the problem.

Professionals do not, or may not, or should not, have a personal relationship with a patient; the relationship should be a professional–client relationship; the person may even be a "stranger." Using pragmatic utility, the main characteristics of social support were identified, and the presence of these social support characteristics was compared between "social support" relationship and a "professional support" relationship (Table 19.6).

TABLE 19.6
Comparison of the Major Characteristics of Social Support and Professional Support

CHARACTERISTICS	SOCIAL SUPPORT	PROFESSIONAL SUPPORT
Type of service provided	Open	Delimited
Duration	Must be developed	Instantly available
Trust	Reciprocal (shared)	Unilateral
Obligation	Kinship/friendship	Based on role expectations
Expectations of the relationship	Based on congruent expectation	Based on role expectations
Reciprocal action	Equivalent	Not required, services "purchased" or financially compensated

Source: Hupcey and Morse (1997).

From this analysis, it was concluded that professional support was very different from social support in many dimensions. Despite this, professionals were considered to have provided social support in many studies. Further, Hupcey observed that despite a consistent definition of social support, the concept of social support itself had not been used consistently in the same way over time. Hupcey, therefore, continued her analysis to compare the theoretical definitions and how social support was conceptualized in the literature (Hupcey, 1998a, 1998b). She first determined that the provider must determine the need and give appropriate support; the recipient must also perceive a need for the support and accept the support (Hupcey, 1998a).

Hupcey's work on social support explored the subtle changes that occurred with the conceptualization of social support in research. By exploring the *patterns* of interaction as used by researchers in exploring social support a myriad of patterns considered to be social support were revealed. For example, the usual pattern of social support was one person supporting another (Figure 19.5a). However, in nursing, the supportive relationship was frequently the nurse supporting the caregiver, and indirectly supporting the patient in a provider–secondary provider model (Figure 19.5b). If more than one provider was meeting the needs of a recipient, we have a multiprovider model as shown in Figure 19.5c (Hupcey, 1998b).

When interactions are considered, the relationship increases in complexity (Figure 19.6a–19.6g). The direct reciprocation model is shown in (a), the delayed reciprocation model in (b). The secondary reciprocation model is shown in (c), a "pay it forward" model, as used for instance by Alcoholics Anonymous. The recipient does not reciprocate, with the provider providing

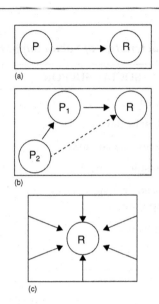

FIGURE 19.5
Present models of social support. (a) Provider–recipient model: one provider meets all the needs of the recipient. (b) Primary–secondary provider model: secondary provider assists primary provider in meeting the needs of the recipient. (c) Multiple provider model: more than one provider involved in meeting the needs of the recipient.
Source: Hupcey (1998b). Reprinted with permission.

more support than is received (d), or does not reciprocate (e). Sometimes the support is provided under duress, even though the exchange is intended to be supportive (f). The last example (g) is when the support is negative, is perceived as negative, or the outcome is negative (Hupcey, 1998b).

Changes Incurred From Different Contexts

Concepts in use are context-bound, and it is the concept's relationship with the context that makes it so difficult to remove the context to discern the features of the concept from the features of the context, or "decontextualizing the concept."

What changes or adaptations occur within the concept themselves when placed in another context? Remember, in order for the concept to remain a concept, all of the attributes must remain and be present regardless of context, and the strength of concept analysis is being able to recognize the stability of these attributes regardless of context. However, changes that occur within the concept themselves are the strength of the attributes, with some

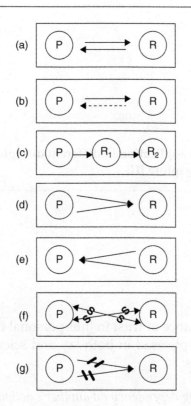

FIGURE 19.6

Proposed models of social support interactions. (a) Direct reciprocation model: recipient provides direct reciprocal acts toward the provider. (b) Delayed reciprocation model: recipient reciprocates at a later time or because of past relationship with the provider does not need to reciprocate. (c) Secondary reciprocation model: recipient reciprocates to a second person in need of support (Alcoholics Anonymous model). (d) Nonreciprocal recipient model: recipient receiving more support than is reciprocated. (e) Nonreciprocal provider model: recipient providing more support than received. (f) Stressful interaction model: interaction between the provider and recipient is stressful, even though behaviors may be intended to be supportive. (g) Negative provider support model: support provided is negative, perceived as negative, or the outcome is negative.

Source: Hupcey (1998b). Reprinted with permission.

becoming less dominant than others as the context changes. In the new context, when the concept changes its role and function, the concept may adapt its form or appearance to the new context (Figure 19.7) by emphasizing some attributes and de-emphasizing others. In the example of hope discussed previously, we saw the form of hope change with circumstances (context). Here we examine a comparison of trust across disciplines (Hupcey, 2002).

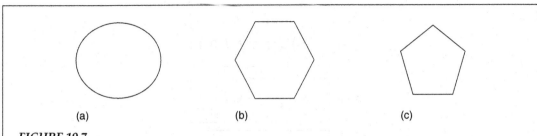

FIGURE 19.7
**Concepts are changed with application in different disciplines: (a) Discipline I;
(b) discipline II; and (c) discipline III.**

THE EXAMPLE: TRUST

Judith E. Hupcey

Despite the significance of trust in interpersonal relations, trust is a relatively undeveloped concept, used in both lay and scientific literature. Analysis of trust was defined as:

> *Trust is a willing dependency on another's actions, but is limited to the area of need and is subject to overt and covert testing. The outcome of trust is an evaluation of the congruence between expectations of the trusted person and actions.* (Hupcey, Penrod, Morse, & Mitcham, 2001, p. 290)

The structure of the concept of trust (Hupcey et al., 2001, pp. 286, 290) was as follows:

Antecedents:

1. A need that cannot be met without the help of another
2. Prior knowledge and/or experience with the other
3. Some assessment of risk or what is at stake

Attributes:

1. Dependency on another individual to have a need met
2. Choice or willingness to take some risks
3. An expectation that the trusted individual will behave in a certain way
4. Limited focus to the area or behavior related to the need
5. Testing of the trustworthiness of the individual

Boundaries: Trust is no longer present when:

1. The decision to place oneself in a dependent or vulnerable position is not based on some assessment of risk
2. There is no perception of choice
3. The risks outweigh the benefits

Outcomes:

1. There is a positive outcome; the trustee's expectation is met or exceeded.

Next, to explore the use of trust in the disciplines of medicine, psychology, sociology, and nursing, the literature was searched, read, and analytic questions developed. Using a huge matrix, these questions were then asked of each discipline. You will notice that there is no direct correspondence between the attributes and the analytic questions.

The major results are summarized in Table 19.7 (see also Hupcey et al., 2001, pp. 286–289). In each column, the values of each discipline were reflected in the way they considered trust to be defined, was developed between individuals and in the work and social setting, how trust was interpreted, and what the positive outcomes were. Look at this table: Does trust appear as the same concept in all of these contexts?

Next, as well as comparing the answers of our analytic questions across disciplines, we also compare the components of trust with the responses to our analytic questions.

Conceptual Components of Trust

The preconditions of trust are: a need within the individual that cannot be achieved without the assistance of another person, a personal friend acquaintance or even a stranger, or a professional. Trusting that person puts the person in a position of vulnerability or dependency, so that prior experience of knowledge of the selected person (or their societal role) is necessary. Finally, the individual must be aware of the risk and consequences of choosing to trust or not to trust (Hupcey et al., 2001, p. 286). All disciplines met the "need" criteria.

- Attribute 1: The necessity of dependence on another in order to have a need met: Question 2 (Table 19.7) shows that all disciplines noted that an individual must have a *need* in order to trust.
- Attribute 2: The decision to trust is a *choice* and that trusting places one at *risk*: Question 3 (Table 19.7) reveals agreement among the disciplines that trusting puts one at *risk*, in order to

TABLE 19.7
Summary Comparing Trust in the Disciplines of Medicine, Sociology, Psychology, and Nursing

ANALYTIC QUESTIONS	DISCIPLINE			
	MEDICINE	SOCIOLOGY	PSYCHOLOGY	NURSING
1. Can/may an individual develop trust instantaneously or is it built over time?	Over time Using active strategies	Built or established, included influence of milieu and personal experience	Over time, through repeated interactions; some role trust is instantaneous	Instantaneous trust = "Naïve trust"; built over time, using strategies; component of relationship building
2. Is "need" a precondition to trust?	Yes	Independent of need; trust is a choice	Trust is a developmental need	Precondition; need for health services
3. By trusting another, does the individual place him or herself at risk?	Risk: breach of confidentiality; abandonment	Calculated risk; will risk—confident of good outcome	Trust enables risk; trusting puts one at risk; or trust implies vulnerability	Risk is incurred
4. Does an individual choose to trust or not to trust?	Choice is not to trust	Decision; a cognitive choice	Trust is a choice; willing; negotiated	Decision; choice
5. Is trust an inherent or learned trait?	N/A	N/A	Learned; personality trait; experience, education; practice	Mix of inherent and learned; education and practice
6. Does an individual trust another person by role or personal characteristics?	Differentiates interpersonal trust vs. social trust (of an institution)	Of society and professionals by role; both individuals and professionals	Specific person; category of strangers; target persons; individual peers	Early—related to role, then individuals. Part of complex systems

(continued)

TABLE 19.7
Summary Comparing Trust in the Disciplines of Medicine, Sociology, Psychology, and Nursing (continued)

	DISCIPLINE			
ANALYTIC QUESTIONS	MEDICINE	SOCIOLOGY	PSYCHOLOGY	NURSING
7. Is trust unilateral, bilateral, or reciprocal?	Mutual; bilateral in counseling relationships	Unilateral. Based on exchange; not necessarily returned	Bilateral or reciprocal; may be potentially unilateral	Unilateral (patient to nurse); reciprocal; mutual
8. Does trust between individuals involve testing behaviors?	N/A	Testing with increased knowledge	Evaluates testing for congruence; once trust established, testing ends	Testing behaviors described
9. Are there different kinds of trust?	Interpersonal vs. social	Personal trust vs. system trust	Interpersonal trust; some generalized. Feelings of trust versus. trusting behaviors	Intimate relationships versus. professional caregiving relationship
10. What are the ramifications/ manifestations of loss of trust?	Focuses on distrust rather than loss of trust. Impacts on health and well-being	May be disrupted	Trust may be broken; reconstruction difficult	Fragile; may be lost. Reestablishment a long and tenuous process.
11. What is the expected outcome of trust: Is trust a means to an end?	N/A	Expectations included in definitions	Expected positive results; outcomes intrinsic and extrinsic; increases coping and control	Trust as a means to an end. Benefits: positive patient outcomes

Adapted from Hupcey et al. (2001).

have the need met. Individuals are aware of the consequences of not trusting and the trusting also places them in a vulnerable position. Further, Question 4 shows that there is agreement that trusting is a *choice*, with the exception of medicine, where patients often feel they have no choice but to trust.

- Attribute 3: The individual expects that the person will behave in a certain way. All disciplines differentiated between individual trust and role/professional trust. We expect trusted individuals to maintain confidentialities or keep promises. We expect professional codes of conduct to be met by professionals (Question 6). Nevertheless, sociology, psychology, and nursing literature all described "testing" behaviors of individuals to ensure trustworthiness. In medicine this was not addressed (Questions 8)—perhaps, if patients have no choice but to trust the physician, testing becomes a moot point.
- Attribute 4: Trust is targeted to the area of need.
- Attribute 5: Testing the trustworthiness of the individual. Our analytic questions did not directly address this attribute, although it is implied that individuals target their trust and select individuals according to the ability of these individuals to meet their needs. Question 6 includes this in the role of the trusted persons.

The boundaries of trust are closely related to the absence of the attributes, and again have significance for medicine.

The outcomes, Attributes 1 and 2 relate to the expectations of trusting and the congruence between expectations of the trustee and the behaviors of the trusted person. Question 11, "Is trust a means to the end?" is important to sociology, psychology, and nursing, but again, had not been addressed in the medical literature. Considering the ramifications of loss of trust is clearly problematic for nursing and psychology, and disruption is noted in sociology. However, the focus on *distrust*, rather than loss of trust, suggests in medicine, with the exceptions of counseling situations, that trust was never gained.

The comparison of trust in these four disciplines was interesting. Trust has greater importance in nursing and psychology. Very problematic to this analysis was the way that trust was reflected in medicine. When we look, from this distance, patient trust in the physician is expected, but not always present. From the perspective of the medical profession, we note that distrust is almost ingrained: When charting, for instance, physicians write: "The patient . . ." or, "The patient denies (smoking/drinking . . .)," so that their professional stance is not one of acceptance or trust, or even testing to build physician–patient trust. Concepts such as compliance (measured as degree of compliance or noncompliance) in the monitoring of patient following (or not) their instructions and treatments are concepts of distrust. This is clearly an important area for further study.

Several Allied Concepts May Actually Be the Same Concept

The last problem we have to solve is the case in which one concept label may be used to cover several concepts. In this case, the concept is too broad to account for the differences in concepts A and B and the associated phenomenon (Figure 19.8).

It is usually the case, when there is such concept confusion, that all of the concepts are immature, and therefore unsuited for analysis using techniques of pragmatic utility and concept comparison. Often, solving this problem is the purview of qualitative researchers, and requires the conduct of fieldwork with careful delineation of each concept or development of the phenomenon. Sometimes this research requires more microanalytic work to delineate the attributes in the subconcepts, so they may be properly identified and named. On the other hand, these competing concepts may be left to those developing scientific concepts to define and delineate as many concepts that they consider useful and to sort out the confusion that way.

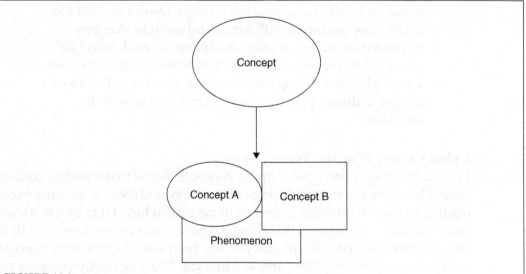

FIGURE 19.8
The main concept label refers to several concepts or phenomena, which may be the same concept under different names, or allied concepts.

TO DO 19.1. IDENTIFYING COMPETING CONCEPTS

Make lists of competing concepts found in nursing. Include lay and scientific concepts in your list.

RECOGNIZING WHEN IT IS GOOD: CRITERIA FOR EXCELLENCE IN CONCEPT DEVELOPMENT

We just need enough to hang ourselves
—Nancy Savage, Snowbird (1979)
(on accepting a corded microphone,
to lead the doctoral students' responses
to Leininger's keynote address)

HINTS FOR GETTING IT RIGHT

When doing concept analysis, the essence of success rests in three factors:

1. Identifying the type of concepts selected and the identification of the level of maturity of the concept selected, both of which determine your approach to the analysis.
2. Your selection of literature to be used as data. This selection must include the major "schools of thought" or primarily researchers who have used the concept. Do not make it too narrow nor too broad without careful thought. Are you interested in *nursing* or other disciplines as well. Why? Or why not? Be purposeful in your delineation of the literature.
3. Developing and asking astute analytic questions. Before you can get to this step, you must be very familiar with the literature.

Using Concepts of the Wrong Type

Pragmatic utility is best used with lay concepts. Recall that scientific concepts should have been perfected during construction, and there is no sense in conducting analysis with them, unless, as in the case of Judy Hupcey's work with social support, you suspect that there has been some conceptual drift. In the literature we see that concept analysis has been used for scientific concepts, such as human ecology (Huyanh & Alderson, 2009) or family-centered care (Mikkelsen & Frederiksen, 2011). Using pragmatic utility for scientific concepts does not make any sense, as the components of the concept should have been described in the literature when the concept was introduced. In other words, there is nothing to uncover.

Remember that if you have an abstract, high-level concept, even if it is a lay concept, a lower level scientific concept may have crept into your model. I fell into this trap only a few years ago. I became interested in transcendence as an outcome of suffering. I was interested in the relationship between emotional suffering (a component of suffering, a high-level lay concept), transcendence, and the interaction of hope, as participants exited the model of suffering. There appeared to be adequate literature on transcendence to use pragmatic utility, but I forgot that *transcendence* was a scientific concept and became frustrated when I could not find any variation to scope the concept. I am a slow learner—I was using a beautiful and large analytic chart, and I would put it down and pick it up again a few months later to continue to work on it—but with no progress. Eventually, I realized my mistake—that *self-transcendence* is a scientific concept. We revised analysis, with insights, and it is published here in Chapter 20.

Use the Best Literature as Data

Do not let data overwhelm the project by pulling data that replicate and reiterate the information of the concepts in one publication after another. This occurs mainly in the literature where researchers have used the same definition of the concept or the same theory for their research, and often the same instruments. Too much data will overwhelm and exhaust you—it is better to choose fewer key articles and think long and hard about them, than to work superficially with a large stack.

Ask Astute Analytic Questions

The key to excellent research is in the identification and development of clear and astute analytic questions. It is this process that separates pragmatic utility from a meta-analysis, and it is via this process that the unique and original insights into the concept are attained.

"WHAT ABOUT RELIABILITY AND VALIDITY?"

I am dodging those terms, despite the risk of public scorn echoing across the land. Remember, we are talking about *perceptions*, not concrete phenomena. And, in light of this, we could nothing better than *perceived validity*—which, after all, may be what validity is, 9 times out of 10. And let us forget about *truth* and its various forms, for it is also a ridiculous criterion for something that we are deliberately manipulating to describe something that may be so temporally intangible that we may not even be able to agree what it is. The correctness of concept development is not a matter of evangelical or political persuasion.[1]

---

[1] In quantitative inquiry, researchers also deal with perceptions of phenomena, but they transform these perceptions, giving them the semblance of solidarity in the processes of quantification.

I prefer to discuss quality in concept development in terms of *adequacy*. Concept development is adequate if it meets your needs, is intelligible, and is something that is generally in agreement with the literature.

CRITERION FOR *ADEQUACY*

Most importantly, the results of various methods of concept development should *move the concept toward maturity*. We must see in the author(s) work, some development of the concept. That means that the research conducted must make a contribution toward our understanding of the concept, making it more useful in research and practice.

Specific criteria are:

- **The concept is representative of the phenomena:** We must be able to recognize the concept by what it represents. From the abstract and decontextualized description of the concept, we must be able to recognize instances within various contexts and in various forms, and be able to recognize future instances of the concept. This means that the definitions and the attributes must be clear, concise, and plausible. The boundaries must be realistic.
- **The concept description must be comprehensive:** The definitions and the attributes must be *inclusive*. That is, the attributes are applicable to the phenomenon in its entirely. The description does not exclude any examples of the concept; it is not narrow and particular, but is abstract, decontextualized, and generalizes the concept over as many contexts as necessary.
- **The concept description delineates boundaries:** From the descriptions one can identify boundaries and identify cases that are and are not instances of the concept. There is clear demarcation between the concept and allied concepts in the concept cluster.
- **The description of the conceptual anatomy and physiology adds insight:** Insight surprises and delights, but "don't be boring dear." People do not want to read what they already know, yet they must be able to recognize what they read. This is a delicate balance. But if you have not provided insight, you have not "moved the concept along."
- **Your description should endure:** As long as your concept is relevant, your description should endure as a contribution. Some concepts have a short life span: consider "ghetto blaster"—we now blast our individual ears through ear pods, rather than half the beach or ghetto. As we no longer have

ghetto blasters, that concept is passé. But if you are studying a concept with a reasonable shelf life, if it is a concept that is still current and if the meaning has not been altered, your concept analysis should outlast other types of scientific results.

- **Solid foundation of scholarship:** One model for concept development in this book (Chapter 8) shows that concepts may be developed from qualitative inquiry or from the literature using techniques similar to qualitative meta-analysis. Each of these strategies is solidly embedded in nursing research, with developed criteria for appropriateness and adequacy. Concept development is not a trivial exercise, with trivial results; it is solid scholarship that is essential to the development of our profession.

But *you* know it is good when you yourself are pleased, and your instructor is impressed. Now get it published!

SUMMARY

"Why is a raven like a writing desk?"

Don't be frustrated if you could not guess. According to Wikipedia, this is the world's most famous riddle. It is one that has stumped philosophers and nurses alike, because it has no answer.

Look it up.

REFERENCES

Agan, R. D. (1987). Intuitive knowing as a dimension of nursing. *Advances in Nursing Science,* *10*(1), 63–70.

Antonucci, T. C. (1985). Social support: Theoretical advances, recent findings and pressing issues. In I. G. Sarason & B. R. Sarason (Eds.), *Social support: Theory, research and application* (pp. 21–37). Boston, MA: Nijhoff.

Antonucci, T. C., & Jackson, J. S. (1990). The role ofreprrocity in social support. In B. R. Sarason, I. G. Sarason, & G. R. Pierce (Eds.), *Social support: An interactional view* (pp. 173–209). New York, NY: Wiley.

Benner, P., & Tanner, C. (1987). How nurses use intuition. *American Journal of Nursing, 87*(1), 23–31.

Caplan, G. (1974). *Support systems and community mental health.* New York, NY: Behavioral Publications.

Carroll, L. (1865/2010). *Alice in wonderland.* Glascow, GB: Collins.

Cassel, J. (1976). The contribution of the social environment to host resistance. *American Journal of Epidemiology, 104*(2), 107–123.

Cobb, S. (1976). Social support as a moderator of life stress. *Psychosomatic Medicine, 38*(5), 300–314.

Cohen, S., Melmstein, R., Karmarck, T., & Hoberman, H. M. (1985). Measuring the functional components of social support. In I. G. Sarason & B. R. Sarason (Eds.), *Social support: Theory, research and applications* (pp. 73–94). Boston, MA: Nijhoff.

Corcoran-Perry, S. A., & Bungert, B. (1992). Enhancing orthopedic nurses' clinical decision making. *Orthopedic Nursing, 11*(3), 64–70.

Correnti, D. (1992). Intuition and nursing practice implications for nurse educators: A review of the literature. *The Journal of Continuing Education in Nursing, 23*(2), 91–94.

Dreyfus, S. E., & Dreyfus, H. L. (1980). *A five-stage model of the mental activities involved in directed skill acquisition* (No. ORC-80-2). Berkeley, CA: University of California, Berkeley Operations Research Center.

Gadow, S. A. (1982). The body and self: A dialectic. In F. Victor (Ed.), *The humanity of the ill.* Knoxville, TN: The University of Tennessee Press.

Gadow, S. A. (1983). Toward a critical gerontology: Curriculum design in the philosophy of aging. *Gerontology & Geriatrics Education, 4*(1), 67–74.

Gadow, S. A. (1989). Clinical subjectivity: Advocacy with silent patients. *Nursing Clinics of North America, 24*(2), 535–541.

Geach, B., & White, J. (1974). Empathic resonance: A countertransference phenomenon. *American Journal of Nursing, 74*(7), 1282–1285.

Gerrity, P. L. (1987). Perception in nursing: The value of intuition. *Holistic Nursing Practice, 1*(3), 63–71.

Gladstein, G. A. (1983). Understanding empathy: Integrating counseling, developmental, and social psychology perspectives. *Journal of Counseling Psychology, 30*(4), 467–482.

Hammond, K. R. (1966). Clinical inference in nursing. II. A psychologist's viewpoint. *Nursing Research, 75*(1), 27–37.

Hammond, K. R., Kelly, K. J., Schneider, R. J., & Vancini, M. (1966). Clinical inference in nursing: Information units used. *Nursing Research, 15*(3), 236–243.

Heller, K., Swindle, R. W. Jr., & Dusenbury, L. (1986). Component social support processes: Comments and integration. *Journal of Consulting and Clinical Psychology, 54*, 466–470.

Hilbert, G. A. (1990). Measuring social support in chronic illness. In O. L. Strickland & C. F. Waltz (Eds.), *Measurement of nursing outcomes: Measuring client self-care and coping skills* (Vol. 4, pp. 79–95). New York, NY: Springer.

Hughes, J. R., Carver, E. J., & MacKay, R. C. (1990). Learning to use empathy. In R. C. MacKay, J. R. Hughes, & E. J. Carver (Eds.), *Empathy in the helping relationship* (pp. 107–119). New York, NY: Springer.

Hupcey, J. E. (1998a). Social support: Assessing conceptual coherence. *Qualitative Heath Research, 8*, 304–318.

Hupcey, J. E. (1998b). Clarifying the social support theory research linkage. *Journal of Advanced Nursing, 27*(6), 1231–1241.

Hupcey, J. E. (2002). Maintaining validity: The development of the concept of trust. *International Journal of Qualitative Methods, 1*(4). Retrieved from http://goo.gl/94Nk5x

Hupcey, J. E., & Morse, J. M. (1997). Can a professional relationship be considered social support? *Nursing Outlook, 45*(6), 270–276.

Hupcey, J. E., Penrod, J., Morse, J. M., & Mitcham, C. (2001). An exploration of the advancement of the concept of trust. *Journal of Advanced Nursing, 36*(2), 282–293.

Huyanh, T., & Alderson, M. (2009). Concept analysis of human ecology. *Nursing Forum, 44*(2), 115–128.

Kahn, R., & Antonucci, T. (1980). Attachment, roles and social support. In P. Baltes & O. Brim (Eds.), *Life-span development and behavior* (pp. 253–286). New York, NY: Academic Press.

Kelly, K. (1966). Clinical inference in nursing: I. A nurse's viewpoint. *Nursing Research, 15*(1), 23–26.

La Monica, E. L. (1983). Empathy can be learned. *Nurse Educator, 8*(2), 19–23.

Lin, N. (1986). Conceptualizing social support. In N. Lin, A. Dean, & W. Ensel (Eds.), *Social support life events and depression* (pp. 17–21). New York, NY: Academic Press.

MacKay, R. (1990). What is empathy? In R. C. MacKay, J. L. Hughes, & J. E. Carver (Eds.), *Empathy in the helping relationship* (pp. 3–12). New York, NY: Springer.

Mikkelsen, G., & Frederiksen, K. (2011). Family-centered care of children in hospital— A concept analysis. *Journal of Advanced Nursing, 67*(5), 1152–1162. doi:10.1111/j.1365 -2648.2010.05574.x

Miles, M., & Morse, J. M. (1995). Utilizing the concepts of transference and countertransference in the consultation process. *Journal of the American Psychiatric Nurses Association, 1*(2), 42–47.

Morse, J. M. (1994). "Emerging from the data." The cognitive processes of analysis in qualitative inquiry. In J. Morse (Ed.), *Critical issues in qualitative research methods* (pp. 23–43). Newbury Park, CA: Sage.

Morse, J. M., Anderson, G., Bottorff, J., Yonge, O., O'Brien, B., Solberg, S., & Mcllveen, K. (1992). Exploring empathy: The conceptual fit for nursing practice. *Image: Journal of Nursing Scholarship, 24*(4), 1–25.

Morse, J. M., Bottorff, J., Anderson, G., O'Brien, B., & Solberg, S. (1992). Beyond empathy: Expanding expressions of caring. *Journal of Advances in Nursing Science, 17*, 809–821.

Morse, J. M., Miles, M. W., Clark, D. A., & Doberneck, B. M. (1994). "Sensing" patient needs exploring concepts of nursing insight and receptivity used in nursing assessment. *Scholarly Inquiry for Nursing Practice, 8*(3), 233–254.

Morse, J. M., & Mitcham, C. (1997). Compathy: The contagion of physical distress. *Journal of Advanced Nursing, 26*, 649–657.

Paley, J. (1996). Intuition and expertise: Comments on the Benner debate. *Journal of Advanced Nursing, 23*(4), 665–671.

Paley, J. (1997). Husserl, phenomenology and nursing. *Journal of Advanced Nursing, 26*(1), 187–193.

Paley, J. (2006). Nursing theorists and their work [Book review]. *Nursing Philosophy, 7*(4), 275–280.

Pilisuk, M. (1982). Delivery of social support: The social inoculation. *American Journal of Orthopsychiatry, 52*, 20–31.

Procidano, E., & Heller, K. (1983). Measure of perceived social support from friends and from family: Three validation studies. *American Journal of Community Psychology, 11*, 1–24.

Pyles, S. H., & Stern, P. N. (1983). Discovery of nursing gestalt in critical care nursing: The importance of the gray gorilla syndrome. *Image: Journal of Nursing Scholarship, 15*(2), 51–57.

Rew, L. (1986). Intuition: Concept analysis of a group phenomenon. *Advances in Nursing Science, 8*(2), 21–28.

Rew, L. (1988a). Intuition in decision-making. *Image: Journal of Nursing Scholarship, 20*, 150–154.

Rew, L. (1988b). Nurses' intuition. *Applied Nursing Research, 1*(1), 27–31.

Rew, L. (1989). Intuition: Nursing knowledge and the spiritual dimension of persons. *Holistic Nursing Practice, 5*(3), 56–68.

Rew, L. (1991). Intuition in psychiatric-mental health nursing. *Journal of Child and Adolescent Psychiatric and Mental Health Nursing, 4(3),* 110–115.

Rew, L., Agan, W., Emery, M. R., & Harper, S. C. (1991). Intuitive skills in crisis management. *Nursing Connections, 4*(2), 3–12.

Rogers, C. R. (1957). The necessary and sufficient conditions of therapeutic personality change. *Journal of Consulting Psychology, 21*(2), 95–103.

Rogers, C. R. (1962). The interpersonal relationship: The core of guidance. *Harvard Educational Review, 32*(4), 416–429.

Schraeder, B. D., & Fischer, D. K. (1987). Using intuitive knowledge in the neonatal intensive care nursery. *Holistic Nursing Practice, 1*(3), 45–51.

Schroder, P. (1985). Recognizing transference and counter transference. *Journal of Psychosocial Nursing and Mental Health Services, 23*(2), 21–26.

Schumaker, S. A., & Brownell, A. (1984). Toward a theory of social support: Closing conceptual gaps. *Journal of Social Issues, 40,* 11–36.

Tanner, C. A. (2006). Thinking like a nurse: A research-based model of clinical judgment in nursing. *Journal of Nursing Education, 45*(6), 204–211.

Tanner, C. A., Benner, P., Chesla, C., & Gordon, D. R. (1993). The phenomenology of knowing the patient. *Image: Journal of Nursing Scholarship, 25*(4), 273–280.

Tanner, C. A., Padrick, K. P., Westfall, U. E., & Putzier, D. J. (1987). Diagnostic reasoning strategies of nurses and nursing students. *Nursing Research, 36*(6), 358–363.

Thoits, P. A. (1985). Social support and psychological well-being: Theoretical possibilities. In L. G. Sarason & B. R. Sarason (Eds.), *Social Support: Theory, research, and application* (pp. 51–72). Boston, MA: Nijhoff.

Tilden, V. P. (1986). New perspectives on social support. *The Nurse Practitioner, 11*(8), 60–62.

Travelbee, J. (1972). *Interpersonal aspects of nursing.* Philadelphia, PA: F. A. Davis.

Westfall, U., Tanner, D., Putzier, D., & Padrick, K. (1986). Activating clinical inferences: A component of diagnostic reasoning in nursing. *Research in Nursing and Health, 9,* 269–277.

Wheeler, K. (1988). A nursing science approach to understanding empathy. *Archive of Psychiatric Nursing, 2*(2), 95–102.

Zderad, L. T. (1969). Empathic nursing: Realization of a human capacity. *Nursing Clinics of North America, 4*(4), 655–662.

SELF-TRANSCENDENCE AND SELF-REFORMULATION: ONE CONCEPT OR TWO?

> *I could tell you my adventures—beginning from this morning," said Alice a little timidly: "but it's no use going back to yesterday, because I was a different person then.*
>
> —Lewis Carroll, *Alice's Adventures in Wonderland* (1865/1977, p. 140)

For individuals who face life-threatening or terminal illness, two concepts are used in research to account for the altered affect and behaviors that occur when they emerge from suffering. The first concept is *self-transcendence*; the second, self-reformulation or the *reformulated self*. These two concepts compete to explain what has been characterized as the peaceful affect that occurs in the later stages of serious illness, and are sometimes used interchangeably. Therefore the purpose of this chapter is to explore the confusion associated with these concepts. Are they the same concept with two names, or are they different? As these concepts have been broadly applied in a variety of health care contexts, such as in individuals facing a terminal diagnosis and in rehabilitation from serious illness, it is, therefore, important to carefully compare self-transcendence and the reformulated self for differences, diagnostic potential, and possible ramifications for therapeutic intervention. By exploring the "concepts in use" literature, we will compare the course, attributes, and outcomes of each concept, with the aim of identifying overlap (if any) and the variations between the two concepts.

SELF-TRANSCENDENCE

The term self-transcendence has come to be widely used to refer to a process whereby individuals encounter life-altering or threatening events that compel a dramatic change in self-perception and culminate in an improved sense of well-being, acceptance, and an expanded worldview. The concept of self-transcendence has a lengthy history in psychology and philosophy. This section covers some of the central definers of this experience.

Viktor Frankl (1966) developed the concept from his observations as a prisoner in a Nazi concentration camp. He observed that some prisoners exhibited a capacity to transcend and find meaning in life despite living in life-threatening and appalling conditions. He posited that self-transcendence means, "that being human always points, and is directed, to something, or someone other than oneself—be it a meaning to fulfill or another human being to encounter. The more one forgets himself—by giving himself to a cause to serve or another person to love—the more human he is and the more he actualizes himself" (1959, p. 110). Frankl believed that transcendence was central to human existence.

Psychologist Abraham Maslow positioned self-transcendence at the pinnacle of his *Hierarchy of Needs*, claiming it represents "the very highest and most inclusive or holistic levels of human consciousness, behaving and relating, as ends rather than means, to one-self, to significant others, to human beings in general, to other species, to nature, and to the cosmos" (1969, p. 66). According to Daniels (2001), Maslow identified 35 aspects of self-transcendence including, "loss of self-consciousness, mystical fusion, letting be, letting things happen, unselfish love, getting off the merry-go-round, enjoying the cosmos, being self-determined, surpassing one's limitations, being independent of culture, being fully accepting of the self, doing one's duty, accepting death, having intrinsic conscience, being absorbed in what one is doing, integrating dichotomies, and being metamotivated" (pp. 3–4). Maslow's characterization of transcendence is not a point of inevitable arrival, but a state that only very few of the most optimistic people would intermittently achieve.

Religious scholar David Chidester identifies four philosophical orientations of transcendence that characterize the ways in which death has been imagined and attended to by human culture: *ancestral, cultural, mythic,* and *experiential transcendence* (Chidester, 2001). Ancestral transcendence recognizes the lineage inheritance of past ancestors living on through their children. Cultural transcendence places emphasis on the surviving community's collective memory of the dead. Dying rituals sustain the link between those who have passed and their continuity with the living community. Mythic transcendence appears in narratives about death and the afterlife (Chidester, 2001, pp. 40–41). It is the fourth pattern, experiential transcendence, that resembles the clinical understanding of the concept. Experiential transcendence reflects "profound and often intense psychological experiences that embrace death in acceptance or ecstasy. Death may be embraced by accepting it as the end of life; perhaps such an acceptance results in an experience of psychological tranquility" (2002, p. 14).

In the course of the past three decades, self-transcendence has emerged as an important scientific concept in nursing theory and research. As a concept, transcendence was brought to the attention of nursing through oncology and spirituality, and first used in the field in the mid-1980s. Reed, in her earlier studies on well-being and health, based her understanding of transcendence on Martha Roger's theory (Reed, 1991a, 1991b, 1996), developing the concept deductively. In this way, transcendence came to be viewed as "a characteristic of developmental maturity, expansions of self-boundaries and an orientation toward broadened life perspectives and purposes" (1991b, p. 64). At this time, Reed also developed an instrument derived from her early clinical practice to measure the experience referred to as the *self-transcendence scale* (*STS;* Reed, 1987; 2009). This 15-item, 4-point Likert survey aimed to measure the extent to which an individual expressed the qualities considered to be associated with transcendence. For example, participants ranked their level of acceptance of aging, changes in physical ability, finding meaning in past experiences, and acceptance of death as a natural part of life. Over the years, Reed developed and expanded her definition so that by 2003 she defined self-transcendence as:

> The capacity to expand self-boundaries intra-personally
> (toward greater awareness of one's philosophy, values,
> and dreams), inter-personally (to relate to others and
> one's environment), temporally (to integrate one's past
> and one's future in a way that has meaning for the
> present), and trans-personally (to connect with
> dimensions beyond the typically discernable world).
> (Reed, 2003, p. 147)

Intrapersonal aspects of the transcendence experience were considered those directed toward self. Accordingly, a crisis event, such as life-threatening illness, can be understood as a catalyst for enhanced self-awareness. Under such circumstances, individual relations and an increased sense of connectedness with others reflected the interpersonal aspects of transcendence. The transpersonal element of transcendence is experienced as a heightened awareness of God, spirituality, or a *higher* power. In 2008 and 2010, Reed presented self-transformation as a mid-range theory, moving from vulnerability to self-transcendence, with an outcome of well-being. Self-transcendence is expressed through "sharing wisdom with others, integrating the physical changes of aging, accepting death as a part of life" (2010, p. 108).

The second researcher influencing the development of the concept of self-transcendence was Coward, who completed her dissertation in 1991, and was a student of Reed. Coward's (1990) research was quantitative, showed a correlation between the STS and emotional well-being, which Reed considered as evidence of construct validity for the STS (Reed, 2009, p. 398). Importantly, Coward (1990) subsequently conducted a qualitative phenomenological study with breast cancer patients describing transcendence as "a sense of being healed, to increased valuing of self, to easing the fear and pain of loss, and to savoring of the small moments of life" (p. 167). Four themes emerged from this study that Coward believed to be the basis for the transcendent experience:

1. "an incident that generates intense negative feelings and emotions" (physical and emotional pain, fear of death, anger, despair over personal losses, which encourage one to look for ways to "find new meaning in ands purpose for living";
2. "great effort" and risk to acquire new skills to overcome and "confront one's fears";
3. emotional sense of healing and well-being, a "sense of physical lightness and relief of burden"; and
4. both helping another and accepting help from others, and a "sense of receiving, in return more than what has been given" (Coward, 1990, p. 167).

Similar findings were found in her phenomenological study with women with AIDS (Coward, 1995).

Despite this important descriptive work, research continued primarily quantitatively using the STS. The scale has been applied to numerous populations across a variety of illness scenarios, as well as to healthy adults. Self-transcendence has been associated with well-being (Coward, 1996), positive mental health outcomes, and inversely correlated with depression (Ellermann & Reed, 2001; Nygren et al., 2005; Stinson & Kirk, 2006; Reed, 2009), and cognitively intact nursing home patients (Haugan, Rannestad, Hammervold, Garasen, & Espnes, 2012). Self-transcendence was regarded as an effective coping strategy for individuals experiencing a range of chronic illnesses, such as rheumatoid arthritis (Neill, 2002), HIV (Mellors, Coontz, & Lucke, 2001; Ramer, Johnson, Chan, & Barrett, 2006), survivors of cancers (Chin-A-Loy & Fernsler, 1998; Farren, 2010; Pelusi, 1997; Thomas, Burton, Quinn, & Fitzpatrick, 2010), liver transplant patients (Bean & Wagner, 2006), and homelessness (Runquist & Reed, 2007). High levels of self-transcendence were found among residents in long-term care facilities who experienced positive nurse–patient interactions (Haugan & Innstrand, 2012) and among caregivers of patients with dementia (Acton & Wright, 2000) and terminal illnesses (Enyert & Burman, 1999). High self-transcendence has been described in nurses' experience caring for others (Park, 2005) and work engagement among nurses in acute care settings (Palmer, Quinn, Reed, & Fitzpatrick, 2010). A negative correlation was found between self-transcendence and burnout among nurses (Hunnibell, Reed, Quinn-Griffin, & Fitzpatrick, 2008). Several studies reported a correlation between increased age and self-transcendence.

Reed has considered the wide application of the STS to be confirmation of the content validity of the STS; "based on a thorough literature review to specify the domain of content with careful attention to construction and refinement of items" (Reed, 2009, p. 398). Yet, at the time that the scale was developed (1987), Reed did not identify the literature used, and the concept had not been previously addressed in the nursing literature. Construct validity was "demonstrated by correlation with a measure of emotional well-being" from Coward's 1990 dissertation (Reed, 2009, p. 398). Recent independent confirmatory factor analysis of the STS with a Norwegian nursing home population showed a two-factor solution with 35.3% of the variance (Haugan et al., 2012, p. 155).

In this section we have attempted to identify the central definers of this complex phenomenon, with specific emphasis on its usage in health care. Comparatively, the concept of self-reformulation has had limited exposure in the research literature. As noted previously, there is considerable overlap and important defining differences that distinguish these experiences and warrants further examination.

SELF-REFORMULATION

Self-reformulation, also a scientific concept but developed qualitatively, was identified by Carter (1994) in her study of long-term survivors of breast cancer patients. Characterizing the process as one that constitutes a "reinterpretation of self," Carter noted at that time that the changes that she was seeing in her study did not fit self-transcendence as it was described. Self-reformulation results from the experience of a self that is mortal, accompanied by a loss of one's previous identity associated with health, career, and relationships. An attendant awareness of a self that is vulnerable to a relapse of cancer is present, as is a shift in focus toward one's self and close relationships. An acquired sense of self as a survivor is definitive of reformulation in this context.

In subsequent qualitative studies, self-reformulation was characterized by a disregard for material things; a changed affect characterized by an ability to reorder life priorities, an appreciation for one's own abilities and the exiting of unsatisfying relationships (Mayan, Morse, & Eldershaw, 2006, pp. 20–26).

Self-reformulation was most apparent when the person emerged from suffering, more specifically, when they faced death and subsequently recovered (Morse & Carter, 1996). The concept was used to describe the state when one emerged from emotional suffering, hope "seeped in," and the person began to assemble a revised and enhanced sense of self (Morse, 2001, 2011). Self-reformulation is considered the ideal goal of rehabilitation and a state of health.

Similarly to the concept of transcendence, self-reformulation has been applied in a variety of contexts, from patients suffering chronic illnesses (Elofsson & Öhlén, 2004; Ohman, Söderberg, & Lundman, 2003) to survivors of cancer (Carter, 1994; Frank, 2003; Kinney, 1996; Vachon, 2001), severe burn trauma (Russell et al., 2013), individuals with multiple sclerosis (Pollock & Sands, 1997), coronary artery disease (CAD; Lukkarinen, 1999), to caregivers (Enyert & Burman, 1999; Hall, 2001), hospital patients (Woogara, 2005); those recovered from serious illness (Mayan, Morse, & Eldershaw, 2006) and to individuals experiencing homelessness (Boydell, Goering, & Morrell-Bellai, 2000).

COMPARING THE CONCEPTS

As the foregoing summary demonstrates, to date, there has been a lack of consensus about the definition of each concept and about the attributes that distinguish the associated experiences. At the same time, there has been scant critical appraisal of existing definitions. Assuming the two experiences are distinct, the manner in which they have been utilized in the clinical and research literature has convoluted these two concepts and confused researchers. The lack of attention to the definitions of these concepts has resulted in their misapplication: they are sometimes used interchangeably; the attributes assigned shift from one to another, and their definitions overlap. Therefore, the purpose of this article is to analyze each of these concepts by exploring existing definitions of self-transcendence and self-reformulation as they are used in the nursing literature, and if necessary, to refine their definitions and to evaluate their utility for clinical application.

METHOD

On the Derivations of Concepts

Behavioral concepts are clusters of behaviors that usually appear together and work to achieve a certain function. They may be derived from common use (as a lay concept) or developed purposefully in research (as a scientific concept). While *lay concepts* are formed from everyday observations, through consensus, labeling, and usage, they are defined in the dictionary, are not static, and their meaning may change over time. *Scientific concepts*, on the other hand, may be quantitatively derived for use in quantitative inquiry, developed with tight, operational definitions, according to the standards of replication, are judged to have validity, and are measurable. *Quantitatively derived concepts* are operationalized, measurable, generalized through randomized sampling strategies, and the outcome is measurement of the concept, often correlated with other variables. Alternatively, they may be *qualitatively derived scientific concepts*, closely linked to reality, observable or recognizable, and have been identified, delineated, and developed through qualitative inquiry, and the outcome is a well-developed concept that may even be incorporated into abstracted explanatory model or theory through which the concept or theory generalized.

Analyzing Concepts

From the initial reading of the literature, a table was prepared so that the major definitions could be compared and contrasted both within each concept and between concepts. The table also lists the context of the study, the characteristics or attributes and circumstances, and outcomes. Next, we asked questions of these two concepts:

- Is there a difference in context in which each was used, or do they apply to the same phenomena?
- Are there similarities in the course of the illnesses (i.e., the timing) in which the concepts are applied?
- Is there a difference in the structure (attributes) of the concepts?
- Is there a difference in the outcomes for each concept?

RESULTS

In each of these concepts, researchers have stipulated distinct indicators that define the process of self-transcendence or self-reformulation. Therefore, our task is to compare each concept as they are described and used in the nursing literature.

Table 20.1 contains a detailed list of the descriptors for each concept as identified in the literature.

TABLE 20.1
Comparison of Definitions, Characteristics, and Outcomes of Self-Transcendence and Self-Reformulation Literature

SELF-TRANSCENDENCE LITERATURE

AUTHOR (Y) AND CONTEXT OF STUDY	DEFINITION/DESCRIPTION	CONDITIONS	KEY ATTRIBUTES AND OUTCOMES
Reed (1991b) Oldest-old adults: mental health symptomology	"A characteristic of developmental maturity, expansions of self-boundaries and an orientation toward broadened life perspectives and purposes" (p. 64).	High rates of depression among the 80+ population: mental health problems found to be related to chronic illness, diminished capacity, institutionalized care and suicide.	Enhanced awareness of the self-boundaries in older adults. Generativity (feeling of productivity), introjectivity (well-being, spiritual focus), temporal integration (positive view of past, present, and future) and body transcendence (acceptance of physical limitations).
Haase, Britt, Coward, Leidy, and Penn. (1992) Concept comparison	The experience of extending one's self inwardly in introspective activities, outwardly through concerns about the welfare of others, and temporally such that the perceptions of one's past and anticipated future enhance the present.	Authors identify various antecedents that lead to self-transcendence (ST) including moving beyond self-preoccupation, having a spiritual perspective, pivotal life event or stressor, acceptance of the inescapable situation, which may inspire a broader perspective, purpose, and activities.	Well-being Self-worth Connectedness Personal growth Purpose and meaning Sense of being healed.
Coward (1995) Women with AIDS	"Reaching out beyond the boundaries of the self to achieve broader perspectives and behaviors that make life meaningful … a source of mental health at end of life" (p. 314).	Experiencing fear and loneliness Experiencing uncertainty Using others as role models Finding inner strength Reaching out to receive and give Making a difference, having purpose. Viewing AIDS as an opportunity. Having hope.	Increased feeling of self-worth and purpose. Emotional well-being. Sense of connectedness to their world, and feelings of self-confidence and purpose.

(continued)

TABLE 20.1

Comparison of Definitions, Characteristics, and Outcomes of Self-Transcendence and Self-Reformulation Literature (continued)

SELF-TRANSCENDENCE LITERATURE

AUTHOR (Y) AND CONTEXT OF STUDY	DEFINITION/DESCRIPTION	CONDITIONS	KEY ATTRIBUTES AND OUTCOMES
Coward and Reed (1996) Advanced breast cancer	"The ability to extend one's self beyond personal concerns and take on a broader life perspective and purpose" (p. 276).	End-of-life experiences are transformed into healing. Spiritual perspective transforms to subjective well-being. Work: "doing for others" led to a sense of well-being, that lessened their pain, fear, regrets associated with dying.	"How to live while dying" Transcendence "is a resource for healing" when persons' "health status for condition is typically not curable or reversible" (p. 281). "Pandimensional experience that facilitates healing" (p. 280).
Coward (1998) Breast cancer support group attendees	Expansion of personal conceptual boundaries through sharing common experience and identity, giving support, having a common purpose.	Diagnosis is a life-threatening event evoking severe emotional distress that may lead one to search outside oneself for information and support.	After the intervention, authors noted an increased well-being, purpose in life, and interconnectedness with others.
Acton and Wright (2000) Family caregivers of adults with dementia	"Ability to move beyond the self and present difficulties, to extend concern to others and to find personal meaning and wholeness in the context of life changing events" (p. 143).	The challenges and grief involved in caring for family members with dementia moves one beyond self with the potential to develop self-reflection, connections with others, and a larger perspective.	Deeper connection with self and others. Spiritual sense of relatedness to God. Knowing one is not alone gives one an enlarged perspective. This helps them deal with the difficulties of caregiving.

(continued)

TABLE 20.1
Comparison of Definitions, Characteristics, and Outcomes of Self-Transcendence and Self-Reformulation Literature (continued)

(continued)

AUTHOR (Y) AND CONTEXT OF STUDY	DEFINITION/DESCRIPTION	CONDITIONS	KEY ATTRIBUTES AND OUTCOMES
	SELF-TRANSCENDENCE LITERATURE		
Ellermann and Reed (2001) Depression among middle-aged adults	ST is a "resource"—a "basic developmental process that emerges during significant life events"(p. 699). The "capacity to expand personal boundaries intrapersonally, interpersonally and transpersonally to acquire a perspective that exceeds ordinary boundaries and limitations" (p. 699).	ST is resource, not tied to chronological age that involves an extension of perspective beyond self and life problems that could decrease depression in this age group. Feelings of meaninglessness, lack of concern for self and other negative feelings impede the transcendent potential during this life phase.	Parenting role, acceptance of current life situations and spirituality were indicators of transcendence and inversely correlated with depression among adults.
Mellors Coontz, and Lucke, (2001) Persons living with AIDS	Existential experience of moving beyond self despite suffering.	Awareness of personal mortality has the potential to evoke ST and well-being.	Creating meaningful life pattern, connectedness and self-care.
Coward and Kahn (2004) Breast cancer support group	Defines ST as "expanding personal boundaries beyond the immediate or constricted view of self and the world as well as extending oneself beyond personal concerns and taking on broader life perspectives and purpose" (p. E24).	Diagnosis causes spiritual disequilibrium, fear of dying, loneliness, threatened self-identity.	Reaching out, finding support and information. Helping others, feeling needed, defining new normal self-identity, and changing priorities and connections with God and others.

TABLE 20.1
Comparison of Definitions, Characteristics, and Outcomes of Self-Transcendence and Self-Reformulation Literature (continued)

	SELF-TRANSCENDENCE LITERATURE		
AUTHOR (Y) AND CONTEXT OF STUDY	**DEFINITION/DESCRIPTION**	**CONDITIONS**	**KEY ATTRIBUTES AND OUTCOMES**
Bean and Wagner (2006) Liver transplantation	Uses the self-transcendence scale (STS). A "developmental process reflecting spiritual growth and maturity; broaden personal perspectives to validate meaning and purpose in life" (p. 47).	Life crisis provides an opportunity for transcendence. Transplant recipients face the possibility of organ rejection and death that can lead to heightened awareness of spirituality, broadened personal awareness beyond self.	ST normalization (acceptance) of death, identification of meaning in life, identification of meaning in death, and value of one's life beyond the physical, psychological and social self" (p. 48). STS scores were higher among recipients who were facing end-of-life issues. Over time, as life normalized and death was no longer a threat, ST scores declined.
Hunnibell, Reed, Quinn-Griffin, and Fitzpatrick (2008) Burnout among hospice and oncology nurses	Uses the STS. Defines ST as an "awareness of the spiritual aspects of self, one's relationship to others and the environment, and relationship to a higher being, or purpose greater than self" (p. 172).	Burnout among nurses—emotional distress due to exposure to repeated patient deaths and suffering. Demands of job, continual need to keep abreast of new skills, technology, lack of preparedness for caring for the needs of the dying, lack of spiritual training.	Spiritual connection, increased age, and part-time work were associated with high STS scores and lower levels of burnout. "Self-transcendence may be restorative, enabling nurses to endure, diminish or rise above burnout" (p. 177).

(continued)

TABLE 20.1
Comparison of Definitions, Characteristics, and Outcomes of Self-Transcendence and Self-Reformulation Literature (continued)

SELF-TRANSCENDENCE LITERATURE

AUTHOR (Y) AND CONTEXT OF STUDY	DEFINITION/DESCRIPTION	CONDITIONS	KEY ATTRIBUTES AND OUTCOMES
Teixeira (2008) Concept analysis	Defines ST as "the feeling of connection with others and the universe" and two allied concepts "spirituality" and "personal transformation" (p. 26).	Identified antecedents of hope, acceptance, and spiritual perspective. Uses the Rogers (2000) method of concept analysis, which draws on the literature to identify attributes of the concept: (1) awareness, defined as awakening to one's own consciousness, surroundings, family, and environment; (2) interconnectedness with self, others, and the universe; (3) expanding consciousness is the ability to relate to self, others, and the environment without limitations; and (4) creative energy that may include feelings of intuition, spirituality, and mysticism (p. 28).	The outcomes were adaptation, finding meaning and purpose in life, a feeling of well-being, and a sense of being healed.

(continued)

TABLE 20.1

Comparison of Definitions, Characteristics, and Outcomes of Self-Transcendence and Self-Reformulation Literature (continued)

| AUTHOR (Y) AND CONTEXT OF STUDY | SELF-TRANSCENDENCE LITERATURE | | |
	DEFINITION/DESCRIPTION	CONDITIONS	KEY ATTRIBUTES AND OUTCOMES
Farren (2010) Breast cancer survivors	Uses the STS. Defines ST as "a profound awareness of one's wholeness . . . looking inward, reaching out towards others, and an ever-changing experience of time where past, present, and future are one" (p. 63).	Throughout survivorship, issues of well-being and quality of life persist. In the face of uncertainty, breast cancer survivors have the capacity to participate in life change that may transcend into new ways of being and larger awareness of self and the world.	Findings "confirmed that power was present in this sample of breast cancer survivors, who were dealing with continued uncertainty in the intermediate stage of survivorship, and they were engaging with their capacity for self-transcendence for quality of life" (p. 69).
Palmer, Quinn, Reed, and Fitzpatrick. (2010) Acute care nurses	Uses the STS. ST is defined as the "ability of human beings to find meaning in their lives by being directed toward something or someone, other than themselves" (p. 138).	ST is tied to "power" and the active participation in maintaining well-being by sharing experiences, awareness of self, making choices reaching out and helping others. "Exposure to human suffering, illness and death can lead to meaning and fulfillment or to emotional overload and burnout" (p. 146).	Positive association between work engagement and ST. As STS scores increased, work engagement increased. "Nurses who engage in self-transcendence are better, happier, more content, and more able to help their patients" (p. 144).

(continued)

TABLE 20.1
Comparison of Definitions, Characteristics, and Outcomes of Self-Transcendence and Self-Reformulation Literature (continued)

SELF-TRANSCENDENCE LITERATURE

AUTHOR (Y) AND CONTEXT OF STUDY	DEFINITION/DESCRIPTION	CONDITIONS	KEY ATTRIBUTES AND OUTCOMES
Willis and Griffith (2010) Middle school boys who have been bullied	Defines ST as opening out beyond self.	Being bullied associated with adjustment difficulties, somatic and psychological health problems, negative self-esteem, depressive symptoms, suicidal thinking.	ST in this population was described as "healing in which boys opened out beyond self to experience a world more expansive, as they (a) felt empathy for others and valued respectful relationships with others, (b) sought out others for help, and (c) learned new things and engaged in fun creative hobbies" (p. 128).
Haugan and Innstrand (2012) Depression among nursing home residents	Uses the STS. Definition: ST is "a resource for well-being among vulnerable populations and at the end of life . . . a psycho-social-spiritual force toward personal maturity that is distinct from the more self-absorbed strivings for self-esteem and intimacy typical in earlier developmental phases" (p. 2).	Impairment, diagnosis, and somatic symptoms tied to depression among Nursing Home (NH) patients. Frailty, mortality, disability, powerlessness, and dependency.	Identified interpersonal activities such as personal interests, learning, involvement with others, connectedness, sharing one's wisdom, and helping others to be associated with low depression. Intrapersonal qualities such as self-acceptance of aging, adjusting well to declining physical abilities and living in NH, finding meaning in past experiences were also correlated with low depression.

(continued)

TABLE 20.1
Comparison of Definitions, Characteristics, and Outcomes of Self-Transcendence and Self-Reformulation Literature (continued)

SELF-TRANSCENDENCE LITERATURE

AUTHOR (Y) AND CONTEXT OF STUDY	DEFINITION/DESCRIPTION	CONDITIONS	KEY ATTRIBUTES AND OUTCOMES
Williams (2012) Stem cell transplant recipients	ST is defined as an inner resource and capacity to move beyond the self and find meaning in the midst of adverse circumstances. The result is reduced suffering (p. E41).	ST arises from great suffering, such as "debilitating symptoms" despair, and the possibility of death. "Self-transcendence emerged as a process of 'rebirth,' a journey from intense suffering to the manifestation of new life" (p. E43).	ST involves mentally becoming disembodied to survive. Contemplation of death and "the ultimate separation not only from their bodies, but from others and from life itself" (p. E43). Survival and ST involved the use of imagery as a source of inspiration, and the caring support of others. Involves a spiritual influence that "lifted participants out of despair and provided a sense of hope" (p. E45). ST reflects a rebirth, a change in self "beyond the physical to the discovery of a deeper sense of the self" . . . a broadened perspective, to view life from a "new vantage previously not apparent" (p. E45). Characterized by a deeper connection to self and others, the desire to give back, and a greater capacity to accept life's challenges.
McCarthy (2013) Successful aging	Uses the STS scale as a measurement of transcendence.	Losses associated with aging. Successful aging is defined as "low risk for chronic disease, independent physical and cognitive function and productive engagement with life" (p. 179).	ST and proactive coping were associated with successful aging. Precursors and attributes of ST include contemplation, introspection, spirituality, creativity, altruistic activities, and relationships.

(continued)

TABLE 20.1
Comparison of Definitions, Characteristics, and Outcomes of Self-Transcendence and Self-Reformulation Literature (continued)

SELF-REFORMULATION LITERATURE

AUTHOR (Y) & CONTEXT OF STUDY	DEFINITION/DESCRIPTION	CONDITIONS	OUTCOME
Carter (1994) Long-term survivors of breast cancer	Reformulating represents a "reinterpretation of self."	Life threatened with breast cancer; expect to die; multiple losses, diminished and vulnerable; emotional distress; recognition of survival; desire to help others.	A process of "reordering your life priorities and making deliberate decisions" to change.
Kinney (1996) Bilateral mastectomy	Reconstructing one's self.	Author's personal journey of recovery from breast cancer.	A sense of exceeding one's usual limits, surpassed or gone beyond material existence. Interweaving of the mind, body, and spirit and an evolving and integrating process that is ongoing and ever-building.
Morse and Carter (1996)	Reformulation of the self.	When worked through suffering "enough," emerge using processes of hoping.	Views life with a renewed perspective. Reorders his or her values and priorities about life and living. Appreciative of joy; help others who are suffering.
Pollock and Sands (1997) Clients with multiple sclerosis	A change in perspective from that of trauma and tragedy to one of challenge and opportunity.	physiological, psychological and sociological changes and losses.	Found meaning in their illness and were "able to grow from it and benefit from their experience" p. 184). It gave them a "deeper meaning to life" that led to a change in perspective from "challenge to opportunity" (p. 184). Finds meaning in suffering. This causes a change in perspective to "challenge and opportunity" (p. 184).

(continued)

TABLE 20.1
Comparison of Definitions, Characteristics, and Outcomes of Self-Transcendence and Self-Reformulation Literature (continued)

SELF-REFORMULATION LITERATURE

AUTHOR (Y) & CONTEXT OF STUDY	DEFINITION/DESCRIPTION	CONDITIONS	OUTCOME
Lukkarinen (1999) Coronary artery disease (CAD) patients	Reorganization of roles and restructuring of one's identity.	CAD causes a transformation from healthy self to the role of patient; disrupted life course.	For Group a: showed "drastic change in their values and attitude towards everyday life"; "new way of life"; "new meaning and structure to life."
		For Group a: accepting, progressive life change, Being close to death altered values and life's goals. Connected with others. With the threat of death, this group found new value and meaning in everyday life and relationships. Acceptance and irreversibility of condition. Vow to live fully, better with a positive attitude. Group b: Nonaccepting regressive. Found it difficult to accept physical limitations, depression, and dissatisfaction, denial of causes of illness. Reluctant to alter lifestyle.	
Enyert and Burman (1999)	Caregiver finds meaning in the caregiving experience.	Distress among caregivers; decline in caregiver morale and possibly depression. Hardship of caregiving: ongoing grief and loss, fatigue, financial, multiple challenges.	Experience somehow changed how they experience reality. They experienced meaning and the perceived ability to transcend adversary. They "described a new life view and were able to reach out to help others as result of their caregiving" (p. 455).
Caregivers of a family member who had died 6–12 months earlier.	Labeled "self-transcendence."		

(continued)

TABLE 20.1
Comparison of Definitions, Characteristics, and Outcomes of Self-Transcendence and Self-Reformulation Literature (continued)

AUTHOR (Y) & CONTEXT OF STUDY	SELF-REFORMULATION LITERATURE		
	DEFINITION/DESCRIPTION	CONDITIONS	OUTCOME
Boydell, Goering, and Morrell-Bellai (2000) Homeless persons	Identity transformation that is "focused on individual capacity and the promotion of health and well-being" (p. 26).	Homelessness that leads to loss of identity, self-worth and self-efficacy. Social marginalization, depersonalization, and stigmatization.	Reevaluation, renewal of self through choices and actions. Sense of pride in past self. Presentation of a present self as resourceful and unlike stigmatized homeless persons. Self-acceptance. Helping others. Deeper understanding of life and its meaning.
Vachon (2001) Cancer survivors	A new way of defining ourselves.	Loss of personal control, loss of self-esteem, changes in body image, reduced social status, and disruption of personal relationships.	"Cancer represents a turning point; an opportunity to reflect on life, change what needs to be changed, move in new directions, new definition of self. Cancer is a spiritually transformative experience" (p. 282).
Hall (2001) AIDS volunteers	Transformative suffering.	Experiencing the suffering, accepting, and focusing on the present; containing the suffering; transformative suffering.	Constructing meaning from loss. Surviving suffering gives an intense need to give back and help others; they alter their lives irreversibly (p. 52).
Morse (2001, 2011)	Reformulated self.	Suffering is a necessary stage in recovery allowing acceptance of the lost past and the altered future; emotional suffering is a healing agent. Hope seeps in.	Revalue their lives; live life more deeply. Have an urge to give back and help others get through the experience.

(continued)

TABLE 20.1
Comparison of Definitions, Characteristics, and Outcomes of Self-Transcendence and Self-Reformulation Literature (continued)

SELF-REFORMULATION LITERATURE

AUTHOR (Y) & CONTEXT OF STUDY	DEFINITION/DESCRIPTION	CONDITIONS	OUTCOME
Frank (2003) Long-term survivors after illness	Finding meaning in illness, then finding ways in that meaning to change one's life.	Cancer instigates a "turning point," a "restitution story of illness"; the person's life is restored and the "illness can be forgotten" (p. 252).	Illness survivors respond to "others' suffering with a self-consciousness of their own" (p. 248). "A heightened self-consciousness of the web of reciprocity" (p. 253).
Ohman et al. (2003) Serious chronic illness	Use Morse and Carter (1996): "Once people have suffered enough and are able to accept the changed reality they gain new insight and appreciate for life as the reformulated self" (p. 540).	Experiencing the body as hindrance. Being alone in illness, hopeless, threat to identity, loss of independence. Struggle for normalcy. Trying to integrate the changes. Being at home. Striving for palliation.	Trying to understand life and integrate changes to limitations. Finding ways to manage pain and conserve energy. Preserving independence. Feelings of well-being and happiness.
Elofsson and Öhlén (2004) Older adults living with chronic obstructive pulmonary disease (COPD)	Uses Morse (2001). Enduring enables day-to-day functioning. Emotional suffering necessary for release, recovery, and reformulation of self.	Living with COPD entails daily struggle, severe fatigue, dependence on medication and oxygen. Regret, longing for former life.	Letting go of former identity and lifestyle. Recovery involves acceptance of altered life and future. Reconfigures life within the confines of body's limitations. Content, connected, and independent. Suggests that reformulation may entail periods of endurance and periods of emotional suffering.

(continued)

TABLE 20.1
Comparison of Definitions, Characteristics, and Outcomes of Self-Transcendence and Self-Reformulation Literature (continued)

AUTHOR (Y) & CONTEXT OF STUDY	SELF-REFORMULATION LITERATURE		
	DEFINITION/DESCRIPTION	CONDITIONS	OUTCOME
Woogara (2005) Dignity and privacy of hospital patients	Uses the term reformulated self.	Staff prioritizes medical treatment to privacy and dignity. Patient's dignity and privacy is compromised by hospital setting: wearing gowns, bed/room position, shared rooming, toileting facilities, sleeping patterns, eroded personal identity, individuality, control, and choice.	The clinical staff's individual "self" is reshaped by culture and demands of hospital unit. "Care" becomes habituated and routinized in response to demands of a busy unit. The patient's self is reformulated by the hospital environment: accept a degree of compromise to privacy and dignity in exchange for treatment. Actions of staff and acceptance of patients to infringements of personal dignity and space in lieu of treatment "creates a feedback loop to the reformulated selves of staff and patients."
Mayan, Morse, and Eldershaw (2006) People who faced death and subsequently recovered	Self-reformulation.	Facing death forced people to reconsider their lives. People emerge from suffering with a newfound attitude and wisdom.	Ability to reorder priorities. Disregard for material things. Exit from unsatisfying relationships. Appreciating one's own abilities. A need to reciprocate. Valuing the experience of suffering.
Russell et al. (2013) Pediatric burn patients in adulthood	No theory of reformulation.	Trauma of being burned and social stigma of disfigurement. Leads to identity disruption: nostalgia for the past led to negative sense of well-being, deflated esteem, underachievement, behavior and mood problems.	Adjust to de-emphasize the importance of appearance and emphasize personal attributes unrelated to appearance. This reformulation results in a positive self-concept. Social support from family and friends tied to positive self-concept.

Is There a Difference in Context in Which Each was Used, or Do They Apply to the Same Phenomenon?

As the table bears out, these two separate bodies of research overlap considerably in terms of context of study. Both fields examine individuals who have encountered a threat to their mortality, as well as those who have survived this threat. Both bodies of literature also explore the lives of individuals experiencing a range of chronic illnesses, such as CAD, depression, chronic obstructive pulmonary disease (COPD), AIDS, and groups whose self has undergone change as a result of threat to a loved one and the demands of caregiving, or the experience of displacement (homelessness) or marginalization (bullied, long-term care residents).

When comparing the contexts, we may ask: Is the shock and/or degree of the threat a pivotal criterion? If so, how do contexts that do not directly attack the self, such as caregiving, lead to a life altering change in self-identity? Do the experiences of being bullied, displaced, or caring for and losing a loved one have similar self-altering characteristics as in the case when one's own mortality is threatened?

Are There Similarities in the Course of the Illnesses (i.e., the Timing) in Which the Concepts are Applied?

There are similarities in the course of the illnesses, particularly at the onset. Both experiences are initiated by a traumatic event, such as a diagnosis that threatens the self. This is responded to with fear, disbelief, and grief. Even at this early stage, the event has an altering effect. They are no longer who they once were. The key to the transformative path is their subsequent response to this encounter. The real dissimilarities show when we consider the latter course of the illnesses that compels the potential for self-transformation. In this respect, some of the research provides more descriptive insight than others.

In the literature identified as self-transcendence:

- *Initially*: Loss of physical health, loss of social relationships, loss of self, and loss of meaning
- *Later*: Extending self-boundaries, connecting with others, spirituality, acceptance of event, altruistic activities, healing, increases in self-worth, and receive support

In the self-reformulation research:

- *Initially*: Facing mortality, loss of self, loss of control, loss of normalcy, loss of meaning, altered self/struggle to preserve self

- *Later:* Reevaluations of priorities; meaning finding/making sense, connecting/reconnecting with others, sharing experiences, reevaluating priorities, prayer, spirituality, regaining control, letting go of self, expanding self-boundaries, altruism, and healing

From the above table and data, it is clear that the two concepts are similar at the beginning of the process; thus, what has been called transcendence is initially experienced by both groups. However the responses to the threat (usually of serious illness) change soon after, with the transcendent group moving beyond the condition and above the loss, and the self-reformulation group "letting go" of former self and dramatically remaking/changing their lives.

Is There a Difference in the Structure (Attributes) of the Concepts?

In our assessment of the two bodies of literature, some of the defining attributes that distinguish these two states are portrayed in Figure 20.1.

In the literature identified as self-transcendence, notable features include acceptance, having a spiritual base of support, and connections with others. These three features were characterized in all but two of the transcendence articles. Acceptance involves recognition of new limitations on life and/or physicality. Spirituality is a quality that has been closely associated with the

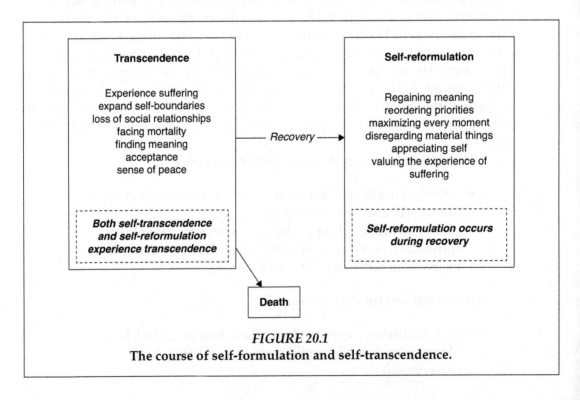

FIGURE 20.1
The course of self-formulation and self-transcendence.

concept since its inception and may provide the wellspring that cuts through fear and enables acceptance. Spirituality, as characterized in the literature on transcendence, is also associated with connections with others and a deeper awareness of self and purpose. A question we ask: Does having a traumatic life event bring one to a spiritual perspective, or does having a spiritual orientation give one hope in the face of suffering that is crucial for transcendence? Also too, if people survive crises, are they still in a transcendent state? Bean and Wagner (2006) report high transcendent states in the face of possible death, but as survival became likely, this state declines.

In the literature identified as self-reformulation, the overriding theme of this state portrayed in the research is that of change and life re-visioning. The people described in this body of research felt gratitude for the encounter that compelled a dramatic reordering of life. A "new life" is pronounced (Enyert & Burnam, 1999), and a "letting go of former identity" (Elofsson & Öhlén, 2004) and a reordering of life priorities (Mayan et al., 2006) characterize this transformation. The development of self-reformulation presents as an appreciation for one's innate abilities, the exiting of unsatisfying relationships, and the ability to reorder life priorities. Those who reformulate have gratitude and appreciation toward life and a desire to give to others (Mayan, Morse, & Eldershaw, 2006).

Is There a Difference in the Outcomes for Each Concept?

The literature examined here shows some similarities in outcomes making us again ask the question: Are these one in the same experience? Or, do they represent unique life-changing events that warrant distinct identifiers?

The notable outcomes of each state as characterized in the literature are reflected in their respective definitions and identified attributes. Both states represent a positive transition, whether acceptance of unchangeable conditions, as in the case of terminal illness, or a feeling of growth that emerges after having survived a traumatic life event. From the existing literature, transcendence represents a sense of closure, peace, a self beyond physical boundaries and connectedness with others, with God, or a spiritual source. In self-reformulation, there is growth, change, renewal: a new lease of life.

Thus, despite their apparent similarities at the onset, the two states represent strikingly different outcomes that, in our reading of the research findings, make them distinct experiences. One state represents an ideal coming to terms and acceptance, while the latter represents regeneration.

It is also noteworthy that some authors characterize self-transcendence as a "resource" (Ellermann & Reed, 2001; Haugan & Innstrand, 2012). This would suggest that it is already present prior to the traumatic event. Or that such a state can be taught or facilitated. Can one "engage" in self- transcendence (Palmer et al., 2010)? Is this something that can be willfully chosen or is it a response that is matured into out of circumstances? Williams (2012) proposes, as Frankl himself observed, that some individuals have an inner capacity to find meaning in the face of great suffering, further suggesting that through suffering there is a potential for peace, rebirth, or positive renewal. More insight into these states of individuals *prior* to these traumatic events could conceivably shed light on this potential.

A serious gap in the literature is a discussion on those who fail to transcend or reform.

Lukkarinen's (1999) study of CAD patients adds some information into these contrary responses to chronic illness and physical decline. A variable identified in this study that distinguishes the two paths is acceptance. Without acceptance of the new conditions and limitations of life that result from the diagnosis, positive reformulation is unlikely.

From the present analysis, we must therefore ask the research question that has not been satisfied in the literature: *Why do some people reformulate or transcend while others do not?* To attempt to answer this, a future line of research might consider exploring resiliency (Earvolino-Ramirez, 2007) as a potential antecedent that enhances the likelihood of positive transformation following life-threatening or challenging events. It may also be the case that individuals choose to remain in suffering and are not able to accept the "changed reality."

In addition, we need to be cautious about definitions that restrict the concepts. Certainly, the elements that characterize these ideal states can experientially mean different things to different people. Some authors have incorporated spirituality into transcendence (e.g., Coward & Kahn, 2004), and it is probable that those who believe in the hereafter transcend more easily than those with "spiritual disequilibrium."

DISCUSSION

It is evident that the research literature to date serves to bring to light two very remarkable life experiences. However, as presently discussed in the literature, the path to this transformation is murky. There is a lack of specificity in populations studied that has led to an overlap in their application. We credit Reed and Coward's path-breaking work in the health care field for their development of a comprehensive definition of *self-transcendence*. Carter (1994) and Mayan et al. (2006) have taken up the charge in defining self-reformulation; however, the abundance of this literature neglects to work toward the development of a theory for this transitive state.

From this review, we recommend that the term self-transcendence be reserved for conditions that threaten one's mortality, whereas self-reformulation be used in cases in which individuals live and thrive as a result of the experience. Further, we question the application of the concept of transcendence to contexts outside serious, life-threatening events (e.g., bullying, homelessness). As life challenging as these circumstances can be, in such cases, we propose the term reformulation as more suitable to describe individuals who thrive beyond adverse conditions.

The general application of this concept to both the healthy and the ill is due, we believe, in part to the wide use of the STS. Despite claims that repeated application of the STS demonstrates validity, there is no support that the instrument has content validity. In our estimation, it does not measure self-transcendence as it has come to be defined in the literature. The replication of this scale serves only to support the scale itself and does not add insight into the processes involved in the state. Self-transcendence is a unique and rare experience, and the particular items presented frame this complex concept, and ultimately minimize the uniqueness and complexity of this state. The research using the STS fails to represent the processes of transformation, lacks in-depth insight, and poorly represents the concept as obtained from qualitative description.

The present literature in self-transcendence has been developed deductively. Further, some of the research has been conducted within support groups (e.g., Coward, 1998; Coward & Kahn, 2004) for the purpose of "teaching" self-transcendence or proposes that nurses can facilitate this experience (Teixeira, 2008), rather than using methods of inductive naturalistic inquiry. This seriously biases the research, placing it at great risk of excluding further learning about the nature of transcendence itself (see Chapter 7).

It is of concern that many authors define self-transcendence by the outcome of the concept, rather than using the attributes more descriptively. We ask: Do the findings inform the definitions, or do the definitions define the findings? This seems to be circular reasoning, but the lack of longitudinal qualitative studies is of great concern. Such close work would surely illuminate this phenomenon beyond a static set of indicators. Finally, individuals who are enduring (Morse, 2011) and suppressing emotion are not transcending. In the *Praxis Theory of Suffering*, individuals must exit emotional suffering and regain hope before reformulating. The similarity between the initial stages of reformation and transcendence makes it possible that there is conceptual confusion between these two states.

It is probable that the commonalities that do occur between self-transcendence and self-reformulation may occur because of "sampling errors." Although those who were researching self-transcendence were unaware of self-reformulation, their samples may have included participants who were actually self-reformulating. Indeed some studies that are more open-ended, for instance, studying the "meaning of illness" (Vachon, 2001) and the "life course of people with coronary artery disease" (Lukkarinen, 1999) both report on transformative life experiences and "drastic change in values and attitudes," which gave them "new meaning and structure to life" (Lukkarinen, 1999, p. 709).

Given the similarities and the differences between transcendence and self-reformulation, we are suggesting that both concepts are relatively immature in development and need further investigation using qualitatively rich description. In addition to further descriptive research, we are therefore suggesting that we must consider if:

- Self-transcendence and self-reformulation are similar processes of transformation in the face of a life threatening encounter. Transcendence occurs when death is imminent and reformulation when life continues.
  or
- They are different concepts, arising from different contexts or situations.
  or,
- The two concepts are the same process that gives rise to different responses in different individuals. These differences may be due to spirituality and religiosity.

Given the lack of clarity of these concepts, there is need for serious qualitative descriptive research into both phenomena, and to continue this comparative work between transcendence and self-reformulation. One option that might be considered is a one-group design, comparing the affects of those who died (Are these self-transcendent?) with those who recovered (Did these patients self-reformulate?). This would be an exceptional study, clarifying a murky area, and one that has much potential for care of the seriously ill.

The last problem is that both self-transcendence and self-reformulation have been "siloed" in the nursing literature. Meanwhile, researchers in psychology have observed the phenomena, and an independent stream of qualitative inquiry describing self-reformulation has emerged. However, this descriptive research has not yet labeled the concept (or even labeled it as self-reformulation), so it is difficult to identify this literature from the databases. For instance, psychologists Skeath et al. (2013) provide a vivid description of "life-transforming changes among cancer survivors" and present their results within a 4-stage learning model. Level 1 (nonlearning), level 2 (nonreflective learning), and level 3 (which extends to posttraumatic growth) result in a coping response within the individual. But the fourth level, *transformative learning*, resembles our description of self-reformulation, and is described as resulting in the "generalization of new ways applied to unrelated domains of the learner's life" (p. 1162).

Perhaps our only clear finding from this study is that further qualitative research is urgently needed. Meanwhile, this study illustrates the problems we have in working with scientific concepts that lack a rigorous base. It illustrates the importance of critical examination of the literature, and this is an exercise in patience, when the hoped-for results are not as clear as one would wish. Exposing confusion and further developing both concepts is what science is all about.

REFERENCES

Acton, G. J., & Wright, K. B. (2000). Self-transcendence and family caregivers of adults with dementia. *Journal of Holistic Nursing, 18*(2), 143–158.

Bean, K. B., & Wagner, K. (2006). Self-transcendence, illness distress, and quality of life among liver transplant recipients. *Journal of Theory Construction & Testing, 10*, 47–53.

Boydell, K., Goering, P., & Morrell-Bellai, T. L. (2000). Narratives of identity: Re-presentation of self in people who are homeless. *Qualitative Health Research, 10*(1), 26–38.

Carroll, L. (1865/1977). *Alice's Adventures in wonderland*. Norwalk, CO: The Easton Press.

Carter, B. J. (1994). Surviving breast cancer. *Cancer Practice, 2*(2), 135–140.

Chidester, D. (2001). *Patterns of transcendence: Religious, death and dying*. Belmont, CA: Wadsworth Thomson Learning.

Chin-A-Loy, S. S., & Fernsler, J. I. (1998). Self-transcendence in older men attending a prostate cancer support group. *Cancer Nursing, 21*(5), 358–363.

Coward, D. D. (1990). The lived experience of self-transcendence in women with advanced breast cancer. *Nursing Science Quarterly, 3*, 162–169.

Coward, D. D. (1995). The lived experience of self-transcendence in women with AIDS. *Journal of Obstetric, Gynecologic & Neonatal Nursing, 24*(4), 314–318.

Coward, D. D. (1996). Self-transcendence and correlates in a healthy population. *Nursing Research, 45*(2), 116–121.

Coward, D. D. (1998). Facilitation of self-transcendence in a breast cancer support group. *Oncology Nursing Forum, 25*(1), 75–84.

Coward, D. D., & Kahn, D. L. (2004). Resolution of spiritual disequilibrium by women newly diagnosed with breast cancer. *Oncology Nursing Forum, 31*(2), E24–E31.

Coward, D. D., & Reed, P. G. (1996). Self-Transcendence: A resource for healing at the end of life. *Issues in Mental Health Nursing, 17*, 275–288.

Daniels, M. (2001). On transcendence in transpersonal psychology. *Transpersonal Psychology Review, 5*(2), 3–11.

Earvolino-Ramirez, M. (2007). Resilience: A concept analysis. *Nursing Forum, 42*(2), 73–82.

Ellermann, C. R., & Reed, P. G. (2001). Self-transcendence and depression in middle-aged adults. *Western Journal of Nursing Research, 23*(7), 698–713.

Elofsson, L. C., & Öhlén, J. (2004). Meanings of being old and living with chronic obstructive pulmonary disease. *Palliative Medicine, 18*, 611–618.

Enyert, G., & Burman, M. E. (1999). A qualitative study of self-transcendence in caregivers of terminally ill patients. *American Journal of Hospice & Palliative Medicine, 16*(2), 455–462.

Farren, A. T. (2010). Power, uncertainty, self-transcendence, and quality of life in breast cancer survivors. *Nursing Science Quarterly, 23*(1), 63–71.

Frank, A. (2003). Survivorship as craft and conviction: Reflections on research in progress. *Qualitative Health Research, 13*(20), 247–255.

Frankl, V. (1966). Self-transcendence as a human phenomenon. *Journal of Humanistic Psychology, 6*, 97–106.

Haase, J. E., Britt, T., Coward, D. D., Leidy, N. K., & Penn, P. E. (1992). Simultaneous concept analysis of spiritual perspective, hope, acceptance and self-transcendence. *Journal of Nursing Scholarship, 24*(2), 141–147.

Hall, V. P. (2001). Bearing witness to suffering from AIDS: Constructing meaning from loss. *Journal of the Association of Nursing in AIDS Care, 12*(2), 44–55.

Haugan, G., & Innstrand, S. T. (2012). The effect of self-transcendence on depression in cognitively intact nursing home patients. *International Scholarly Research Network Psychiatry, 2012*, 10. Retrieved from http://dx.doi.org/10.5402/2012/301325

Haugan, G., Rannestad, T., Hammervold, R., Garåsen, H., & Espnes, G. A. (2012). Self-transcendence in cognitively intact nursing-home patients: A resource for well-being. *Journal of Clinical Nursing, 21*, 3429–3441.

Hunnibell, L. S., Reed, P. G., Quinn-Griffin, M., & Fitzpatrick, J. J. (2008). Self-transcendence and burnout in hospice and oncology nurses. *Journal of Hospice & Palliative Nursing, 10*(3), 172–179.

Kinney, C. K. (1996). Transcending breast cancer: Reconstructing one's self. *Issues in Mental Health Nursing, 17*, 201–216.

Lukkarinen, H. (1999). Life course of people with coronary artery disease. *Journal of Clinical Nursing, 8*(6), 701–711.

Maslow, A.H. (1969). Various meanings of transcendence. *Journal of Transpersonal Psychology. 1*(1), 56–66.

Mayan, M., Morse, J. M., & Eldershaw, L. P. (2006). Developing the concept of self-reformulation. *International Journal of Qualitative Studies on Health and Well-being, 1*(1), 20–26.

McCarthy, V. L., Ling, J., & Carini, R. M. (2013). The role of self-transcendence: A missing variable in the pursuit of successful aging? *Research in Gerontological Nursing, 6*, 178–186.

Mellors, M. P., Coontz, P. D., & Lucke, K. T. (2001). Transcending the suffering of AIDS. *Journal of Community Health Nursing, 18*(4), 235–246.

Morse, J. M. (2001). Toward a Praxis Theory of Suffering. *Advances in Nursing Science, 24*(1), 47–59.

Morse, J. M. (2011). The Praxis Theory of Suffering. In J. B. Butts & K. L. Rich (Eds.), *Philosophies and theories in advanced nursing practice* (pp. 569–602). Burlington, MA: Jones & Bartlett.

Morse, J. M., & Carter, B. (1996). The essence of enduring and the expression of suffering: The reformulation of self. *Scholarly Inquiry for Nursing Practice, 10*(1), 43–60.

Neill, J. (2002). Transcendence and transformation in the life patterns of women living with rheumatoid arthritis. *Advances in Nursing Science, 24*, 27–47.

Nygren, B., Alex, L., Jonsen, E., Gustafson, Y., Norberg, A., & Lundman, B. (2005) Resilience, sense of coherence, purpose in life and self-transcendence in relation to perceived physical and mental health among the oldest old. *Aging and Mental Health, 9*, 354–362.

Ohman, M., Söderberg, S., & Lundman, B. (2003). Hovering between suffering and enduring: The meaning of living with serious chronic illness. *Qualitative Health Research, 13*(4), 528–542.

Palmer, B., Quinn, M. T., Reed, P., & Fitzpatrick, J. J. (2010). Self-transcendence and work engagement in acute care staff registered nurses. *Critical Care Nursing Quarterly, 33*(2), 138–147.

Park, E. J. (2005). Self-sacrifice, self-transcendence and nurses' professional self. *Nurse Philosophy, 6*(4), 247–254.

Pelusi, J. (1997, September). The lived experience of surviving breast cancer. *Oncology Nursing Forum, 24,* 1343–1353.

Pollock, S. E., & Sands, D. (1997). Adaptation to suffering. *Clinical Nursing Research, 6*(2), 171–185.

Ramer, L., Johnson, D., Chan, L., & Barrett, M. T. (2006). The effect of HIV/AIDS disease progression on spirituality and self-transcendence in a multicultural population. *Journal of Transcultural Nursing, 17*(3), 280–289.

Reed, P. G. (1987). Spirituality and well-being in terminally ill hospitalized adults. *Research in Nursing & Health, 10,* 335–344. doi:10.1002/nur.4770100507

Reed, P. G. (1991a). Self-transcendence and mental health in oldest-old adults. *Nursing Research, 4*(1), 5–10.

Reed, P. G. (1991b). Toward a nursing theory of self-transcendence: Deductive reformulation using developmental theories. *Advance Nursing Science, 13*(4), 64–77.

Reed, P. G. (1996). Transcendence: Formulating nursing perspectives. *Nursing Science Quarterly, 9*(1), 1–4.

Reed, P. G. (2003). The theory of self-transcendence. In M. J. Smith & P. Liehr (Eds.), *Middle range theories in nursing* (pp. 145–165). New York, NY: Springer.

Reed, P. G. (2008). Theory of self-transcendence. In M. J. Smith & P. L. Liehr (Eds.), *Middle-range theory for nursing* (2nd ed., pp. 105–129). New York, NY: Springer.

Reed, P. G. (2009). Demystifying self-transcendence for mental health nursing practice and research. *Archives of Psychiatric Nursing, 23,* 397–400.

Reed, P. G. (2010). Theory of self-transcendence. In M. J. Smith & P. R. Lier (Eds.), *Middle range theory for nursing* (2nd ed., pp. 105–129). New York, NY: Springer.

Rodgers, B. L. (2000). Concept analysis: An evolutionary view. In B. L. Rodgers & K. Knafl (Eds.), *Concept development in nursing: Foundations, techniques, and applications* (pp. 77–117). Philadelphia, PA: Saunders.

Runquist, J., & Reed, P. G. (2007). Self-transcendence and wellbeing in homeless adults. *Journal of Holistic Nursing, 20*(2), 118–122.

Russell, W., Robert, R. S., Thomas, C. R., Holzer, C. E., Blakeney, P., & Meyer, W. J. (2013). Self-Perceptions of young adults who survived severe childhood burn injury. *Journal of Burn Care & Research, 34*(4), 394–402. doi:10.1097/BCR.0b013e3182700198

Skeath, P., Norris, S., Katheria, V., White, J., Baker, K., Handel, D., . . . Berger, A. (2013). The nature of life-transforming changes among survivors. *Qualitative Health Research, 23*(9), 1155–1167.

Stinson, C. K., & Kirk, E. (2006). Structured reminiscence: An intervention to decrease depression and increase self transcendence in older women. *Journal of Clinical Nursing, 15*(2), 208–218.

Teixeira, E. M. (2008). Self-transcendence: A concept analysis for nursing praxis. *Holistic Nursing Practice, 22*(1), 25–31.

Thomas, J. C., Burton, M., Quinn, M. T., & Fitzpatrick, J. J. (2010). Self-transcendence, spiritual well-being, and spiritual practices of women with breast cancer. *Journal of Holistic Nursing, 28*(2), 115–122.

Vachon, M. L. S. (2001). The meaning of illness to a long-term survivor. *Seminars in Oncology Nursing, 17*(4), 279–283.

Williams, B. J. (2012). Self-transcendence in stem cell transplantation recipients: A phenomenologic inquiry. *Oncology Nursing Forum, 39*(1), E41–E48.

Willis D. G., & Griffith C. A. (2010). Healing patterns revealed in middle school boys' experiences of being bullied using Roger's Science of Unitary Human Beings (SUHB). *Journal of Child and Adolescent Psychiatric Nursing, 23*(3), 125–132.

Woogara, J. (2005). Patients' privacy of the person and human rights. *Nursing Ethics, 12*(3), 273–287.

SECTION V

TOWARD MID-RANGE THEORY

The latest quandary for nursing doctoral students is how to form the required three chapters for their dissertation. It is nonsense, under the guise of holism, to create a beautiful mid-range theory, only to chop it up into concepts or portions according the stages of the process, simply to have three articles to defend.

So keep it whole, write it as one or two articles, and find a journal that accepts longer articles.

21

FROM CONCEPT DEVELOPMENT TO QUALITATIVELY DERIVED THEORY: ETHICAL SENSITIVITY IN PROFESSIONAL PRACTICE

> *The signs – sometimes imperceptible, at others very clear – are all around us. But they require careful interpretation if they are to be transformed into a road map.*
>
> —Coelho (2007)

The literature lacks clear guidelines for synthesizing results of concept analysis beyond conceptual categories toward the development of theory to guide practice. Except for the most simplistic models, concept development rarely leads to theory development. Pragmatic utility (Morse, 2000b), a balanced and systematic method to develop concepts, enables the examination of the interactions between attributes, modeling, and theory development. Depending on the state of science within a particular discipline or a combination of disciplines, the results of exploring pragmatic utility bring new knowledge into the conceptual bases to guide research, theory, and practice. In this chapter, I explore the processes used for taking analyses to a beginning level of qualitatively derived theory. I describe using pragmatic utility for examining the concept of ethical sensitivity in nursing and other professional practices to develop qualitative theory, and the methodological tools and processes involved in abstraction beyond the limits of concept analysis toward theory.

OVERVIEW

An extensive critical appraisal of relevant available literature on ethical sensitivity in professional practice was undertaken to inform ethical practice in the care and treatment of those with complex, poorly understood conditions (such as eating disorders). The inquiry was needed because clients and their families perceived their experiences with health services as traumatic, rather than as healing, despite professional expertise and good intentions (Weaver, 2012; Weaver, Wuest, & Ciliska, 2005). Furthermore, this perceived jeopardy was associated with care across multiple disciplines and posed as much a threat to client well-being as the health challenge itself. I wanted to learn how to deal with this perception and the situations that give rise to it. To begin to find answers for how nurses and other professionals might better address the moral complexities encountered in providing care and services, I needed a clearer understanding of the quality of ethical practice that enables professionals to accurately recognize and sensitively respond to the needs of those they serve. These aspects could potentially impact professions by influencing a professional's behavior in a given situation.

As a scientific concept, ethical sensitivity has been explicitly defined within professional disciplines including nursing, medicine, dentistry, philosophy, business, education, psychology, bioethics, law, theology, journalism, and social and political sciences. Despite the volume of this work and the common definitions used, the available literature provided a clutter of competing descriptors for the concept of ethical sensitivity and only limited understanding of its nature, associated negative consequences, and the role of education in preparing professionals to develop their ethical sensitivity. Validity has been compromised through practices of not matching samples to the population (e.g., convenience rather than randomly selected samples), including only students as study participants, cueing participants to the presence of an ethical problem versus allowing them to recognize it on their own, failing to ensure accurate conclusions about relationships studied, and using inadequate underlying theoretical frameworks and definitions. Validity of this qualitative research was to some extent preserved because participants were asked to describe their own experiences of making decisions when working with vulnerable clients. However, without agreement about the core features and definition of ethical sensitivity, findings from individual studies could not be consolidated and further research would not significantly contribute to knowledge development.

CONCEPT ANALYSIS USING PRAGMATIC UTILITY

In seeking greater knowledge of the concept, I applied the guiding principles within the Morse criterion-based method for exploring pragmatic utility to clarify study purpose, selecting adequate and appropriate literature, comprehending the topic, and synthesizing results. The purpose of the inquiry was to:

- Understand the perspectives of professionals in providing care and services to clients, and
- Construct a basic foundation for ongoing and future investigation through exploring the usefulness and implications of the concept ethical sensitivity

This analysis used as data the published literature from a number of professional disciplines, and 200 published reports meeting the study's inclusion criteria were included. Validity in selection of literature was attained through restricting search fields to articles with such related terms as *ethical sensitivity, moral sensitivity, ethical perception, moral perception, ethical sensibility, moral sensibility,* and *ethical intuition* in titles or abstracts. Inclusion criteria were accessibility, relevancy (i.e., publication contains an explicit or inferred definition of the concept), and usefulness to the emerging conceptualization. Additional data were included through ongoing searches and primary sources.

To comprehend the topic, publications were sorted and color-coded by discipline. Each publication was first read without coding to begin to holistically understand the concept and identify its dimensions without losing the connections between these dimensions and their context. Data were then coded, sorted into predetermined analytic categories of concept anatomy (internal structure) and physiology (action), and examined for *fit* within and across categories. Fit is used for identifying and matching characteristics of one entity with those of another entity to determine if similar characteristics are present (Morse & Singleton, 2001). In analyzing the anatomy and physiology of ethical sensitivity, fit determined if an entity was considered a component of these dimensions, and fit allowed data to be linked together to enable analysis, organization, conceptualization, and summarization while raising the level of abstraction.

As extensive knowledge was built about the concept, questions were formulated and asked of the literature to develop new insight and information. Results from such questioning were synthesized to produce a more comprehensive definition and interpretation of the concept of ethical sensitivity in professional practice that would better represent the phenomenon (Weaver, Morse, & Mitcham, 2008). Exploring pragmatic utility pulled knowledge beyond concept analysis to inform a mid-range theory beyond the expectations of the initial project.

EXPLICATING CONCEPT ANATOMY

Assessing anatomy involves examining the internal dimensions of the concept: its theoretical definition(s), preconditions, attributes, boundaries, and outcomes (Morse, 1995b). These dimensions form the categories for sorting data to enable the concept's anatomy to be explicated and illustrated (Table 21.1).

Examination of concept anatomy revealed incomplete and diverse theoretical definitions for ethical sensitivity. It had been scientifically defined by
researchers for use in specific studies with limited agreement of definitions
across different studies. The conditions under which ethical sensitivity
occurs were not fully explicated. Attributes of moral perception, affectivity,
and dividing loyalties were identified but relationships between these attributes and their components were not clear. Ethical sensitivity was used
interchangeably with its allied concepts (e.g., moral sensitivity, ethical intuition) indicating a need to clarify the concept's boundaries. Positive outcomes of client comfort and well-being, professional learning, and
integrity-preserving compromise were found in the professional literature;
yet, negative consequences, which could reasonably include emotional over-
load, exploitation, and personal and moral distress, were meagerly considered with regard to ethical sensitivity.

TABLE 21.1
Anatomy of the Concept of Ethical Sensitivity

DIMENSION	DEFINITION	ILLUSTRATIONS OF ETHICAL SENSITIVITY
Theoretical definition	Degree to which concept is communicated, which enables different people or the same person at different times to agree that something is an instance of the concept (Berthold, 1964).	Competing/incomplete definitions that involve one or more components of care, knowledge, affect, skill, and responsibility.
Preconditions	Circumstances that must be present for the concept to develop or the behaviors that distinguish the characteristics to occur.	Suffering and vulnerability cues, relationship, receptivity, responsiveness, and uncertainty precede incidents of ethical sensitivity.
Attributes	Features always present in instances of the concept. Must be abstract enough to define the concept regardless of the context yet unique enough to differentiate concept from allied (similar) concepts.	Attributes: moral perception, affectivity, and dividing loyalties are identified in all instances of concept.
Boundaries	Separateness of the concept from others. Boundaries may be fuzzy or merge or overlap with other concepts (and thus share attributes).	Used interchangeably with allied concepts (e.g., moral sensitivity, ethical intuition, ethical perception, ethical sensibility).
Outcomes	Results or consequences from utilization of the concept.	Outcomes are client comfort and well-being, professional learning, and integrity-preserving compromise.

Adapted from Weaver and Morse (2006).

MOVING FROM ANATOMY OF THE CONCEPT TO ITS PHYSIOLOGY

Physiology or action of the concept was explored as described by Morse (1995a, 2000b) via examining its conceptualizations, perspectives, measurement, and applications in research and practice settings. In contrast to decontextualizing the concept's anatomical dimensions, analyzing physiology recontextualized the data to understand the concept's action in its various applications. Table 21.2 portrays the physiology of the concept across disciplines of nursing, medicine, business/accounting, theology, and dentistry.

Differences are revealed in how ethical sensitivity was conceptualized within and across these disciplines (e.g., as cognition and responsibility in dentistry compared to affect, cognition, skill, responsibility, and knowledge in nursing and theology). Different settings and perspectives (e.g., client and lay views in theology and business/accounting) were provided. Of the various measurement instruments used, the Lutzen Moral Sensitivity Questionnaire (MSQ; Lutzen, Johansson, & Nordstrom, 2000) was developed from qualitative nursing research and the Dental Ethical Sensitivity Test (DEST; Bebeau, Rest, & Yamoor, 1985) from hypothesized practice scenarios. Ethical sensitivity was most often evaluated quantitatively through scored responses to real life or hypothetical dilemmas (e.g., a choice between two or more equally good or bad options) or violations (e.g., infringement on rights and harm to stakeholders). The scenarios portrayed ethical sensitivity as a *negative* concept, that is, ethical sensitivity would not be applied to a situation if people were behaving ethically. Missing was conceptualization of ethical sensitivity as a positive, proactive component of practice.

EVALUATING CONCEPT MATURITY

Maturity or readiness of a concept for research is evaluated by establishing the degree of the concept's coherence with the following principles: *epistemological* (clear description of definition, preconditions, attributes, boundaries, and outcomes), *pragmatic* (how well the concept is operationalized; its usefulness to and fit with other phenomena of interest to the discipline), *linguistic* (the consistency of the concept's use in and across contexts), and *logical* (how well the concept holds its boundaries through integration with other concepts).

The evaluation of the maturity of ethical sensitivity was detailed in Chapter 11. Briefly, using the literature, evaluate the epistemological, pragmatic, linguistic, and logical dimensions of the concept. If the concept is immature, epistemologically there are no (or inadequate) definitions; the pragmatic criterion is not operationalized and fits poorly; the linguistic aspects are confused, and logically, it does not hold its boundaries.

TABLE 21.2
Physiology of the Concept of Ethical Sensitivity Across Five Disciplines

DISCIPLINE	HOW CONCEPTUALIZED	WHOSE PERSPECTIVE	SETTING	INSTRUMENTS	RESEARCH METHODS
Nursing (n = 47)	Affect Cognition Skill Responsibility Knowledge	Bedside nurses, nurse practitioners, students	Psychiatric-mental health, medicine, surgery, emergency room	6 scenarios: 3 dilemmas, 2 violations, 1 control. Moral Sensitivity Questionnaire (attitude survey)	Qualitative (Grounded Theory, phenomenology) Case study Philosophical Quantitative (descriptive, correlational)
Medicine (n = 19)	Cognition Skill Knowledge	Students in all but 1 study	General practice	15 scenarios: 9 dilemmas, 5 violations, 1 control	Quantitative (experimental, descriptive) Philosophical
Accounting and business (n = 15)	Cognition Affect Responsibility	Accountants, auditors, managers, students, clients	Small-, mid-, large-sized organizations Various cultures	62 scenarios: 41 dilemmas, 21 violations	Quantitative (experimental, descriptive, correlational)
Theology (n = 9)	Affect Cognition Skill Responsibility Knowledge	Jewish leaders, Catholic priests, Christian lay counselors, divinity students	Places of worship Academic settings	Bibliotext examples discussed 1 "Good Samaritan" scenario	Philosophical Case study Quantitative (quasiexperimental)
Dentistry (n = 6)	Cognition Responsibility	Dentistry students	Office practice	Dental Ethical Sensitivity Test: 4 hypothetical scenarios based on practice dilemmas	Quantitative (experimental, descriptive, correlational)

n = number of reports examined.
Source: Weaver (2005). Reprinted by permission of the author.

If the concept is partially mature, epistemologically there will be multiple competing definitions; it will be partially operationalized; linguistically, partially linked with context, and linkages with other concepts will be partially developed.

Mature concepts are well defined epistemologically; they pragmatically fit with other phenomena and are operationalized; linguistically, they are integrated into other texts, and logically used in theory (Morse, Mitcham, Hupcey, Tasón, 1996; Weaver & Morse, 2006).

Establishing its maturity illuminates the current state of the science concerning a concept of interest (Penrod & Hupcey, 2005b). From this baseline assessment of maturity, ethical sensitivity was shown to typify a partially mature, emerging scientific concept that lacked consensus about its meaning, structure, and use. Introduced as a concept by Rest in 1982, ethical sensitivity is interchanged with its allied concepts (e.g., moral sensitivity). Although it was beginning to be used in research (e.g., measuring ethical sensitivity levels in various professional groups; Bebeau & Brabeck, 1989; Lutzen, Johansson, & Nordstrom, 2000), it has not been logically linked with other concepts. Epistemologically, ethical sensitivity presented as many definitions and needing greater explication and integration of its preconditions, attributes, and outcomes. Pragmatically, ethical sensitivity was conveyed as an aspect of a professional's decision making; however, the focus of the decision making varied within and across disciplines. To illustrate, business, law, and nursing reported concern with client satisfaction; nursing and education with attrition; theology and philosophy with client comfort. The multiple descriptors for ethical sensitivity evident across disciplines could indicate linguistic immaturity; however, that is not the case if all these descriptors are components of ethical sensitivity. For this concept to be useful for theory, research, and practice, its plethora of definitions, descriptors, and differing perspectives required further development.

ADVANCING THE CONCEPT OF ETHICAL SENSITIVITY USING CRITICAL APPRAISAL

Described by Morse (2000b) as a process of formulating and asking a series of increasingly complex questions of the literature, critical appraisal enables analysis and synthesis of assumptions underlying the concept's application in research and theory. Arising from and driven by in-depth understanding of the literature (as achieved through assessing the concept's anatomy, physiology, and maturity), critical appraisal stimulates "thinking outside the box." It provokes intense examination and direction beyond the limits of isolated findings and individual disciplines, and contributes to advancing the development of a partially mature concept by synthesizing new or hitherto unexplored tacit knowledge.

Analytic Questions

Carefully constructed questions are used to stimulate inquiry into aspects of the concept that are incomplete, confusing, or uncritically accepted. The questions must be clearly understood by all readers and singularly focused toward a significant line of inquiry within a substantive area and discipline. The questions have breath (able to address a wide range of application) and depth (ability to penetrate beyond obvious surface knowledge) to promote insight and illuminate the concept's complexity. Prepared as a set, the analytic questions fully and completely address the concept in ways that permit a fair and comprehensive comparison of concept characteristics across disciplines by treating all perspectives respectfully and as equally important (Weaver & Morse, 2006). The analytic questions designed to examine the nature of ethical sensitivity, its requirements, and preparation for ethically sensitive practice are included in Box 21.1.

In comparing the answers to the analytic questions, the sample of literature was at times expanded to clarify emerging ideas. For instance, in examining the component of reflexivity as a quality for ethically sensitive practice (Analytic question # 7, Box 21.1), literature concerning whistle-blowing and moral distress was included in light of reports that professionals did not always act with ethical sensitivity despite having comprehensive knowledge of the situation (e.g., Austin, Bergum, & Goldberg, 2003; Cherrington, 2002; Ulrich, Soeken, & Miller, 2003). New information and insights emerging while examining the responses to the analytic questions were integrated using the principle of fit (explained in the section "Concept Analysis Using Pragmatic Utility") and negative case analysis. Negative cases are examples of conflicting data that do not initially fit the pattern being discovered in the data (Glaser & Strauss, 1967). Negative cases rekindle researcher thinking about the data, often in new ways that round out and contribute to denser conceptualization.

Synthesizing Results

Critical appraisal guided induction and abstraction, facilitating data transformation from concrete individual study findings to new knowledge and comprehensive results. The answers to the analytic questions are synthesized through comparing and reducing the data. In the ethical sensitivity study, a large (6 foot by 8 foot) paper matrix was constructed with the analytic questions forming rows and individual disciplines forming columns. Arranging the data to be viewed as a whole facilitated the process of synthesizing results. Characteristics of the data were compared to help describe their relationships. Overarching themes, hypotheses, and conclusions about the concept were generated and explored by moving between description and verification of

---

BOX 21.1. ANALYTIC QUESTIONS USED IN CONCEPT ANALYSIS OF ETHICAL SENSITIVITY

Nature of Ethical Sensitivity

1. Is ethical sensitivity applied in all practice situations or just in particular ones?
2. Does ethical sensitivity have a futuristic or anticipatory function or does it emerge only within ongoing dilemmas?
3. Are there variations in types of ethical sensitivity? Is ethical sensitivity graduated (e.g., continuum from low to high) or absolute (e.g., present or absent in particular situations)?
4. Does the nature of ethical sensitivity change with the level of the professional's involvement in the situation (e.g., if the professional is an observer or an actor in the setting)? Can a professional have ethical sensitivity if it does not translate into an action or behavior?
5. Is ethical sensitivity innate or acquired?
6. What is the relationship between technical competency and ethical sensitivity (e.g., Must a professional be competent to be ethically sensitive? Can a professional be ethically sensitive without being competent? Could a physician be able to recognize ethical content in an accounting situation?)

Ethical Requirements for Praxis

7. What personal and interpersonal characteristics are required for developing ethical sensitivity in professional and interdisciplinary praxis?
8. Do employing organizations foster ethical sensitivity?

Preparation for Professional Practice

9. Assuming that ethical sensitivity or at least some aspect of it can be taught or learned, what if any strategies best prepare professionals to develop ethical sensitivity?

Source: Weaver and Morse (2006). Reprinted with permission.

---

possibilities. Results were confirmed by returning to the original data set, thereby enhancing rigor and validity of results.

TOWARD CLEARER UNDERSTANDING OF THE CONCEPT

Analytic questions about the nature and requirement of ethical sensitivity pushed deeper examination of the concept's attributes, theoretical definitions, and boundaries. Attributes are the essential characteristics that define instances of the concept within a specified phenomenon (Morse, 1995a). Attributes identified through analyzing concept anatomy are decontextualized or considered "abstract of time, place, and person." When the concept is recontextualized, its attributes appear in different combinations and strengths. For instance, the finding that business clients recognized the culpability of managers who employed deceptive packaging trials (Bone & Corey, 2000) accentuated the core feature of responsibility, whereas teachers treated ethical sensitivity as a skill in recognizing ethical dilemmas that could be acquired via student participation over a 4- to 12-week term (Clarkeburn, 2002a, 2002b). Attributes are stronger in the most obvious examples of the concept (Morse, Hupcey, Penrod, & Mitcham, 2002). Identified from these relevant sources, the attributes of the concept of ethical sensitivity—moral perception, affectivity, and dividing loyalties—are summarized in Box 21.2. Together, these attributes denote how professionals appraise the client situation and act to promote client welfare.

The theoretical definitions for ethical sensitivity conveyed numerous conceptualizations and descriptors for the concept. Sorted and content analyzed, these descriptions roughly fit within a core domain comprising basic features of affect, cognition, skill, knowledge, and responsibility (Weaver, 2007). Comparing these basic features with the concept's attributes (Box 21.2) explicated the following defining features of ethical sensitivity as (a) caring affectivity oriented toward excellence in practice, public-mindedness, compassion, and otherness; (b) means for knowing a particular situation through exploring the competing perspectives of relevant stakeholders including clients, colleagues, organizations, and professional associations as well as the

---

BOX 21.2. SUMMARY OF ATTRIBUTES OF ETHICAL SENSITIVITY

MORAL PERCEPTION: Intuitive discrimination of cues and patterns enabling the professional to perceive the ethical nature of a situation that could negatively influence client well-being. Two aspects of moral perception are *awakening* (initial intrusive gut level response akin to worry or alarm) and *particularizing* (perceptual processing of client's actual or potential distress cues). Awakening and particularizing draw largely on intuition (combined affect and cognition) and knowledge (from experience and professional values). Skill is required for reading the situation to identify the particular ethical issue and client interests. Responsibility materializes as concern for the client.

AFFECTIVITY: Emotional response (affect) of feeling the client's distress while cognitively gaining information about what hurts or threatens the client (cognition, knowledge). Emotions enable access to the moral conditions clients experience by pinpointing salient cues (skill) and registering facts (knowledge) with resonance and depth. Professionals are responsible for examining affectivity. Affectivity prevents blindness and hardness to the client's plight. Ethical sensitivity cannot be expressed unless the professional has the skill to connect with personal vulnerabilities and particular emotions.

DIVIDING LOYALTIES: Consideration of the situation from the perspectives of relevant stakeholders and other sources of knowledge to determine one's moral agency. Strategies involve *interpretation* (eliciting multiple perspectives, particularly those most affected and vulnerable), *justification* (comparing the situation's immediate and long-term demands, choices, and consequences against external knowledge/standards to determine legitimacy), and *reflexivity* (examining individually held goals, commitments, and ideals regarding the needs of the situation and greater good in reaching a decision the professional can endorse). Interpretation draws mainly on communication and language skills; justification on cognitive processing; and reflexivity on responsibility and affect as the professional acts or chooses to not take action.

Source: Weaver, Morse, and Mitcham (2008). Used with permission.

knowledge from academic, clinical, and ethical insights; (c) obligation to pursue responsible action; (d) skill development to respond in the situation; and (e) decision making by perceiving, interpreting, and evaluating the ethical import of the situation.

Saturation of data within these defining features enabled a synthesizing transdisciplinary definition of ethical sensitivity as a type of practical wisdom in pursuit of client comfort and professional satisfaction with care delivery. Specifically, the synthesized definition for ethical sensitivity is put forward as:

> Capacity to decide with intelligence and compassion, given
> uncertainty in a care situation, drawing as needed on a critical
> understanding of codes for ethical conduct, clinical experience,
> academic learning and self knowledge, with an additional
> ability to anticipate consequences and the courage to act.
> (Weaver, Morse, & Mitcham, 2008, p. 610)

Having proposed a synthesized theoretical definition for the concept, attention went to the boundaries to further distinguish the concept's scope and meaning. The presence of competing concepts indicated a need to clarify the boundaries given that attributes may weaken at the boundaries where competing or allied concepts may share some attributes with the concept of interest (Morse et al., 2002). To clarify boundaries, I examined allied concepts of moral perception, moral sensitivity, clinical perception, clinical sensitivity, ethical or moral sensibility, and ethical intuition alongside the concept of ethical sensitivity. My approach involved comparing (a) moral, ethical, and clinical and (b) sensitivity, sensibility, intuition, and perception in terms of etymology, scope, and focus. Although ethical sensitivity, moral sensitivity, ethical perception, clinical perception, clinical sensitivity, ethical intuition, and moral or ethical sensibility share some features (e.g., particularizing [moral perception], interpreting and justifying [dividing loyalties]), they do not necessarily represent the same phenomenon. For example, the difference between ethical sensitivity and moral sensitivity is that ethical sensitivity describes the goodness or rightness of decisions and conduct by their conformity to values and codes established by professional organizations (Beauchamp & Bowie, 1997), whereas moral sensitivity is concerned with goodness or rightness embodied in daily life and applied to lay contexts (Lutzen, 1993).

BEYOND CONCEPT ANALYSES TO SYSTEMATIC CLASSIFICATION AND THEORY CONSTRUCTION

The new knowledge from synthesizing the answers for the analytic questions was used in further exploring the concept's dimensions. This resulted in the generation of a taxonomy distinguishing the limits of ethical sensitivity. In addition, the rigorous techniques of pragmatic utility assisted theory construction.

Taxonomy

Concept components were precisely defined, illustrated using examples from the synthesis, and classified. Taxonomies improve description and evaluation of phenomena by allowing diverse, complex dimensions to be summarized and compared (Bradley, Curry, & Devers, 2007). The taxonomy generated from the concept analysis of ethical sensitivity (Table 21.3 and Box 21.3) clearly explicated the preconditions, attributes, and outcomes by clarifying what is and what is not considered as ethical sensitivity. For example, ethical sensitivity is absent if others must point out the presence of an ethical problem (lacking in moral perception), if one is not in touch with one's own humanities and vulnerabilities or is robotically doing one's job (lacking affectivity), and if one remains uncommitted to a plan of action to address the problem (lacking reflexivity of dividing loyalties).

TABLE 21.3
*Taxonomy of Ethical Sensitivity Characteristics**

	ETHICAL SENSITIVITY	NOT ETHICAL SENSITIVITY
Preconditions		
Suffering and vulnerability cues	Ethical sensitivity triggered by watching suffering of others (Malone, 2000)	Moral blindness (Not see/hear/detect cues; Gastmans, 2002)
Uncertainty	Moral doubt and dissonance (Hawkins, 2001; McPhail, 2001) *Not know rules in advance * Situation of ambiguity—above and beyond technical competency * Sense of own vision as limited and that own beliefs may not hold true (Bracci, 2001; Georges, 2002; Scott, 2000; Walker, 1991)	Moral certainty * Knows in advance what is right to do (Wurzback, 1999) * Addresses situation as technical (Kane, 2003; Oddi et al., 1995; Shaner, 1989) * "Cognitive conservation" (seeks information consistent with own beliefs; Payne & Giacalone, 1990)
Relationship	Engagement (Punzo, 1996; Sarat, 1991) Cooperative (Wallace, Reed, Pasero, & Olsson, 1995), nonhierarchical (Canon, 1985; Keenan, 2002)	Detachment (Jaeger, 2001; Lerman, 1998; Mahone, 2000) * Autocratic, repressive or coercive (e.g., managed care; Ulrich et al., 2003)

(continued)

TABLE 21.3
Taxonomy of Ethical Sensitivity Characteristics* (continued)

	ETHICAL SENSITIVITY	NOT ETHICAL SENSITIVITY
Receptivity	Open-mindedness toward possible ethical issues (Branch, 2000; Vetlesen, 1994)	Indifference (Nortvedt, 2001) "Survivalist" mentality (Shaner, 1989) False front/hard shell (Hueber, 1996)
Responsiveness	Feels responsible for impact of own actions or potential actions (Rest, 1982) Internal locus of control (Aharony & Geva, 2003) Internalized commitment to others	Insensitive of potential for harming others, nature, and environment (May, 1992) External locus of control (Aharony & Geva, 2003) Doing one's duty as externally prescribed (Steinkraus, 1987)
Courage	Acting consistently with own opinions (Mohr & Horton-Deutsch, 2001; Naden & Eriksson, 2004; Stark, 2001)	Passivity
Attributes		
Moral perception awakening	Spontaneous (unassisted) recognition (Clarkeburn, 2002b; Simpson & Garrison, 1995)	Others must point out ethical problem
Particularizing	Accurate decoding of nonverbal cues (i.e., identifies components of discrimination, abuse, extreme pain, illness in situation; Bebeau & Brabeck, 1989)	Incorrect recognition of ethical components (related to inexperience, emergency situation; Abdolmohammadi & Owhoso, 2000; Narvaez, 1991)
Affectivity	In touch with/protects own humanity and vulnerability (i.e., not a "robot"; Flannery, 1995)	Desensitized to own needs (i.e., "wounded healer" who lives vicariously through others; Greene, 2004)
Dividing loyalties interpretation	Inclusion of relevant others to gain broad view Interdisciplinarity (Crowden, 2003, 2004) Open public forums (Conway, 2000)	Exclusion or mere tolerance of relevant stakeholders Blind partiality or impartiality
Justification	Long-term public commitment (Canon, 1992) Examines referent community values with respect to the ethical principles being sustained (Canon, 1992)	Short-term private advantage (Procario-Foley & McLaughlin, 2003) May not consider referent community values. May ignore if sanctions are not clear or enforceable

(continued)

TABLE 21.3
Taxonomy of Ethical Sensitivity Characteristics* (continued)

	ETHICAL SENSITIVITY	NOT ETHICAL SENSITIVITY
Reflexivity	Moral and developmental maturity Commitments are "identity-conferring" (i.e., cannot live with self if break them; McFall, 1987) Autonomy to influence quality of care (Yarling & McElmurry, 1986)	Lack of maturity Deception/moral hypocrisy (Batson et al., 1999; Kitchener, 1992) Commitments are "identity-defeasible" (may delegate to others; McFall, 1987) Limited autonomy (Granstrom, 1995; Huebner, 1996; Jaeger, 2001; Lutzen, 1990)
Outcomes		
Client comfort and well-being	Client satisfied—feels heard and that issues matter to the professional (Sarat, 1991)	Client dissatisfied Moral neglect of client (Sherwin, 2001)
Professional learning and transcendence	"Becomes" ethically sensitive/noble (Fowers, 2003) Practices appropriate self-care (e.g., obtains support; Layman & McNamara, 1997)	Unable to transfer skills to future/unfamiliar situations (requires ongoing guidance and preparation) May practice self-neglect (e.g., exhaustion; Holland, 1998)
Integrity-preserving compromise (Benjamin, 1991)	Directs care to common good (Baron, 1991; Layman & McNamara, 1997; Simpson & Garrison, 1995), preventing harm (Robson, 2002; Scheyer, 1991), and global salvation (Bouley, 1984; Pawlikowski, 1984)	Ignores common welfare by placing individual/private over public/collective interest: * Pure "client" perspective (Bailey, 1999) * Self-interest (Canon, 1992; Garrod, 1989; Mudrack et al., 1999; Rest et al., 1997) Ignores client welfare (Banja, 1994; May, 1992; Symonds, 1995): * Routine-oriented care—focus on profession, organization, or society

* For references, see Box 21.3.
Source: Weaver and Morse (2006). Reprinted with permission.

This taxonomy (Table 21.3) has intuitive and logical grasp (i.e., the results resonate with the expectations of professional practice). In sum, when the professional perceives the client's suffering and vulnerability, the professional may be uncertain about what to do. The uncertainty is maintained until the professional achieves an adequate understanding of the situation. Professional characteristics of receptivity (being open-minded), responsiveness (being aware of the impact the professional's actions could have on the

BOX 21.3. REFERENCES FOR TAXONOMY OF ETHICAL SENSITIVITY CHARACTERISTICS IN TABLE 21.3

Abdolmohammadi, M. J., & Owhoso, V. (2000). Auditors' ethical sensitivity and the assessment of the likelihood of fraud. *Managerial Finance, 26*(11), 21–32.

Aharony, J., & Geva, A. (2003). Moral implications of law in business: a case of tax loopholes. *Business Ethics: A European Review, 12*(4), 378–393.

Bailey, F. L. (1999). Ethical abuse of technicalities: A comparison of prospective and retrospective legal ethics. *Harvard Law Review, 112,* 1082–1099.

Banja, J. D., & Banes, L. (1993). Moral sensitivity, sodomy laws, and traumatic brain injury rehabilitation. *Journal of Head Trauma Rehabilitation, 8*(1), 116–119.

Baron, M. (1991). Impartiality and friendship. *Ethics, 101,* 836–857.

Batson, C. D., Thompson, E. R., Seuferling, G., Whitney, H., & Strongman, J. A. (1999). Moral hypocrisy: Appearing moral to oneself without being so. *Journal of Personality & Social Psychology, 77,* 525–537.

Bebeau, M. J., & Brabeck, M. M. (1989). Ethical sensitivity and moral reasoning among men and women in the professions. In M. M. Brabeck (Ed.), *Who cares? Theory, research, and educational implications of the ethic of care* (pp. 144–163). New York, NY: Praeger.

Benjamin, M. (1990). *Splitting the difference: Compromise and integrity in ethics and politics.* Kansas, KS: University Press of Kansas.

Bouley, A. (1984). Response: Liturgy and moral sensitivity between the Holocausts. *Worship, 58,* 330–332.

Bracci, S. L. (2001). Managing health care in Oregon: The search for a civic bioethics. *Journal of Applied Communication Research, 29*(2), 171–194.

Branch, W. T. (2000). The ethics of caring and medical education. *Academic Medicine, 75,* 127–132.

Cannon, K. G. (1985). Resources for a constructive ethic in the life and work of Zora Neale Hurston. *Journal of Feminist Studies in Religion, 1*(1), 37–51.

Canon, H. J. (1992). Psychologist as university administrator: Visible standard-bearer. *Professional Psychology Research & Practice, 23*(3), 211–215.

Conway, R. (2000). Ethical judgements in genetic engineering: The implications for technology education. *International Journal of Technology and Design Education, 10,* 239–254.

Clarkeburn, H. (2002). A test for ethical sensitivity in science. *Journal of Moral Education, 31,* 439–453.

Crowden, A. (2003). Ethically sensitive mental health care: Is there a need for a unique ethics for psychiatry? *Australian and New Zealand Journal of Psychiatry, 37*(2), 143–149.

Crowden, A. (2004). The debate continues: Unique ethics for psychiatry. *Australian and New Zealand Journal of Psychiatry, 38,* 111–114.

Flannery, E. J. (1995). One advocate's viewpoint: Conflicts and tensions in the Baby K case. *Journal of Law, Medicine & Ethics, 23,* 7–12.

Fowers, B. J. (2003). Reason and human finitude: In praise of practical wisdom. *American Behavioral Scientist, 47*(4), 415–426.

Flannery, E. J. (1995). One advocate's viewpoint: Conflicts and tensions in the Baby K case. *Journal of Law, Medicine & Ethics, 23,* 7–12.

Gastmans, C. (2002). A fundamental ethical approach to nursing: Some proposals for ethics education. *Nursing Ethics: An International Journal for Health Care Professionals, 9*(5), 494–507.

Georges, J. J., Grypdonck, M., & Dierckx de Casterle, B. (2002). Being a palliative care nurse in an academic hospital: A qualitative study about nurses' perceptions of palliative care nursing. *Journal of Clinical Nursing, 11,* 785–793.

Granstrom, K. (1995). Accounts and explanations in group decisions concerning students with learning and social disabilities. *Learning and Instruction, 5,* 125–141.

Green, B. (2004). Attitudes toward mental illness in medical students. *Medical Education, 34,* 166–167.

Hawkins, G. (2001). The ethics of television. *International Journal of Cultural Studies, 4,* 412–426.

(continued)

BOX 21.3. REFERENCES FOR TAXONOMY OF ETHICAL SENSITIVITY CHARACTERISTICS IN TABLE 21.3 (*CONTINUED*)

Holland, M. G. (1998). Touching the weights: Moral perception and attention. *International Philosophical Quarterly, 38*, 299–312.

Huebner, D. (1996). Teaching as moral activity. *Journal of Curriculum & Supervision, 11*(3), 267–275.

Jaeger, S. M. (2001). Teaching health care ethics: The importance of moral sensitivity for moral reasoning. *Nursing Philosophy, 2*, 131–142.

Keenan, J. P. (2002). Comparing Indian and American managers on whistleblowing. *Employee Responsibilities & Rights Journal, 14*(2), 79–89.

Kitchener, K. S. (1992). Psychologist as teacher and mentor: Affirming ethical values throughout the curriculum. *Professional Psychology Research & Practice, 23*(3), 190–195.

Layman, M. J., & McNamara, J. R. (1997). Remediation for ethics violations: Focus on psychotherapists' sexual contact with clients. *Professional Psychology Research & Practice, 28*(3), 281–292.

Lerman, L. G. (1998). Teaching moral perception and moral judgment in legal ethics courses: A dialogue about goals. *William & Mary Law Review, 39*, 457–487.

Lutzen, K. (1990). Moral sensing and ideological conflict. *Scandinavian Journal of Caring Sciences, 4*(2), 69–76.

Malone, R. E. (2000). Dimensions of vulnerability in emergency nurses' narratives. *Advances in Nursing Science, 23*(1), 1–11.

May, L. M. (1992). Insensitivity and moral responsibility. *Journal of Value Inquiry, 26*(1), 7–22.

McFall, L. (1987). Integrity. *Ethics, 98*, 5–20.

McPhail, K. (2001). The other objective of ethics education: Re-humanising the accounting profession - a study of ethics education in law, engineering, medicine and accountancy. *Journal of Business Ethics, 34*, 279–298.

Mohr, W. K., & Horton-Deutsch, S. (2001). Malfeasance and regaining nursing's moral voice and integrity. *Nursing Ethics, 8*, 19–35.

Mudrack, P. E., Mason, E. S., & Stepanski, K. M. (1999). Equity sensitivity and business ethics.

Journal of Occupational and Organizational Psychology, 72, 539–560.

Naden, D., & Eriksson, K. (2004). Understanding the importance of values and moral attitudes in nursing care in preserving human dignity. *Nursing Science Quarterly, 17*(1), 86–91.

Narvaez, D. F. (1991). Counseling for morality: A look at the Four-Component Model. *Journal of Psychology & Christianity, 10*(4), 358–365.

Nortvedt, P. (2001). Clinical sensitivity: The inseparability of ethical perceptiveness and clinical knowledge. *Scholarly Inquiry for Nursing Practice, 15*(1), 25–43.

Pawlikowski, J. T. (1984). Worship after the Holocaust: An ethician's reflections. *Worship, 58*, 315–330.

Payne, S. L., & Giacalone, R. A. (1990). Social psychological approaches to the perception of ethical dilemmas. *Human Relations, 43*, 649–665.

Procario-Foley, E. G., & McLaughlin, M. T. (2003). A propaedeutic for a framework: Fostering ethical awareness in undergraduate business students. *Teaching Business Ethics, 7*, 279–301.

Punzo, V. A. (1996). After Kohlberg: Virtue ethics and the recovery of the moral self. *Philosophical Psychology, 9*(1), 7–23. Retrieved March 2, 2004, from the World Wide Web: EBSCO Host

Rest, J. (1982). A psychologist looks at the teaching of ethics. *Hastings Centre Report, 12*(1), 29–36.

Rest, J., Thoma, S., & Edwards, L. (1997). Designing and validating a measure of moral judgment: Stage preference and stage consistency approaches. *Journal of Educational Psychology, 89*(1), 5–28.

Robson, E. (2002). "An unbelievable academic and personal experience": Issues around teaching undergraduate field courses in Africa. *Journal of Geography in Higher Education, 26*, 327–344.

Schneyer, T. (1991). Sympathy for the hired gun. *Journal of Legal Education, 41*, 11–27.

Sarat, A. (1991). Lawyers and clients: Putting professional service on the agenda of legal education. *Journal of Legal Education, 41*, 43–53.

(*continued*)

BOX 21.3. REFERENCES FOR TAXONOMY OF ETHICAL SENSITIVITY CHARACTERISTICS IN TABLE 21.3 (*CONTINUED*)

Scott, P. A. (2000). Emotion, moral perception, and nursing practice. *Nursing Philosophy, 1*(2), 123–133.

Shaner, A. (1989). Asylums, asphalt, and ethics. *Hospital & Community Psychiatry, 40*(8), 785–786.

Sherwin, S. (2001). Moral perception and global visions. *Bioethics, 15*(3), 175–188.

Simpson, P. J., & Garrison, J. (1995). Teaching and moral perception. *Teachers College Record, 97*(2), 252. Retrieved March, 2004 from Academic Search Premier.

Stark, S. (2001). Virtue and emotion. *Nous, 35*(3), 440–455.

Steinkraus, W. E. (1987). The spiritual life as ethical sensitivity. *Scottish Journal of Religious Studies, 8*(2), 103–108.

Symonds, B. R. (1995). The origins of insane asylums in England during the 19th century: A brief sociological review. *Journal of Advanced Nursing, 22*, 94–100.

Ulrich, C. M., Soeken, K. L., & Miller, N. (2003). Ethical conflict associated with managed care: Views of nurse practitioners. *Nursing Research, 52*(3), 168–175.

Vetlesen, A. J. (1994). *Perception, empathy, and judgment: An inquiry into the preconditions of moral performance*. University Park, PA: Pennsylvania State University Press.

Walker, M. U. (1991). Partial consideration. *Ethics, 101*, 757–774.

Wallace, K. G., Reed, B. A., Pasero, C., & Olsson, G. L. (1995). Staff nurses' perceptions of barriers to effective pain management. *Journal of Pain & Symptom Management, 10*(3), 204–213.

Wurzbach, M. E. (1999). Acute care nurses' experiences of moral certainty. *Journal of Advanced Nursing, 30*, 287–293.

Yarling, R., & McElmurray, B. (1986). The moral foundation of nursing. *Advances in Nursing Science, 8*(2), 63–73.

client), and courage (acting in line with beliefs and feelings despite resistance or adverse conditions) foster ethical sensitivity. Attributes of moral perception, affectivity, and dividing loyalties enable the professional to appropriately respond to the client's plight by thoughtfully taking into account the needs of the client, the perspectives of various stakeholders, and situational resources. Outcomes include (a) client comfort, well-being, and satisfaction; and (b) professional learning and self-transcendence that enable self-care and becoming ethically sensitive. Through integrity-preserving compromise, professional care can be directed toward a common good based on consideration of collective client, professional, and organizational perspectives.

The taxonomy provides clear, parsimonious description, elucidating the futuristic role of ethical sensitivity in preventing ethical problems (e.g., moral maturity, public-mindedness), and the role of organizations in influencing ethical sensitivity (e.g., routine care, focus on the organization). However, taxonomies in general risk oversimplification, exaggerating differences and reducing complexity through rendering poorly understood entities concrete (Eppler & Mengis, 2011). The taxonomy of ethical sensitivity does not illuminate a process for how the professional self-transcends to develop ethical sensitivity in practice.

Qualitatively Derived Theory

An initial straw frame depicting the implicit ordering of preconditions, attributes, boundaries, and outcomes was constructed (Figure 21.1). The frame is based on a view of concepts as miniature "theories themselves in that they embody explanations of the relations between their constituents, of their origins, and of their relations to other clusters of features" (Keil, 1989, p. 281). Concepts as theories are tools to be used with awareness of how they are being used. To explain, a concept can be a theory, a model, or a category depending on the level of abstraction chosen by the researcher. The difference between a concept and a theory is complexity. As a useful tool for visualizing overall complexity and sequencing relationships within and among the dimensions, the frame would be fleshed in to reflect advanced understanding of the concept and to establish a theoretical basis for future studies on ethical sensitivity in professional practice.

It was possible to generate a model of ethical sensitivity in professional practice through infusing the straw frame with results from the analytic questions and linking results to the concept dimensions. I began by examining the interactions of the set of defining attributes. As described earlier (Box 21.2), these attributes (moral perception, affectivity, and dividing loyalties) concern professional decision making and share core features of affect, cognition, skill, knowledge, and responsibility. Importantly, the attributes are concepts in their own right that pragmatically fit with the phenomenon of ethical sensitivity.

The attribute of dividing loyalties (process of in-depth elicitation and appraisal of information to decide the plan of action) is familiar to professionals and has the most relevance for professional practice. In determining the fit of one attribute to another, dividing loyalties was the foundational attribute with which the other attributes (moral perception and affectivity) fit.

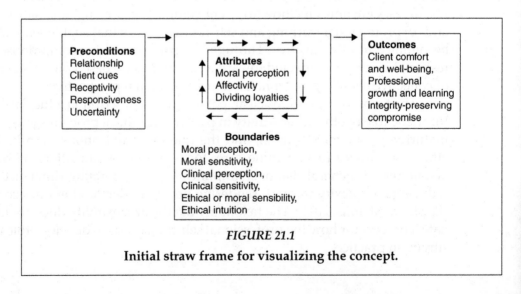

FIGURE 21.1

Initial straw frame for visualizing the concept.

It was logical to link the attributes of affectivity and dividing loyalties, given their related characteristics. For example, reflexivity (aspect of dividing loyalties) and affectivity (embodied response) each involve the professional responding to the situation; however, the attributes of reflexivity and affectivity differ in their combinations of affect, cognition, and responsibility. To explain, affectivity is composed primarily of emotional response (affect) without conscious effort (cognition) directed toward agency (responsibility). In contrast, reflexivity may involve processing of one's affectivity while primarily engaging intellectual processing (cognition). Both reflexivity and affectivity require skill in reading situations and knowledge of self. Although affectivity may begin immediately within or following a situation, reflexivity often occurs later on as information about the situation and those affected within and outside of the professional–client relationship is solicited and weighed. Affectivity may be denied or suppressed, but reflexivity necessarily culminates in a decision to act or not act to address the situation.

In comparison to the attributes of affectivity and dividing loyalties, the attribute of moral perception shared different strengths of affect and cognition, which comprised its intuitive nature, knowledge (from personal/professional experience and professional values), skill in reading the situational cues to identify ethical import, and responsibility for the client's welfare. The awakening aspect of moral perception closely linked with affectivity; the particularizing aspect (determining the particular ethical prototype relevant to the client's distress) fit logically and coherently with the reflexivity of processing of one's "bottom line" decision.

Based on the shared core features, the attributes were linked with each other and with the other dimensions of the concept. The resulting mid-range theory of ethical sensitivity in professional practice (Figure 21.2) portrays the interaction of necessary skills and prerequisites, realization of the need for preserving as much as possible the welfare and well-being of those most affected by the decision making, and client/professional outcomes. The components of the theory fit together logically with minimal overlap. Linkages between the components were verified in the data (professional literature). The theory recognizes the compromising nature of professional decision making—that social, institutional, and personal circumstances can influence professionals' enactment of ethically sensitive behaviors. The model captures an aspect of ethical sensitivity not obvious in the taxonomy (Table 21.3)—that is, the model conveys a paradigm for understanding the professional role in learning from past situations wherein the professional experienced moral distress from being unable to act in ethically sensitive ways but subsequently transforms previously held views concerning one's role within the situation in such a way that the professional builds capacity to approach new situations and future ethical issues through developing ethical sensitivity.

In evaluating the model, a clearer understanding of the sequencing of the attributes would be helpful to inform practice. However, it was not

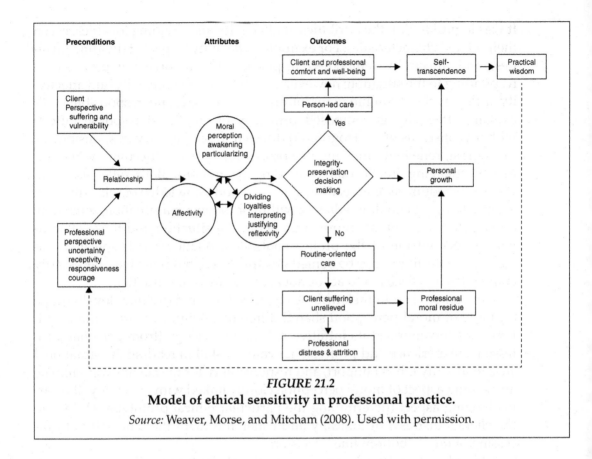

FIGURE 21.2
Model of ethical sensitivity in professional practice.
Source: Weaver, Morse, and Mitcham (2008). Used with permission.

possible to more clearly express the ordering of the attributes from the available data of the published professional literature. Although there is an intuitive fit of moral perception and affectivity preceding dividing loyalties (After all, would one address a problem that one did not identify or feel as a problem?), examples located in the medical, legal, and theological literature do not support this fit. Instead, these bodies of literature provide evidence that physicians and lawyers are often socialized to reduce their affectivity. For example, medical students learned to ignore feelings to reduce their distress in working with suffering clients and horrific situations in clinical practice (Smith III & Kleinman, 1989); the law faculty's emphasis on linear thinking and reason was associated with law students losing connection with their feelings, personal morals, values, and sense of self (Hess, 2002; Sheldon & Krieger, 2004). Because of the high trust level that clients/parishioners show to their priests or clergy persons through full disclosure of problems without prompting, the use of moral perception to apprehend the ethical component in the client/parishioner's problem may not come into play until these religious leaders engage in the decisional processes (dividing loyalties; Haug, 1999). In these examples, the professional's emotional response (affectivity) and recognition of the ethical nature of the problem (moral perception) followed or accompanied the decision making of dividing loyalties. Difficulty in ordering the attributes of ethical sensitivity related to the literature having reached the "glass ceiling" effect, meaning that the level of science was inadequate to answer the question and a different type of data through a different method (e.g., interview, observation) is needed to serve study purpose.

The model developed from analysis of the concept of ethical sensitivity in professional practice (Figure 21.2) is, according to the specifications put forward by Morse et al. (2002), a disclosive or mid-range theory that expresses complexity. This theory begins to identify causal relationships. For example, when institutional rules preempt the client as the focus of the professional's attention, client outcomes of comfort and satisfaction are thwarted and professional moral distress may occur. The resultant theory from the analyzed concept sensitizes readers to see a pattern in a phenomenon represented by the concept that makes them feel they understand and can explain what they see.

SUMMARY

In this chapter, I described analysis of the concept of ethical sensitivity that resulted in the development of a beginning mid-range theory describing complexity. Building from careful baseline evaluation of the concept's anatomy, physiology, and maturity, a clearer understanding was explicated using pragmatic utility's analytic tool of critical appraisal along with complementary standard qualitative research techniques of data coding, sorting, clustering, and saturation; fit; and negative case analysis. Critical appraisal directed lines of inquiry and synthesis of results in asking data-driven questions of a large body of interprofessional literature. Such direction enabled comprehensive definition and systematic classification of the concept's essential characteristics beyond a single discipline perspective that exceeded current knowledge about ethical sensitivity, thereby contributing unique information to meet disciplinary needs. Exploring pragmatic utility increased the comprehensiveness, scope, and level of abstraction of the concept to the level of theory that demonstrated the concept in all the forms in which it was manifested throughout various contexts. The pragmatic utility method pulled knowledge beyond concept analysis to descriptive theory beyond the expectations of the initial project. The concept analysis denotes a pattern carefully developed through questioning and fitting many incidents of data until conceptual dimensions explain fundamental patterns in the phenomenon represented by the concept of ethical sensitivity in professional practice.

REFERENCES

Austin, W., Bergum, V., & Goldberg, L. (2003). Unable to answer the call of our patients: Mental health nurses' experience of moral distress. *Nursing Inquiry, 10*(3), 177–183.

Beauchamp, T. L., & Bowie, N. E. (1997). Ethical theory and business practice. In T. L. Beauchamp & N. E. Bowie (Eds.), *Ethical theory and business* (5th ed., pp. 1–49). Upper Saddle River, NJ: Prentice Hall.

Bebeau, M. J., & Brabeck, M. M. (1989). Ethical sensitivity and moral reasoning among men and women in the professions. In M. M. Brabeck (Ed.), *Who cares? Theory, research, and educational implications of the ethic of care* (pp. 144–163). New York, NY: Praeger.

Bebeau, M. J., Rest, J. R., & Yamoor, C. M. (1985). Measuring dental students' ethical sensitivity. *Journal of Dental Education, 49*, 225–235.

Berthold, J. S. (1964). Prologue: Symposium on theory development in nursing. *Nursing Research, 17*(3), 196–197.

Bone, P. F., & Corey, R. J. (2000). Packing ethics: Perceptual differences among packaging professionals, brand managers and ethically-interested consumers. *Journal of Business Ethics, 24*(3), 199–213.

Bradley, E. H., Curry, L. A., & Devers, K. J. (2007). Qualitative data analysis for health services research: Developing taxonomy, themes, and theory. *Health Services Research, 42*(4), 1758–1772. doi:10.1111/j.1475-6773.2006.00684.x

Cherrington, D. J. (2002). Whistleblowers. *Administrative Science Quarterly, 47*(2), 381–384.

Clarkeburn, H. (2002a). A test for ethical sensitivity in science. *Journal of Moral Education, 31*, 439–453.

Clarkeburn, H. (2002b). The aims and practice of ethics education in an undergraduate curriculum: Reasons for choosing a skills approach. *Journal of Further & Higher Education, 26*, 307–315.

Coelho, P. (2007). From "Manual of the Warrior of Light." In *Life: Selected quotations* (p. 84). New York, NY: HarperCollins.

Eppler, M. J., & Mengis, J. (2011, July). *Drawing distinction: The visualization of classification in qualitative research* (=mcm working paper, No. 2/2011). St. Gallen, Switzerland: =mcm institute, University of St. Gallen. Retrieved from www.knowledge-communication.org

Glaser, B. G., & Strauss, A. L. (1967). *The discovery of grounded theory: Strategies for qualitative research*. Chicago, IL: Aldine Atherton.

Greene, J. A. (2004). 2002 Roy Porter memorial prize essay: Therapeutic infidelities: "Noncompliance" enters the medical literature, 1955–1975. *Social History of Medicine, 17*(3), 327–343.

Haug, I. E. (1999). Boundaries and the use and misuse of power and authority: Ethical complexities for clergy psychotherapists. *Journal of Counseling & Development, 77*(4), 411–418.

Hess, G. F. (2002, March–June). Heads and hearts: The teaching and learning environment in law school. *Journal of Legal Education, 52*, 75–111.

Keil, F. C. (1989). *Concepts, kinds, and cognitive development*. Cambridge, MA: MIT Press.

Lutzen, K. (1993). *Moral sensitivity: A study of subjective aspects of the process of moral decision making in psychiatric nursing* (Doctoral dissertation). Solna, Sweden: Karolinska Institute.

Lutzen, K., Johansson, A., & Nordstrom, G. (2000). Moral sensitivity: Some differences between nurses and physicians. *Nursing Ethics, 7*(6), 520–530.

Morse, J. M., Mitcham, C., Hupcey, J. E., & Tasón, M. C. (1996). Criteria for concept evaluation. *Journal of Advanced Nursing, 24*, 385–390.

Morse, J. M. (1995a). Exploring the theoretical basis of nursing using advanced techniques of concept analysis. *Advances in Nursing Science, 17*(3), 31–46.

Morse, J. M. (1995b). The significance of saturation [Editorial]. *Qualitative Health Research, 5*(2), 147–148.

Morse, J. M. (2000a). Theoretical congestion [Editorial]. *Qualitative Health Research, 10*(6), 715–716.

Morse, J. M. (2000b). Exploring pragmatic utility: Concept analysis by critically appraising the Literature. In B. Rodgers & K. Knafl (Eds.), *Concept development in nursing* (pp. 333–352). Philadelphia, PA: Saunders.

Morse, J. M., Hupcey, J., Penrod, J., & Mitcham, C. (2002). Integrating concepts for the development of qualitatively-derived theory. *Research and Theory for Nursing Practice: An International Journal, 16*(1), 5–18.

Morse, J. M. & Singleton, J. K. (2001). Exploring the technical aspects of fit in qualitative health research. *Qualitative Health Research, 11*, 841–847.

Penrod, J., & Hupcey, J. E. (2005b). Enhancing methodological clarity: Principle-based concept analysis. *Journal of Advanced Nursing, 50*, 403–409.

Sheldon, K. M., & Krieger, L. S. (2004). Does legal education have undermining effects on law students? Evaluating changes in motivation, values, and well-being. *Behavioral Sciences and the Law, 22*, 261–286. doi:10.1002/bsl.582

Smith III, A. C., & Kleinman, S. (1989). Managing emotions in medical school: Students' contacts with the living and the dead. *Social Psychology Quarterly, 52*(1), 56–69.

Ulrich, C. M., Soeken, K. L., & Miller, N. (2003). Ethical conflict associated with managed care: Views of nurse practitioners. *Nursing Research, 52*(3), 168–175.

Wallace, K. G., Reed, B. A., Pasero, C., & Olsson, G. L. (1995). Staff nurses' perceptions of barriers to effective pain management. *Journal of Pain & Symptom Management, 10*(3), 204–213.

Weaver, K. (2005). *Analysis of the concept of ethical sensitivity* (PhD Thesis). Edmonton, AB, Canada: University of Alberta.

Weaver, K. (2007). Ethical sensitivity: State of the science and needs for further research. *Nursing Ethics, 14*(2), 141–155.

Weaver, K. (2012). Loving her into well-being one day at a time: Parents' narratives of caring for daughters with eating disorders. *Open Journal of Nursing, 2*, 406–419. doi:10.4236/ojn.2012.24059

Weaver, K., & Morse, J. M. (2006). Using pragmatic utility to analyze the concept of ethical sensitivity. *Research and Theory in Nursing Practice, 20*(3), 191–214.

Weaver, K., Morse, J. M., & Mitcham, C. (2008). Ethical sensitivity in professional practice: Concept analysis. *Journal of Advanced Nursing, 62*(5), 607–618. doi:10.1111/j.1365-2648.2008.04625.x

Weaver, K., Wuest, J., & Ciliska, D. (2005). Understanding women's journey of recovering from Anorexia Nervosa. *Qualitative Health Research, 15*(2), 188–206.

LINKING AND ORDERING CONCEPTS

The First Rule of Conceptualization

It must be possible

And it should be probable

And then

If it can be verified, even if it is extraordinary, you can keep it

But if it is extraordinary and not verifiable, it is probably wrong

Throughout this book we have discussed how to improve research by developing "solid," clear, and appropriate concepts. However this is not our end goal. These concepts are not isolated in the context. They may be connected—linked and ordered—and by identifying these connections, we may develop mid-range theory. This theory may at whatever level of mid-range abstraction and scope that is needed.

THE PROCESS OF QUALITATIVELY DEVELOPING MID-RANGE THEORIES

Qualitative inquiry does not always begin with raw data, and the researchers are never without an agenda. Often researchers deliberately select a concept, and explore that concept in a particular situation, with the concept of interest used as a conceptual scaffold or skeleton, as we discussed in Chapter 9. In these cases the researchers build the concept(s) using inductive inquiry within that identified structure. For instance, if the researcher is creating a program on traumatic childbirth (Beck, 2015, 2016), systematic investigation of the phenomenon in a different setting does not mean that each study ignores the findings of those studies that came before. Rather, the investigator usually uses his or her own work (or that of others) and own data to systematically enhance and validate the developing theoretical concepts and components in each sequential study, linking concepts and expediting the development of mid-range theory. As Beck (2015) notes, there is a distinct advantage in using your own work for such theory development—you have all of the data and have systematically conducted the necessary studies; the disadvantage is that it takes a long time.

On occasions, this process of inquiry is not an in-depth examination into the same phenomenon or concept, but rather *developing theory by working from minor to major concepts*, or laterally across the dimension of a phenomenon in scope or over time as a process, or horizontally from minor to major concepts, that engulf the minor concepts. Sometimes inquiry into two related concepts may be linked at the theoretical level to produce an even larger theory. For instance, we do this in Chapter 35 by linking theories of suffering using theoretical coalescence (Chapter 34).

To proceed, in this chapter we discuss ways to *link* concepts by identifying shared attributes and creating a larger theory. We discuss how to *order* concepts hierarchically by scope and level of abstraction. Then, we talk about how to identify all of the concepts within a phenomenon and order those concepts. This is a method of theory development commonly used when organizing a process as, for instance, when one moves through a trajectory. In these ways we move toward mid-range theory.

LINKING CONCEPTS

Although the complexity of a particular context demands that the researcher focus on a single concept of interest within a particular study, the process of such a focus actually delineates the concept from the context and simplifies the study. It gives the researcher a tunnel vision—but a necessary one. Reality is complex, and qualitative research is slow and cumbersome, when done well. However, this does not mean that the researcher is ignorant about the conceptual components in the setting, nor of their significance. It usually is a matter of what is feasible within the complexity of the setting, the limitations of qualitative methods, and limitation of the researcher's analytic ability; or a compromise between that and understanding something in depth and comprehending the entire setting in a superficial manner. Nevertheless, often we have previous work sitting on the shelf, or even published, and the concept of interest at least partially already developed.

Such was the case when we were concluding our studies on the *Praxis Theory of Suffering*. We understood emotional suffering, but not how the transition to the reformulated self occurred, except that "hope seeped in." We lacked a conceptual understanding of this transition. Yet we previously conducted as study of hope, and incorporated these theoretical insights.

How Was This Done?

Simply, we:

1. Identified the two concepts of interest
2. Identified the dominant concept
3. "Opened" the concepts to reveal the attributes
4. Looked for common (shared) attributes. We asked: Is there temporal order in the "strength" of the attributes?

Wherever two attributes were shared in each concept, that is where the concepts linked.

LINKING CONCEPTS IN THE PROCESS OF INQUIRY

Frequently, however, once into data collection and analysis, it becomes clear that one cannot focus on a single concept as originally intended. The first concept may be intricately intertwined with another allied concept, and only by exploring both concepts will the study make sense. Recall the case of privacy and interpersonal relationships discussed in Chapter 12?

CONTEXT DEPENDENCY AND LINKING CONCEPTS

When conducting qualitative inquiry either within a project or by combining two projects, linking allied concepts is a way to validly create a larger model. The trick is to determine that the two concepts are indeed allied concepts that co-occur constantly within the same context. If this can be ascertained, they are probably a part of the same process within a larger concept or phenomenon.

DETERMINING LINKAGES BETWEEN CONCEPTS

The process of linking consists of determining which of the two concepts is dominant; opening the concepts, determining if any of the attributes are shared, or common, and then describing the nature of the linkages.

Opening Concepts to Determine Relationship

Opening the concepts refers to the process of listing all of the attributes within each concept. If the concepts are *mature*, the attributes should be easily identified in the authors' descriptions. If several authors have described the concept, and if their descriptions are *good*, there should be some consistency in the attributes listed, although sometimes the attributes are named differently.[1] Because of the theoretical level of maturity, both concepts will have been decontextualized, and data that may contribute as evidence have been removed. Therefore, if the authors have access to the original data for each concept, this may provide additional support for the comparison of the attributes. Verify each notion, by selecting interview text or observations that may confirm, refute, or provide additional insights into observations in the situations in which the two concepts link. If necessary, collect additional data to inform situations in which data are not available. Such an iterative process contributes to the rigor of the process (Morse, Hupcey, Penrod, & Mitcham, 2002).

Reformulate the Expanded Theory

Once the linkage has been established, and the nature of the connections of the new concept is determined, the researcher describes the expanded theory. If the new linkage contains a full intermediate concept linking the first two concepts, then the researcher, following the demands of created concept, defines the boundaries, defines, names and defines the attributes of the new concept.

ORDERING CONCEPTS

Determining Dominance

The first decision is to determine which concept is dominant; that is, determine which concept is of a higher level of abstraction or precedes or dominates over the other. This concept is the one that is dominant; the other butts against, or fits into. This is done by asking analytic questions and ordering your concepts, making notes with stickies as you work.

Ordering Concepts According to Scope and Level of Abstraction

Q: Is "scope" the same as "level of abstraction?"
A: Yes and no and maybe.

---

[1] Finding consistency of attributes between concepts is particularly important if you are conducting a meta-synthesis.

Scope is the expansiveness of theory. It is how spread out, or how much area the concept covers. Usually the greater the scope, the less specific the concept is, and therefore the greater number of instances it represents. For example, if the concept were something like "emotions," the concept would include all instances of all emotions (sad, happy, forlorn, joy, etc.). We would not differentiate between types of emotions and would keep them all in the same category.

Level of abstraction is the distance from the data. If a concept is highly abstract it will be some distance from the data, and contain within it lower level categories of different types of examples. For instance, if we were using "emotion" as an *abstract concept*, it could contain a lower level concept of bereavement, which in turn could contain lower level concepts of "grief," "sorrow," and so forth, which in turn connect our abstract concept, "emotions," with particular data.

Given this hierarchical situation, when *ordering concepts* by level of abstraction, one should place the concepts according to which concept is a part of another concept. For instance, grieving may be considered a part of, or type of, bereavement, but bereavement is not considered a part of, or type of, grieving. Use colored sticky labels, each with a concept written on, so that you can move them around, asking the "order questions": "Is this a part of that?"; "Is this a type of that?"

Ordering Concepts Temporally

Ordering concepts within a process may be a little easier. Some concepts occur at a certain point in trajectory, but not in others, thereby logically preceding or following or coinciding with certain events. For instance, one gets into bed, lies down, and then gets out of bed in an "ingress–egress" sequence. But at another time, the same concept follows through the process in the same form or slightly changed. A runner running in a race may have an energy level "fresh" and then "exhausted." Our concept "energy level" changes both quantitatively and qualitatively.

When organizing concepts temporally, again using sticky labels, the changes in the main concept may have other concepts that change concurrently, or may have transitions between the stages and phases that result in the change.

Yes, basic model building.

Simple.

CONCEPTUAL DEVELOPMENT: THE MATURITY OF THE THEORY

The level of analysis achieved by the investigator before developing the theory schematically will determine the quality or level of maturity of the theory. If the researcher does not develop concepts within the theory, the theory will remain low level, particular to the context from which it was developed (and therefore not generalizable). Therefore, good mid-range theory must have the following characteristics.

The Concepts Must Be Developed to Fit in With Current Literature

"Fitting" into the literature means that the concept labels are not "emic" labels, but the researcher has taken time to compare the emerging concepts with those already published in the literature, and has made a case for adopting (or for not adopting) the concept labels that are currently used in nursing or other social sciences. For instance, does the coping that you are seeing in your data and developing concept fit the definitions and descriptions of coping in the literature? Why or why not? If it does, then adopt the labels presently used. Not everything you identify in your study will be unique or new. Keeping your own (or the participant's) labels will result in too many labels for the same concept, and result in "theoretical congestion" (Morse, 2000)—researchers will not find your work when they search the literature, and your work will fall into oblivion, and the results will become cluttered with so many studies describing the same thing; we will all die of fatigue trying to sort it out, or it will be used as a blade of grass in the fodder used in a meta-analysis. Any of these routes are less desirable for you: the strength of your contribution in your mid-range theory in the whole, as well as the particular.

The Descriptive Fit of Your Mid-Range Theory With Your Own and Multiple Contexts

Your theory must enlighten, surprise, and yet make sense to those who are familiar with your setting. It seems contradictory that they must, at the same time, recognize yet be enlightened by the theory. They will say, "Ah, yes! So that is what is going on!" Others must be both able to recognize the conceptual organization or the processes depicted and see the potential of your work. In this way the familiar is reorganized as a "new" insight.

The Utility of Your Theory

Usually a standard criterion of theory is to predict. This criterion may or may not be pertinent for qualitatively derived mid-range theory. It will be pertinent, if for instance, with a theory of comforting, by explaining comforting processes, predicts how comfort is attained: It is *predictive*. On the other hand, if the theory explains and makes sense of suffering, it does not necessarily predict the outcome of suffering for any one individual, but by illustrating and making sense of the processes of suffering, clinicians will be able to also understand the process, categorize individuals they see, and move toward identifying appropriate interventions.

Clarity, Parsimony, and Scope

Other criteria used to evaluate all theories pertain to their description and presentation. You must be clear—brief and succinct. Diagramming will assist you in this process. Finally, it must be clear about what the theory does and does not pertain to. Mid-range theories are limited and do not describe everything; they do, however, describe certain processes, and can be applied to new situations that do not exceed the parameters of the theory.

OTHER TECHNIQUES FOR DEVELOPING CONCEPTS TO THEORY

As we link and order concepts, our theory becomes increasingly generalizable, and, of course, is broader in scope. Techniques of meta-synthesis and meta-analysis are reviewed fully in later chapters and are just included here as a reminder.

Meta-Synthesis

A meta-synthesis is a project that compares, synthesizes, and combines concepts or theories related to the same topic (usually studies conducted by different authors on different populations), that are *synthesized* into theory that combined the commonalities of the theories, hence developing a theory that is stronger than any of the original theories. The model in Figure 22.1,

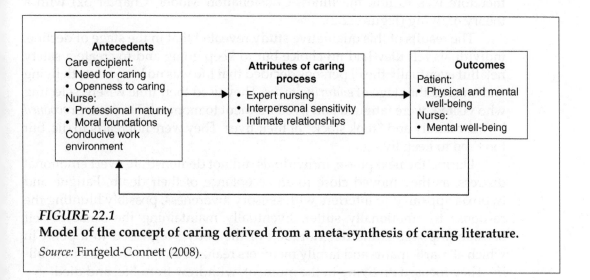

FIGURE 22.1
Model of the concept of caring derived from a meta-synthesis of caring literature.
Source: Finfgeld-Connett (2008).

from a meta-synthesis of the concept of caring conducted by Finfgeld-Connett (2008), shows that caring is a combination of technical tasks, sensitivity, and intimate relationships (see Chapters 30 and 31).

Developing a Model by Fitting Two or More Concepts Together

Several authors have developed a model by fitting two (or more) concepts together. They have simultaneously analyzed the concepts in the process of comparison or analyzed them separately and then compared the results. For instance, Finfgeld-Connett (2008) compared and synthesized nursing presence and caring, concluding that both concepts were a part of an "intentional therapeutic process that involved nursing practice and intimate interpersonal activity," with outcomes that "improved physical well-being among recipients and well-being among nurses" (p. 111). By integrating presence into caring, she expanded her model on caring.

Haase, Britt, Coward, Leidy, and Penn (1992) simultaneously analyzed concepts of spirituality, self-transcendence, hope, and acceptance, to develop a conceptual model. This process simultaneously developed each concept, as well as refining the theoretical definitions for each concept, and from their interrelationships, developed a model.

Linking Illness and Dying Trajectories

This association between two allied concepts linked in a trajectory was identified by Olson, Morse, Smith, Mayan, and Hammond (2000–2001) and was studied using qualitative methods. The authors argued that despite the large numbers of theories about illness or about death and dying, these two areas have not been theoretically linked. The purpose of this research therefore was to link the Illness-Constellation Model (Chapter 32) with a theory of dying (Figure 22.2).

The results of this qualitative study revealed that in the stage of decline, individuals felt they had no choice but to keep going and to create a safety net. But eventually the ill persons decided that life was no longer worth living and entered the stage of *enduring to die.* They used their time wisely, selecting who visited, were fatigued and lived moment to moment. They were *cocooned* by their family and "took stock" of their lives. They were not ready to die, but too tired to keep living.

During the next phase, individuals did not demonstrate overt emotional distress, as they moved close to an acceptance of their death. Fatigue and hypoxia appeared to interfere with sensory awareness, possibly blunting the response to emotionally suffer. Eventually maintaining the sense of self became impossible; the deterioration of the body progressed to a point in which all participants and family members realized that death was a possibility. They focused on living in the moment, withdrew from life, and died.

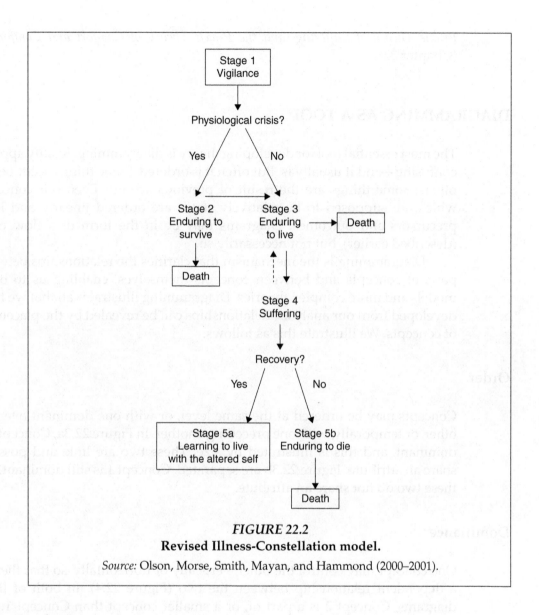

FIGURE 22.2
Revised Illness-Constellation model.
Source: Olson, Morse, Smith, Mayan, and Hammond (2000–2001).

Meta-Analysis

A meta-analysis, on the other hand, consists of studies that are combined into higher level concepts or meta-theory. The concepts are "opened," compared and contrasted, and reconceptualized. The result is a higher level theory, with broader application. This is addressed in Chapter 32.

Theoretical Coalescence

Theoretical coalescence is a method of combining studies of different topics (but within the same general focus), using different methods, and at different levels of abstraction to develop a mid-range theory. Examples are the

Praxis Theory of Suffering, and the Praxis Theory of Comfort and Comforting (Chapter 37).

DIAGRAMMING AS A TOOL

The most essential tool for developing theory is diagramming. Reality appears confusing—and it usually is. But often it is ordered. Some things occur before others; some things are the result of previous actions. Even our concepts, which are supposed to be relatively static, are ordered linearly and have precursors and outcomes. Diagrams may be in the form of a flow chart (described earlier), but not necessarily so.

Diagramming is the mechanism that clarifies the relationships between parts of concepts and between concepts themselves, enabling us to build models and more complex theories. Diagramming illustrates all that we have developed from our analysis: Relationships can be revealed by the placement of concepts. We illustrate this as follows.

Order

Concepts may be ordered at the same level, or with one dominant over the other, or temporally, with one preceding another. In Figure 22.3a, Concept 1 is dominant, and this is illustrated by size. These two are link, and possibly share an attribute. Figure 22.3b are separated. Concept 1 is still dominant, but these two do not share an attribute.

Dominance

One concept may control the other, vertically or horizontally, so that there is a dependent relationship between the two (Figure 22.4). In both of these diagrams, Concept 2 is a part of, or a smaller concept than Concept 1. For instance, contentment may be part of happiness.

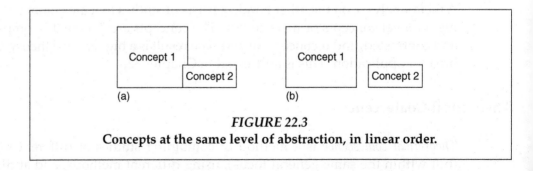

FIGURE 22.3
Concepts at the same level of abstraction, in linear order.

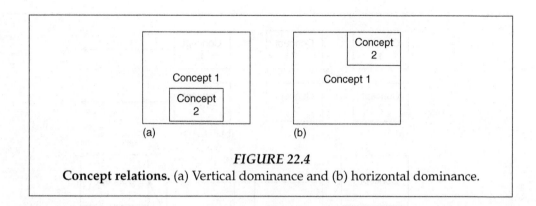

FIGURE 22.4
Concept relations. (a) Vertical dominance and (b) horizontal dominance.

Temporality

One concept may always precede another. In this case two concepts are linked, and Concept 1 always precedes Concept 2 (Figure 22.5). Something *funny* precedes *laughter*.

Interaction

In a temporal model, concepts may (a) *intersect*, (b) *parallel*, (c) *merge* (altering one or both concepts), and (d) *split* (Figure 22.6, a–d). The minor concept may also *bounce, disintegrate,* or may even be *subsumed/absorbed* by the dominant concept.

Intersection

The Venn diagram: A Venn diagram consists of two or three concepts that intersect. A new concept is formed at the point of intersection, in which shared attributes appear (Figure 22.7). These form either a new concept, or a new form of the most dominant concept. The attributes unique to each concept are in the surrounding areas where the concepts do not link.

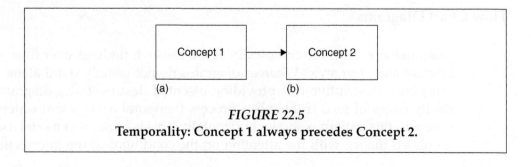

FIGURE 22.5
Temporality: Concept 1 always precedes Concept 2.

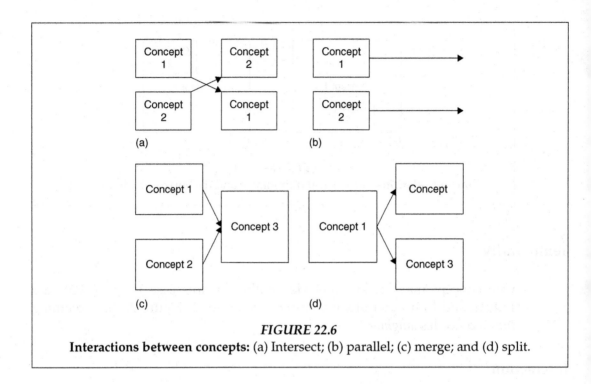

FIGURE 22.6
Interactions between concepts: (a) Intersect; (b) parallel; (c) merge; and (d) split.

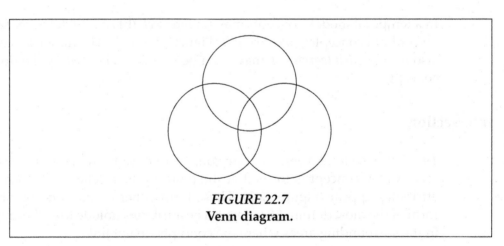

FIGURE 22.7
Venn diagram.

Flow Chart Diagrams

Diagraming reveals the complexity of the research findings over time, in an efficient and clear style. Whereas diagrams do not usually stand alone, they must have descriptive text providing essential details—but a diagram can clarify pages of text. If there is a process (temporal aspect) that orders the concepts, this pattern is shown horizontally. This is a common model used in grounded theory, with the attention on the conditions at the intersection of stages, or transitions, resulting in the changes in the process. In grounded theory, the addition of a core variable or basic social process runs through the model, holding the theory together and giving the theory purpose.

These diagrams become more complicated as concepts (variables) are added as cells, and arrows linking the cells display various "routes" or conditions or pathways that may be taken through the model. When developing a diagram that shows changes over time, the main direction is from left to right or from top to bottom. There should be a starting point and an end point. Flow chart notation (and software) is invaluable for diagramming, and standardizes notation.

In qualitative models the pathways are usually participants' behavioral choices or decisions identified by the researcher during the process of data analysis. Although the researcher may illustrate subprocesses schematically, in the diagram of the complete theory, the boundaries of the theory should be evident in the complete diagram.

The complexity of these diagrams appears to be proportional to the complexity of details of the analysis. Regardless of the details in the text that accompany the diagram, the rule is that the diagram must be understandable, and the relationships evident, without the text. That is, a reader scanning the article must be able to interpret the relationships without reading the text. An example of such as complex figure may be found in Figure 22.8.

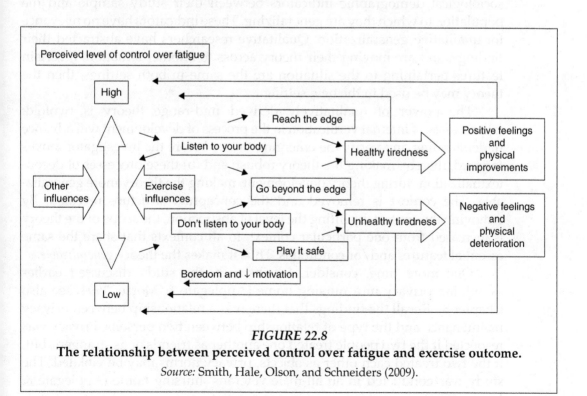

FIGURE 22.8
The relationship between perceived control over fatigue and exercise outcome.
Source: Smith, Hale, Olson, and Schneiders (2009).

TO DO 22.1. IDENTIFYING TRUST

Write a paragraph describing developing role of *trust* in the nurse–patient relationship. Then download the article:

Weaver, K., Morse, J. M., & Mitcham, C. (2008). Ethical sensitivity in practice: Concept analysis. *Journal of Advanced Nursing, 62*(5), 607–618.

Now compare what you have written with the authors' description of the model.

QUALITATIVE GENERALIZABILITY

Because of the limited scope of qualitative research, these theories are usually *small*, and often developed from few participants. Because of the nature of saturation, because the researcher is usually working alone, the study is small in scope and narrow. However, the same time there's great confusion about the ability of these mid-range theories to generalize. Applying quantitative criteria to *qualitative* inquiry, researchers erroneously write that their findings are not generalizable, because of the limitations, the sample size, ethnic composition, and so forth. However, these quantitative criteria have been developed because quantitative researchers are attempting to match certain sociological demographic indicators between their study sample and the population to which they are generalizing. These indicators have no relevance for qualitative generalization. Qualitative researchers have abstracted their findings, and are moving their theory across to another situation. *If* certain features pertaining to the situation are the same in both settings, then the theory may be used in the new setting.

The power of qualitatively derived mid-range theory is twofold: (a) processes of internal verification in the process of development will advance understanding and verify the emerging theory before the investigator moves forward, thereby making the theory robust; and (b) these processes of decontextualization during theory development, making the theory more generalizable. The context is removed and the conceptual structure revealed. By removing the context, by lifting the level of abstraction, the scope of the theory is increased from one particular context, to all contexts that share the same essential features and/or conditions. Thus it makes the theory *generalizable*.

One more time, consider, for instance, the study discussed earlier examining privacy in a nursing home (Applegate & Morse, 1994; see also Chapter 8). Recall the findings that there was a relationship between privacy maintenance and the type of relationship between two persons. Privacy was respected if the two people treated one another as friends or as strangers; but, if the two treated each other as objects, privacy norms may be violated. The study was conducted in an all-male veterans' nursing home (Applegate & Morse, 1994).

The demographics have little to do with the generalizability of the study. What must be considered are situations in which privacy maintenance is at risk and in which people have the opportunity to treat one another differently. I can think of several situations in which the findings would be pertinent, and I am certain you would add to this list: a gynecological or obstetrics unit; a boarding school; a prison.

This is directly opposite to generalizability in quantitative inquiry, in which processes of generalizability are determined by the *similarity of the population* (as determined by comparing the demographics of each group). *Do not forget*, for these statements are the most "crossed out" part of articles submitted to *Qualitative Health Research* (Morse, 1999), and qualitative researchers appear to be the biggest culprits delimiting their own studies by using quantitative criteria, apologizing for the small sample size, and applying quantitative criteria for delimiting generalization. They write: "Because of the small, purposeful sample, these findings cannot be generalized . . ." Yet in qualitative inquiry we generalize through the theory (not the sample) to situations that have essential characteristics in common. Qualitative research is generalizable.

Theoretical Generalization Over Time

How long does theory "last" in the literature? Does the 5-year or 10-year expiration date apply?

The "shelf life" of a theory, of course, depends on the topic, the quality of the theory, and its origin (qualitatively or quantitatively derived).

First the topic: Is it a behavioral theory? Is it related to a basic process essential to our humanness? Or is it related to something that is time-limited, such as the use of a technology (e.g., a theory relating to cell phone use when driving will only last as long as the cell phone is in use). Second, is it good theory? By now, you can evaluate theory.

In 1963, Ervin Goffman published *Stigma: Notes on the Management of Spoiled Identity.* According to Google Scholar, as of December 2015 it has been cited 22,924 times, and the book was last reprinted in 2009. As you know, the theory has been applied to (i.e., generalized to) numerous health care conditions, in particular to our understanding of AIDS. Goffman's work has been tremendously influential and is certainly not outdated 45 years later.

THE LAST THOUGHT

Concept analysis in nursing has been treated as an end result in itself. In this chapter we examined relationships between concepts, and how these concepts could be ordered and linked to build theory. This makes concept development, in itself, a much more important activity.

REFERENCES

Applegate, M., & Morse, J. M. (1994). Personal privacy and interaction patterns in a nursing home. *Journal of Aging Studies, 8*(4), 413–434. doi:10.1016/0890-4065(94)90012-4

Beck, C. T. (2015). Middle range theory of traumatic childbirth: The ever-widening ripple effect. *Global Qualitative Nursing Research, 2.* doi:10.1177/2333393615575313

Beck, C. T. (2016). *Developing a program of research.* New York, NY: Springer.

Finfgeld-Connett, D. (2008). Meta-synthesis of caring in nursing. *Journal of Clinical Nursing, 17*(2), 196–204.

Haase, J. E., Britt, T., Coward, D. D., Leidy, N. K., & Penn, P. E. (1992). Simultaneous concept analysis of spiritual perspective, hope, acceptance and self-transcendence. *Journal of Nursing Scholarship, 24*(2), 141–147.

Morse, J. M. (1999). Qualitative generalizability [Editorial]. *Qualitative Health Research, 9*(1), 5–7.

Morse, J. M. (2000). Theoretical congestion [Editorial]. *Qualitative Health Research, 10*(6), 715–716.

Morse, J. M., Hupcey, J., Penrod, J., & Mitcham, C. (2002). Integrating concepts for the development of qualitatively-derived theory. *Research and Theory for Nursing Practice: An International Journal, 16*(1), 5–18.

Olson K., Morse, J. M., Smith, J., Mayan, M., & Hammond, D. (2000–2001). Linking trajectories of illness and dying. *Omega, 42*(4), 293–308.

Smith, C., Hale, L., Olson, K., & Schneiders, A. G. (2009). How does exercise influence fatigue in people with multiple sclerosis? *Disability and Rehabilitation, 31*(9), 690.

23

MAKING USEFUL THEORY: MAKING THEORY USEFUL

> *There was a dean at my university who was a scientist with high intelligence but low boiling point. One day at the faculty meeting, after I said something that displeased him, he replied. "Peter, you have never made a contribution of interest to scientists." Naturally, my first thought was to take offence. But trying to maintain a generous spirit, and believing that a highly intelligent dean offers personal insults only in private, I decided what he really meant was not the singular "you", but the plural one. "You philosophers of science," he meant, "have nothing to offer us scientists."*
>
> *This interpretation at least took some of the sting out of his remarks and enabled me to think about them more clearly. Perhaps the dean is right, I now speculated. Although philosophers of science have carefully worked out views about a range of general concepts scientists employ— such as, evidence, explanation and law, to name just three of many— scientists seem to take little heed of them.*
>
> —Peter Achinstein (2001, p. 3)

In this chapter, I address the *why* and *how* of theory development in qualitative inquiry. Let us explore the processes of constructing mid-range theory, modeling, and moving toward the certainty of our models; most important, let us explore modes of clinical application for theory. First, we discuss "Making Useful Theory"—rather than esoteric theory, or theory for its own sake—and in the second part of the chapter, "Making Theory Useful," we deal with some of the clinical applications of theory itself.

MAKING USEFUL THEORY

Qualitative research methods are usually implemented by targeting a particular concept or group of concepts. An exception to this less focused approach may be a researcher who wants to find out "what is going on" in a particular setting, or a researcher who is interested in a particular phenomenon (but not in a concept per se). However, the majority of researchers are interested in some *thing*—that is, a concept at some level of development. Of course, concepts in the research setting do not occur in isolation— but rather occur with other concepts that influence the target concept's "performance."

WHAT IS MID-RANGE THEORY?

A mid-range theory is a theoretical scheme that reveals, enlightens, and provides understanding clinically. It is the analysis of data and organization of the subsequent derived concepts into a network that explains reality, predicts future actions and outcomes, and guides actions. Mid-range theory ranges in the level of abstraction from a theory that is closely associated with the data, to one that is reasonably abstract. It ranges from theory that is quite narrow in scope to those that are quite comprehensive, broad, and abstract. If the theory is developed from linked and interrelated concepts[1] (as in Chapter 22), the theory may itself range from connected small concepts, to laterally connected studies, to horizontally connected larger concepts. There is no formula dictating how many concepts are required to make a theory, what level of abstraction is "ideal," and how it guides practice. Mid-range theories contain whatever is necessary to understand the phenomenon and fulfill its role, in nursing or elsewhere, for guiding practice. Recall that a concept is anatomically static, an elaborate label of sorts, so it is the physiology of the concepts and the interaction of their components, or the interaction between concepts themselves, which make mid-range theory dynamic—as theory needs to be if it is to fit reality.

The most important feature of mid-range theory is that the theory makes the research potential obvious and exciting, useful, and powerful. Mid-range theories are generally about phenomena of clinical significance, and are sufficiently "applied" enough as to guide care.

Authors have argued about the interrelationship of concepts and theory, and I talked about this in Chapter 7. Some authors considered concepts of the

---

[1] Mid-range theory developed in sociology (Merton, 1949) as a particular type of theory linked to data. It came to nursing through Glaser and Strauss and their work developing grounded theory. Because nursing finds mid-range theory very useful clinically, it remains the most common type of theory used in nursing.

"building blocks of theory" (Walker & Avant, 1995), and Paley (1996a) describes concepts as "notches in theory." These discussions are important for describing quantitative theories, which are deliberately constructed by linking concepts according to the researchers' needs, and are modified in response to subsequent research results. But when developing qualitatively derived theory, these discussions are rather extraneous, for the concepts within a theory, and the theoretical form, are developed as they *need to be* to represent the phenomena, and the necessary conceptual components and the theoretical form may change from project to project. Often the concepts remain identified, but their form is still at the level of description. You cannot always quickly find the anatomical structure of some concepts. In quantitative inquiry it is different. Their concepts have been developed, defined, and operationalized before having been placed in the theory. Therefore, the method used to develop mid-range theory differs between qualitative and quantitative inquiry; here, the discussion focuses on the modes of development of qualitatively derived, mid-range theories.

What, then, is mid-range theory? It is something that is full of enough misgivings and misunderstandings to make a student shudder? Let us start with what it is not.

Mid-range theory is *not*:

- A collection of concepts linked with lines
- Something that must be learned by rote and rigidly applied
- Something that is fence-like, delineates, grabs, dictates
- Something that is fixed, immobile, and perceived to be right

Sometimes, in the process of developing concepts, researchers order the attributes and diagram the results to show a rudimentary process. We will refer to these as a *within-concept theory*. Recall in Chapter 16, by exploring the different patterns of the attributes, or different *strengths* of the attributes, we found different types of *hope* (hoping for a chance for a chance, and so forth). This conceptual scheme was a nice development of a concept working toward a theory, but does not fit our definition of a mature theory.

Definition of Mid-Range Theory

A mid-range theory is a theoretical schema that reveals, enlightens, and shows. It organizes complexity, labels, and thus enables communication and understanding. It shows how "things work," and enables agreement and communication and discussion about complex phenomena. In some cases, as well as enlightening, the development of the mid-range theory will also allow understanding of what will happen (prediction) and sometimes for quantitative testing (Wuest & Hodgins, 2011).

THE ROLE OF THEORY

Burton (1974), succinctly describes the roles and uses of theory from the informal sorting of the "overwhelming number of observations" and "masses of data" that we accumulate in everyday life ("theory as cognition") to formal theory that allows for hypothesis testing and formal knowledge development. Burton also states that theories cause tension and compete with each other in science; or as "counter-nihilism," fills voids of "intellectual nothingness" of that which is not known. Theory as "temporality" is theory that enables us to place things in time (past, present, and future) and account for trends and critical periods in history.

Theories clarify pulling together, and fitting, discrepant data. But in the process, investigators privilege some data and ignore others, invalidating discrepant data so that such theory is "a provisional, imaginative structure" (Burton, 1974, p. 14). It is "on this schema that measurement hangs its hat, and leads the way for still more measurement . . . How one sees it depends on the context and the readiness with which one sees."

Theory as prediction, as a predictive tool, is the most common perception of the use of theory: it is considered valid and a "good" theory if it holds when tested. But, Burton notes, theory does not "rise or fall on its predictive value alone," and the "distinction between fact and theory has always been overdrawn" (p. 14) and the prediction must be valued by society. A theory in itself may "lead to a consequence or away from it; go in several directions simultaneously, or importantly, lead a researcher to new directions" (p. 15). Theory may be "silence"; where no theory necessarily exists or when "a phenomenon requires social incubation necessary for its application" (p. 15). Theories may conceal, rather than being open and direct and, as Burton notes, sometimes this concealment is the direct function of a theory. "The silence of the theory is a salient theory-property, in that society is not ready for the disclosure" (p. 15). Theories may reveal, "show," disclose properties, and every theory has its "showing or disclosing properties, which, even without their propositions or postulates, change something" (p. 15).

The Roles of Mid-Range Theory

Where does mid-range theory fit into Burton's (1974) scheme? Clearly mid-range theory is theory that *shows*, reveals, and organizes lay theories of cognition. Mid-range theory clarifies and, although it is internally verified in the process of construction, qualitatively derived mid-range theories are not usually tested in the quantitative sense (although we discuss this later in the chapter). Mid-range theories sometimes delve into areas of silence, much to the discomfort of others, so that researchers may report explicitly on sexual behaviors about which we may sometimes rather not know the details. Our norms and our values impinge on science when we develop such theory at the personalized, behavioral level.

How Abstract Should a Mid-Range Theory Be?

Mid-range theories range in the level of abstraction from a theory that is closely associated with data, to one that is reasonably abstract. The theory may be one that is quite narrow in scope, or one that is quite comprehensive and abstract. There is no formula—these studies are, in Glaser's (1978) phrase, "whatever is demanded by the concept" to understand the phenomenon. Further, the concept, as we have discussed, is anatomically static; it is the physiology of the concepts and their interaction that make the theory dynamic—as theory needs to be.

However, note that there is a relationship between the level of abstraction and the scope of mid-range theory. If the theory is descriptive and close to data, then the scope is relatively narrow. If the mid-range theory is abstract, it will be broader in scope and have much wider application.

THE STRUCTURE OF MID-RANGE THEORIES

Mid-range theories that are developed usually contain reasonably developed concepts and explicitly show their relationship. Remember, concepts within a theory are developed as they are needed in the theory, and may change from project to project. Usually they are developed directly from data (and this we do that all the time in grounded theory or ethnography). Sometimes the concept is partway developed into a theory by ordering the attributes within a concept, and sometimes they start out by developing concept(s) and then develop those into a mid-range theory in a subsequent study. And sometimes the researcher commences the study with a targeted concept in mind, or one that is partially developed.

The difference between a qualitative project that develops the *concept* and one that directly develops a *theory* is somewhat blurred. The concept-developing qualitative study has as its product a *concept*, which is by definition abstract and somewhat static, but may be an end goal in itself. Qualitatively derived theory is not usually static, and may have *movement* (often describing transitions). Frequently qualitatively derived theory contains broader explanations and is more abstract than concept development research. Qualitatively derived theory may contain more than one concept, and in this case it will explore the relationship between those concepts.

TYPES OF QUALITATIVELY DERIVED THEORY

In Chapter 2, I discussed various types of theory as theories were originally used in nursing research and practice. We discussed philosophy as it gives research a gaze or an agenda, such as feminism, culture, or social justice. We discussed what has become known as "nursing theory," developed by the nurse theorists to give focus or frameworks for practice. We discussed theoretical frameworks that are used to justify your qualitative project (without impeding induction), or for a quantitative study used deductively to organize concepts in preparation for measurement. Finally, we discussed conceptual frameworks used in qualitative inquiry that provide context for qualitative research: that is, research that is intended to develop concepts or mid-range theory. Recall that these frameworks may include a philosophical stance, or concepts or even theories that the researcher is building upon or even using as a scaffold and skeleton.

What Are Theoretical Models?

The term *model* is used in a number of ways: A model may be a schematic diagram that shows the relationships of concepts or attributes within the theory. It may or may not show a part of the theory, or the theory in its entirety. Theoretical models, however, are diagrammed to illustrate results, and depict the form of the theory obtained; often the form of the model represents the type and structure of the method used.

Are models the same as theories? Models come in various types. When they are schematic representations of the attributes within a concept, they are best called a model. If they are to be considered as some type of a theory, they are relatively low-level theory.

THE PROCESS OF QUALITATIVELY DEVELOPING MID-RANGE THEORIES

Mid-range theories are developed either by processes of data analysis and synthesis in the process of qualitative inquiry or, as in quantitative inquiry, by identifying, analyzing, and linking concepts.

PROCESSES OF THEORY CONSTRUCTION

How Is Mid-Range Theory Constructed?

Most commonly, mid-range theory is developed from qualitative data extending qualitative strategies beyond the stage of simple description or developing concepts. Several qualitative methods are designed to bring analysis to the level of mid-range theory—most commonly grounded theory (Glaser, 1978; Corbin & Strauss, 2008; Charmaz, 2006), or some types of ethnography. Other methods of developing mid-range theory are by the linking of concepts, either deliberately looking for shared attributes, or by placing concepts associated with the topic, at different levels of abstraction, and looking for connections.

Continuing Qualitative Inquiry

While it is not my intention to write a textbook on qualitative methods at this point, I will quickly provide an overview listing the major analytic strategies for moving one's study to the level of mid-range theory.

Analytic Strategies

- *Induction, deduction, and abduction*: Cognitive process inherent in qualitative inquiry, induction (i.e., thinking up from data), deduction (for testing conjectures, however small), and abduction (a process of induction–deduction, building and testing and then building again) all play a part in project theory construction. By constantly asking analytic questions of these data, by developing conjectures and "testing" these conjectures both within categories and newly gathered data, the research systematically builds categories and concepts. This constant internal incremental testing ensures validity. Other processes in theory construction are as follows.
- *Processes of synthesis*: As similar data are gathered, they are synthesized within the categories, within attributes, and within concepts. This process of synthesis decontextualizes, meaning that it removes the variation that pertains to individual nuances in the context.
- *Emergence*: Ideas are derived both from the data and from the investigator. Important features within data demand the investigator's attention by occurring over and over until the researcher takes notice and incorporates that finding into the emerging conceptual scheme. Ideas also arise from the researcher's observations and when seeking answers to the analytic questions. These are noted, tested and incorporated into the emerging theory.
- *Category formation*: As data collection continues, data are sorted into broad categories. As these data become dense,

copious, the researcher is able to sort each category and ask: Is this one category or more than one thing? Is this one concept, or different types of the same concept? Or, is this one concept with different attributes in this category?

- *Identification of themes*: Not all data are analyzed with categories. Themes run right through the data, and are sometimes foregrounded; at other times they are backgrounded and must be reached by inference. In grounded theory the core variables for the basic social processes are usually derived from a theme.
- *Fit and fittingness*: As the analysis proceeds, categories and concepts fit together in a cohesive whole. Unlike quantitative data in which linkages are drawn by a line with a + sign for a positive relationship or a – sign for a negative relationship, the theory is linked by logic, by common sense, and by similarity.
- *Micro–macro linkages*: Not all linkages are horizontal; some are vertical, with some processes being a microanalytic analysis of a larger process. Alternatively, several smaller microdescriptive processes may be a part of a larger (macro) process.
- *Identifying relationships*: Recognizing that this goes with that, this is a part of that, and when, why, and how is the essence of fitting the pieces together into a cohesive whole.
- *Indices of causality*: We recognize that *this* causes *that*; and that *that* co-occurs with *that*; when *this* is present, *that* is absent, and so forth.
- *Forming the structure*: Once the researcher can tell the story in a general form, as, for instance, "these people do *this and that*, and on the other hand, these people do *that* because _____" analytic procedure may commence. Being able to address the topic in this narrative-schematic style enables the outline to the theory to be developed. Hold seminars to let the researcher articulate the emerging concepts and relationships, and to recognize where he or she should be theoretically sampling, where the parts that require more thinking or development are, and which parts are rich and well understood.
- *Functions of exemplars*: Exemplars are illustrations only. Excellent theory has descriptive passages that can *stand alone* and convince the reader; the exemplars are representative sections of text that *illustrate* the text. The reason that the text must explain in a self-contained way is that the participants do not speak for themselves—the

analyst/researcher/investigator does that, and if the analysis
is good, then readers will see more in the text than they
would if they had simply read the quotation without the
explanation.

- *Revisiting saturation and negative cases*: Saturation is achieved
  when the investigator is bored; this means when all
  dimensions of the concept have been explicated, when the
  boundaries are clear, when the concepts are well developed,
  and when the definitions hold across numerous instances
  and cases.

- *Issues in validity and verification*: Some researchers think that
  data should be coded by more than one person. Although
  interrater reliability is appropriate for descriptive research,
  elsewhere I argue that such a strategy makes interpretative
  analysis superficial, obvious, and trite—"perfectly healthy but
  dead" (Morse, 1997). Earlier, we spoke of internal
  verification—how ideas are tested in the process of doing
  research, so that as the theory is built, the theory is internally
  solid. But, the constructed theory must always stand up to
  external scrutiny. How?

Some researchers suggest that the theory be returned to the participants
for verification. Again, I argue, "Who's the analyst here?" You have gone to
school for umpteen years and learned social science theory and researcher
methods. If your interpretation is a great theory, synthesized and abstracted
from the context, it is highly likely that they will not recognize their own
interview or story in the analysis.

THE STRUCTURE OF MID-RANGE THEORY

In this section we are talking about how the results of research are presented
once the theory is developed. Of course, this is a product of the research
agenda as justified in the proposal, the kind of phenomenon studied and its
level of development, the method used, and the level of development of the
concepts and the level of abstraction obtained. However, there are "sets" of
ways that researchers present their theoretical results, as models, and here we
discuss the most common ones.

Table Presentation, Comparing and Contrasting Concepts

The most common way to illustrate components of a theory is either to
write descriptive text or describe differences and commonalities between

attributes, or even to list these in a table. The use of a table helps the reader to see the contents and their attributes easily, and therefore improves comprehension. There are examples of such tables throughout this book.

Process Trajectories

Trajectories are major processes, often containing a standard pattern of interconnecting concepts that change over time, such as in the course of illness. In mid-range theory illustrating a trajectory, often transitions (major points between two stages, in which the changes from one stage to another occur) punctuate stages in the course of the trajectory. In grounded theory, for instance, the researcher knows at the beginning of the study that the phenomenon that he or she is interested in is a process; that is why grounded theory has been chosen, is justified in the literature review, and was selected as the method to be used. Although the researcher knows it is a process, the stages and transitions between each stage, and the conditions that lead to the next stage, are unknown at the beginning of the study; they are identified in the process of analysis. In the process of doing grounded theory the researcher develops descriptions of each stage, investigates how the concepts change over time, and identifies the core variable (Corbin & Strauss, 2008), or the basic social process (Glaser, 1978), which is the variable that runs right through the process and accounts for most of the "variance." However, although the structure of the theory in grounded theory may be known, the theoretical content, even how many stages, what the concepts are, and what the core variable is, is not known to the researcher (Figure 23.1). Thus, grounded theorists use a particular way of approaching their interviews and their thinking about their data when coding, and so forth.

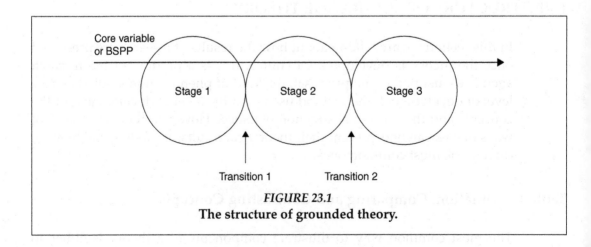

FIGURE 23.1
The structure of grounded theory.

SETTING UP YOUR STUDY TO DEVELOP QUALITATIVELY DERIVED THEORY

Naturalistic Experiments

Multiple projects from a qualitative research program are often formed around a general topic that is a higher level concept. Studies that are conducted around the concept are aimed at obtaining theoretical insights that provide an understanding or enlightening the research program about the concept, rather than providing descriptions about the new setting/incidence. Thus, research programs have a more substantive goal than description of a new setting.

For instance, the invitation to study a "vent camp"—a 1-week summer camp for children who were normally nursed at home and on a ventilator—provided us with the opportunity to study the systematic development of the nurse–patient relationship without new illness variables normally associated with hospitalization (Wilson, Morse, & Penrod, 1998). We asked: "How long does a nurse–patient relationship take to be established?" Our answer: "Until Wednesday" considering various "variables," that is whether or not the nurse and the patient liked each other; knew each other previously; were in a new or familiar environment, and so forth. Qualitative observations enabled us to view testing behaviors, "courting" each other, or on the other hand, rejecting behaviors. This enabled us to develop indices of the stages of the developing relationships, and to appreciate the significance of various types of relationships.

Recently we used a naturalistic experiment design. We developed the *Praxis Theory of Suffering* (which we will talk more about in Chapter 35). In this theory, people who have suffered a loss or faced death initially endured. They suppressed emotions so that they could go about daily activities. This enduring lasted until they were able to face that fact that the loss actually occurred. At this time they stopped enduring and moved into a state of emotional suffering—crying, weeping, and mourning the ir loss.

TO DO 23.1. EXPLORE THE DEVELOPMENT OF A MID-RANGE THEORY

Mid-range theories do not usually arise from a single project (but they can do). More often the theories arise out of thinking that takes place of over many years and the conduct of many projects. This is true for both qualitative and quantitative middle-range theory. Select and read one of the theories listed in Box 23.1. Using the reference list for that article, gather all of the previous articles written by the author.

For our naturalistic experiment, we wanted to know if someone who was enduring (and suppressing emotions) always exited enduring in emotional suffering by releasing those pent-up emotions—that is, by crying, weeping, and mourning their loss. Or could people who were in the state of enduring exit directly without emotional release?

To do this study we had to identify a situation in which participants would be enduring intensely, and explore participants' responses when the stress they were enduring was removed. The situation that fit our conditions was enduring the threat of breast cancer. We would study the experience of women who were undergoing the diagnostic processes for breast cancer. If they were later shown that the biopsy results were negative, they would no longer need to endure the threat of cancer. Did they return to normal life by releasing emotions through emotional suffering? Or would they return to normal without release of pent-up emotions. A study set up in that context fit the criteria to answer our questions, and it is reported in Chapter 24 (Morse et al., 2014). Again, these "naturalistic experiment" studies are designed to elicit information that may contribute to the developing theory, so the setting or the participants are incidental to the study's major purpose.

Positioning Studies According to Level and Scope

In Chapter 27, we talk about the scope and level of abstraction of concepts. We will add one more dimension to this, and that is *time*. Some concepts become (mature into) others; if we are working with a trajectory, they may interact: They may merge, split, transect, or parallel. This is very important, because we are now going to sort the concepts according to their positions in a quantitative theory we are constructing. Qualitatively, this is not so tricky, because the data dictate the position. But if you are building a quantitative model, you have to get their position right, logically, practically, and realistically.

First, we consider the position of the concept in the vertical hierarchy. Ask: Is this concept the same as, a part of, or is the other concept a part of this one? We can test this relationship linguistically:

- Is grief a part of pain?
- Is pain a part of grief?
- Does pain cause grief?

Making Theoretical, Generalized Statements

From the above analysis, which concept is higher level, has greater scope, and is therefore more general? Which concepts are lower level and more specialized? Which concepts are lay concepts; which are scientific concepts? The next step is to make generalized statements.

Generalized statements are overall synthesizing statements that may be applicable for all cases. They are the first step toward abstraction. In this case, the generalized statement will be about each concept; some will be the same and applicable to both concepts, some will be particular to grief, and some will only apply to suffering.

As an example, I will make the first statement:

I observe that both are in response to something. Is the grief and pain in response to an injury, such as to a painful knee or hip, or to "breaking up" a relationship, especially when you are not the partner who wanted to break up? Such examples you may be thinking of may be considered a response to a loss. But a painful hip or knee? Is that "mourning a loss?" We may "wish it would get better" and "that the pain would stop." We wish we could bend and move about as we used to. So in some sense we are mourning the loss of a pain-free knee or hip. If you can buy this argument, the generalized, theoretical statement may be:

Both grieving and suffering occur in response to a loss.

DEVELOPING THEORY USING CONCEPTUAL INQUIRY

Changing Concepts

Is this manipulative ability true for *scientific concepts*? No. Recall that scientific concepts are fixed, defined concretely, and are used the way they are proposed. Any modification must be done carefully, for solid reasons, and preferably via consultation with the original developer.

But this does not always happen. Through use, through carelessness or investigator sloppiness, or through *reflexivity* (Alvesson & Skoldberg, 2009), and perhaps because the way the concept was proposed initially was a poor fit, scientific concepts do change over time. This *conceptual drift* may be deliberate, or as in Hupcey's analysis of social support, change without awareness over time (Hupcey, 1998a, 1998b).

Use of a Skeleton or a Scaffold

As previously noted in Chapter 9, qualitative inquiry may not always begin with raw data; nor do the researchers begin without an agenda. Often researchers deliberately select a concept, and explore that concept in a particular situation, with the concept of interest used as a conceptual scaffold or skeleton. In order to prevent violating processes of induction, these inductive process are still maintained, but are shortcut somewhat. The researcher builds on what is already there. Here is a reminder from Chapter 9:

Skeleton

A skeleton is the "bones," or the internal conceptual scheme, of a study. Think of it as the attributes that are presented, and the task of your study is to place the soft tissue on those bones—to build description for your context.

Scaffold

A scaffold is the structure surrounding the phenomenon that delineates the boundary of the concept you are studying. It targets your observations and reveals the structure (skeleton) of the phenomenon you are studying.

Can one use another's published work as a scaffold? Can qualitative researchers use the research of those who went before, and is already published, as a scaffold? The answer is yes, provided that you are certain that you are using it correctly. Do you have to have permission from the author? It depends on the extent of your use, but certainly you must give credit to the author.

Concepts should be analyzed carefully before using them as stepping-stones in one's own research, for it is not uncommon that even published work may be incorrect, inaccurate, or slightly skewed. The distinct disadvantage of using the work of another is that it is not your work—you do not have the data from which it was developed, and that is a risk when using the work of others as a skeleton or as a scaffold.

Begin Appropriately

Therefore, if you wish to investigate a lay concept about which there has been little inquiry, but which you can recognize, *common sense* should tell you that you do not have to "begin your study at the beginning." Do an armchair walkthrough (Morse, 1999) and think your study through to identify your approach. Use "if" statements: If I do ___ (this), then I will ____ (have this result). And, of course, analyze all concepts you wish to use as a skeleton in your study. Evaluate the concepts as described in Chapter 6. Do not be tempted to build your study on sand. Start where the previous investigators left off to develop their descriptions of the concept (the anatomy, developing the physiology). We do this by moving it into a context (again, as in the example of hope; Chapter 16) and see how it performs in different settings and situations. Look for types of _____ (the concept), and the different roles and strengths of the attributes.

EXAMPLES OF QUALITATIVELY DERIVED MID-RANGE THEORIES

There are examples of qualitatively derived mid-range theories in this text (Chapters 19, 26, 30–31, 33, 35, 37, and 38). Other examples of qualitatively derived mid-range theories from the literature may be found in Box 23.1. Carefully study the titles of these qualitatively derived mid-range theories, and from the titles, can you discern the role of concepts and how it has been applied during inquiry?

TO DO 23.2. EXPLORE A RESEARCH PROGRAM

An outstanding example of moving a research program sequentially through a number of studies, from conception, to understanding, to theory, to developing and then testing an intervention, is the work of Judy Wuest and her collaborators, Marilyn Ford-Gilboe, Marilyn Merritt-Gray and Colleen Varcoe (2013).

Read this and discuss the process from development of the theory, to identification of the interventions, to practice.

Wuest, J., Ford-Gilboe, M., Merritt-Gray, M., & Varcoe, C. (2013). Building on "grab", attending to "fit", and being prepared to "modify": How grounded theory "works" to guide health interventions for abused women. In C. T. Beck (Ed.), *Routledge international handbook of qualitative nursing research* (pp. 32–46). New York, NY: Routledge.

BOX 23.1. EXAMPLES OF QUALITATIVELY DERIVED MID-RANGE THEORIES

Title	Author (Date)
A metaethnography of traumatic childbirth and its aftermath: Amplifying causal looping	Beck (2011). Also see Beck (2015, 2016).
Cultural aspects of early childhood obesity	Clark, Johnson, O'Connor, and Lessetter (2013).
Qualitative research program for the care of ventilator-dependent ICU patients	Happ (2013).
Learning about the nature of fatigue	Olson (2013).
Motherhood in the context of maternal HIV infection	Sandelowski and Barroso (2003).
Empirical development of a middle range theory of caring	Swanson (1991).
Cancer care communication: The power to harm and the power to heal?	Thorne, Hislop, Armstong, and Oglov (2008).
Cultural safety and the socioethical nurse	Woods (2010).
A theoretical understanding of abusive intimate partner relationships that become non-violent: Shifting the pattern of abusive control	Wuest and Merritt-Gray (2008).

THE PLACE OF CONCEPT DEVELOPMENT: UNDERSTANDING ITS CONTRIBUTION IN RESEARCH PROGRAMS AND ITS CONTRIBUTION TO KNOWLEDGE AND PRAXIS

People worry about scholarship in nursing. They have observed an enormous pile of publications—a concept analysis of this or that—but have not seen significant outcomes. They read the end discussion in the concept articles, and find out that more work needs to be conducted developing it. They have not seen "concepts in action," well-developed concepts applied in practice, or used in assessment. They may have used concepts in their quantitative work, but have only noticed concepts generally available and well established, concepts such as coping and grief, which have instruments of measurement associated with them. They have not noticed concepts developed in nursing, for the assessment and measurement of nursing phenomena. And although we have observed nursing philosophy being implemented into hospitals across the country, we are uncertain whether they are making a difference in care.

It is a worry. We have an enormous push for knowledge transfer and instruments to evaluate the clinical readiness for an intervention, and yet we are not certain why research takes 17 years to move into practice (Green, Ottoson, Garcia, & Giatt, 2009).

I can give my own opinion for the lack of knowledge transfer for qualitative inquiry and for well-developed concepts.

First, qualitative research results are not developed far enough for implementation; the findings are not developed by qualitative researchers to the point at which they can be grasped and implemented by the clinician. We leave the research at the stage at which we have developed a concept or a mid-range theory. Then the clinician reads the article on the concept development or the theory, and thinks, "Oh, that is interesting! But what do I do with the information?" Therefore, in this chapter, under the above assumption, I present several strategies for researchers to move their project closer to the clinician and the patient care.

Levels of Completion

Let us consider the various levels of completion of a qualitative project, which may range from descriptive synthesis to a developed theory. All is fine, but when we consider utilization, there is nothing for the clinician to use. We must, therefore, have a two-pronged approach to this problem. In the first place, it should be the responsibility of researchers to move forward with their form of their research findings, and to bring them closer to clinical application. But the other responsibility is for clinicians. They should be willing to move with the findings, to pull them into the clinical arena, and to use them in their practice. Of course, research findings may be used by other researchers, and that is a legitimate reason to be doing a project, so our concept may be incorporated into a theory as a component of another researcher's work, before it makes the clinical move. Regardless, nursing research will always ultimately be conducted for the benefit of the patient, the client, the client's family and support system, the community, and the good of humanity. That is our charge.

Level 1 Description

Descriptive research records what is there. It does not reveal; it does not conceptualize; it does not extend much beyond what can be seen. If used for evaluation, it will provide a good foundation for comparing any future change, or even for making decisions about what should be changed. It shows us what we already see.

However, if the descriptive researcher is working at the microanalytic level, data will reveal to us what is there but cannot be seen, but what is nevertheless information that we need if we are to complete our theory.

INDICES OF THEORETICAL ADEQUACY

How do you tell if a mid-range theory is any good? Let us start with *worth*. Is it *worth* developing? Or publishing? Is it *worth* making the effort to understand it? Or learn it? Is it *worth* the effort of testing? Is it *worth* implementing in practice? Or using in your research?

Grab

"Grab" is a criterion for excellent qualitative theory, proposed by Glaser (1978), but it is a criterion interesting enough to be used for all theory: philosophical, qualitative, or quantitative. For a theory to be worthwhile, it must have intrigue. It must be of interest to you, and fit whatever you are thinking of investigating, applying it to, or using in your practice. In order to have grab, it must provide you with a new way of seeing the phenomenon, or to "unpack" the phenomenon or its concepts so that they are measurable. It must be logical, tight, and *make sense*. Hopefully, it is innovative, and will provide you with something new: a new way of seeing or something new to investigate.

Conceptual Development: The Maturity of the Theory

The level of analysis achieved by the investigator will determine the quality or level of maturity of the theory. Theory that has undeveloped concepts will be at a low level, will be descriptive, and particular to the context from which it was developed. It will not be very abstract, and therefore not generalizable. In this light, a good mid-range theory must have the following characteristics:

The Concepts Must Be Developed and Must Fit in With Current Literature

This means that their labels are not "emic" labels, but that the researcher has taken time to compare the emerging concepts with those in the literature, and has made a case for adopting (or for not adopting) the concept labels that are currently used in nursing or other social sciences. For instance, does the coping that you are seeing in your data and your developing concepts fit the definitions and descriptions of coping in the literature? Why or why not? If it does fit, then adopt the labels presently used. Not everything you identify in your study will be unique or new. Keeping your own (or the participant's label) will result in too many labels for the same concept, and produce "theoretical" (Morse, 2000). Researchers will not find your work when they search the literature, and your work will fall into oblivion. The results will become cluttered with so many studies describing the same thing that we will all die of fatigue trying to sort it out; it will be used as a blade of grass in the fodder used by the meta-analysis folk. Any of these routes are less desirable for you: the weakened strength of your contribution in your mid-range theory in the whole, as well as in the particular.

The Descriptive Fit of Your Mid-Range Theory With Your Own and Multiple Contexts

Your theory must enlighten and surprise, and yet make sense to those who are familiar with your setting.[2]

It may seem contradictory that they must, at the same time, recognize yet be still enlightened by the theory. They will say, "Ah yes! So that is what is going on!" Others must be both able to recognize the conceptual organization or the processes depicted, and see the potential of your work. In this way, the familiar is reorganized to appear as "new" ideas.

The Utility of Your Theory

Usually, a standard criterion of theory is to predict. This criterion may or may not be pertinent for qualitatively derived mid-range theory. If, with a theory of comforting, by explaining comforting processes, it will be pertinent if it predicts how comfort is attained; then, the theory is indeed predictive. On the other hand, if the theory explains and makes sense of suffering, it does not necessarily predict the outcome suffering for any one individual,

---

[2] What is the essential difference between aging and maturity?

but by illustrating and making sense of the processes of suffering, clinicians will also be able to understand the process, categorize what they see, and move toward identifying appropriate interventions.[3]

Clarity, Parsimony, and Scope

Other criteria used to evaluate all theories pertain to their description and their presentation. You must be clear, brief, and succinct. Diagramming will assist you in this process. Finally, it must be clear about what the theory does and does not pertain to. Mid-range theories are limited and do not describe everything; they do, however, describe certain processes, and can be applied to new situations that do not exceed the parameters of the theory.

Internal Consistency

This is usually listed as a criterion for quantitative theory, but the logic and clarity that produce constructs *internal consistency* are important to all theories. Qualitative researchers must be clear about the level of abstraction attained, and that their definitions are not context-bound. Quantitative researchers must develop their operational definitions and predictive hypotheses systematically. All theory should be free of ambiguity and be parsimonious and elegant.

TOWARD CERTAINTY

Verification of Qualitative Inquiry

Qualitative theory is verified stepwise, in the process of construction. During the simultaneous processes of data collection and analysis, while the researcher is trying to ascertain what is going on, conjectures are created, and are verified before the researcher moves on to the next analytic step. This process is often supported by the literature, which the developing theory may agree with or mays even contradict. If the latter occurs, then the researcher returns to data collection, to be absolutely certain, and tries to understand *why* the present findings differ. Once the theory is completed and verified, it is still considered *theory*, or it becomes actual fact. But usually it remains a theory, as it is applied to new circumstances and situations.

---

[3] Can you think of a theory that has aged without maturing? And can you think of a theory that has matured as it has aged?

Verification of Quantitative Inquiry

Quantitative theory is constructed for testing, but once tested, several outcomes are possible: If the theory is supported, further testing may be conducted with replication, in similar or in different populations, and by different research teams. If the theory is not supported, it may be modified and the testing of the theory repeated. If the testing fails totally, the theory may be discarded for a more feasible theory or, now knowing what does not work experimentally, explore a new line of investigation.

RIGOR

Qualitative and quantitative research have different approaches to ensuring rigor in research. For qualitative inquiry, the approaches to rigor also differ according to research that is descriptive and semistructured, and research that is interpretative.

Qualitative Rigor

For descriptive qualitative inquiry the text or the observations are taken at "face value" provided that the researcher has taken care to obtain unbiased information from an adequate and cohesive sample. Rigor in these studies depends on the consistency of definitions, and the coding schemes of the researchers. Care is taken with such standards as definitions of coding schemes, inter-rater reliability, and accuracy in reporting.

For interpretive inquiry, strategies such as inter-rater reliability actually weaken validity (Morse, 1997). Insight depends on in-depth knowledge of the interviews or observations, on the use of interpretative strategies such as the recognition and analysis of metaphors, and of inference, and perception.

Interpretative research therefore relies heavily on internal methods of verification during the conduct of inquiry, and on the phenomenological criteria of agreement and recognition from others, known as the "phenomenological nod" (van Manen, 2014).

Quantitative Rigor

Reliability and validity in quantitative research are intricately involved with measurement. The first concern is with research design, controls, and sampling techniques to ensure that the experiment will be conducted adequately to maximize confidence in the findings. The fit between the variable and the measurement instrument is a validity issue, ensuring that the instrument is actually measuring what it is intended. The collection of the data becomes a reliability issue concerning the stability of the measure. Various statistical techniques are conducted to ensure the adequacy of the sample and the reliability of the measures.

THE PLACE OF CONCEPT DEVELOPMENT

We are often told that "qualitative inquiry goes nowhere" and the gap between research and practice is vast. I will not debate whose responsibility it is to close the "gap": should the researcher go into the clinical arena; the clinicians do research in their spare time; should we develop another specialty, and give this charge to the Doctors of Nursing Practice?

Understanding Patient Behavior

Qualitative theories may be used to enlighten nurses as to what is "going on" with their patients; they may be used to identify particular patient states or responses. But they have not found their way into care plans or formal nursing diagnoses yet. But there are some techniques to make your research more useful.

Understanding Our Conceptualization of Nursing

One of the most important (and perhaps unrecognized) functions of concept analysis and theory development is the way that it exposes, challenges, and even remodels the profession. Consider these examples:

- The identification of infant response to pain:
  Côté, Morse, and James (1991).
- Challenges to how we perceive empathy in nursing:
  Morse, Bottorff, Anderson, O'Brien, and Solberg (1992).
- The reorganization of our perceptions of caring (Chapter 14):
  Morse, Bottorff, Neander, and Solberg (1991).
  Morse, Bottorff, Anderson, O'Brien, and Solberg (1992).

These types of articles result in different types of challenge to practice than a clear-cut statistical evaluation of a nursing procedure, and are a different type of "evidence." How should type be classified? As basic research? As applied research?

Consider: Is this type of inquiry important? How should it be supported (funded)?

Using Concept Inquiry to Develop Assessment Guides

The first technique is to revise your grounded theory model to make an assessment guide. Sometimes this means rewriting your findings as assessment questions. For instance, a grounded theory finding from the stages of hope (Chapter 16) may be:

Stage I: Recognizing the threat: The nursing assessment—using the data from which the stage was derived, we see that people had trouble recognizing what had happened. Therefore the question that would capture this may be:

> *Did the impact of the event sink in?*

The behavioral signs of this incomprehension (also from the data) are:

1. *Reiteration in speech and thoughts connecting with others to reiterate or release (in the sense of emotional suffering)*
2. *Being stressed or overwhelmed with the situation*
3. *There is a one-way information flow, in which the person speaks rapidly and reiterates, or takes in information unquestionably*

The next step, identifying therapeutic strategies for persons in this stage, is to:

> *Provide information and monitor the level of comprehension by teaching or responding to the expressed feelings.*
> (Penrod & Morse, 1997)

Additional Details for Making Assessment Guides

These sources provide additional information for making assessment guides:

Morse and Penrod (2000).
Morse, Hutchinson, and Penrod (1998).
Penrod and Morse (1997).

Identification of Interventions: Observational Research

Qualitative inquiry may be used to identify interventions. Many comforting nursing interactions are implicit, and by carefully observing care, we can identify those strategies that are helpful. An example is the way of "talking through" or the Comfort Talk Register, to help the patient maintain control during trauma care, or while having a nasogastric tube inserted (see Chapter 29).

Fall Interventions

A second example from observational research is watching a patient with an impaired gait walk and move around the room. In this way we identified "furniture walking," or the patient's need for support forcing the person to move from one support to another, using the bed, then the chair, and then the wall for support. If the gap between these supports was too great to reach across, the person would "dive" to the next support.

SUMMARY

In this chapter, I have introduced the various forms of theory that may be used during inquiry to "make useful theory." In the second part of this chapter, I illustrated how theory could be useful in clinical practice. These applications of theory are expanded in Chapters 35 through 38.

TO DO 23.3. IDENTIFYING THE LEVEL OF DEVELOPMENT OF THEORIES

Search for three or four qualitative studies that have resulted in a middle-range theory. Examine the structure of these theories: are the concepts clear and well-developed? Is the theory diagrammed? The attributes well defined? The boundaries? What level of abstraction is the theory?

REFERENCES

Achinstein, P. (2001). *The book of evidence*. New York, NY: Oxford University Press.

Alvesson, M., & Skoldberg, K. (2009). *Reflexive methodology: New vistas for qualitative research*. Thousand Oaks, CA: Sage

Beck, C. T. (2011). A metaethnography of traumatic childbirth and its aftermath: Amplifying causal looping. *Qualitative Health Research, 21*(3), 301–311.

Beck, C. T. (2015). Middle range theory of traumatic childbirth: The ever-widening ripple effect. *Global Qualitative Nursing Research, 2*. doi:10.1177/2333393615575313

Beck, C. T. (2016). *Developing a program of research*. New York, NY: Springer.

Burton, A. (1974). The nature of personality theory. In A. Burton (Ed.), *Operational theories of personality* (pp. 1–19). New York, NY: Brunner/Mazel.

Charmaz, K. (2006). *Constructing grounded theory: A practical guide through qualitative analysis*. London, UK: Pine Forge Press.

Clark, L., Johnson, S. L., O'Connor, M. E., & Lassetter, J. (2013). Cultural aspects of Latino early childhood obesity. In C. T. Beck (Ed.), *International handbook of qualitative nursing research*, pp. 103–118. New York, NY: Routledge.

Corbin, J., & Strauss, A. (1996). Analytic ordering for theoretical purposes. *Qualitative Inquiry, 2*(2), 139–150.

Corbin, J., & Strauss, A. (Eds.). (2008). *Basics of qualitative research: Techniques and procedures for developing grounded theory.* Los Angeles, CA: Sage.

Côté, J. J., Morse, J. M., & James, S. G. (1991). The pain experience of the post-operative newborn. *Journal of Advanced Nursing, 16*, 378–387.

Glaser, B. G. (1978). *Theoretical sensitivity.* Mill Creek, CA: Sociology Press.

Green, L. W., Ottoson, J. M., Garcia, C., & Giatt, R. A. (2009). Diffusion theory and knowledge dissemination, and integration in public health. *Annual Review of Public Health, 30*, 151–174.

Happ, M. B. (2013). Qualitative research program for the care of ventilator-dependent ICU patients. In C. T. Beck (Ed.), *Routledge international handbook of qualitative research* (pp. 86–102). New York, NY: Routledge, Taylor & Francis.

Hupcey, J. E. (1998a). Social support: Assessing conceptual coherence. *Qualitative Heath Research, 8*, 304–318.

Hupcey, J. E. (1998b). Clarifying the social support theory-research linkage. *Journal of Advanced Nursing, 27*, 1231–1241.

Merton, R. K. (1949). The role of applied social science in the formation of policy: A research memorandum. *Philosophy of Science, 16*, 161–181.

Morse, J. M. (1997). "Perfectly healthy, but dead": The myth of inter-rater reliability. *Qualitative Health Research, 7*(4), 445–447.

Morse, J. M. (1999). Qualitative generalizability [Editorial]. *Qualitative Health Research, 9*(1), 5–7.

Morse, J. M. (2000). Theoretical congestion [Editorial]. *Qualitative Health Research, 10*(6), 715–716.

Morse, J. M., & Penrod, J. (2000). Qualitative outcome analysis: Evaluating nursing interventions for complex clinical phenomena. *Journal of Nursing Scholarship, 32*(2), 125–130.

Morse, J. M., Anderson, G., Bottorff, J., Yonge, O., O'Brien, B., Solberg, S., & McIlveen, K. (1992). Exploring empathy: A conceptual fit for nursing practice? *Image: Journal of Nursing Scholarship, 24*(4), 274–280.

Morse, J. M., Bottorff, J., Anderson, G., O'Brien, B., & Solberg, S. (1992). Beyond empathy. Expanding expressions of caring. *Journal of Advanced Nursing, 17*, 809–821.

Morse, J. M., Bottorff, J., Neander, W., & Solberg, S. (1991). Comparative analysis of the conceptualizations and theories of caring. *Image: Journal of Nursing Scholarship, 23*(2), 119–126.

Morse, J. M., Hutchinson, S., & Penrod, J. (1998). From theory to practice: The development of assessment guides from qualitatively derived theory. *Qualitative Health Research, 8*, 329–340.

Morse, J. M., Pooler, C., Vann-Ward, T., Maddox, L., Olausson, J. M., Roche-Dean, M., . . . Martz, K. (2014). Awaiting the diagnosis of breast cancer: Strategies of enduring for preserving self. *Oncology Nursing Forum, 41*(4), 350–359.

Olson, K. (2013). Learning about the nature of fatigue. In C. T. Beck (Ed.), *Routledge international handbook of qualitative research* (pp. 64–74). New York, NY: Routledge.

Paley, J. (1996a). How not to clarify concepts. *Journal of Advanced Nursing, 24,* 572–578.

Penrod, J., & Morse, J. M. (1997) Strategies for assessing and fostering hope: The hope assessment guide. *Oncology Nurses Forum, 24*(6), 1055–1063.

Sandelowski, M., & Barroso, J. (2003). Classifying the findings in qualitative studies. *Qualitative Health Research, 13,* 905–923.

Swanson, K. M. (1991). Empirical development of a middle range theory of caring. *Nursing Research, 40*(3), 161–165.

Thorne, S. E., Hislop, T. G., Armstrong, E. A., & Oglov, V. (2008). Cancer care communication: The power to harm and the power to heal? *Patient Education and Counseling, 71*(1), 34–40.

Van Manen, M. (2014). *Phenomenology of practice: Meaning-giving methods in phenomenological research and writing.* Walnut Creek, CA: Left Coast Press.

Walker, L. O., & Avant, K. C. (1995). *Strategies for theory construction in nursing.* Norwalk, CT: Appleton-Century-Crofts.

Wilson, S., Morse, J. M., & Penrod, J. (1998). Developing reciprocal trust in the caregiving relationship. *Qualitative Health Research, 8,* 446–465.

Woods, M. (2010). Cultural safety and the socioethical nurse. *Nursing ethics, 17*(6), 715–725.

Wuest, J., Ford-Gilboe, M., Merritt-Gray, M., & Varcoe, C. (2013). Building on "grab", attending to "fit", and being prepared to "modify": How grounded theory "works" to guide health interventions for abused women. In C. T. Beck (Ed.), *Routledge international handbook of qualitative nursing research* (pp. 32–46). New York, NY: Routledge.

Wuest, J., & Hodgins, M. J. (2011). Reflections on methodological approaches and conceptual contributions in a program of caregiving research: Development and testing of Wuest's theory of family caregiving. *Qualitative Health Research, 21*(2), 151–161.

Wuest, J., & Merritt-Gray, M. (2008). A theoretical understanding of abusive intimate partner relationships that become non-violent: Shifting the pattern of abusive control. *Journal of Family Violence, 23*(4), 281–293.

MODES OF RELEASING IN THE *PRAXIS THEORY OF SUFFERING:* THE RESPONSES OF WOMEN TO THE RESULTS OF BREAST BIOPSY

> *For the next thirty-six hours this situation was precarious. They would answer none of my questions. They said only, "Let's wait a couple of days," with little pats on the shoulder that filled me with dread.*
> —Martha Lear (1980, p. 334)

The experience of suffering is extremely common, yet as a process or an emotional response, it has not been carefully explored and described by researchers. In fact, more careful descriptions appear in the literature and movies. Over the past 15 years, Morse and her colleagues have conducted a number of descriptive studies into the experience of suffering and developed the *Praxis Theory of Suffering* (Morse, 2001, 2011; Morse & Carter, 1995, 1996; see also Chapter 35).

Despite these studies, several important questions remain. The *Praxis Theory,* as conceived, has individuals entering a stage of enduring (in which emotions are suppressed) and entering a stage of emotional suffering (in which emotions are released) before eventually relinquishing suffering. A question remains: *Must all who suffer exit enduring through emotional suffering, or are there other emotional routes to exit enduring?*[1]

In order to answer this important question, a naturalistic experiment was designed. We identified a situation that placed the participants in profound enduring, and then that which was being endured was removed for some participants and continued for others. Conditions for this

---

[1] This grounded theory is a further analysis of the stages of "Waiting to Hear," a grounded theory of the entire diagnostic process (Morse et al., 2014). Read this with Chapter 35, to understand the full theoretical structure.

naturalistic experiment occur when women undergo diagnosis for breast cancer and the results are negative. Those who receive a positive diagnosis must continue within the experience of suffering, and provide a comparison group. By conducting a grounded theory of women who are *waiting to hear results*, we were able to explore and, if necessary, extend/expand/clarify the *Praxis Theory of Suffering*.

LITERATURE

Finding a breast lump oneself, or receiving the results of a possible abnormal mammogram or breast examination, is a most frightening experience that immediately involves the threat of disabling surgery, long-term sickness from chemotherapy, disability and deformity, and death. Because most women have known others who have had breast cancer, subsequent long-term illness from treatments, and have died, it immediately places women in a state of panic, horror, and profound fear (Montgomery & McCrone, 2010; Novy, Price, Huynh, & Schuetz 2001; Poole et al., 1999; Witek-Janusek, Gabram, & Mathews, 2007).

Therefore, waiting for the diagnostic results of breast cancer is considered one of the most stressful periods ever experienced by women (Lally, 2010; Lally, Hydeman, Schwert, Henderson, & Edge, 2012; Lebel, Jakubovits, & Rosberger, 2003; Poole & Lyne, 2000; Thorne, Harris, Hislop, & Vestrup, 1999; Woodward & Webb, 2001). The emotional state of women during this time confounds practitioners to the extent that there is confusion and uncertainty about how best to support these patients (Haas, Kaplan, & McMillan, 2001). Although this experience has been well described, there is little known about women's responses, and a comprehensive framework of strategies women use when enduring this stress and the effectiveness of these strategies in alleviating distress are lacking in the literature. There is a paucity of information on how the stress is resolved with the news of the biopsy results. The terms used in the literature describing such states as "distress" (Iwamitsu, Shimoda, Abe, & Okawa, 2005; Lowe, Balanda, Del Mar, & Hawes, 1999; Northouse, Jeffs, Cracchiolo-Caraway, Lampman, & Dorris, 1995), "anxiety" (Deane & Degner, 1998), or even "uncertainty" (Montgomery, 2010) appear, from a qualitative experiential perspective, as a profound understatement.

Panic escalates during the diagnostic period, which, in our study, lasted from a few days to 3 weeks. During this period, women typically are called (phoned) to come to the clinic for a repeat mammogram and/or biopsy, and then, following the procedure, must wait for the results. Frequently, negative biopsy results are given on the phone; if the results are positive, then the women is not told the result on the phone, but is given an appointment for a consultation with the physician and asked to "bring someone with her." Thus, women are able to "forecast" if the news is bad (Morse et al., 2014).

How do women control their panic during the diagnostic period? The women's affect has been a constant concern in the literature, being linked with posttraumatic stress disorder (PTSD; Naidich & Motta, 2000), depression (Lampic, Thurfjell, Bergh, & Sjödén, 2001), and psychological distress (Iwamitsu, Shimoda, Abe, & Okawa, 2005). The majority of this research uses quantitative measures (Maxwell et al., 2000), and often women's unexpected flat affect, rather than distress, causes problems for researchers. For instance, Iwamitsu et al. (2005) are puzzled by "emotional suppression" and flat affect manifest in this population, and other researchers concur that women do not report anxiety.

A grounded theory of the process of the entire diagnostic experience from finding a lump or having a suspicious mammogram was developed also from the data used in this study (Morse et al., 2014). It revealed a three-stage process. In Stage I, women faced the idea of cancer by *feeling stunned*, grappling with the idea, and bracing for the biopsy. Stage II, *waiting to hear* the results, contained processes of *enduring*, in which women were *wrapping their minds around it*, were *controlling distress*, and were *keeping going*. Finally, in Stage III, women who heard positive results were *confronting their worst fears*, and were *continuing enduring*; those who had negative results enabled *releasing from enduring* and *sharing the good news*. The core variable was *preserving self*, represented the participants' strategies in minimizing suffering, thereby concealing their distress from others and maximizing day-to-day functioning by normalizing their affect.

In this chapter, we explore in greater detail the women's reported affect and emotional responses to breast cancer diagnosis, primarily in Stages II and III, using the *Praxis Theory of Suffering* (see Chapter 35) as a scaffold, to explore those who had a negative result, and how they exited the state of enduring, compared with those who had a positive result.

The *Praxis Theory of Suffering*

The *Praxis Theory of Suffering* has been developed from qualitative research, including interviews and observations, and encompassing numerous acute and chronic illnesses and injuries, the dying, and bereaved relatives. All interviews have been conducted as unstructured open-ended narratives that enable the person to tell his or her story without interruption (Corbin & Morse, 2003). Observational studies of persons' suffering have been conducted by videotaping in the trauma room and videotaping interviews, thus eliciting behavioral indices of the states of suffering.

Briefly, the *Praxis Theory of Suffering* consists of two major states, enduring and emotional suffering. When *enduring* the person suppresses emotional response to whatever is being suffered. They deliberately block thoughts of the event, and thereby block emotional responses. They maintain an immediate focus, blocking the past and the future, thus controlling thoughts of what the potential outcome of the event may mean. They focus on one step, one task at a time. This cognitive suppression reduces the emotional response, removes panic, and enables day-to-day functioning. However, the suppression requires constant vigilance and effort, and the process of suppressing the events and the motions may also suppress behavior, produce a flat affect, create a monotone voice, and loss of spontaneous movement, probably a lumbering gait. They speak in short sentences, in a monotone, barely moving their lips. They have an unfocused, gaze and little facial expression.

People who are enduring think they are coping well, even though they may make poor judgments (such as driving through red lights and stopping at the green). Others may stand away from them, avoid touching them, or just stand quietly or be with them.

Emotional suffering is a state in which the person recognizes that which is being suffered, and responds with weeping and distress. They have a hunched posture, a distraught expression, and cry and may talk incessantly about their suffering. Other are moved to comfort and support the person, including coming close and using touch.

Problem Statement

We asked: Do women who receive a negative result exit the *Praxis Theory of Suffering* from *emotionally suffering?* Or do those who receive negative results exit the *Praxis Theory of Suffering* from *enduring?*

METHODS

Data Collection

Women who volunteered to be in the study were invited to participate in one or two unstructured, audio-recorded telephone interviews, intended to elicit their experience with minimal direction from the interviewers. Because we were interested in the participant's experience as it occurred, in this study we used narrative unstructured retrospective interviews to avoid "leading" the participant and with the interviewer primarily listening. Following obtaining informed consent (which informed the participant about the study and obtained verbal consent), we asked only: "Tell me . . .," inviting the participants to begin their story at whatever point they wished, and to take as long as they desired in the telling.

Telephone interviews were set up by appointment so that the participants knew they would be on the phone for 1 to 2 hours, and could ensure a private time without distraction. In this way, the participant would be free to express emotions and maintain dignity, for instance, while crying. These interviews were conducted with minimal interruption by the researcher, and emotions were easily identified over the phone. If additional questions or clarifications were required, they were asked at the end of the interview or in a follow-up interview.

With unstructured interviews the emotions of the participants reflect those experienced toward events at the time to which they are relating. This phenomenon, *emotional re-enactment* (Morse, 2002), may be used as an indicator of validity of the interviews. During the interview process, the participants become immersed in their stories and their own emotional responses. *Institutional review board* (IRB) approval for this project was provided by the University of Alberta and the University of Utah. All participants provided written consents, including permission for the release of their images.

Sample

Women who had undergone a breast biopsy and who had received either positive or negative results for breast cancer were solicited from a breast clinic (with the assistance of staff) or from newspaper advertisement, in a large western Canadian city. Thirty-three women participated in the study; 14 learned about the study from the breast cancer clinic, and the remainder responded to an advertisement placed in the health section of the daily newspaper. Women were aged between 32 and 76 years. From this, 11 women received a positive diagnosis of breast cancer and 24 a negative result. We also interviewed two physicians specializing in breast cancer and one clinic nurse, for their general observations of the responses of women who had been given either "good" or "bad" news; all three were female.

Thirty-three tape-recorded first interviews with women participants were conducted by phone. Seven women were interviewed twice. Two interviews with the women participants were conducted face to face by their preference, as were the interviews with the staff.

Data Analysis

Tapes were transcribed, and according to the methods of grounded theory, were coded and theoretical memos were placed directly into the text in capital letters, to identify notes from the participant's text. Categories were formed by copying text with common topics into separate files, and synthesizing the contents.

Expressed emotions, identified by content and expression, were mapped by event, to reveal enduring or emotional suffering, and stages of enduring and emotional suffering were noted on a timeline. Specifically, the researchers were interested in the demonstrated and reported characteristics of enduring, and manifestations of emotional suffering, as follows.

Verbal Indices: (a) *Enduring*: the participants use short sentences, speak in a monotone, and voice lacks expression. Speech is present-oriented; content focuses on events, rather than feelings.

(b) *Emotional Suffering*: emotional tone of distraught distress; crying frequently. Verbal content may be future- or past-oriented.

Emotions were then *mapped* to illustrate major affective responses over time, from the time the breast abnormality was discovered until just after the results of the breast biopsy were learned. Placing the reported major events horizontally across on a "map," using markers for "enduring," "normal," "emotional suffering," and "relief," enabled illustration and sorting of the patterns of responses.

RESULTS

The Experience of Breast Cancer Diagnosis as a *Suffering* Response

When interviewing the participants, they often chose to first relate the "medical" story, often as a rote recitation of events and dates and treatments to the present time. This preoccupation with *facts* rather than *felt emotions* is indeed an indicator of the state of enduring. Once the medical details of the context were related to the interviewer, the interviewer would then ask the participant to return to the beginning to elect her emotional response, with a question such as, "Tell me, what was that like for you?" This question, in addition to the trust that had now developed in the interview, encouraged participants to provide the experiential details of their experiences essential for our analysis. Participants' emotions reflected the felt emotions experienced at the particular stages of the experience. When enduring (for instance when waiting for results), indices of enduring were evident in the tone and verbal content of the participant's story. Similarly in emotional suffering, the emotional state and crying were evident.

Comparison of the Emotional Responses of Participants to Positive and Negative Diagnostic Results

Following responding to "hearing the news," the experiences and responses fell into two broad categories: (a) living with the possibility or probability of cancer; and (b) escaping from the possibility or probability of cancer.

Discovering the Lump/Learning of a Suspicious Finding

Women's narratives during the period that they were forced to wait for confirmation that they did or did not have breast cancer were surprisingly similar. Hearing of an abnormal finding on mammogram or finding a lump in their breasts was one of shock, fear, and dismay:

> *I mean, I; I just, I just knew, there was, there was something. And*
> *I mean, the girls that did the ultrasound, well you know, she just said*
> *there was a spot they wanted to check but you just have a feeling that,*
> *that there's a problem somehow. You just do. It's just a gut feeling.*

> *I really had this fear that I had gone through for a week with a whole*
> *series of tests. A week, week and a half. It was just a real turmoil that*
> *I will never forget. And the fear is still with me. I, I go to, for a*
> *mammogram and I wonder, are they really catching everything.*

Once the initial horror could be controlled, women's attitudes toward the possibility or probability that they did or did not have cancer could be sorted onto two categories: "I probably have cancer" or "I probably do not have cancer." These perceptions were not associated with the confirmed diagnosis of cancer (which the women were waiting to hear), rather they were a decision made by the women in preparation for hearing the actual diagnosis. This decision, that they probably had or a more definite *had* or that they probably did not have or a more definite did *not* have cancer, was a cognitive strategy that enabled them to live through the waiting period and prepare for the actual diagnosis, and largely determined their behaviors and emotional responses during the days of waiting confirmation.

Women came to these decisions about their own diagnosis by reading the behavior of the physicians and other clinic staff; by assessing their own family history of the occurrence of cancer with mothers, siblings, and other close relatives; and assessing their past behaviors (such as: Did I breastfeed? Smoke? Refuse to diet?). For example, one woman described her experience waiting for the news as,

> *[I'm] not being too concerned because they [the clinic staff] are not*
> *being too concerned. A week later, back at my doctor's office, shock.*
> *And you hear that C word, boy! It was, um . . . yeah, it's devastating.*

Importantly, none of the women's attitudes could be classified as *uncertain* about their diagnosis—none said, for instance, that they did not know or that they would wait and see. All women's expected diagnoses fell into a dichotomy from definitely not having cancer to definitely having cancer. The decision was significant enough to be a life-changing event that immediately demanded that they evaluate their lives: The group consisted of those who were certain they had cancer and made plans for the anticipated impending treatments and even dying; those who expected to be told that they did not have cancer intentionally forced any thoughts to the contrary to the back of their minds, and deliberately lived life normally. The emotional responses of each group of women—whether they primarily endured or emotionally suffered—followed their past behaviors, although those who believed they had cancer were more public about their emotional suffering; and those who believed they did not have cancer tended to conceal their distress and tears and publicly endured and kept their day-to-day life normal as possible.

Living With the Possibility/Probability of Cancer

These women conceptually foregrounded the probability that they had cancer, letting themselves envision a future with cancer and prepare their lives accordingly. They imagined various scenarios, tentatively considering alternative trajectories and consequences of a positive diagnosis, *bracing* themselves for the confirmation of the positive diagnosis. This mindful *rehearsing* enabled them to have a glimpse of their future in a limited way, considering the scenario of cancer, treatment, and even death. These processes of *mulling it over* and *dwelling with the feared unknown* enabled them to become stronger, *building resilience*, and to make plans to prepare for the eventual bad news. These participants talked to themselves ("I have the capacity . . ."), trying to convince themselves that they were strong enough, resilient enough, to "get through' the anticipated surgery and the treatments, even though their diagnosis was not confirmed at this time. They requested help to be strong, to endure, in the form of prayer. They tried to find out what to expect by seeking information, both from the web and asking others who had experienced breast cancer.

> *What helped me was the fact that he was so upset I knew I had to have*
> *that strength, even at night when you know you could cry, I didn't.*
> *I thought I've gotta be strong I have to keep that strength cause*
> *I thought of it in the future in the future if I do have cancer I have to*
> *be the strong one and we have to do it a step at a time and its going to*
> *be harder for them but if I could be strong and if they could see I could*
> *handle it.*

> *I mean, at night you know, when you're laying there, of course, bad*
> *thoughts get into your head but you've got to push them out and say*
> *you know, even if this is cancer, we can deal with it. . . I was lucky. It*
> *wasn't, it wasn't bad so uh, but you do find, you do find strength*
> *within you. Especially I think with the kids, you know. You've got to*
> *find that strength cause you can't, you can't break down and you*
> *know, you have to, you have to be strong.*

Several of these women compared themselves to those they knew who had had breast cancer, trying to determine how they in turn would respond.

They tried to find out details and to learn more about what to expect when their time came. They *marked time,* by keeping track of the length of waiting time. They were aware of when their results were due, and took action by phoning physicians to ask for their results if their notification was delayed.

Escaping From the Possibility/Probability of Cancer

The second group believed that *It is unlikely that I have cancer* or more definitely, that *I do not have cancer.* These women blocked information about cancer, deliberately putting any consideration that they may have cancer at the back of their mind. They reminded themselves that in their case, the statistical odds of a positive result was minimal, and their family histories made chances that it was cancer unlikely. Yet, if their minds were not occupied or focused, for instance when they were lying awake in bed at night or taking a shower and aware of their breasts, the threat of cancer would come tumbling back into their consciousness. They would be *sideswiped* by the sudden realization of the threat of cancer, and felt instantly emotionally overwhelmed. Therefore, their "coping" strategies were to remove any thoughts of cancer from their minds and keep their thoughts occupied, thus controlling the intrusive thoughts about cancer.

> *I think my feeling was there's not much I can do about it. It's there,*
> *you know. I was more upset with the doctor in his attitude for*
> *some—And my opinion with some doctors is sometimes they*
> *panic—You know, they, they, they kind of create the panic. But um . . .*
> *I didn't, I guess maybe, **back in my mind**, I thought there is no*
> *history. And, and based on my mom having cysts out, you*
> *know—probably 40 years ago. And she's had a number of them out.*
> *And, I don't think I overly panicked. But mind you, when I went back*
> *this last time and she felt the lump, it was a little scary thinking that,*
> *well maybe it was—but I wasn't, when I went there, I wasn't upset or*
> *anything like that.*

These women focused intensely on living day by day and getting through each day moment by moment. They determinedly *maintained a normal* atmosphere in the home and at work in their daily activities. They *avoided telling* others about their suspected diagnosis, to the extent that they avoided their friends and parents, because they knew they could not conceal their distress.

> *I did not panic. And, and uh, I did not discuss it with anybody. The*
> *only other person that knows other than my husband is my daughter.*
> *I did not tell my son—we had decided we would just not say*
> *anything. If there was something there, we would [tell], we would say.*
> *And then in that case, I would have to inform my sisters and my*
> *mother. But to this day, they know nothing.*

"Telling others" would make the possibility of cancer real for themselves. These women intuitively knew they could not face the emotional responses of others and any advice offered. Self-talk took the form of *chiding*, of trying to convince themselves that their chance of having cancer was unlikely. They persuaded themselves that the "lump" was a cyst—not a tumor—that the physician had expressed doubt that it was cancer, and the biopsy was only to "make sure." If they told someone about the cancer and received unsolicited and unwanted information, they then refused to confide in anyone else.

These women who refused to consider the possibility of cancer deliberately focused on tasks, forcing themselves to concentrate on their work, and sometimes *immersing themselves in activities* that occupied their minds. They pushed the knowledge of the impending cancer to the back of their minds by *focusing* on the needs and health concerns of others. Children's needs and everyday activities came first, filling their days and leaving no opportunity to worry or even to consider cancer. These women kept silent about the cancer; they did not tell others, and by refusing to tell, they avoided having to watch the distress of others, which enabled them to avoid acknowledging the problem themselves and increasing their own distress. These women enjoyed activities such as puzzles, the concentration blocked out cancer. One participant learned biblical Greek; others exercised intensely, gardened, or *distracted themselves* in the evenings by going to the movies, enjoying the company of friends, and laughing about unrelated matters. The intensity of engagement in these tasks silenced the possibility of cancer, consumed their attention, and occupied the women mentally, physically, and emotionally. Even though things did not feel normal, they acted *as if* everything was normal.

> *I kept busy. That's important so that I didn't have too much time to dwell on it. My family was going through other crisis at the time. So I couldn't just think of me. That was important. Um . . . . important not to; not to stop working. I also go to the gym. And uh . . . I found that if I went each day rather than the three times a week that I had been going, that it really helped me . . . . to have exercise, more exercise than a normal working mother has.*

Depending on the success of their efforts of *convincing themselves that they did not have cancer*, when thoughts of cancer broke through, emotional suffering would emerge. Aware that their own emotional response distressed others, these women would hide their emotional suffering, and this is perhaps the reason that they did not reveal what they were going through to even their closest friends—a strategy that denied them the support that these friends could offer.

> *It was a real uh struggle for me to keep the, the tears back. I was just very frightened, you know, that what if something isn't quite right.—I did talk to, to a couple of people, and cried a little bit.*

Styles of Suffering

The success of the above strategies, whether the woman kept the threat of cancer in the foreground or background of her mind, enabled women to endure and to go about their daily lives. However, whether women stayed in enduring or emotional suffering or swung rapidly between these two states was also dependent on the women's usual style of responding to distressful events. If the woman reported that "she usually cried" in response to other stressors and crises, then the woman was likely to respond with emotional distress at this time; conversely if the woman was stoic, she was more likely to endure. We have graphed these emotional responses using the woman's descriptions of her emotions at that time.

Primarily enduring

Those who were primarily enduring are shown in Figures 24.1(a) and 24.1(b). These women who were able to maintain enduring, often with effort, are shown in Figure 24.1(a), reporting transitioning occasionally into emotional distress, which broke through, usually in private places. Figure 24.1(b) shows enduring more successfully, with less effort; although they also reported some breakthrough emotional distress, it was not as overwhelming as the first group.

Primarily Emotional Suffering

Emotional distress is shown in Figure 24.1(c) and 24.1(d). These women were not able to endure for very long periods, and those who were a "basket case" reported emotional distress—crying—most of the time, transitioning for only short periods into enduring:

> *I'm quite a fun-loving sort of person. And uh you know, the host asked you know, whether I was not well that day and what not. We were sitting out in the patio and I just burst into tears. You know, I was just sobbing. And um . . . you know, because at that particular point in time, I didn't know whether I had cancer or not. And um . . . you know, I, I really felt quite alone, quite isolated. . . I was you know, really quite frozen for awhile. I thought um . . . I didn't know what to do. I was really terrified at that point.*

One of the physicians reported that when giving the patient diagnostic news, "we see more tears from those who are negative." Of importance, is Figure 24.1(d), which shows that emotional suffering continued, despite negative results. There was evidence that these women believed that they "really had cancer" and that the doctor had "just not found it yet." The tentative nature of the physician's language ('We will continue to follow

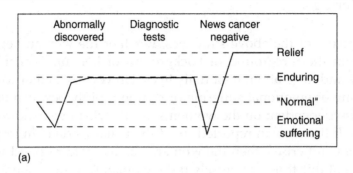

(a)

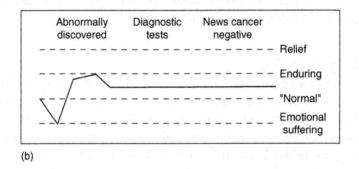

(b)

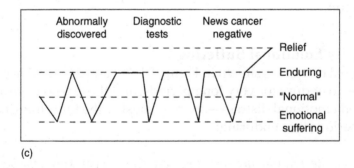

(c)

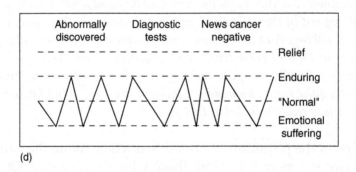

(d)

FIGURE 24.1
Patterns of releasing from enduring: (a) enduring, exit through suffering and relief;
(b) optimal enduring; (c) enduring with sporadic emotional suffering; exit through
relief; and (d) emotional suffering continues—even after receiving the diagnosis.

you") and the request for repeated mammograms in 6 months endorsed these participants' beliefs.

> *My doctor at the_____ [clinic] just to get it checked out. And when she,*
> *when I went in to see her and she gave me the examination, she was*
> *concerned because she said she wasn't, she couldn't give me any*
> *assurances that it, that it was nothing.*

Emotional Responses to Receiving the Diagnosis

Again, there was no apparent association between these styles of suffering and how these women perceived and responded to the threat of cancer. Again, the women's style of enduring was most closely associated with their own personality—as they had "coped" with previous losses emotionally in the past. However, if the woman was cognitively "backgrounding" cancer, she tended to endure in public as a part of concealing their fear from others.

Can One Exit the Suffering Model From Enduring, or Must One Release Emotions Through Emotional Suffering?

When examining participant emotions on receiving news of a negative biopsy, some participants release enduring through emotional suffering and cried, followed by relief. Others did exit the *praxis model of suffering* directly from the state of enduring and did not experience emotional suffering, releasing pent up emotions as relief and joy.

> *Relief, just finally knowing, just it's almost like you can breathe again*
> *without that tightness and your heart racing. You almost feel*
> *weak-kneed and that was the good news like what would I have done if*
> *it was bad?*

Relief was reported as a "giddy high" and often women had a formal celebration with their husbands and family. This group provided the information that the emotions that were suppressed during enduring could be released without the person entering emotional suffering. Within the context of the suffering model, this supports our conjecture that the emotions must be released, and may be released either through emotional suffering or directly from enduring as relief. The model of suffering was revised accordingly (see Figure 24.2).

We examined the strategies for enduring, and how enduring was maintained. During the period of waiting through the diagnostic tests, women fell into two broad categories, and the prognostic beliefs were not related to their actual diagnosis of cancer (Chi Square = X^2, 3.84' df = 1, NS).

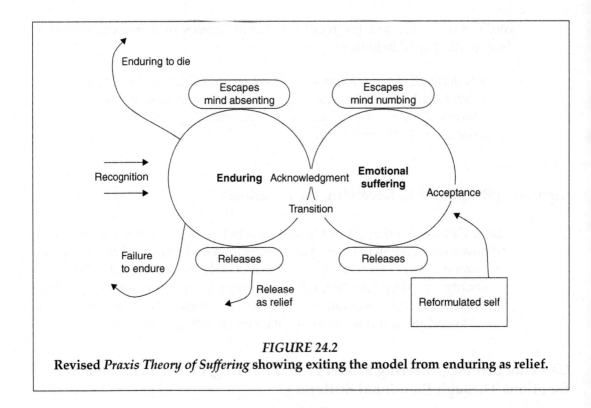

FIGURE 24.2
Revised *Praxis Theory of Suffering* showing exiting the model from enduring as relief.

Participants were sorted by their descriptions of whether or not they believed they had cancer. The first group was *Living with the probability of cancer,* and this group included the range of responses of women who reported *"I have cancer"* or *"I probably have cancer."* The second was labeled *Escaping from the possibility of cancer,* and this group included the range of responses from *"I probably do not have cancer"* to *"I do not have cancer."* Whereas the modes of enduring for each of these two groups were different, it must be noted that we were examining *patterns of responses.* In each case there were exceptions, and even those who *backgrounded* cancer had moments when cancer forced its way into the *foreground.* Of importance, the beliefs of these two groups about their own susceptibility to cancer were not related to their pattern of emotional responses.

DISCUSSION

In this study, women's emotional responses to the threat of cancer appear as a good explanatory fit with the *Praxis Theory of Suffering* (Morse, 2001, 2011). Women develop cognitive and behavioral ways to support and maintain their enduring behaviors, and transitioned into emotional suffering when they were unable to contain the enduring. Friends and relatives support women in their style of suffering. Those who are enduring are supported in their enduring strategies, and those who are emotionally suffering are allowed to cry and be comforted, but are also bolstered into enduring by countering their fears and terror. While waiting for biopsy results, those women who were enduring did maintain control, focused on the present, used distraction and kept busy, and avoided thoughts that would trigger emotional distress.

The study also taught us more about the experience of suffering, which is a fundamental response to threats and losses. The *Praxis Theory of Suffering* provides understanding behavioral indices of enduring or emotional suffering, and these are evident in this context. Caregivers can easily "read" these behavioral cues and know how well a woman is coping and the effective strategies for her to do so. Given the difficulty in accurately measuring distress psychometrically with the *Distress Thermometer* (Shimizu et al., 2010), it is recommended that some thought be given to using behavioral assessment and the indices described in the chapter. Professionals could easily assess suffering by following the cues of the women, evaluating observed behaviors, and making recommendations to others. It is important that health care providers recognize the impact of the information, its timeliness and delivery.

REFERENCES

Corbin, J., & Morse, J. M. (2003). The unstructured interactive interview: Issues of reciprocity and risks. *Qualitative Inquiry, 9*(3), 335–354.

Deane, K. A., & Degner, L. F. (1998). Information needs, uncertainty, and anxiety in women who had a breast biopsy with benign outcome. *Cancer Nursing, 21*(2), 117–126.

Haas, J., Kaplan, C., McMillan, A., & Esserman, L. (2001). Does timely assessment affect the anxiety associated with an abnormal mammogram result? *Journal of Women's Health & Gender-Based Medicine, 10*(6), 599–605.

Iwamitsu, Y., Shimoda, K., Abe, H., & Okawa, M. (2005). Anxiety, emotional suppression, and psychological distress before and after breast cancer diagnosis. *Psychosomatics, 46*(1), 19–24.

Lally, R. M. (2010). Acclimating to breast cancer: A process of maintaining self-integrity in the pretreatment period. *Cancer Nursing, 33*(4), 268–279. doi:10.1097/NCC.0b013e3181d8200b

Lally, R. M., Hydeman, J. A., Schwert, K., Henderson, H., & Edge, S. B. (2012). Exploring the first days of adjustment to cancer: A modification of acclimating to breast cancer theory. *Cancer Nursing, 35*(1), 3–18. doi:10.1097/NCC.0b013e318227ca62

Lampic, C., Thurfjell, E., Bergh, J., & Sjödén, P. O. (2001). Short-and long-term anxiety and depression in women recalled after breast cancer screening. *European Journal of Cancer, 37*(4), 463–469.

Lear, M. W. (1980). *Heartsounds: The story of a love and loss.* New York, NY: Simon & Schuster.

Lebel, S., Jakubovits, G., Rosberger, Z., Loiselle, C., Seguin, C., Cornaz, C., . . . Lisbona, A. (2003). Waiting for a breast biopsy: psychosocial consequences and coping strategies. *Journal of Psychosomatic Research, 55*(5), 437–443.

Lowe, J. B., Balanda, K. P., Del Mar, C., & Hawes, E. (1999). Psychologic distress in women with abnormal findings in mass mammography screening. *Cancer, 85*(5), 1114–1118.

Maxwell, J. R., Bugbee, M. E., Wellisch, D., Shalmon, A., Sayre, J., & Bassett, L. W. (2000). Imaging-guided core needle biopsy of the breast: Study of psychological outcomes. *The Breast Journal, 6*(1), 53–61.

Montgomery, M. (2010). Uncertainty during breast diagnostic evaluation: State of the science. *Oncology Nursing Forum, 37*(1), 77–83.

Montgomery, M., & McCrone, S. H. (2010). Psychological distress associated with the diagnostic phase for suspected breast cancer: Systematic review. *Journal of Advanced Nursing, 66*(11), 2372–2390. doi:10.1111/j.1365-2648.2010.05439.x

Morse, J. M. (2001). Toward a Praxis Theory of Suffering. *Advances in Nursing Science, 24*(1), 47–59.

Morse, J. M. (2002). Emotional re-enactment [Editorial]. *Qualitative Health Research, 12*(2), 147.

Morse, J. M. (2011). The Praxis Theory of Suffering. In J. B. Butts & K. L. Rich (Eds.), *Philosophies and theories in advanced nursing practice* (pp. 569–602). Burlington, MA: Jones & Bartlett.

Morse, J. M., & Carter, B. J. (1995). Strategies of enduring and the suffering of loss: Modes of comfort used by a resilient survivor. *Holistic Nursing Practice, 9*(3), 33–58.

Morse, J. M., & Carter, B. J. (1996). The essence of enduring and the expression of suffering: The reformulation of self. *Scholarly Inquiry for Nursing Practice, 10*(1), 43–60.

Morse, J. M., Pooler, C., Vann-Ward, T., Maddox, L., Olausson, J. M., Roche-Dean, M., . . . Martz, K. (2014). Awaiting the diagnosis of breast cancer: Strategies of enduring for preserving self. *Oncology Nursing Forum, 41*(4), 350–359.

Naidich, J. B., & Motta, R. W. (2000). PTSD-related symptoms in women with breast cancer. *Journal of Psychotherapy in Independent Practice, 1*(1), 35–54.

Northouse, L. L., Jeffs, M., Cracchiolo-Caraway, A., Lampman, L., & Dorris, G. (1995). Emotional distress reported by women and husbands prior to a breast biopsy. *Nursing Research, 44*(4), 196–201.

Novy, D. M., Price, M., Huynh, P. T., & Schuetz, A. (2001). Percutaneous core biopsy of the breast: Correlates of anxiety. *Academic Radiology, 8*(6), 467–472.

Poole, K., & Lyne, P. A. (2000). The "cues" to diagnosis: Describing the monitoring activities of women undergoing diagnostic investigations for breast disease. *Journal of Advanced Nursing, 31*(4), 752–758. doi:10.1046/j.1365-2648.2000.01345.x

Poole, K., Hood, K., Davis, B. D., Monypenny, I. J., Sweetland, H., Webster, D. J., . . . Mansel, R. E. (1999). Psychological distress associated with waiting for results of diagnostic investigations for breast disease. *The Breast, 8*(6), 334–338.

Shimizu, K., Ishibashi, Y., Umezawa, S., Izumi, H., Akizuki, N., Ogawa, A., . . . Uchitomi, Y. (2010). Feasibility and usefulness of the 'distress screening program in ambulatory care in clinical oncology practice. *Psycho-Oncology, 19*(7), 718–725.

Thorne, S. E., Harris, S. R., Hislop, T. G., & Vestrup, J. A. (1999). The experience of waiting for diagnosis after an abnormal mammogram. *Breast Journal, 5*(1), 42–51. doi:10.1046/j.1524-4741.1999.005001042.x

Witek-Janusek, L., Gabram, S., & Mathews, H. L. (2007). Psychologic stress, reduced NK cell activity, and cytokine dysregulation in women experiencing diagnostic breast biopsy. *Psychoneuroendocrinology, 32*(1), 22–35.

Woodward, V., & Webb, C. (2001). Women's anxieties surrounding breast disorders: A systematic review of the literature. *Journal of Advanced Nursing, 33*(1), 29–41. doi:10.1046/j.1365-2648.2001.01635.x

SECTION VI

MIXED- AND MULTIPLE-METHOD APPROACHES

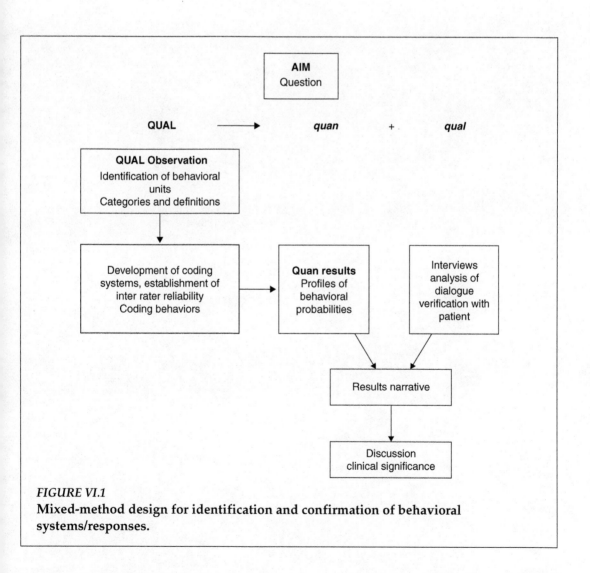

FIGURE VI.1

Mixed-method design for identification and confirmation of behavioral systems/responses.

EXPANDING THEORY USING MIXED METHODS

*A comparison of **apples and oranges** occurs when two items or groups of items are compared that cannot be practically compared.*

The idiom, comparing apples and oranges, refers to the apparent differences between items, which are popularly thought to be incomparable or incommensurable, such as apples and oranges. The idiom may also be used to indicate that a false analogy has been made between two items, such as where an apple is faulted for not being a good orange.

—Wikipedia (n.d.)

So far in this book, we have focused our discussion on the advantages of developing theory—inductively, using qualitative methods; and deductively, using quantitative measures. By now it should be clear that there are advantages and disadvantages to both approaches. The advantage of developing qualitative theory from data is that the theory is relatively valid, but because these theories are so close to the data, they may not be generalizable. The deductive quantitative theory has the advantage of being verifiable and generalizable (at least, in a way that most understand). The problem is that when working deductively, it is a circular process of developing—conducting the research—testing the research—modifying the theory—testing research—modifying theory—testing research—modifying research, and so forth.

In the past 20 years, a movement of using both qualitative and quantitative research in the same project has developed with the intent of overcoming the limitations of both qualitative and quantitative research for theory/knowledge development. This movement is called mixed-method design and it is most frequently the utilization of both qualitative and quantitative methods with the same project (Morse & Nichaus, 2009). Here we will not discuss how to "do" mixed-method research but rather discuss its role in theory development.

MIXED-METHOD APPROACHES

There are three approaches to mixed-method research. The first two designs, qualitatively driven mixed-method design and quantitatively driven mixed-method design, use a core (main project) of either qualitative or quantitative methods and attach a supplementary strategy of either qualitative or quantitative research to obtain data that could not be elicited by the core method alone. Note that the supplemental project cannot stand alone, nor is it publishable with the core component. Therefore, mixed methods may be conceived as "one-and-a-half projects."

Multiple-Method Design

The other major type of design is called multiple-method design, consisting of several projects of qualitative and quantitative designs, all addressing the same project aim. Again, multiple-method design has a theoretical thrust of either induction (qualitative) or deduction (quantitative), determined by the project aims that run across all projects. The theoretical thrust leads the project, despite the fact that there may be qualitative and/or quantitative projects within the same research program. A theoretical framework for multiple-method study holds the entire research program together. As each project is conducted, the framework may be revisited and even revised, but it serves to hold the project together with a common goal. A third article, combining results of the first two projects, is then published.

Let us discuss each mixed-method design in detail.

Qualitatively Driven Mixed-Method Design

Qualitatively driven designs are inductive. They consist of a *core project* that is a major qualitative method: grounded theory, ethnography, phenomenology, narrative inquiry, and so forth. These studies are conducted as a complete project and are publishable alone. However, what makes the project a mixed-method design is that there are some aspects of the study question that are not accessible to the core qualitative study. This additional data may be either qualitative or quantitative and is called the supplemental component. If a qualitative supplement combined with a qualitative core, so there are two sets of qualitative data, this is also mixed-method design. The two components may be a different level of analysis, or contain different types of qualitative analysis, or different data sets, and this is known as a QUAL–*qual* design. For instance, it may be conversational analysis data that will illustrate some aspect of the qualitative project. If quantitative data is used, QUAN–*quan* design, the supplement may consist of scores from the core sample itself that provide quantitative data (how much, how far, how often) that further illustrate the qualitative data. If the core component is quantitative (QUAN), the supplementary is qualitative (QUAN–qual) or quantitative (QUAN–*quan*). The supplementary components may be conducted at the same time as the core project (simultaneous mixed-method design) or follow the core project, to answer a question that has arisen during the conduct of the qualitative project (i.e., sequential mixed-method design).

Quantitatively Driven Mixed-Method Design

The primary research question for a quantitatively driven mixed-method design is a deductive theory-testing question. The core project is a standard quantitative research study. However, in designing the project, the researcher becomes aware that the project is inadequately scoped using quantitative methods alone: For instance, there may be some aspect that the researcher cannot incorporate into the quantitative design because not enough is known about that particular area. In this case, the researcher will add a qualitative supplement, such as questions or observations of participants pertaining to that area QUAN–*qual*. Because the study is quantitatively driven, the core quantitative project forms the basis of the results with the qualitative supplemental data providing additional description. If the researcher needs to add additional quantitative information, perhaps from a different data set, the project is conceived as a QUAN–*quan* design.

Theoretical Frameworks for Qualitatively Driven Mixed-Method Research

These frameworks follow the conventions of inductive frameworks in that a theoretical context may be used to provide justification for the inquiry. Again, as with qualitative research, these frameworks should not guide the inquiry to the extent that they direct the researcher toward "seeing" but rather sensitize the researcher to what may be possibly present. Processes of reflexivity are extremely important so that if some aspect arises during qualitative inquiry that would be amenable to measurement, and make the research stronger, such measures should be added as a supplementary component.

As with all inductive research, the researcher is "diving into" the area, and if questions arise during the conduct of the core component, the researcher may add a supplemental component to the end of the study. However, as the supplemental project may not be anticipated at the beginning of the study, it may not necessarily be included in the preliminary theoretical framework.

Theoretical Frameworks for Quantitatively Driven Mixed-Method Research

In contrast to the qualitative theoretical frameworks, the quantitatively driven theoretical framework for mixed-method research must be well developed. According to the criteria presented in Chapter 25, the quantitative method proposed must fit the aim of the study and be well developed. The theory must be explicated, logically developed, and persuasive. The researcher should list variables, justify measurement, and diagram the study.

The researcher must also be aware of the need to conduct a mixed-method study. The researcher will be aware that there are some data that will increase the validity of the study but cannot be included in the quantitative design. Thus, the rationale for including a qualitative supplementary component is justified at this time and within the study.

EXAMPLE OF QUALITATIVELY DRIVEN MIXED-METHOD DESIGN: PATTERNS OF ATTENDING

One of the most common qualitatively driven mixed-method designs is derived from human ethology, an approach used to explore behaviors. It is conducted in two phases: The first phase is qualitative, in which close observation assists in determining the *behaviors of interest*, definitions of these behaviors are developed, and a microanalytic coding system developed. The behaviors are then coded using some time frame: continuous movements or some set time frame. Videotaping permits microanalytic coding as the movement may be slowed or even stopped; dialogue transcribed; and field notes recorded. It is therefore a qualitatively driven, QUAL→*quan* design.

The quantitative phase uses multivariate statistics to explore relationships between clusters of variables and actions, confirming hypothesized relationships and enabling the determination of the more significant behavioral clusters. In this way, theoretical statements may be developed.[1] The result is a very strong theory developed from micro-observations confirmed quantitatively.

In Chapter 26, Joan Bottorff uses this QUAL→*quan* design (see Figure VI.1) to study the nurse–patient interactions in an oncology unit. Her results, "Patterns of Attending" form a very strong model for providing care.

---

[1] A second example for QUAL→*quan* was used to explore infants' responses to pain. Conducted at a time in which it was believed that infants' neurological systems were too immature to feel pain, this is an incredibly important nursing study (Côté & Morse, 1991).

REFERENCES

Côté, J. L., & Morse, J. M. (1991). The pain experience of the post-operative newborn. *Journal of Advanced Nursing, 16*, 378–387.

Morse, J. M., & Niehaus, L. (2009). *Mixed method design: Principles and procedures.* Walnut Creek, CA: Left Coast.

Wikipedia. (n.d.). Apples and oranges. Retrieved from https://en.wikipedia.org/wiki/Apples_and_oranges

FURTHER READING

Morse, J. M., & Neihaus, L. (2009). *Mixed-method design: Principles and procedures.* Walnut Creek, CA: Left Coast Press.

Morse, J. M. (2016). *The essentials of qualitatively-driven mixed-method designs.* New York, NY: Routledge.

Joan L. Bottorff

DEVELOPING THEORY USING MIXED METHODS: PATTERNS OF ATTENDING IN NURSING

> *The amount of relief and comfort experienced by the sick after the skin has been carefully washed and dried, is one of the commonest observations made at a sick bed.*
>
> —Nightingale (1860, p. 93)

Caregiving in nursing is a complex phenomenon. Descriptions of nurse caregiving as a process of interaction began with early theorists (Orlando, 1961; Peplau, 1952; Travelbee, 1966; Wiedenbach, 1964). In response, researchers began to describe, operationalize, and measure nursing interactions. In 1977, Diers and Schmidt classified the rapidly expanding research on nurse–patient interaction (NPI) as: (a) descriptive or correlational studies, (b) studies that measure the indices of nursing using hypothetical interactions, and (c) studies that describe or evaluate nursing interaction using conceptual frameworks and measurement tools from other disciplines (Diers & Schmidt, 1977). Some researchers recognized the problems inherent in using borrowed frameworks and instruments to capture relevant clinical data. To obtain findings more germane to nursing theory and practice, researchers were challenged to design instruments and studies specifically for examining NPIs.

Investigators continued to study those aspects of NPI that were quantifiable using predominately deductive approaches with increasingly sophisticated techniques. However, the results were often discouraging. In general, although some researchers continued to provide indications of the positive effects of various types of NPIs, others reported that NPIs were seriously limited in practice and that nurses lacked effective communication skills (Bottorff & Morse, 1994). Although many factors influence the quality of NPIs in clinical practice, two important limitations of this research must be considered: First, the focus of this research has been on single channels of communication (verbal or nonverbal) despite the fact that a multichannel perspective is necessary to capture the variations in interactions. Second, it is unlikely that insightful accounts of the unique styles of interaction that are characteristic of nursing practice can be obtained using deductive accounts when the context that influences NPIs is ignored, the complexity of encounters is not taken into account, and research is based on communication theories that are derived from contexts that differ from nursing practice in important ways.

Influenced by the acceptance of qualitative research methods, researchers began to explore NPIs using a variety of new approaches. These methods compensated for the limitations of earlier studies in that more comprehensive accounts of the dynamics of the interaction and context are facilitated and a means for obtaining insight from both the patient's and nurse's perspective is provided. The result was that in the early 1990s, descriptions of NPIs that are closer to the day-to-day realities of nursing and the identification of previously unrecognized competencies emerged (Estabrooks, 1989; Estabrooks & Morse, 1992; Hunt & Montgomery-Robinson, 1987; Hunt, 1991; McIntosh, 1981; Morse, 1991; Pepler, 1991; Pepler & Lynch, 1991).

Developments in audiovisual technology provided the opportunity to capture rich permanent records of NPIs that could be obtained for subsequent frame-by-frame, and real and slow-time analysis. This made it possible to simultaneously analyze a wide range of verbal and nonverbal behaviors. The use of audiovisual technology along with qualitative research methods enabled a comprehensive approach to the study of NPIs, and the means to study the details of the encounters to advance the development of theory regarding NPIs. The purpose of this chapter is to describe a study that took advantage of these developments to develop a model of NPI and in doing so demonstrate the value of qualitatively driven, mixed-method approaches in theory building in nursing.

THE STUDY OF NURSE–PATIENT INTERACTIONS

The focus of this study was on exploring and describing NPIs that involved touch episodes. Video-ethological methods were used to inductively identify the types of NPIs in which touching behaviors were used (Bottorff, 1994a). Ethology is a method used to identify complex behavioral patterns through systematic observation and description under natural conditions (Morse & Bottorff, 1990), characteristically beginning with an inductive phase. Ethologists often build on this phase to conduct more structured deductive and quantitative investigations. The objectives of this mixed-method study using this approach were to: (a) inductively derive a comprehensive description of NPIs from naturalistic videotaped observations, (b) to verify and extend qualitative descriptions of NPIs by conducting semistructured interviews with patients and nurses using videotaped data to prompt discussion, (c) to develop a detailed coding system based on the qualitative findings to capture significant verbal and nonverbal behaviors in NPIs, (d) to evaluate the use of the coding scheme to determine whether the patterns of NPIs can be identified in different samples of NPIs, and (e) to demonstrate the utility of the identified patterns of NPIs by exploring variations in response to patient state and transitions in patterns of NPIs.

Capturing Routine Nurse–Patient Interactions

Data Collection

First, videotaped data of NPIs were collected. To maximize observations of various types of interactions involving touch, patients who required a high proportion of nurse–patient contact (e.g., patients who experienced pain and nausea) were invited to participate. The convenience sample included 8 cancer patients (three females, five males) and 32 nurses who were assigned to provide care (Bottorff, 1994b). Informed consent was obtained from all participants who were told that the observations would focus on verbal and nonverbal behaviors of nurses without emphasizing the researchers' interest in touch.

Videotaping was done in a private room on an active treatment oncology ward. The cameras ran continuously at slow speed for 72 hours for each patient. Taping was only discontinued for brief periods at the request of patients (usually to provide privacy during particular caretaking activities) or when staff members who did not wish to be involved in the study entered the room. A total of 1,085 interactional units delineated by the entry and exit of the nurse (average duration 1.9 min) were collected. Tape-recorded unstructured interviews with patients and selected nurses were conducted to complement the videotaped, observational data. One nurse who cared for each patient was selected to be interviewed to explore segments of the videotape in which he or she appeared to elicit perceptions of the interaction and, specifically, the purpose of the nurse–patient touch and the perceived effect of the touch. Following completing of the videotaping, eight nurses were interviewed. With the exception of the first two patients who were part of a pilot study and were not interviewed, the remaining six patients participated in a similar interview 3 to 10 days after each was videotaped.

Data Analysis

Data analysis of the videotapes began with the development of an ethogram, which is a detailed textual description of the behavior patterns under study were identified qualitatively (Eibl-Eibesfeldt, 1989; Martin & Bateson, 1986). Videotaped interactions were played and replayed to observe major behavior clusters in interactions involving touch. The researchers assumed an inquiring attitude toward the data in order to delineate distinct interactional segments, asking themselves questions such as, "What is going on here?", "How does this interaction differ from that interaction?", and "What are the characteristics of this interaction?" Intensive examination of the videotaped interactions enabled other instances of similar interaction patterns to be located. Specific recurring behavioral patterns were then delineated by continuing to compare and contrast interactional segments. For example, it was noted that NPIs differed by the amount of nurse–patient proximity, the degree to which the nurse focused on a patient and caretaking tasks, and the way in which patients participated in the interactions. Units of interaction that shared particular characteristics were grouped and the properties of each group were listed and described. In addition to the characteristics of behavior, the descriptions included interpretations of the functions, conditions, and consequences of each behavior and variations in techniques.

Four patterns of behavior, referred to as "types of attending" were identified as the structural units of NPI (Bottorff & Morse, 1994). These patterns were *doing more*, *doing for*, *doing with*, and *doing tasks*. The types of attending used by a nurse could change several times during a single interaction simulated by a patient's behavior. Factors influencing type of attending were the perceived needs of the patient, the nature of the task, time constraints, and the sensitivity of the nurse. With the exception of *doing for*, the types of attending were not task specific. The characteristics of each type of attending were distinct in terms of focus, eye gaze, intent, nurse–patient relationship, time/task ratio, nature of the dialogue, tone of voice, and type of touch (see Table 26.1). Although nurses and patients were not asked to comment on the types of attending during interviews, data from these interviews provided some support for this classification and insight into these types of attending from the perspective of both patients and nurses. Transcripts of verbal interactions captured on videotapes were used to demonstrate how the characteristics of each type of attending were played out in everyday interactions between nurses and patients. Although these examples are limited to the extent that they emphasize the verbal interaction and underplay the contribution of nonverbal behaviors, they provide helpful exemplars. Five types of touch were also identified and described: comforting touch, connecting touch, working touch, orienting touch, and social touch (Bottorff, 1993).

A MODEL OF NURSE–PATIENT INTERACTIONS

The four types of attending identified from the videotaped interactions provide a model for describing the interactional context of the touch events (Bottorff & Morse, 1994). Each is described below.

TABLE 26.1
Types of Attending

	TYPE OF ATTENDING			
CHARACTERISTIC	**DOING MORE**	**DOING FOR**	**DOING WITH**	**DOING TASKS**
NURSES' BEHAVIORS				
Nurse's focus	Primarily focused on patient as a person	Focused on the patient	Focused equally on task and patient	Focused on task to exclusion of patient
Nurse's eye gaze	Frequent sustained eye gaze toward patient's face	Very few periods of sustained eye gaze	Occasional periods of sustained eye gaze	No sustained eye gaze, may be occasional, brief glances toward patient
Tone of nurse's voice	Concerned	Conversational	Conversational or concerned	Rote, uninterested, absent-minded
Type of touch	Comforting, connecting, and working touch	Working touch and some connecting and social touch	Working touch with some orienting and connecting touch	Little physical contact, limited working touch
BEHAVIORS DESCRIBING THE INTERACTION				
Nurse's intent	To understand patient's experience of illness/treatment	To give patient opportunity to direct own care	To involve patient in care	To get job done
Time/task ratio	More time spent with patient than simply required to complete task	Time spent with patient determined by time required to complete task; however, nurse is not hurried	Time spent with patient determined by time required to complete task, although extra time may be spent with patient at times	Time with patient determined by time required to complete task, nurse appears hurried
Nurse–patient dialogue	Intensive or in-depth discussion about care, with emotionally supportive statements by the nurse	Superficial talk about care or social talk	Two-way discussions about care, inquiries about patient needs, instructions	Silence or very brief task-related communication with patient
Relationship	Engaged	Helper/helpee	Cooperative	Distanced

Adapted from Bottorff and Morse (1994).

Doing More

The first pattern of behavior, *doing more* (making contact), was a type of attending in which the nurse "did something" beyond what is usually required to complete care. It was characterized by an engaged relationship between a patient and nurse, and was used when the nurse was making contact or trying to "reach out" to the patient. The nurse might have been physically closer or have taken more time than was usually required, although attending interactions of this type may be brief. This type of attending could occur with or without a task and was characterized by an intense focus on the patient. The nurse's attention often provided the patient with an opportunity to confide in the nurse. Videotaped observations indicated that this type of attending was also characterized by concerned acknowledgment of patient concerns and symptoms, and an attempt to understand a patient's experience in order to provide more care. It was frequently, but not always, associated with patient distress or discomfort.

As nurses were providing care, working touch occurred frequently in all four types of attending. However, in *doing more*, the tone of the interaction was different. It was more intimate, and more focused on the patient, as evidenced by the use of comforting, connecting, and orienting touch along with working touch. The following excerpt from one interaction provides an example of a *doing more* type of attending.

> [The nurse begins to rub powder on radiation area on patient's neck]
>
> Nurse: It's sore? Is it sore now?
> Patient: No. It just kind of burns.
> Nurse: Yeah
> Patient: Burns, burns and itchy. [Pause] Oh well. Just two shots to go.
> Nurse: Mm hmm. How many, how long has it been?
> Patient: Thirty-four shots.
> Nurse: You've sure done well.
> Patient: Yeah. Considering.
> Nurse: Mm hmm. [She continues to rub powder on patient's neck and lower face.]
> Patient: I didn't think it would be this bad. I guess maybe a lotta people are maybe worse off than I am when it comes to that.
> Nurse: That's right. There are. There's always something, isn't it? There's always someone worse off than yourself.
> Patient: Yeah. Yeah. I'm not gonna complain. I've never complained since the day . . .

Nurse: I bet you haven't.
Patient: No. [pause] What for?
Nurse: Ah, well sometimes it makes you feel good. It makes
          me feel good sometimes.
Patient: Yeah. Well thank you for the opportunity. That
          sounds strange but, that's O.K.

During this brief interaction, the nurse made herself available to the patient, showed concern, and provided support and encouragement. She provided the opportunity for the patient to express feelings by allowing him to complain indirectly by "not complaining."

Interview data about similar interactions with patients fit with a *doing more* type of attending. These data underlined the importance of focusing on the patient as well as the factors that influenced engagement with patients.

I think it is really important to try to direct as much as you can
towards them [patients] . . . and I know in nursing it's really
hard because you have so many demands . . . . You've got to be
careful you don't get caught up in nursing technicalities.

The engaged interaction that was characteristic of *doing more* was often referred to by nurses as being "close" to patients. Nurses identified the following factors that influenced how close they were able to get to patients: how well they knew the patient, how comfortable the patient was with them, the intimacy of the nursing procedure that they provided, their workload, whether the patient had any immediate family to support them, and the level of patient distress. Interview data with patients provided evidence that patients recognized and appreciated this type of personalized care.

Doing For

The second type of attending, *doing for*, was evident when the nurse was primarily occupied in responding to patient requests and needs that were not treatment-related. It was characterized by a personalized approach to assistance. It often involved extras, such as organizing the patient's room so that things were in easy reach. However, the time a nurse spent with the patient was limited to that necessary to complete a task. These activities sometimes led to interactions in which a pleasant, considerate nurse attempted to understand a patient's personal experience of illness, but these interactions were not part of *doing for*. *Doing for* attending was characterized by the use of working and connecting touch, although comforting and orienting touch occurred in rare instances.

The following excerpt reflects the type of interaction that was characteristic of *doing for*:

[Nurse tides up room a little and helps patient pull his shirt down.]

Patient: That's a beautiful day out there today.
Nurse: It's crisp, but it's nice.
Patient: Oh boy.
Nurse: And I will get a little thing for you to spit the tooth-paste in, O.K.?
Patient: Yeah. Right.
           [Nurse returns with a kidney basin]
Nurse: There ya be.
           [Nurse tidies up room a bit more.]
Nurse: Is there anything else for now, or . . . ?
Patient: Uh, nope.
Nurse: O.K.

Here the dialogue was more superficial and focused on the procedures or the assistance being given to a patient rather than on a patient's feelings, although there was opportunity for friendly social talk, for example, about the weather. In *doing for*, the dialogue served as a distraction and diversion from illness.

In the interviews, nurses talked about trying to be "more personable and friendly" by doing "a lot of little things" for patients. They tried to keep the patients' surroundings neat and uncluttered, put things within easy reach, helped them find comfortable positions, assisted with their grooming, provided extras such as colourful quilts, rubbed their legs or back, or just took time to chat. Nurses explained that during these interactions they tried to give patients as much control as possible, a point that some nurses believed was very important considering that much of the time patients had very little control over the care they were receiving. Patients appreciated the friendly way nurses did things for them and the time, no matter how short, that nurses spent "just chatting."

Doing With

The third type of attending, *doing with*, was evident when nurses focused equally on the task and patient. This type of attending was characterized by a willingness to work cooperatively with patients. For example, the nurse may have actively engaged a patient by seeking or attending to his or her opinions, thoughts, and perceptions. The nurse often used eye gaze to focus on the patient and reinforce interest in the patient; however, the gaze might have been broken to attend to activities or tasks. In this type of interaction the patient was alert and able to cooperate. The nurse was friendly and used a tone of voice that was conversational. In this type of attending, working touch predominated, although orienting touch was most likely of all the other touches to be used along with working touches. Connecting touches occurred less often than orienting touch and comforting touch was seldom used.

In the following excerpt, the patient had requested a hot pack for abdominal discomfort and the nurse returned with the hot pack and a sphygmomanometer:

Nurse: Feeling any better?
Patient: Oh yeah. Some yeah.
Nurse: Need this? [referring to the hot pack]
Patient: Oh, ya. It's just, just ah, it comes upon you, eh?
       [The nurse applies hot pack to patient's abdomen.]
Nurse: Just have to take your blood pressure and
       temperature.
       [The nurse starts to put on the BP cuff.]
Nurse: When did this last happen?
Patient: Oh, it happens, well, almost every day.
Nurse: You think it's related to your feeding?
Patient: Oh yeah.
Nurse: You think it's because you're getting overloaded?
       [The nurse proceeds to take patient's blood pressure.]
Nurse: It's O.K. anyway.
Patient: Oh yeah. It's just I feel kinda finicky. [The nurse nods
       and removes BP cuff. The patient rubs his forehead.]
Nurse: Feel as if you want to throw up?
Patient: No
Nurse: No? Just sweaty.

The verbal interaction was accompanied by sustained eye gaze, and although physical contact was limited to that associated with nurse care procedures, the touches were substantially more than just a few brief contracts. For example, when the nurse placed the blood pressure cuff on the patient's arm, she provided extra support by cradling the arm.

Nurses believed it was important to keep patients informed about issues related to their care, and at the same time, they encouraged patients to keep them informed about how they were feeling, how the treatments were affecting them, or the effectiveness of symptom management strategies. This sense of working together was most clearly reflected in the *doing with* type of attending. Some patients indicated they could recognize whether the nurses were sincere in the concern they showed by the degree to which and the way that nurses involved them in their care. At times, their comfort depended on it. For example, one patient with a pathological fracture of the hip was frequently asked about how moving from bed to chair should be done. Even though she would let nurses know how it worked best, she still appreciated being informed about the nurse's plans for the next step.

They tell you exactly what they're going to do and why they're
going to do it . . . It makes you feel so much more comfortable
and confident, that you know everything's going to be all right
. . . [If they do not tell you] it makes you nervous because . . .
you sort of tense up and wonder how much it is going to hurt.

Doing Tasks

In this last type of attending, *doing tasks*, the nurse focused on equipment,
treatment, and getting the job done. This type of attending was characterized
by an indifferent, apathetic, or routinized approach. The nurse appeared to be
preoccupied with the task at hand or other commitments. There was little or
no attempt to engage the patient; in fact, patient's comments or concerns were
ignored sometimes in an attempt to concentrate on the task. The nurse spoke
in a rote, uninterested, absent-minded way to the patient. This type of attending was often characterized by no eye gaze or only brief glances toward the
patient. The nurse appeared to hurry, and the time spent with the patient was
determined by the length of time required to do the task. When nurses
touched patients during this type of attending, it was predominantly working touch. Connecting and orienting touches were seldom used, and comforting touch did not occur at all.

The exclusive focus on tasks, often to the exclusion of the patient, is
reflected in the following excerpt. In this example, a nurse focused on transferring a patient from the mobilizer to her bed, an interaction which was
classified as *doing tasks*:

[The patient is in the hallway on the mobilizer. The nurse comes
into the room to make sure there is a clear pathway to the bed.]

Patient: I hope my lunch won't be cold.
Nurse: We have a microwave.
Patient: I have been through this quite a few times. Either my
          breakfast or my lunch ends up [cold].
Nurse: That seems to happen.
Patient: Oh yeah.
Nurse: Unfortunately . . . .
Patient: No problem.
          [Silence as the nurse slowly moved patient into the
          room and then put down side rails.]
Nurse: Now does this foam and everything go . . .
Patient: They're all attached. Yes. Everything goes with me.
          Quite a bundle.
Nurse: Yeah.
          [Silence as nurse got everything ready for the transfer
          back to the bed.]

Patient: I'm probably due for a breakthrough soon. It's that
terrible pain in my leg and shoulders.
[Silence as the nurse continued to prepare to transfer
patient. She checked over the controls and then gave
them a try. Nothing worked.]

Nurse: What am I doing wrong?
[Nurse checked over mobilizer, put side rail up and
exited the room.]

While at times a focus on tasks was critical, it seemed to distance the
nurse from the patient; consequently nurses were less sensitive to patient
concerns or distress. The distancing is evident in the verbal interaction in this
example as well as in the accompanying nonverbal behaviors, including the
lack of any sustained eye contact with the patient and the absence of any
physical contact except for brief accidental bumps as the nurse checked
bedding on the mobilizer.

During interviews with nurses, some of their comments could be linked
to the exclusive focus on tasks that is characteristic of this type of attending,
labeled *doing tasks*. They legitimized this focus in several ways, the first being
in relation to workload. Nurses explained that some days all they had time to
do was to get the work done. Nurses also indicated that when procedures
become routine for patients and they were no longer apprehensive about
them, the procedures became something that just had to be done. In these
instances, explanations or emotional support were viewed as no longer necessary. What nurses did not mention was that sometimes the nature of the
task demanded their full attention. They also focused on tasks when patients
were asleep or when they did not want to interrupt conversations with visitors. The type of touch was also different when nurses were concentrating on
the task *as a task*. At these times, nurses were less likely to give an extra caress,
stroke, or tap; instead, skin-to-skin contact was limited to that required to
complete the task.

DEVELOPMENT OF A CODING SCHEME TO EXPLORE
PATTERNS OF NPI

Using the descriptions of the types of attending and touch, important behaviors were identified that could be included in a coding scheme (Bottorff,
1994a). Because some of the behaviors of interest were used in prior observational schedules (Porter, Redfern, Wilson-Barnett, & Le May, 1986; Weiss,
1990) these were assessed; and when appropriate, some components of previous observation schedules were adapted for use in this study. To be sure that
meaningful patterns of behavior could be identified the unit of analysis was
type of attending. From initial observations of the videotapes, it was noted

that during any one interaction the type of attending used by nurses could change several times. Therefore, each interaction was divided into attending units based on the number of times the nurse changed the type of attending he or she used. The length of each attending unit varied from 30 sec to several minutes.

Mutually exclusive and exhaustive codes were developed and explicitly defined for the categories of behavior represented in attending units (see Box 26.1). These included six categories of behavior that described the

---

BOX 26.1. SUMMARY OF CODING SCHEME

1. Identifying codes: patient code, patient sex, type of caregiver, staff code, observer code
2. Type of attending: doing more, doing for, doing with, doing tasks, other
3. Categories describing the interactional context

   a. Proximity to patient: unable to determine; intimate zone: close; intimate zone: not close; personal zone; and social/public zone
   b. Nurse–patient dialogue: unable to determine, silence, emotional support, care talk, self-talk, social talk, other
   c. Nurse activity: unable to determine, adjusting environment, checking, giving medications, nonpharmacological symptom management, starting/maintaining intravenous and subcutaneous sites, caring for skin, assisting with dressing, grooming and toileting, assisting and supporting movement, providing environment for leisure activities, approaching the patient, departing/leaving patient, visiting, other
   d. Eye gaze: unable to determine, prolonged direct eye gaze, inferred eye gaze, brief glance, or no eye gaze
   e. Patient condition: unable to determine, enduring physical pain/distress, enduring emotional pain/distress, no apparent distress and awake, no apparent distress and eyes closed, other
   f. Others in room: unable to determine, no one else in room, visitors in room, other nursing staff in room, other

4. Categories describing the touch event

   a. Initiator: able to determine, caregiver, patient, mutual, simultaneous combination
   b. Location of touch: unable to determine, face, head, neck, fingers, palm/back of hand, forearm, elbow, upper arm, shoulder, upper trunk, lower trunk, thigh, knee, lower leg, foot/toes, other
   c. Form of touch: unable to determine, nonmoving, pressing, palpating, rubbing holding/grasping sticking (i.e., a momentary contact), wrapping, other
   d. Intensity: unable to determine, weak, moderate, firm
   e. Verbal comment associated with touch (by initiator): unable to determine, no talk, talk related to touch, talk unrelated to touch, talk related to one or two types of simultaneous touch
   f. Type of touch: unable to determine, comforting touch, connecting touch, working touch, social touch, orienting touch, other
   g. Duration: length of contact to nearest second

Source: Bottorff (1994a).

interactional context (i.e., proximity to patient, nurse–patient dialogue, nurse activity, nurse's eye gaze, patient condition, and whether others were in the room) and seven categories of behavior that described the touch event (i.e., initiator, location of touch, form of touch, intensity, verbal comment associated with touch, type of touch, duration of touch). Codes were used to represent mutually exclusive (only one can be scored at any one time) and exhaustive (no time can pass without a codable event taking place) classes of behavior within each category. Because codes represented discrete behaviors, patterns of concurrent and sequential behaviors could be represented. In addition, by using mutually exclusive and exhaustive codes, the onset of one behavior marks the offset of another; thus the duration and frequency of all behaviors could be captured within each attending unit.

Coding Procedure

The procedure for using the observational schedule was to view each videotaped interaction at least twice. During the first pass, the observer identified the type(s) of attending and noted where touch events occurred on the transcript of the interaction. During the second pass, using continuous coding, types of attending were recorded with their respective start times. When a type of attending that included one or more touch events commenced, detailed continuous coding for the remaining dimensions of the coding scheme began. In essence, this required that coding be initiated the exact second that any behavior of interest changed. Times recorded on the videotapes (in hours, minutes, and seconds) were used for this purpose. Observers repeatedly reviewed segments (often in slow motion or using frame advance) in which behaviors of short duration occurred or several behaviors were changing at once in order to identify precise start times and/or to determine the exact nature of the behaviors being observed. Detailed continuous coding concluded when the nurses exited the room or when the type of attending changed and the next unit did not include a touch event. Interactions were coded once by one of three trained nurse observers. Acceptable levels of inter- and intraobserver agreement were established and maintained, and the observers discussed their observations frequently with each other in order to reduce coding errors.

Evaluating the Coding Scheme

Focal observations that could be used to evaluate the observational schedule were sampled in two ways. The first 15 NPIs that clearly represented each type of attending and included touch events were purposefully selected from the total sample of videotaped interactions. This selection method was used to ensure that each of the four types of attending was adequately represented. Four of the 60 interactions were later eliminated because on closer inspection they did not meet selection criteria. The remaining 56 interactions (total duration 236.56 min) were coded. For the purpose of comparison and to evaluate the sensitivity of the measure to the same behaviors in a different sample of NPIs, a second sample of 60 NPIs (total duration 245.71 min) was then selected randomly from the remaining videotaped interactions that included scorable touch events and coded. A total of 116 NPIs were coded. Interactions ranged from 36 sec to 19.16 min, with a mean of 4.18 min (s.d. = 3.45) in data set #1 and 4.08 min (s.d. = 3.62) in data set #2.

To compare patterns of observed behavior in the two samples of NPIs, frequencies (i.e., the number of units of attending in which at least one touch behavior occurred) and the mean total duration of touch in seconds for types of touch were calculated for each sample. In total, only seven social touch events (0.1%) were observed in the interactions selected for coding. Because these touches were most similar to connecting touches, they were combined with these touches for data analysis. As shown in Table 26.1, touch varied with the type of attending in ways that were consistent with the inductively developed model of attending in both study samples. There were some differences between the two samples. The mean time spent touching with any type of touch in units of attending classified as *doing more* was longer in sample #1 (13.6 sec) than in sample #2 (6.5 sec). During the *doing more* types of attending, the total durations of comforting and working touches in sample #1 (17.4 and 22.8 sec, respectively) on average were longer than in sample #2 (10.8 and 4.2 sec, respectively). In part, this may be explained by the relatively small number of units classified as *doing more* in sample #2 (n = 7 or 6% of the total number of observed units of attending). The overall duration of touch when the unit of attending was classified as *doing tasks* was also longer in sample #2 (sample #1= 12.85 sec; sample #2 = 34.20 sec). The difference can be largely attributed to a longer duration of working touch in sample #2 (sample #1 = 13.42 sec; sample #2 = 37.85 sec). The relative proportions of types of attending and types of touch are likely to be more accurately reflected in the randomly selected sample (#2). In both samples, standard deviations are large, suggesting that the scores range widely.

Patterns of Attending, Touch and Nurse Dialogue

Using the combined data set, NPIs were further explored by examining relationships among types of attending, each type of touch and five types of nurse dialogue (silence, emotional support, care talk, talk to self, and social talk; Bottorff, 1992). Several patterns were evident (see Table 26.2). Of all the types of nurse dialogue, care talk had the highest probability of occurring concurrently with each type of touch. Although emotional support had the highest probability of occurring concurrently with comforting touch, it could occur with connecting and working touches; but admittedly, the probabilities were low at .013 and .016, respectively. When the type of attending was considered, the pattern of conditional probabilities for each type of dialogue with

TABLE 26.2
Concurrent Dialogue With Type of Touch and Type of Attending

Types of Attending	COMFORTING					CONNECTING					ORIENTING					WORKING					ALL TYPES				
	n	1	2	3	4*	*n*	1	2	3	4	*n*	1	2	3	4	*n*	1	2	3	4	*n*	1	2	3	4
DOING MORE																									
Frequency	55	14	10	30	1	39	2	1	35	1	2	-	-	2	-	85	10	6	53	16	181	26	17	120	18
Probability**		.26	.18	.55	.12		.06	.03	.90	.03		-	-	1.00	-		.12	.07	.62	.19		.14	.09	.66	.10
DOING FOR																									
Frequency	2	-	-	2	-	17	-	-	7	10	3	-	-	3	-	308	85	9	157	54	327	85	9	169	64
Probability		-	-	1.00	-		-	-	.41	.59		-	-	1.00	-		.28	.03	.51	.18		.26	.03	.52	.20
DOING WITH																									
Frequency	5	1	2	2	-	15	1	-	10	4	25	-	-	25	-	682	165	9	430	78	727	167	11	467	82
Probability		.20	.40	.40	-		.07	-	.67	.27		-	-	1.00	-		.24	.01	.63	.11		.23	.02	.64	.11
DOING TASKS																									
Frequency	-	-	-	-	-	4	1	-	3	-	1	-	-	1	-	394	321	-	72	-	399	322	-	76	1
Probability		-	-	-	-		.25	-	.75	-		-	-	1.00	-		.82	-	.18	-		.81	-	.19	.00
ALL TYPES																									
Frequency	62	15	12	34	1	75	4	1	55	15	31	-	-	31	-	1466	581	24	712	149	1634	600	37	832	165
Probability		.24	.19	.55	.02		.05	.01	.73	.20		-	-	1.00	-		.40	.02	.49	.10		.37	.02	.51	.10

* 1 = silence, 2 = emotional support, 3 = care talk, 4 = social talk; ** row probability.

Source: Bottorff (1992). Reprinted with permission.

all types of touch was most similar for *doing for* and *doing with* types of attending. The pattern for touches occurring in *doing more* types of attending departed from this in that the probability for silence was lower than in the previous types of attending and that emotional support and social talk were equally likely to occur concurrently with touch (although the probabilities were small). Last, in units of attending categorized as *doing tasks*, touches were most likely to occur concurrently with silence (probability = .81), followed by care talk (probability = .19). Emotional support did not ever occur with any touch in this type of attending and social talk only occurred once.

Patterns of Attending and Touch in Response to Patient Distress

Three categories describing patient state were coded: uncomfortable, comfortable—eyes open, and comfortable—eyes closed. When the two data sets were combined and all types of touch were considered in relation to all types of attending, the probability of touch events occurring concurrently with a comfortable, awake patient was the highest (probability = .63), followed by an uncomfortable, awake patient state (probability = .32; Bottorff, 1992). This pattern was consistent for all touch types, except for comforting touch. If the touch was comforting, it was most likely to occur concurrently with an uncomfortable patient state (probability = .83). When the context in which the touch took place was considered, in the units of attending classified as *doing more* and *doing with*, the probability that touch occurred concurrently with an uncomfortable patient state was higher than in the other units of attending (probabilities = .44 and .41, respectively).

Transitions in NPIs

The number of units of attending within each interaction ranged from 1 to 10 (mean = 2.36). Using a combination of both samples, 152 transitions from one type of attending to another were identified (Bottorff & Varcoe, 1995). Transitions originated within each of the four types of attending: *doing more* (n = 13), *doing for* (n = 17), *doing with* (n = 65), and *doing tasks* (n = 57). From these origins, transitions were made to each other type of attending with one exception (*doing for* to *doing more*). The number of transitions between types of attending varied from 3 instances of *doing more* to *doing for*, to 47 instances of *doing with* to *doing tasks*. Transitions were grouped according to type (e.g., *doing with* to *doing for* were grouped) for comparative analysis using videotaped observations. These transitions were explored and described to determine the usefulness of the types of attending in extending our understanding of NPIs.

Three transition patterns were identified (see Table 26.3). Weaving proficiency with presence was the most predominant pattern, and was

TABLE 26.3
Patterns in Transitions in Nurse–Patient Interactions

TRANSITION PATTERN	TYPES OF ATTENDING	CONTEXT	INTENT
Weaving proficiency with presence	*Doing with* ⇔ *Doing tasks* *Doing tasks* ⇔ *Doing for* *Doing for* ⇔ *Doing with*	Provision of treatment-related care or assistance	Common work pattern for prevision of routine care that: • Engages the patient • Provides foundation for nurse–patient relationship
Sensitive responses	*Doing tasks* or *Doing with* → *Doing more*	Patient need evidenced by: • Anticipated or actual cues of distress • Cues indicating need for teaching or support	Response to individual, immediate needs that interrupts common work pattern to allow: • Further assessment • Promise or offer of assistance • Direct intervention
Creating openings	→ *Doing with* or *Doing more*	Anticipation of patient needs	Provision of opportunity for patient to express concerns, ask questions, or obtain assistance to: • Provide appropriate intervention • Ensure leave taking is not premature • Further develop nurse–patient relationship

Adapted from Bottorff and Varcoe (1995).

punctuated with a second pattern of transition that allowed sensitive response to immediate needs, and a third pattern of transition that created openings for patients to express concerns, ask questions, or to obtain assistance or information. In some instances apparent patient cues did not result in transitions expected based on the patterns identified. These were described as missed opportunities.

Weaving Proficiency With Presence
The most common pattern involved the nurse working simultaneously to complete a task and engage with the patient, with periodic shifts of central focus between the two. This pattern involved three of the four types of attending. In this pattern *doing tasks* alternated with either *doing with* or *doing for*.

Most of the NPIs were within the context of treatment-related care and were, therefore, characterized by a series of shifts back and forth between *doing tasks* and *doing with*. For example, a nurse actively engaged a patient by asking about her pain and then shifted focus to fixing a drainage tubing. Rather than being an abrupt change, this transition represented a shift in central focus from the patient to the task, with attention on the patient being merely suspended for brief time. This "pause" in the interaction was sometimes related to the nurse's need to refocus on the task at hand. Less frequently, patients appeared to suspend their participation. For example, in one situation the patient seemed to have exhausted his questions and stopped talking.

The shift back to *doing with* was initiated by either the patient or the nurse. While fixing the drainage tubing, the nurse re-engaged the patient by asking if the tubing was leaking, reflecting a change in attending from *doing tasks* to *doing with* initiated by the nurse. In another instance, a patient initiated the transition by asking a nurse about his blood pressure as she was taking vital signs.

Transitions between *doing tasks* and *doing for* were similar except that they occurred in the context of the provision of assistance with activities of daily living rather than treatment-related activities. Furthermore, these transitions did not appear unexpected in the context of the particular task and, because of the relatively brief duration of the *doing tasks* type of attending, did not seem to substantially disrupt the continuity of the interaction.

A variation of this common pattern of transition occurred between *doing for* or *doing with* types of attending. These transitions represented natural changes in attending that accompany the shifts between assistance in daily living and treatment-related tasks, discussions, or both. For example, after discussing the effects of morphine while giving an injection, the nurse offered to give the patient a back rub. At this time the nature of their interaction changed, reflecting a transition from *doing with* to *doing for*. Toward the end of the back rub, the nurse responded to questions the patient posed about her medications, representing a shift back to *doing with*.

The transitions back and forth between *doing tasks* and either *doing with* or *doing for* and the transitions between *doing with* and *doing for* were important patterns that characterized nurses' work such that patients were engaged, at least episodically, during the provision of care. These patterns provided a foundation for the development of nurse–patient relationships. Furthermore, the patterns allowed nurses to integrate expertise associated with nursing presence with the provision of prescribed treatments and assistance with activities of daily living in a proficient manner.

Sensitive Responses

A second pattern of transition was characterized by a change to *doing more* from either a *doing tasks* or *doing with* type of attending. This pattern of transition occurred in response to particular types of patient cues. The majority of cues indicated distress or discomfort, such as grimaces of pain, whimpering, vomiting, shortness of breath, or statements of pain. In a few instances nurses anticipated distress or discomfort associated with particular treatments before patient cues were presented. Alternatively, cues suggesting a need for support or teaching were embedded in patients' statements and social conversation.

The cues appeared to be important triggers following which the nurse intently focused on the patient and his or her concerns. This focus was accompanied by further assessment, a promise or offer of assistance, direct intervention, or both. However, it is interesting to note that patients' verbal statements indicative of a need for support or teaching were often followed by direct intervention rather than any further assessment. For example, when a patient casually remarked that he was trying to do without pain medication, the nurse responded by explaining how the medication worked and that he should not be concerned about addiction. The nurse appeared to intervene without exploring the basis of the patient's statement or validating that the information provided was relevant, although prior knowledge of the patient may have influenced her interaction.

The *doing more* type of attending ended with satisfactory resolution of the immediate concern or by the patient limiting the type of attending by refusing the assistance offered. Rather than creating recurring patterns with other types of attending, transitions to *doing more* reflected a complete unit of sensitive response to patient needs. These transitions to *doing more* were significant in that they allowed nurses to interrupt their common work patterns to respond to specific patient cues that required immediate attention.

Creating Openings

Nurses created openings for patients to express their concerns, ask questions, or to obtain assistance or information. These openings precipitated transitions to a *doing with* type of attending. Usually within the context of preparing to leave the patient's room after providing the patient with some assistance typical of *doing for*, the nurse asked in an open, inviting manner: "Is there anything else?", "Can I get you anything more?", and so forth. These openings could also be based on specific observations or prior knowledge of the individual patient. For example, before leaving a patient who has been nauseated, the nurse offered an antiemetic. This resulted in the patient sharing her concerns about her medication.

There are several significant features of this type of transition. Unlike the transitions labeled as sensitive responses, these transitions usually occurred in the absence of obvious patient distress or discomfort. These proactive openings offered the nurse the opportunity to identify patient needs, invited patients to express concerns and direct care, and further the development of nurse–patient relationships. The openings also served to ensure that leave taking was not premature. In examples that did not include openings before the nurse left, there was a sense of awkwardness or incompleteness in the final phase of the interaction and the patient often called the nurse back to provide additional care.

Missed Opportunities

Although infrequent, nurses sometimes missed or ignored patient cues that in other instances would precipitate a change in the type of attending. Overlooked or ignored patient cues were often subtle, and sometimes missed because they were embedded in social conversation with the nurse. For example, during a conversation involving social banter and laughter about the fact that the nurse was unable to find a pair of pajamas with a fly, a new graduate nurse did not pick up on subtle cues as the patient disclosed that the need for hospitalization for pain control caught him completely off-guard and unprepared. Rather, the nurse continued the conversation on a social level by asking the patient if he had any family in the city. Although it is impossible to speculate what might have transpired if the nurse had picked up on these cues, when this did occur in similar instances with other nurse–patient dyads the type of attending changed to *doing with* or *doing more.* In other cases missed or ignored patient cues were more obvious. For example, in one instance a patient's statement that she needed something for pain was completely ignored by a nurse who was focused on transferring the patient to her bed using an electric mobilizer, a piece of equipment she was unfamiliar with.

Another type of missed opportunity occurred when nurses responded to patient cues with a type of attending that was not optimal. This was exemplified by the situation in which it appeared that the nurses' transition from *doing for* to *doing tasks* was a protective response. In an interaction characterized by a *doing for* type of attending, the patient indicated to the nurse that he had many questions. The nurse responded in a patronizing tone asking if they were "hard" questions and focused on the task she was completing, representing a shift to *doing tasks*. Her subsequent answers to his questions were curt and matter-of-fact. It appeared that as a result of the nurse's response the patient had trouble thinking of his questions and ultimately asked very few. The transition to *doing tasks* appeared to protect the nurse from dealing with potentially difficult issues that face terminal cancer patients and could be viewed as a missed opportunity to engage in either a *doing with* or *doing more* type of attending.

DISCUSSION

An ethological approach in combination with videotaped data facilitated the systematic observation of a wide range of behaviors, in conjunction with important contextual variables, using a qualitative and quantitative mixed-method design to explore NPIs. This provided a unique opportunity to uncover some of the otherwise invisible aspects of nursing practice and to enhance our understanding of important features of NPIs during the provision of routine nursing care.

The model of nurse attending identified in this study provides an important contribution to our understanding of nursing practice and stands in contradiction to the linear problem-solving or textbook examples of interpersonal skills (Bottorff & Varcoe, 1995). Rather nurses involved patients in unique, albeit often episodic ways, as they completed tasks and responded openly to patients' active and passive negation for different types of involvement in relation to a range of activities.

It is evident that the dynamic quality of NPIs is not only an internal experience on the part of the patient or the nurse, but that important differences can be observed by focusing on verbal and nonverbal behaviors of nurses and patients. It is proposed that the four types of attending form the structure of NPIs and, in part, reveal the significance and purpose of an interaction. An important underlying assumption of the concept is that single behaviors do not define a type of attending; instead, they are defined in combinations of behavior that occur across a wide range of activities. By focusing on such behaviors, these types of attending can be recognized irrespective of the individual characteristics of the nurse, patient, or situations.

Individual nurses were also observed to use the full range of attending types and make smooth transitions from one to the other (Bottorff & Varcoe, 1995). The use of attending types and identified patterns of transition would, therefore, seem to be less dependent on the personal characteristics of the nurse than other factors, such as the needs of the patient or work-related demands or levels of expertise. It may be that more experienced nurses are more variant in the use of types of attending than novice nurses. Focused more intently on the tasks to be performed, it is not unreasonable to expect that the novice would be less sensitive or aware of patient cues, less able to intermittently or simultaneously engage with patients as they complete tasks, or to provide appropriate openings for patients to discuss their concerns or needs. However, it appeared that workload and the need for nurses to shield themselves from patient suffering could influence flexibility in attending, potentially lead to missed opportunities, and decrease nurses' effectiveness in meeting patient needs and achieving desired patient outcomes.

Other nurse theorists have proposed typologies of NPI that occur in nursing practice and these have some features in common with the types of attending identified in this research. Data for these theories were obtained through interviews with patients, parents and professionals (Swanson, 1991), nurses (Benner, 1984; Benner & Wrubel, 1989), or from personal experiences and observations in clinical settings (Orem, 1991). The sources of data are significant as they delimit the type of information obtained and shape the resulting descriptions of nursing care. First, from interviews with nurses who were asked to recount critical incidents, Benner (1984) identified and developd the domain of the helping role. Although significant, the eight characteristics inherent in the domain range from the very general (e.g., "the healing relationship: creating a climate for and establishing a commitment to healing") to the more specific (e.g., "providing comfort and communication through touch").

Swanson (1991) developed a mid-range theory of caring from a meta-analysis of three studies in which she interviewed women who miscarried: neonatal intensive care unit (NICU) nurses and parents, and socially-at-risk mothers under the care of public health nurses. Meta-analysis of these three studies revealed five caring processes: knowing, being with, doing for, enabling, and maintaining belief (Swanson, 1991). However, the subprocesses are described as psychosocial dispositions and strategies used by caregivers that may be difficult to identify in the clinical setting. Again, perhaps because it is a theory of caring (focusing on the nurse, rather than the nurse and the patient), these dimensions address only the extraordinary caring practices of nurses and exclude the everyday routine work of nurses that forms the foundation of interactions that may lead to significant caring events. Furthermore, as Swanson's and Benner's typologies do not provide a complete compendium of nurses' work, they are not always useful for documentation of everyday work of nurses. Using videotaped data as observations provided a more "balanced" perspective of the nurse–patient caregiving interaction than reliance on interviews with nurses. In the study reported here, the quantitative verification of the types of attending was an important step in validation.

Nurses were observed to be capable of applying the range of attending types and often used several during any single interaction, suggesting that the use of types of attending is not solely dependent on the personal characteristics of a nurse, but rather is related to the needs of patient or the nurse's work. Others have attributed differences in the ways nurses practice to developing expertise (Benner, 1984; Melia, 1987). For example, it has been observed that the novice practitioner needs to focus on the task and is unable to simultaneously attend to a patient's other needs. However, there may be times when the task is of such complexity or that by its nature requires a nurse's full attention that even the expert may need to fully attend to the task at hand. It is possible, though, that expert nurses may be more sensitive to indications that they need to change their attending style and that the range of skills they use in all types of attending is broader than those of the novice. It is important to note that when used appropriately one type of attending should not be seen as more important or more effective than another type. Nurses were observed using each of these types in various situations to effectively provide patient care. The premise that these patterns of NPIs provide a foundation for the development of nurse–patient relationships is supported by Morse and colleagues' (1997) Comforting Interaction-Relationship Model in which NPIs are proposed as a means by which nurses and patients negotiate and establish therapeutic relationships, and the description of interactional patterns leading to the development of a nurse-patient relationship (Lotzkar & Bottorff, 2001).

Similar observational approaches used to explore naturally occurring NPIs in different contexts have also revealed important insights about caregiving interactions that provide further support for understanding different levels and types of interaction for different goals, and the complexities inherent in managing simultaneous interpersonal and caregiving needs. For example, in describing negotiation in NPIs among home care nurses and their patients, Spiers (2002) described six interactional contexts that demonstrate variations in the strategies nurses use to negotiate mutually acceptable levels of distance or intimacy, self-disclosure, privacy, and information exchange. Four different approaches to nurse–patient collaborations during noninvasive ventilation treatment for hospitalized patients also show how nurses adjust to varying situations and the significance of these different approaches (Sørensen, Frederiksen, Groefte, & Lomborg, 2012). And detailed explorations of styles of NPIs in trauma contexts in which nurses are reacting to events as they unfold have resulted in explicit descriptions of different approaches and the effectiveness of various comforting strategies (Morse, Penrod, Kassab, & Dellasega, 2000; Penrod, Morse, & Wilson, 1999; Proctor, Morse, & Khonsari, 1996). In summary, detailed analysis and microanalysis of NPIs have revealed important insights and support that the notion of unique patterns in NPIs in the context of caregiving and that nurses can use these findings to be more deliberate in their interactions with patients in order to respond in ways that optimize patient outcomes.

As efforts to address health care delivery problems have turned to finding better ways to support patient-centred care, increasing attention has turned to NPIs as a critical element of health care (Hobbs, 2009). The model of nurse attending reinforces the notion that patient-centred care requires NPIs go far beyond the collection of information about patient preferences and caring attitudes. Although understanding the personal and contextual factors that shape both nurses' and patients' capacities for connections in health and illness contexts and encouraging nurses to reflect on their own practice is important in developing communication skills (Doane & Varcoe, 2007), the patterns of attending described in this research provide a framework for reflecting on the subtle and complex dynamics of NPIs that influence caregiving. Further exploration of interaction patterns and relational dynamics is critical to demonstrating the inherent value in NPIs in the context of caregiving and the process by which nurses are able to achieve positive patient outcomes.

SUMMARY

A better understanding of the interaction between patients and nurses continues to be important because NPIs are central to providing nursing care and can influence patient outcomes. Changes from one type of attending to another were meaningful junctures in NPIs. Sensitivity to the different types of attending and patterns of transition, and awareness of nurses' ability to strategize their interactions for therapeutic purposes affords nurses increased opportunities to explore different approaches for different patient care contexts. Determining how effective patterns of attending can be better supported is key to enhancing caregiving interactions and patient outcomes. This work demonstrates that observations of naturally occurring interactions using a mixed method design enables exploration of age-old questions about what nurses actually to advance nursing theory development.

REFERENCES

Benner, P. (1984). *From novice to expert: Excellence and power in clinical nursing practice.* Menlo Park, CA: Addison Wesley.

Benner, P. E., & Wrubel, J. (1989). *The primacy of caring: Stress and coping in health and illness.* Menlo Park, CA: Addison-Wesley.

Bottorff, J. L. (1992). *Nurse–patient interaction: Observations of touch* (Unpublished doctoral dissertation). University of Alberta, Edmonton, AB, Canada.

Bottorff, J. L. (1993). The use and meaning of touch in caring for patients with cancer. *Oncology Nursing Forum, 20*(10), 1531–1538.

Bottorff, J. L. (1994a). Development of an observational instrument to study nurse–patient touch. *Journal of Nursing Measurement, 2*(1), 7–24.

Bottorff, J. L. (1994b). Using videotaped recordings in qualitative research. In J. M. Morse (Ed.), *Critical issues in qualitative research* (pp. 244–261). Newbury Park, CA: Sage.

Bottorff, J. L., & Morse, J. M. (1994). Identifying types of attending: Patterns of nurses' work. *Image: Journal of Nursing Scholarship, 26*(1), 53–60.

Bottorff, J. L., & Varcoe, C. (1995). Transitions in nurse–patient interactions: A qualitative ethology. *Qualitative Health Research, 5*(3), 315–331.

Diers, D. K., & Schmidt, R. L. (1977). Interactional analysis in nursing research. In P. J. Verhonick (Ed.), *Nursing research II* (pp. 77–132). Boston, MA: Little, Brown.

Doane, G. H., & Varcoe, C. (2007). Relational practice and nursing obligations. *Advances in Nursing Science, 30*(3), 192–205. doi:10.1097/01.ANS.0000286619.31398.fc

Eibl-Eibesfeldt, I. (1989). *Human ethology.* New York, NY: Aldine de Gruyter.

Estabrooks, C. A. (1989). Touch: A nursing strategy in the intensive care unit. *Heart & Lung, 18*(4), 392–401.

Estabrooks, C. A., & Morse, J. M. (1992). Toward a theory of touch: The touching process and acquiring a touching style. *Journal of Advanced Nursing, 17*(4), 448–456. doi:10.1111/j.1365-2648.1992.tb01929.x

Hobbs, J. L. (2009). A dimensional analysis of patient-centered care. *Nursing Research, 58*(1), 52–62.

Hunt, M. (1991). Being friendly and informal: Reflected in nurses', terminally ill patients' and relatives' conversations at home. *Journal of Advanced Nursing, 16*(8), 929–938.

Hunt, M., & Montgomery-Robinson, K. (1987). Analysis of conversational interactions. *Recent Advances in Nursing, 17*, 150–168.

Lotzkar, M., & Bottorff, J. L. (2001). An observational study of the development of a nurse-patient relationship. *Clinical Nursing Research, 10*(3), 275–294.

Martin, P. R., & Bateson, P. P. G. (1986). *Measuring behaviour: An introductory guide.* Cambridge, UK: Cambridge University.

McIntosh, J. (1981). Communicating with patients in their own homes. In W. Bridge & J. M. Clark (Eds.), *Communication in nursing* (pp. 101–114). London, UK: HM + M Publishers.

Melia, K. M. (1987). *Learning and working: The occupational socialization of nurses.* London, UK: Travistock.

Morse, J. M. (1991). Negotiating commitment and involvement in the patient-nurse relationship. *Journal of Advanced Nursing, 16*, 455–468.

Morse, J. M., & Bottorff, J. L. (1990). The use of ethology in clinical nursing research. *Advances in Nursing Science, 12*(3), 53–64.

Morse, J. M., Penrod, J., Kassab, C., & Dellasega, C. (2000). Evaluating the efficiency and effectiveness of approaches to nasogastric tube insertion during trauma care. *American Journal of Critical Care, 9*(5), 325–333.

Nightingale, F. (1860). *Notes on nursing: What it is, and what it is not.* New York, NY: D. Appleton and Company.

Orem, D. E. (1991). *Nursing: Concepts of practice* (4th ed.). St. Louis, MO: Mosby.

Orlando, I. J. (1961). *The dynamic nurse–patient relationship: Function, process, and principles.* New York, NY: Putnam.

Penrod, J., Morse, J. M., & Wilson, S. (1999). Comforting strategies used during nasogastric tube insertion. *Journal of Clinical Nursing, 8*, 31–38.

Peplau, H. E. (1952). Interpersonal relations in nursing. *The American Journal of Nursing, 52*(6), 765.

Pepler, C. J. (1991). The messages of touch in nursing homes. *Perspectives (Gerontological Nursing Association Canada), 15*(1), 14–19.

Pepler, C. J., & Lynch, A. (1991). Relational messages of control in nurse–patient interactions with terminally ill patients with AIDS and cancer. *Journal of Palliative Care, 7*(1), 18–29.

Porter, L., Redfern, S., Wilson-Barnett, J., & Le May, A. (1986). The development of an observation schedule for measuring nurse–patient touch, using an ergonomic approach. *International Journal of Nursing Studies, 23*(1), 11–20. doi:10.1016/0020-7489(86)90034-9

Proctor, A., Morse, J. M., & Khonsari, E. S. (1996). Sounds of comfort in the trauma center: How nurses talk to patients in pain. *Social Science & Medicine, 42*(12), 1669–1680. doi:10.1016/0277-9536(95)00298-7

Sørensen, D., Frederiksen, K., Groefte, T., & Lomborg, K. (2012). Nurse–patient collaboration: A grounded theory study of patients with chronic obstructive pulmonary disease on non-invasive ventilation. *International Journal of Nursing Studies, 50*(1), 26–33. doi:10.1016/j.ijnurstu.2012.08.013

Spiers, J. A. (2002). The interpersonal contexts of negotiating care in home care nurse–patient interactions. *Qualitative Health Research, 12*(8), 1033–1057. doi:10.1177/104973202129120430

Swanson, K. M. (1991). Empirical development of a middle range theory of caring. *Nursing Research, 40*(3), 161–165.

Travelbee, J. (1966). *Interpersonal aspects of nursing*. Philadelphia, PA: F.A. Davis.

Weiss, S. J. (1990). Effects of differential touch on nervous-system arousal of patients recovering from cardiac disease. *Heart & Lung, 19*(5), 474–480.

Wiedenbach, E. (1964). *Clinical nursing: A helping art*. New York, NY: Springer.

SECTION VII

THE QUANTITATIVE MINDFRAME

In this section, we address "thinking quantitatively" about theory. This very important process is often omitted in research design texts, although such procedures as operationalization were taken very seriously a few decades ago (Waltz, Strickland, & Lenz, 1984). Perhaps the wave of developed instruments has reduced the difficulty of finding a good match for your concepts, and therefore falsely reduced the need to tread carefully in this important step.

SECTION VII

THE QUANTITATIVE MIND FRAME

DEVELOPING QUANTITATIVE THEORY

> *Theories cannot be verified absolutely and forever; however, they can be falsified—i.e., they can be proven to be wrong—given a certain degree of certainty (or probability).*
>
> —Karl Popper (1959)

Quantitative theories are tools developed by the investigator to be deductively tested using particular statistical methods: theories are constructed logically from what is already known about the topic, considering the feasibility of measuring the concepts or variables in the theory. Once tested, the theory may be supported (i.e., statistically significant), or considered "weak" (i.e., having poor results but with some indication toward a positive relationship), or not statistically supported. Importantly, as Popper (1959) stressed, theories are not proven, but may be supported. They do not show us absolute truth, but rather probable truth, with some (not necessarily complete) degree of certainty. However, they can show us when we are wrong. In this way, theories can be modified and retested and positivistic science progresses.

Quantitative research therefore rests upon two components: the development of a theoretical model and the measurement and statistical procedures for testing the model. It is the purpose of this chapter to give you an introduction to the construction of theories and models used in quantitative inquiry. Although the concomitant research design and statistical interpretation are outside of our scope, these matters are discussed in many texts. However, an exception is with factorial designs, which allows the researcher to develop the model directly. The model itself serves as a framework, which is then "tested" in the setting. From these data, significant variables are selected. For example, Bubela et al. (1990) surveyed patients' perceptions of their learning needs on discharge. Seven subscales were identified, including medications, activities of daily living, feelings related to their condition, community, and follow-up. These findings were used by Smith (1999) for a follow-up survey of patients to evaluate nursing discharge teaching.

THE ROLE OF QUANTITATIVE THEORY

Theory in quantitative inquiry has an extremely important role. Theory is the reason for conducting the inquiry in the first place; it is conjecture, with hypotheses to be tested, and therefore it must be worthwhile and linked to what is known. Testing a hypothesis is important. If supported, the findings will enable knowledge to move forward; if not supported, at least the investigator will know what does not work. Therefore, theory must be innovative and contain new ideas, but at the same time must be based on work that has been previously supported. It must be cumulative, logical, and convincing. And, in nursing, we often add another criterion: It must be applicable (i.e., useful to practice), or else lead to a more distant goal that will be applied and improve practice.

The development of the theory and subsequent testing is a deductive process, and sometimes a risky endeavor. The paradigmatic assumptions on which the theory is based may not be correct, yet because of the strength of the prevailing paradigm, the theory may be supported when tested. These "errors" in science are more easily identified in historical documents (e.g., in "The Diseases of Masturbation"; see To Do 5.1) and in class discussion you may think of other examples. But science generally, sooner or later, corrects itself.

"If I Can't Measure It, It Doesn't Exist"

Consider the McNamara fallacy:

> The **McNamara fallacy** refers to Robert McNamara, the United States Secretary of Defense, involves making a decision purely on quantitative data, and ignoring others. The first step is to measure whatever can be easily measured. This is OK as far as it goes. The second step is to disregard that which can't be easily measured or to give it an arbitrary quantitative value. This is artificial and misleading. The third step is to presume that what can't be measured easily really isn't important. This is blindness. The fourth step is to say that what can't be easily measured really doesn't exist. This is suicide. (Daniel Yankelovich, 1972)[1]

Although in this book we are not going to discuss measurement strategies, the role of measurement cannot be put entirely aside. Quantitative theory *must*, by definition, deal with what is measurable. Thagard (1999), a Canadian

---

[1] https://en.wikipedia.org/wiki/McNamara_fallacy

philosopher, writes extensively about theories that may be proposed but cannot be empirically supported (at least initially), and are therefore not considered credible. One recent example is the "bacteria theory of peptic ulcers" proposed by Warren and Marshall (1983) that was "considered preposterous" by his colleagues (Thagard, 1999, p. 41). The research trajectory of Warren and Marshall came in three stages: (a) from serendipitous observation, which they conducted from studies that identified and revealed the presence of bacteria, *Helicobacter pylori,* in the stomach; (b) that which showed that *H. pylori* caused peptic ulcers by locating the bacteria in the ulcers, and (c) that peptic ulcers can be treated with antibiotics. As their research continued, the medical community moved from rejection, to acceptance, to explanatory coherence between hypotheses and evidence, as other researchers replicated their studies. But the road was a little rough whereas the investigators gained credence for their work. [2] The use of antibiotics for peptic ulcers is now standard treatment.

Explanatory coherence is the removal of alternative hypotheses. This is done by processes of logical argument and by statistically ruling out alternative explanations. Therefore to do this, excellent theory is required to be parsimonious, explicit, logical, and often developed by means of many intermediate goals. Explanatory hypotheses are controlled by research designs.

CREATING THEORETICAL FRAMEWORKS

In your research, you will probably create a theoretical framework. Theoretical (conceptual) frameworks are logical explanations and justifications to guide quantitative inquiry methodologically. Basically, the theory makes a case for conducting the research, the scope and variables to be included, and the selection of the sample and type of analysis to be conducted. Without such theory, the research becomes a descriptive "fishing trip" in which researchers explore large data sets for significant correlations; such correlations, in large data sets, may turn out to be *spurious.* In such cases, with exploratory data analysis, the researchers create possible explanations for the results (often spurious correlations) and subsequently conduct further confirmatory research.

The process of developing the conceptual framework for a quantitative study begins with (a) evaluating the literature, (b) identifying a quantitative question, (c) identifying the concepts, (d) operationalization, (e) determining measurement, and (d) developing appropriate research design. As the entire process is dependent on your question and the research designs are the purview of many texts, here I will address steps 1 to 5, and provide examples of several quantitative designs.

---

[2] In 1983, Marshall submitted a paper to the Australian Gastroenterology Society contending the bacteria may be responsible for ulcers. Fifty-nine of the 67 submissions were accepted for the meeting: Marshall's was not (Thagard, 1999, p. 41).

EVALUATING THE LITERATURE

Reading the literature to identify a topic is the most crucial part of the process, for it gets you started—and for many, "getting started" is the greatest hurdle. First, you must decide on a topic, which is a general area of interest, for without that you will not know where to start reading. Think through what you are really interested in, or think of clinical problems you have encountered in practice when you were hunting for something else online.

Think about what you often think about.

Identifying a topic or an area may be enough for now. Pull the literature and start reading. Think while you are reading. Do not skim; read broadly within your area. As you read, sort the literature into groups, according to the "schools of thought," types of questions asked and answered, or the author's theoretical perspective.

It is very helpful, at this point, to conduct a review or a meta-synthesis or meta-analysis, for a class paper. This may develop into an article that may even "do" as one of your articles for your dissertation, or even be publishable. But the most important thing is that it enables you to discuss the literature with authority. Sounding as though you know what you are talking about is a trait that can never be underestimated or undervalued.

Identifying the Research Question

This step is often a nightmare for students because it signifies a commitment. Therefore, the more you try to think of an original question (one that will make a contribution and hopefully fits in your advisor's research program) and one that is the right size for a dissertation (which may be completed in a year, and does not require a huge sample or fancy instrumentation), and has the right price (affordable, cheap, and does not require outside grant funding), the more your minds becomes completely blank. So, step back and identify your aim or aims.

Identifying Your Aim(s)

You do this by thinking backward. Start thinking about the end of the project and try to identify what you want to know when you finish the project, which is your goal. That is the aim of your study (or those are the aims, if you may have more than one).

Now comes the question—or questions.

A question may just "pop" into your mind in the middle of the night. Grab it, research it, refine it . . .

Or, you may have to deliberately sit and write it down. Give yourself some leeway by asking "If I ask this _____, then I will have to _____."

"If I ask *that*_____, then I will have to _____."

"If I ask *thus and so*_____, then I will have to _____."

Looking at the problem from different directions opens your mind and makes things appear less rigid, less narrow.

Now select the best question for your purposes, and refine it. Refining your question may be tricky for quantitative research. First you may have to narrow the question by making it smaller, breaking it into several subquestions.

IDENTIFYING THE CONCEPTS

Often your questions and your reading will have provided you with many concepts in your area. List these. You will have a nice collection of scientific concepts, all with operational definitions with means of measurement. This is more likely to be so if you have a physiological question. But with a social or psychological question, often you will have descriptors rather than concept labels, or lay concepts. Look at these labels analytically: what does the description represent? Are there concepts available in the literature that would account for these descriptions?

If concepts are available, at this point *revisit your question(s)* and substitute phrases in your questions with the concepts. Once you understand *operationalization,*[3] you will see that this step will be one giant step in the right direction for your project, for your project will probably be closely linked to an instrument that will enable measurement. Here is the great secret: The concept may be your variable. Alternatively, the attributes within the concept may serve as *indicators* for the concept, that is, serve as variables. Either way, what you have learned so far about the anatomy of concepts will be very helpful at this point.

If a concept is *not* available, or you cannot think of a concept that will address or fit into your question, then things will be a little more difficult, but not impossible. It may be that you have a question that needs to be addressed qualitatively, and the concepts developed. Or you may have to develop the concept. Quantitative researchers do not usually develop concepts qualitatively as we have described in Chapter 6. Rather, they often move directly to developing the concept as a scientific concept. They develop a label that fits the phenomenon they have listed in their question, develop a definition, and operational definitions as a means to measure the concept, and move directly to quantitative research.

For example, if you have a description that reads:

"Patient disagreeing with treatment." Think—is that an example of noncompliance? Or is it an antecedent to noncompliance? (McDonald, 2013)

---

[3] Operationalization is defining something in terms of the way it can (or will) be measured.

Using your knowledge of the anatomy of concepts (Chapter 7), analyze the concept of noncompliance as in the literature. Does it fit? Continue with this process of exploring scientific concepts until you find an appropriate concept to fit your statement.

The result of this process will probably be one of the following:

- You find a concept that is defined, operationalized, and has a selection of measurement tools that fits the phenomenon you are seeing. You accept that concept and move forward, creating your conceptual framework.
- You find a concept that is defined, operationalized, and has a selection of measurement tools, one of which fits your needs but does not have a measurement instrument associated with it for your context. This is not very good news, for creating an instrument is too much work and requires a much higher level of expertise than is required for a dissertation. Discuss it with your advisor: Either you will have to find another concept or accept the less than "ideal" match between your concept and the measure.
- You find a concept that is defined but is not operationalized. You may go ahead and operationalize it to fit your needs, if there is a tool that will then measure the concept.
- You do not find a concept label that fits your phenomenon. This is not a good sign. If you cannot find a concept, can you create one? No, that is not a poor idea for your first project. If you decide to continue this line of investigation, you may have no alternative than to change your question slightly and retarget the phenomenon. Discuss the problem with your advisor.

OPERATIONALIZATION

Operationalization is the process of defining something in terms of measurement. We consider our variables (concepts or attributes) in a way that they can be measured. Measurement may be by means of a survey questionnaire, a psychological instrument, a physiological measure, an observed behavior, and so forth.

How do you operationalize? Operationalization differs from a definition: A definition provides the meaning of the concept; when operationalizing, one develops an *empirical* meaning for the concept. From this operational definition, the variables may be identified. Ask yourself: What indicators, or observations, will show the presence of the concept? If concepts have operational definitions that fit into theory, then they are useful. The operational definition must link to measures that are accurate and precise.

If you have found a concept that is defined, there are two schools of thought about the next step. The first is to identify the concepts, operationalize variables, and locate an instrument that fits the operationalization (Geering, 2012; Loseke, 2013; Figure 27.1a). The second is to operationalize by identifying the question, and from there identify measurement instruments, and refine the definition of your variables to fit the instrument (LoBiondo-Wood & Haber, 2014; Remler & van Ryzin, 2011; Figure 27.1b). All of these authors agree that research consists of interconnected parts, and there must be a logical flow from one step to the next. Loseke (2013) reminds us that it is the research question that drives the process of writing the literature review, identification of the concepts, and further, what data to collect, and how to interpret these data.

Let us walk through an example: Suppose the concept is "disagreeing with treatment." Our description tells us that the patient did not argue with the physician, but you saw he had not been prescribed the medication that he expected, wanted, or requested. You doubt that he will bother to fill the prescription, or if he does, you guess he will not take the medicine. Noncompliance is defined as "failure or refusal to comply," but at the point the patient has been prescribed the medication, then he has not refused to comply, according to the definition. If we do decide to use "noncompliance" as our concept, we could define it as "reluctant acceptance of treatment." Alternatively, we could reject noncompliance as a concept and label the concept as "pending noncompliance" or "pre-noncompliance." Because that concept does not exist, the choice (and the appropriate operational definition) is yours.

But now you have to *operationalize the concept.* This consists of translating the concept into observable or measurable events, so that it can be:

- Consistently recognized by others
- Measured

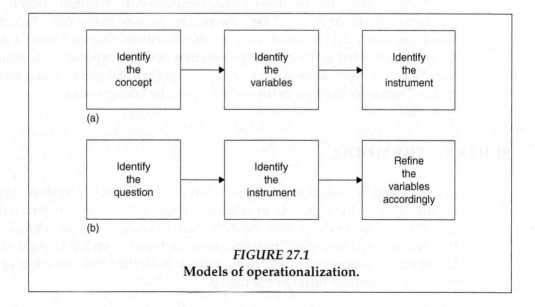

FIGURE 27.1
Models of operationalization.

Measurement may be direct or indirect: Direct measures have a one-to-one association with the outcome; indirect measures are *indicators* of the outcome. If the concept may be directly measured, then your task is easy. You may decide that your concept of *pending noncompliance* is directly measured by:

- Refusal to take the prescription from the prescriber
- Tossing it in the trashcan on leaving
- Failure to have the prescription filled

Indirect measures of *pending noncompliance* may be:

- Pulling a face when the prescriber tells the patient what medication will be ordered
- No signs of improvement on the next visit; if the patient has taken the medication, it was not therapeutic

These indictors leave some doubt; that is why they are *indirect*.

Indirect measures are therefore weaker indicators of the concept, as they leave a possibility of doubt. Our patient may appear reluctant but may get the prescriptions filled and may take the medication "to see if it works." Therefore, the disagreeable face is not an ideal measure of *pending noncompliance.*

PLANNING YOUR RESEARCH DESIGN

Now the questions, and how they are asked, lead directly to your research design.

Your model may be descriptive, correlational or causal. Descriptive questions ask: What is ____? Or how much___, how many of___? Correlational questions ask: Is there an *association* between this and that? Causal questions ask what is the *effect of* this on that, and are experimental designs, usually based on randomization, with an experimental group and a control group. Therefore, the sign to the path you will be taking is clear.

BUILDING THE MODEL

The next step is to decide on the position of your concepts to show logical organization of the concepts in relation to one another and, if you have a causal question, to determine the anticipated linkages in your model. The final model must be logical, parsimonious, and read from left to right or top to bottom, whenever possible, with arrows indicating the direction of the effects or movement through the model.

Map your model by writing the concept names and variables on small sticky notes that may be moved around on your desk. Position the concepts, considering the type of concept in your model.

Descriptive Research

The most basic level of quantitative research is description of a phenomenon, process, procedure, group, population, or so forth, which is determined by the researcher's interest. From the literature, from qualitative inquiry (such as focus groups), or from the researcher's observations, a conceptual framework is constructed that justifies the research and which will guide the construction of survey questions.

The results of the survey will determine the presence or frequencies of the items (or variables) of interest. Some of these variables may be correlated, but the results are generally used to describe the population in frequency counts.

Research Questions That Show Association or Causality

These types of relationships are evident in your question. Does your question ask for correlation (Is *this* associated with *that*?) or "What is the effect of *this* on *that*?"

Independent Variables

Independent variables are the variables that are considered to cause or to influence the dependent variable, and they usually placed on the first level or left-hand column of your model. Examples of independent variables are often demographic variables, such as age or gender, and other independent variables that would have influence on your model. According to the researcher's theoretical framework, other concepts may be added and linked with lines to indicate the direction of relationship or causation. The dependent variable is usually depicted on the right side of the map. For instance, in our study of *pending noncompliance*, patient history (defined as whether or not the patient has had the desired medication previously) is an independent variable.

At this stage, you should have identified your research design, and your study will be very organized on paper. Now is the time to write your theoretical framework, and once you have that, to prepare your proposal.

THE THEORETICAL FRAMEWORK

Quantitative conceptual frameworks are established at the beginning of the study to guide inquiry, and are used to illustrate results. The theoretical framework fulfills several functions: (a) it identifies the problem, concepts, and variables; (b) it justifies their theoretical linkages of the concepts and variables; (c) it builds an argument for the significance of the question. The theoretical framework generally is an argument for conducting the study. It starts out broadly and systematically funnels logically down to the question.

Theoretical frameworks are constructed from the work of others. They are well cited, and it is your questions that will extend this framework of knowledge a little further, so that until you get almost to the end of the framework, it is a solid construction of knowledge. Two things make it theory: (a) the original piecing together of the theory concepts and prior knowledge from the literature to build the argument and (b) the logical progression in structure from asking your question and hypotheses.

The theoretical framework is crucial to your study. Diagram it if possible. If you are using a descriptive survey, your theoretical framework justifies the scope of your study, and the concept and variables you have decided to include. It will also direct the items (questions) on your survey.

If you have a study that looks at association or correlation, the theoretical framework justifies the concepts and variables that are being associated and the type of correlations expected. In other words, it is the foundation of your study.

If you have a study that qualifies as causal design, it is the theory—your conceptual framework—that is being tested when you conduct your research. Therefore, it is the most important part of your study and is the one that will be scrutinized at your examination prior to commencing your study.

Now, once all of these decisions are made and components prepared, you are ready to write your proposal.

EXAMPLES OF MODELS FOR MULTIVARIATE RESEARCH

Developing Causal Models

When building the model, the concepts/variables are placed in order, in a format that fits the method of analysis. The simplest cause and effect model is:

Cause → effect.

Once the theoretical components of the study are identified, these are diagrammed in a model according to their hypothesized relationship with other concepts. The measurement instrument for each concept is identified, and the scores are hypothesized to show anticipated results. The complexity of the diagram and the relationships between variables, and the level of measurement determine the type of analysis. Other independent variables, such as gender, ethnicity, and educational status, that may also influence results. The linkages between the concepts are dependent on measurement scores. Quantitative conceptual frameworks are established at the beginning of the study, to guide inquiry, according to their hypothesized relationship with other concepts. The diagram for a conceptual framework therefore consists of concepts linked by hypothesized relationships, in addition to other independent variables, such as gender, ethnicity, and educational status, that may also influence results. The measurement instrument of each concept is identified, and the scores are hypothesized to show the developing results. The complexity of the diagram and the relationships determine the type of analysis.

Theory for Multivariate Analysis

Causal modeling approaches define correlations within a network. Exemplars are regression analysis or structural equation modeling (SEM). Rules for path tracing are:

1. You can pass through each variable only once
2. You cannot go forward and then back

A simple example of a regression model is shown in Figure 27.2.

Path Analysis

Path analysis is an extension of the simple regression model, which allows for indirect causal paths. The independent variables are called "exogenous

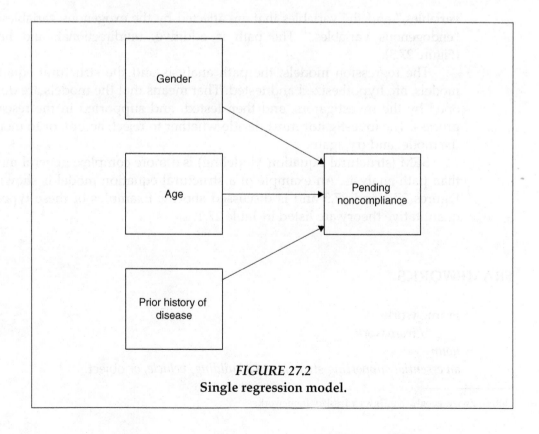

FIGURE 27.2
Single regression model.

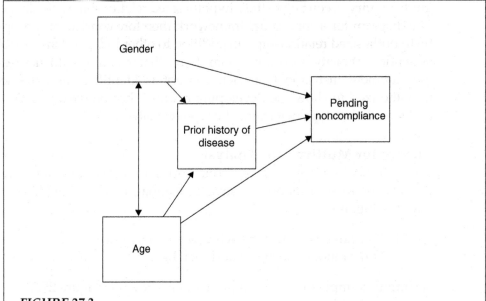

FIGURE 27.3
Model for path analysis, predicting gender, age and prior history of disease,
and indirect paths of gender and age through prior history of disease on
pending noncompliance.

variables," and the variables that are affected by the exogenous variables are "endogenous variables." The path is additive, unidirectional, and linear (Figure 27.3).

The regression models, the path analysis and the structural equation models, are hypothesized and tested. That means that the models are developed by the investigators, and then tested, and supported in the research process. The investigator must decide whether to reject, accept, or to modify the model and try again.

SEM (structural Equation Modeling) is a more complex, general model than path analysis. An example of a structural equation model is shown in Figures 27.4 and 27.5 and is discussed shortly. Examples of these types of quantitative theory are listed in Table 27.1.

FRAMEWORKS

Frame·work
    [4]/ˈfrāmˌwərk/
noun
an essential supporting structure of a building, vehicle, or object.

——————————
[4] https://www.google.com/?gws_rd=ssl#q=framework

TABLE 27.1
Examples of Quantitatively Derived Theory

REGRESSION ANALYSIS

Grummer-Strawn, L. M., & Mei, Z. (2004). Does breastfeeding protect against pediatric overweight? Analysis of longitudinal data from the Centers for Disease Control and Prevention Pediatric Nutrition Surveillance System.	*Pediatrics, 113*(2), e81–e86.
Gobbens, R. J., van Assen, M. A., Luijkx, K. G., & Schols, J. M. (2012). Testing an integral conceptual model of frailty.	*Journal of Advanced Nursing, 68*(9), 2047–2060.

PATH ANALYSIS

Arnetz, J. E., Arnetz, B. B., & Petterson, I. L. (1996). Violence in the nursing profession: Occupational and lifestyle risk factors in Swedish nurses.	*Work & Stress, 10*(2), 119–127.
Tourangeau, A. E., Doran, D. M., Hall, L. M., O'Brien Pallas, L., Pringle, D., Tu, J. V., & Cranley, L. A. (2007). Impact of hospital nursing care on 30-day mortality for acute medical patients.	*Journal of Advanced Nursing, 57*(1), 32–44.

PATH ANALYSIS

Fried, T. R., & Mor, V. (1997). Frailty and hospitalization of long-term stay nursing home residents.	*Journal of the American Geriatrics Society, 45*(3), 265–269.
Conn, V. (1998). Older adults and exercise: Path analysis of self-efficacy related constructs.	*Nursing Research, 47*(3), 188–189.
Resnick, B., Palmer, M. H., Jenkins, L. S., & Spellbring, A. M. (2000). Path analysis of efficacy expectations and exercise behavior in older adults.	*Journal of Advanced Nursing, 31*(6), 1309–1315.

STRUCTURAL EQUATION MODELING

Beckstead, J. W. (2002). Modeling attitudinal antecedents of nurses' decisions to report impaired colleagues.	*Western Journal of Nursing, 24*(5), 537–551.
De Jonge, J., & Schaufeli, W. B. (1998). Job characteristics and employee well-being: A test of Warr's Vitamin Model in health care workers using structural equation modeling.	*Journal of Organizational Behavior, 19*(4), 387–407.
Demerouti, E., Bakker, A. B., Nachreiner, F., & Schaufeli, W. B. (2000). A model of burnout and life satisfaction amongst nurses.	*Journal of Advanced Nursing, 32*(2), 454–464.
Musil, C., Jeanblanc, A. B., Burant, C. J., Zausniewski, J. A., & Warner, C. B. (2013), Longitudinal analysis of resourcefulness, family strain, and depressive symptoms in grandmother caregivers.	*Nursing Outlook, 61*(4), 225–233.

Frameworks are large conceptual schemes that organize ideas; often grand ideas, which provide direction to education, research, and policy. Frequently, they are not intended to be researched per se, but rather give direction for a research program that is conducted within the framework and over time, using many projects. A collection of studies conducted by various authors (or in Solberg's case, even by international groups, as a review of the Social Determinants of Health; Chapter 28) eventually results in a paradigm shift. The use of a framework of this type is almost a grand theory. These frameworks keep research on a certain topic focused within the same area. It is different from a "theoretical framework that you may use to frame your research project or a term paper." These frameworks are conceptually *much* larger and greater in scope.

Frameworks are generally quite abstract. This means that the components of the framework have not usually been operationalized for measurement, but rather may be represented by a number of measures. In nursing, we have several frameworks, such as Leininger's (1991) *Sunrise Model,* and Ray's (2001) *Model of Bureaucratic Caring.*

In nursing, Nola Pender (1982) proposed a framework for health promotion. Briefly, this model posits *individual characteristics and experiences* (prior related behavior, and research has been personal, biological, psychological and sociocultural factors) and lead to *behavior-specific cognitions and affect, commitment to a plan of actions* (moderated by *competing demands and preferences*) resulting in *health-promoting behavior* (see Figure 27.4).

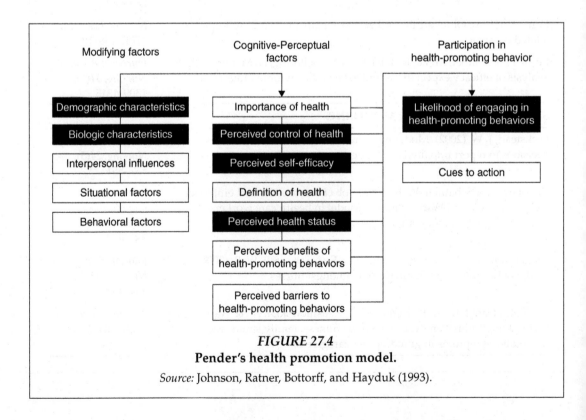

FIGURE 27.4
Pender's health promotion model.
Source: Johnson, Ratner, Bottorff, and Hayduk (1993).

Although frameworks are not intended to be tested directly, as is a type of theory, a group of researchers did test Pender's Model using a large data set and SEM (Bottorff, Johnson, Ratner, & Hayduk, 1996; Johnson, Ratner, Bottorff, & Hayduk, 1993; Ratner, Bottorff, Johnson, & Hayduk, 1994). Their results are included in Figure 27.5. They concluded:

> Despite the fact that the model proved to fit the data, little of the variance in the health-promoting behavior concepts was explained and all significant effects were found to be weak . . . Thus, little of the variance in the health-promoting behaviors was explained, calling into question the explanatory power of the model. (Johnson, Ratner, Bottorff, & Hayduk, 1993, p. 138)

Because these results were not very positive, Pender subsequently revised her model, and it has been subject to several iterations since (Ronis, Hong, & Lusk, 2006), and her book is now in the sixth edition (Pender, Murdaugh, & Parsons, 2011). This is important because although frameworks are relatively abstract, this does not mean they are not subject to testing. Pender had participated in testing her model with other investigators (McCullagh, Lusk, & Ronis, 2002; Pender, Walker, Sechrist, & Frank-Stromborg, 1988, 1990; Pender, Bar-Or, Wilk, & Mitchell, 2002; Shin, Yun, Pender, & Jang, 2005; Walker, Sechrist, & Pender, 1987; Wu & Pender, 2002); it was used in nursing education (Pender, Barkauskas, Haymen, Rice, & Anderson, 1991) and applied to subpopulations (Srof, & Velsor-Friedrich, 2006).

One of the most influential frameworks for organizing health in recent decades is the *Social Determinants of Health* reviewed in Chapter 28 by Shirley Solberg. This model is used in research, to direct policy internationally, and now appears in nursing texts.

EVALUATING QUANTITATIVE THEORY

The main characteristic of an excellent quantitative theory is *coherence*. There must be consistency among all of the components of the project, or *fit* among the question, the theoretical framework, the concepts and their operationalization, the variables and measurement, data analysis, and the way that the theory is addressed in the results and discussion.

The adequate design of quantitative theory is evaluated in the process of *testing*. Included in testing adequacy are such features as sampling adequacy and appropriateness, selection of adequate tool and measures, and so forth. Results of the statistical analyses will reveal the support (or lack of support) for the hypothesized relationships, and the model is then accepted or revised.

LoBiondo-Wood and Haber (2014, p. 87) present an additional criterion: Is the theory consistent with a nursing perspective?

What do you think?

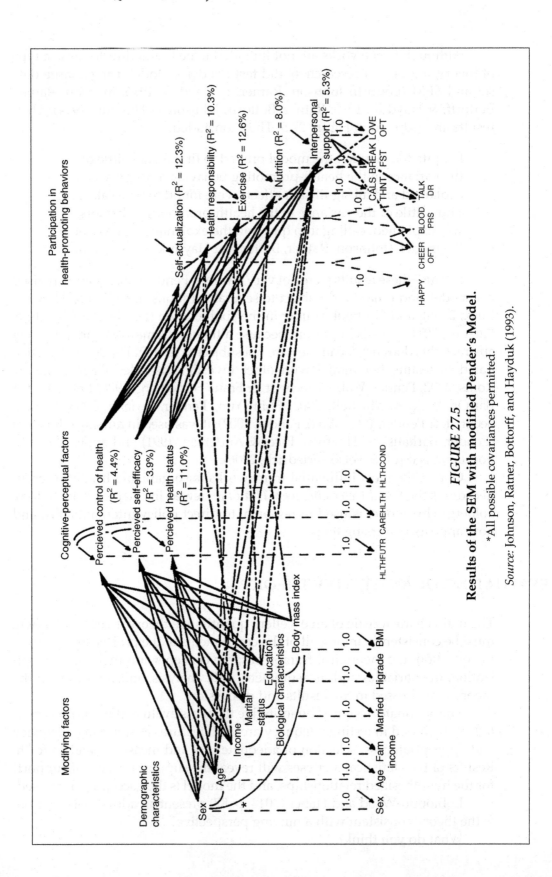

FIGURE 27.5

Results of the SEM with modified Pender's Model.

*All possible covariances permitted.

Source: Johnson, Ratner, Bottorff, and Hayduk (1993).

Substruction

Substruction is the valuation of the structure of quantitative theory by the deconstruction of design structures. This is done by identifying the design structures (how the variables are quantified) and the analysis structure (how the collection of quantitative data and the processes of analysis are treated).

Hinshaw (1979) noted that for a quantitative theory to be valid there must be logical consistency among three research structures: the theoretical structure (that is the theoretical framework), the structure of the research design, and the structure of the analysis. These three components within the project must be consistent and logically flow from one structure to the next.

1. Identify and isolate the major concepts/constructs on the study,
2. Specify the relationships between the concepts given in the study's theoretical explanation,
3. Hierarchically order the concepts and relationships according to their level of abstraction, and
4. Portray the identified concepts and relationships in a pictorial structure. (Hinshaw, 1979, p. 319)

For an example, see (Bekhet and Zauszniewski [2008]).

SUMMARY

Operationalization and measurement are the keys to quantitative modeling. The concepts and variables used must be measurable or converted so that they are measurable. The form of the model is highly dependent on the nature of the statistical analysis. These conceptual issues regarding quantitative modeling are integrated into your research design classes; therefore, this chapter provides the basics to help you start thinking theoretically about your project and about the issues in quantitative modeling. The form of the model developed is dependent on the aims, the type of question asked, what is known about the topic, the nature of the concepts the variables identify, how they are operationalized, the measurement instruments available, the type of research design, and statistical analysis to be conducted. All of this relies on the quality of development of your theoretical framework.

REFERENCES

Bekhet, A., & Zauszniewski, J. A. (2008). Theoretical substruction illustrated by the theory of learned resourcefulness. *Research and theory for Nursing Practice*, 22(3), 205–214. doi:10.1891/0889-7182.22.3.205.

Bottorff, J. L., Johnson, J. L., Ratner, P. A., & Hayduk, L. A. (1996). The effects of cognitive-perceptual factors on health promotion behavior maintenance. *Nursing research, 45*(1), 30–36.

Bubela, N., Galloway, S., McKinnon, A., Nagel, L., Pringle. D., Ross, E., & Shamian, J. (1990). The patient learning needs scale: Reliability and validity. *Journal of Advanced Nursing, 15*(10), 1181–1187.

Geering, J. (2012). *Social Science methodology* (2nd ed.). New York, NY: Cambridge University Press.

Hinshaw, A. S. (1979). Problems in doing research. *Western Journal of Nursing Research, 1,* 319–324. doi:10.1177/019394597900100410

Johnson, J. L., Ratner, P. A., Bottorff, J. L., & Hayduk, L. A. (1993). An exploration of Pender's health promotion model using LISREL. *Nursing Research, 42*(3), 132–138.

Leininger, M. M. (1991). *Caring an essential human need*. Thorofore, NJ: Charles B. Slack

LoBiondo-Wood, G., & Haber, J. (2014). *Nursing research: Methods and critical appraisal* (8th ed.). St Louis, MO: Mosby.

Loseke, D. E. (2013). *Methodological thinking: basic issues in social research design*. Thousand Oaks, CA: Sage.

McCullagh, M., Lusk, S. L., & Ronis, D. L. (2002). Factors influencing use of hearing protection among farmers: A test of the Pender health promotion model. *Nursing Research, 51*(1), 33–39.

McDonald, D. (2013). Trialing to pain control: A grounded theory. *Research in Nursing & Health, 37*(2), 107–116. doi:10.1002/nur.21584

Pender, N. (1982). *Health promotion in nursing practice*. New York, NY: Appleton-Century-Crofts.

Pender, N. J., Walker, S. N., Sechrist, K. R., & Frank-Stromborg, M. (1990). Predicting health-promoting lifestyles in the workplace. *Nursing research, 39*(6), 326–332.

Pender, N. J., Barkauskas, V. H., Hayman, L., Rice, V. H., & Anderson, E. T. (1991). Health promotion and disease prevention: toward excellence in nursing practice and education. *Nursing Outlook, 40*(3), 106–112.

Pender, N. J., Walker, S. N., Sechrist, K. R., & Frank-Stromborg, M. (1988). Development and testing of the health promotion model. *Cardio-vascular nursing, 24*(6), 41.

Pender, N. J., Bar-Or, O., Wilk, B., & Mitchell, S. (2002). Self-efficacy and perceived exertion of girls during exercise. *Nursing Research, 51*(2), 86–91.

Pender, N., Murdaugh, C. L., & Parsons, M. A. (2011). *Health promotion in nursing practice* (6th ed.). Boston, MA: Pearson.

Popper, K. (1959). *The logic of scientific discovery*. New York, NY: Harper Tourchbooks.

Ratner, P. A., Bottorff, J. L., Johnson, J. L., & Hayduk, L. A. (1994). The interaction effects of gender within the health promotion model. *Research in Nursing & Health, 17*(5), 341–350.

Ray, M. A. (2001). The theory of bureaucratic caring. In M. Parker (Ed.), *Nursing theory and nursing practice* (pp. 421–444). Philadelphia, PA: F. A. Davis.

Remler, D. K., & Van Ryzin, G. G. (2011). *Research methods in practice: Strategies for description and causation*. Thousand Oaks, CA: Sage.

Ronis, D. L., Hong, O., & Lusk, S. L. (2006). Comparison of the original and revised structures of the health promotion model in predicting construction workers' use of hearing protection. *Research in Nursing & Health, 29*(1), 3–17.

Shin, Y., Yun, S., Pender, N. J., & Jang, H. (2005). Test of the health promotion model as a causal model of commitment to a plan for exercise among Korean adults with chronic disease. *Research in Nursing & Health, 28*(2), 117–125.

Smith, J. (1999). *Patient education practice: A study of patient's perceptions* (Unpublished report). University of Utah Hospitals and Clinics, Salt Lake City, UT.

Srof, B. J., & Velsor-Friedrich, B. (2006). Health promotion in adolescents: A review of Pender's health promotion model. *Nursing Science Quarterly, 19*(4), 366–373.

Thagard, P. (1999). *How scientists explain disease*. Princeton, NJ: Princeton University Press.

Walker, S. N., Sechrist, K. R., & Pender, N. J. (1987). The health-promoting lifestyle profile: Development and psychometric characteristics. *Nursing Research, 36*(2), 76–81.

Waltz, C. F., Strickland, O. L., & Lenz, E. R. (1984). *Measurement in nursing research*. Philadelphia, PA: F. A. Davis.

Warren, J. R., & Marshall, B. (1983). Unidentified curved bacilli on gastric epithelium in active chronic gastritis. *The Lancet, 321*(8336), 1273–1275.

Wu, T. Y., & Pender, N. (2002). Determinants of physical activity among Taiwanese adolescents: An application of the health promotion model. *Research in Nursing & Health, 25*(1), 25–36.

Yankelovich, D. (1972). *Corporate priorities: A continuing study of the new demands on business*. Stanford, CA: Yankelovich.

Shirley M. Solberg

THE SOCIAL DETERMINANTS OF HEALTH: AN EXPANDED CONCEPTUAL FRAMEWORK FOR NURSING

> *If our goal is to reduce health disparities rather than to just study them, nursing research must include a major focus on resources such as income, education, access to care, social and political power, and human rights. We will not achieve this goal by focusing on individual behaviours and risk factors alone. We need a new paradigm that recognizes societal factors as primary pathogenic forces in the major health problems facing the U.S. today.*
>
> —Flaskerud and Nyamathi (2002, p. 139)

More than a decade ago in a guest editorial in Nursing Research, Flaskerud and Nyamathi (2002) essentially called on nurse researchers to expand their thinking about health and the environment by embracing a new paradigm that would enable them to move beyond what were traditional approaches to nursing research, in order to reduce health disparities. This was not the first in recent times that nurses were asked to think more broadly about how the environment might have an impact on health. In a call to approach theory development in a new way Chopoorian (1986) believed that nurses' "lack of consciousness of environment" (p. 43) limited nurses' abilities "to turn their attention to the conditions that control, influence, and produce health or illness in human beings" (p. 53). Stevens (1989) advocated a critical social theory approach so that "nurses may reconceptualize their understanding of the environment to encompass social, political, and economic worlds" (p. 59) to improve nursing care. Likewise, Butterfield (1990) suggested that "upstream" thinking was needed for nurses to address "social, environmental, and political determinants of health" (p. 1). More recently, some concrete approaches have been put forward on how to broaden the conceptualization of the environment and health. Reutter and Kushner (2010) suggested nurses tackle health inequities through a critical approach using the social determinants of health (SDH) as a guide.

The centrality of the concepts of health and the environment to nursing as a practice and a discipline has been well recognized beginning with Nightingale and continuing to the present day (Risjord, 2010). Health and the environment are core concepts in most, if not all, theories and frameworks of nursing and a clear conceptualization of health, and the environment remains central to what we do as nurses in practice, education, and research (Meleis, 2012). However, in many of the nursing models and frameworks, the concept of the environment has been limited, or at least interpreted to be somewhat limited, to the more immediate environment of the individual or family. Even in many models or frameworks that present a broader view of the environment, there is no account taken of the many structural factors in society (economic, political, and social), that as the SDH frameworks have illustrated, produce a huge impact on health. How the concepts of health and the environment are understood and used can be limiting or enabling, not only for improving health of individuals and populations, but in reducing health disparities and inequities.

Health disparities and health equities are important because nurses are ethically mandated to help individuals, families, communities, and populations by protecting, promoting, and restoring health in the many interactions that nurses have with the client, however defined (American Nurses Association, 2015; Canadian Nurses Association, 2008; International Council of Nurses, 2012). Additionally nurses have both an ethical requirement and a social responsibility for broader actions around equity, fairness, and social justice when it comes to responding to the health and social needs of human populations on a local, national, international, and increasingly a global scale (Anderson et al., 2009; Canadian Nurses Association, 2010; Pauly, 2013). To fulfill this mandate requires a framework that is capable of providing a solid understanding of health and the factors that influence health within an environmental context that can inform our thinking and thus practices. Equally important is an understanding of what accounts for the differences or disparities in health that exist. Understanding individual health and its distribution in populations is complex because of the many factors that have an indirect or direct impact on health, so a comprehensive framework is required: one that takes into account the various interacting factors and conditions that influence health (Solar & Irwin, 2010). An SDH framework is a good fit for understanding the myriad of influences on health because it more closely mirrors the environment in which health and illness, including health disparities and inequities, are created and experienced and thus could enhance nurses in their ability to fulfill their professional mandate (Canadian Nurses Association, 2005; Mahony & Jones, 2013; Reutter & Kushner, 2010).

An SDH framework is evidence-based and broadly addresses the many factors that affect health (Braverman, Egerter, & Williams, 2011; Commission on the Social Determinants of Health [CSDH], 2008; Muntaner, Ng, & Chung, 2012; Marmot & Wilkinson, 2006; Raphael, 2004). The SDH framework has evolved over the past four decades as evidence for and knowledge of the SDH has accumulated (Irwin & Scali, 2007; Marmot & Wilkinson, 2006; Raphael, 2004), the concepts clarified (Braverman, 2006; Chang, 2002; Dahlgren & Whitehead, 2006; Kelly, 2010; Williams, 2003), and the knowledge translated and promoted as a means to address the health of individuals and populations (Canadian Nurses Association, 2013; CSDH, 2008; Muntaner, et al., 2012). A SDH framework or elements of this framework have been widely advocated, adapted, and used as a policy framework by a number of governments (King, 2000; Turrell, Oldenburg, McGuffog, & Dent, 1999) and organizations (Canadian Nurses Association, 2013; Centers for Disease Control and Prevention [CDC], 2010; Royal College of Nursing, 2012; Solar & Irwin, 2010). The SDH have been adopted as the basis for conceptual frameworks in education programs in nursing (Cohen & Gregory, 2009; Gillis & MacLellan, 2013), as well as for public health and community health programmes (Villarruel, Bigelow, & Alvarez, 2014) and community health initiatives internationally (Blas & Kurup, 2010). SDH frameworks have been used in nursing research (Wuest, Merritt-Gray, Berman, & Ford-Gilboe, 2002) and for conducting and translating research into policy (Ommer, 2006; Ommer With the Coasts Under Stress Research Project Team [Solberg], 2007). The purpose of this chapter is to present the SDH framework as a basis for nursing practice, education, and research.

WHAT ARE THE SOCIAL DETERMINANTS OF HEALTH?

There are a number of conceptualizations and definitions of the SDH and the categories or elements that are to be included in the list of determinants (Graham, 2004; Raphael, 2004). In some of the conceptualizations, the terms determinants of health and SDH are used interchangeably. In other definitions, the SDH are considered as a subset of the determinants of health or of population health and used more particularly to refer to societal factors, which usually do not include individual factors such as biology or genetics (MacDonald, Newburn-Cook, Allen, & Reutter, 2013; Williams, 2003). The role of health care systems/access to health care as a determinant of health has been much contested, with some definitions and lists of the SDH including it (Dahlgren & Whitehead, 2006; Public Health Agency of Canada, 2013), others not (Wilkinson & Marmot, 2003), and some authors advocating for its inclusion (McGibbon, Etowa, & McPherson, 2008).

Some of the variation in conceptualization represents a developmental stage in how to best conceptualize the SDH (WHO, 1986). Early definitions or conceptualizations of the SDH encompassed societal factors that were thought to contribute to or determine the overall health of a population or a country (Wilkinson & Marmot, 2003). Other variations in definitions embody more ideological or political differences. Raphael (2011) illustrated the importance of ideological differences through an examination of discourse in six different SDH concepts, and the willingness or not, of the proponents of the definition to link the concept of the SDH with broad policy implications or development that would address inequities in the health of the population. Over the past decades, definitions of the SDH have been refined and broadened to include the phenomena of health inequities, inequalities, or disparities (Solar & Irwin, 2010). Based on research evidence, the SDH and health inequities have been found to be strongly linked and this link is encompassed in the WHO framework for SDH and social determinants of health inequities (CSDH, 2008). The latest WHO (2014) definition of the SDH that is in widespread use is:

> The social determinants of health are the conditions in which people are born, grow, live, work and age. These circumstances are shaped by the distribution of money, power and resources at global, national, and local levels. The social determinants of health are mostly responsible for health inequities—the unfair and avoidable differences in health status seen within and between countries. (WHO, para. 1, 2014)

EVOLUTION OF SOCIAL DETERMINANTS OF HEALTH

This section is an overview of the evolution of the SDH as a concept and framework. See Table 28.1 for some of the main milestones in the development of the SDH. It is not meant to be a comprehensive account because that is well beyond the scope of this chapter. Many countries have their own history incorporating and adapting the SDH within more local contexts (Edwards & Cohen, 2012), and some of these developments may or may not have contributed to the overall development of the SDH as a conceptual framework. It is difficult to trace when the first use of the term "social determinants of health" came into common use. One of the challenges is that the word "determinant" has a number of meanings, for example "a factor that decisively affects the nature or outcome of something" ("Determinant," 2014). Other meanings of determinants are causal factors or influences. Nevertheless, as some authors have indicated, the idea of health being rooted in social circumstances is not new, with a gradual shift from thinking about health strictly as a biomedical concept that is linked to the absence of disease to a social concept that links health to life circumstances and determined by social, political, and environmental factors (Graham, 2004; Raphael, 2004;

TABLE 28.1

Key Phases and Milestones in the Evolution of the Social Determinants of Health (SDH) and Social Determinants of Health Inequities as a Basis for Practice, Policy, and Research

PHASE	KEY DEVELOPMENTS
Phase 1: Broadening the debate	1. Development of social medicine as a division within medicine with the goal of understanding social influences on health in the early 20th century (Porter, 2006).
	2. Development of subdiscipline in sociology, sociology of medicine, which extended the focus to examining societal influences on health (Williams, 2003).
	3. McKeown (1976; 1979) introduced the "thesis" that the medical approach is limiting for improving health and that behavioral and environmental factors are more important.
	4. Lalonde (1974) took up McKeown's thesis and suggested the traditional view of health and dependence on the current health care system based on a curative model would not improve health to the extent needed in Canada.
	5. The Black Report released in Great Britain in 1980 (Townsend, Davidson, Whitehead, 1992).
	6. Declaration of Alma-Ata in 1978 (WHO, 1978) that attainment of health "requires the action of many other social and economic sectors in addition to the health sector" (p. 1).
	7. *The Health Divide* (Whitehead) is published in 1987 (Townsend et al., 1992).
	8. European states agree on *"Health for All"* strategy proposed by WHO in 1984. Other countries adopt this strategy, for example, Canada and *Achieving Health for All: A Framework for Health Promotion* (Epp, 1986).
	9. The First International Conference on Health Promotion (WHO, 1986) is held and the adoption of the *Ottawa Charter for Health Promotion*, which contains a list of requisites for health and redefining health as a positive concept emphasizing "*social* (my emphasis) and personal resources, as well as physical capabilities" (p. 1).
	10. The Acheson Report *Independent Inquiry Into Inequalities in Health* is released in 1998. This report shows that inequalities in health persist in Great Britain.
	11. WHO Regional Office for Europe's Centre for Urban Health launches a social determinants campaign in 1998 with an emphasis on healthy cities. Other countries launch similar campaigns.
	12. The United Nations Millennium Campaign is launched in 2002 with a series of Millennium Development goals (MDG). This is a global strategy to address many of the SDH with a strong recognition of the interdependence between social conditions and health. Details of MDG can be found online (http://www.un.org/millenniumgoals/bkgd.shtml).
	13. "Strengthening the social determinants of health: The Toronto Charter for a healthy Canada" is adopted at a conference in 2002 and brought together a number of experts to discuss the determinants of health (Raphael, 2004).
	14. The Commission on Social Determinants of Health (2008) and the document *Closing the gap in a generation: Health Equity through action on the social determinants of health. Final Report.*
	15. Rio Political Declaration on Social Determinants of Health at World Conference on Social Determinants of Health in 2011(WHO, 2011) reaffirms the importance of SDH approach to reduce inequities in health and called for global actions.

(continued)

TABLE 28.1
Key Phases and Milestones in the Evolution of the Social Determinants of Health (SDH) and Social Determinants of Health Inequities as a Basis for Practice, Policy, and Research (continued)

PHASE	KEY DEVELOPMENTS
Phase 2: Identifying concepts	1. Health field—four broad elements as causes or factors in morbidity and mortality: human, biology, environment, lifestyle, and health care organization (Lalonde, 1974). 2. Prerequisites for health—peace, shelter, education, food, income, stable ecosystem, sustainable resources, social justice, and equity from the *Ottawa Charter for Health Promotion* (WHO, 1986). This was the first attempt at delineating a comprehensive list of the determinants of health. 3. Social determinants of health—broadly refers to social and economic conditions that influence the health status of groups or populations. (WHO, 2014; Raphael, 2004). See Table 28.2 for various social determinants. 4. Health inequities—the systematic disparities in health (or in the SDH) that exist between more or less advantaged social groups. Black Report (Marmot, 2001). 5. Social gradient (in health)—"life expectancy is shorter and most diseases are more common further down the social ladder in each society" (Wilkinson & Marmot, 2003, p. 10).
Phase 3: Providing evidence	1. *Inequalities in Health* (Townsend, Davidson, & Whitehead, 1992)—an updated edition of *The Black Report* and *The Health Divide*. 2. The Acheson Report (1998). *Independent inquiry into inequalities in health.* 3. *Social determinants of health* (Marmot & Wilkinson, 2006). 4. *Why are some people healthy and some people not?* (Evans et al., 1994). This was aimed at understanding population health, but frequently cited in the SDH literature. 5. *Social determinants of health: Canadian perspectives* (Raphael, 2004).
Phase 4: Developing a conceptual framework	1. Model depicting the relationship between social and individual factors and human well-being and prosperity (Evan & Stoddart, 1994, p. 53). The model broadly identifies the determinants of health as structural (social and physical environments) and individual factors (genetic endowment) with individual responses (behavior and biology) affecting health and function, disease, and health care and ultimately well-being and prosperity. The model is based on a series of feedback loops from the various components. 2. Social determinants of health (Brunner & Marmot, 2006, p.9). This is a multilevel pathway model that demonstrates the links between social structure and health and well-being of populations, taking into consideration many of the SDH as mediating factors. The model was originally in the first edition of the book, published in 1999. 3. Rainbow or Social Model of Health (Dahlgren & Whitehead, 2006). The model is a socioecological model of health that illustrates the SDH as multilevel and interacting at various levels. The model was introduced in the early 1990s. This is one of the most frequently used and adapted models for SDH. 4. Committee on the Social Determinants of health and health inequities conceptual framework (Solar & Irwin, 2010, p. 6). This occurred in a number of stages until it evolved into a multilevel framework that illustrates the links between structural determinants of the social determinants of health inequities and intermediate determinants of the SDH to impact equity in health and well-being.

Williams, 2003). This shift has been one of evolution and has had a number of influences or developmental milestones. The work conducted under the leadership in the WHO has had a huge impact on the development of the SDH as a way to think about health and health inequities and as a framework for health policy (Irvine, Elliott, Wallace, & Crombie, 2006). A description and analysis of the main events that contributed to this history is presented by Irwin and Scali (2010) and by Irvine et al., (2006). Irwin and Scali traced this development from the first WHO constitution in 1946 that included a goal to address "social roots of health problems" (p. 5) to the 1960s and 1970s, with an increasing emphasis on how social, economic, and political factors affected health, to the concentrated work on the SDH in the 1990s. This culminated in the setting up of the CSDH by the WHO in 2005 and a final report (CSDH, 2008). The work by the WHO on the SDH continues. Throughout these developments and in keeping with principles of the WHO, there was an emphasis on health as a human right and promoting strategies to reduce the health inequities that have been identified within countries, between countries, and globally; hence a link to social justice.

Some of the groundwork for the development of an SDH framework predates the work of the WHO and has emerged from developments in medicine and sociology in the early 1920s and 1930s with the creation of a division within medicine known as "social medicine" now referred to as "public health medicine" (Young, 2005) and development of the subdiscipline medical sociology within sociology known as sociology of health (Segall & Fries, 2011). As Porter (2006) indicated in a brief history of social medicine, the early goals in the 1930s in North America and Great Britain "were overtly linked to political programs of social reform" (p. e39). The main area of concern within medical sociology gradually evolved from a focus on the medical professions and organization of health systems to incorporate the roles that society and social structures played in health and illness, with a more recent interest in SDH (Williams, 2003). Others describe it as evolving from early social reform movements and public health, with the focus on living conditions and the environment (Irwin & Scali, 2007). Although all these developments no doubt were influential, the rise of epidemiology and social epidemiology in the past several decades with a focus on distribution and determinants of disease, and later on the determinants of health, helped to establish not only strong evidence in this area, but powerful quantitative methods for researching the SDH (Honjo, 2004; Young, 2005). Integration of such techniques as geographical information systems into health research is promising for providing more evidence for the SDH because it provides the ability to map out areas of greater disparities in health (Bloch, 2011). Other approaches are critical as well in order to more fully understand pathways and explanations of the social phenomena inherent in an SDH framework (Williams, 2003). In some ways the evidence has outstripped our understanding, particularly in how causal pathways work between the broader determinants to the level of population and individual health (CSDH, 2008).

BEGINNING THE DEBATE

A number of authors are credited with beginning the debate about determinants of health. An early use of the term was by McKeown (1976; 1979), who presented strong evidence for the role that behavioral and environmental factors had in the improvement in health. He examined the decline in mortality rates in England and Wales between 1700 and 1971 and linked reduction in mortality to improved social factors, such as access to improved nutrition and living in healthier environments. Healthier environments were marked first by greater hygienic measures than existed previously, improved housing, and later cleaner atmospheres and improved working conditions. In contrast, he suggested medical interventions contributed little to improved health. McKeown (1979) concluded that "in order of importance the determinants of health, at least in the past were nutritional, environmental, and behavioural" (p. 164). His writings are cited as influential in development of the Lalonde Report in 1974 and the health field concept (Crighton, Robertson, Gordon, & Farrant, 1997; Irvine et al., 2006), and the SDH (Frank & Mustard, 1994).

Selected government directions and debates on public health policy have been credited with influencing the development of the SDH as a concept and approach (Graham, 2004). Although the WHO provided much of the leadership on an SDH framework, the recognition of the importance of this approach and developments in other countries were equally important. Some key studies carried out in the 1970s and 1980s in Canada and Great Britain, either as parallel developments or in collaboration with the WHO, are noteworthy in that they are cited as influential in developing our understanding of and the importance of emphasizing the SDH. Western European countries, Australia, and New Zealand were also important contributors to developments in SDH (Irwin & Scali, 2010). Research funding and institutes established in Canada, Great Britain, the United States, and no doubt other countries provided key resources, both financial and human, to carry on the critical work of providing evidence and knowledge creation, transfer, translation, and implementation critical to the further development of the SDH.

Canada

In the early 1970s, the Canadian government released a white paper titled *A New Perspective on the Health of Canadians* (Lalonde, 1974), usually referred to as the Lalonde Report, which was widely distributed. The new perspective introduced was the "health field concept" consisting of four broad elements: human biology, environment, lifestyle, and health care organization (p. 31). This framework broadened thinking within Canada on what determined health and influenced work on health promotion within the Canadian health system and beyond (Crighton et al., 1997; Pederson, Rootman, & O'Neill, 2005). The report also influenced a debate on an international scale and is widely attributed to beginning a discussion on the SDH (Irwin & Scali, 2010; Robertson, 1998) and public policies to address health inequities (Irvine et al., 2006; Graham, 2004). A second major milestone was the release of the Canadian policy paper *Achieving Health For All: A framework for health promotion* (Epp, 1986) in conjunction with the WHO's First International Conference for Health Promotion held in Canada that year (Pederson et al., 2005). In this paper, Epp identified "reducing inequities in the health of low- versus high-income groups" (p. 4) as one of the main challenges to achieving health for all. This conference resulted in the *Ottawa Charter for Health Promotion*, which identified eight prerequisites believed important for health (WHO, 1986). Later, these factors were modified and described as the SDH (Canadian Nurses Association, 2013). These events were also considered the beginning of a "new health promotion" or "new public health" that was based on a broad conceptualization of health and what influenced health (Robertson, 1998; Scriven & Garmin, 2005). The Ottawa Charter reaffirmed the WHO (1978) Alma-Ata Declaration of "Health for All" and the goal of health equity. In practice and service delivery, health promotion became the main paradigm and thus health promotion and the SDH developed as "two solitudes" (Jackson, Birn, Fawcett, Poland, & Schultz, 2013). Nevertheless, the work of Lalonde (1974) planted the ideas of the SDH as a focus in health circles and they were translated into at least some of the health discourse in Canada, used for health education programs, and eventually adopted by the Canadian Nurses Association (2013) and the Public Health Agency of Canada (2013).

Within Canada, both inside and outside of academic circles, Raphael (2004, 2010) has promoted the concept of SDH defined as "the economic and social conditions that influence the health of individuals, communities, and jurisdictions as a whole" (2004, p. 1). Through work with other academics and individuals in public policy and based on research evidence within Canada, he identified a number of SDH. Raphael's work on the SDH is widely cited. Funding for research on the SDH is supported mainly through the Canadian Institutes of Health Research (CIHR) established in 2000, but especially the Institute for Population and Public Health (2014), which has as a mandate to "support research into the complex biological, social, cultural, and environmental interactions that determines the health of individuals, communities, and global populations" (para. 1). A core pillar of the CIHR for Gender and Health and Aboriginal People's Health is social and cultural dimensions of health, and this pillar supports health equity research on the SDH as it applies to gender and aboriginal people (Edwards & Cohen, 2012). In 2005, the Public Health agency of Canada established six National Collaborating Centers (NCCs); one in eastern Canada for the Determinants of Health (Edwards & Cohen, 2012) tasked with knowledge translation, developing networks, and identifying gaps in research.

Great Britain

In Great Britain, a working group was appointed in 1977 to examine and report on the health disparities evident in that country. The work of this group resulted in the release of the 1980 Report on the Working Group on Equalities in Health (better known as the Black Report) (Townsend, Davidson, & Whitehead, 1992). This event was followed by Whitehead's *The Health Divide* published in 1987 and later the Acheson Report into inequalities in health (Acheson, 1998); both of which provided updated evidence on inequalities in health because the Black Report indicated the need for an SDH approach. Unlike the Lalonde Report in Canada, which was widely distributed, the Black Report received little attention by the British government (Marmot, 2001; Townsend, et al., 1992). It did garner widespread academic interest and later attention by the WHO and in other countries, most notably the Netherlands, Spain, and Sweden (Irwin & Scali, 2007). One of the important concepts established was that of social inequalities in health (Marmot, 2001). A second and related concept also important was that of a gradient in health status, illustrating that those in lower socioeconomic positions had lower health status than those occupying increasingly higher socioeconomic positions; the higher up in socioeconomic position the better the health status. These were important findings, not only for understanding the SDH but also for identifying the social determinants of health inequities and how health is distributed across populations. At first, the two constructs, the SDH and social determinants of health inequalities, were used interchangeably and frequently confused, resulted in a blurring of "the distinction between the social *factors* that influence health and the social *processes* that determine their unequal distribution" [emphasis added]; (Graham, 2004, p. 107). Separating these two major constructs conceptually is particularly important for researchers, practitioners, and policy makers (CSDH, 2008; Whitehead & Dahlgren, 2006).

Marmot and Wilkinson (2006) and academic colleagues in Great Britain produced two editions of the book *Social Determinants of Health*. This work synthesized the evidence on important SDH, such as early life, labor market disadvantages (unemployment, nonemployment, and job security), psychosocial work environment, transport, social support and social cohesion, food, social exclusion, and neighbourhoods and housing. Their work for the WHO on *Social Determinants of Health: The Solid Facts* (Wilkinson & Marmot, 2003) was used as a guide for identifying the SDH in many countries that adopted this approach. Although they have been criticized for not including health systems and personal health behaviors in their determinants, they certainly acknowledged the importance of both factors and in an early model of the SDH (Brunner & Marmot, 2006, p. 9) health behaviors were depicted within the model. They asserted that "access to medical care is clearly one of the social determinants of health" (Wilkinson & Marmot, 2003, p. 7), however their purpose in identifying the SDH was to try and understand what caused people to be ill in the first place, or the "cause of causes" as this phenomenon became more widely known, and why others remained healthy. Work on the SDH has continued in Great Britain with an emphasis on advocating the development of policy that would address health inequalities related to these determinants (Marmot, 2010).

United States

In the 1970s and 1980s, the United States had a quite divergent approach to health promotion and determinants of health than that adopted by Canada and other European countries because of the very different structure of the health system and the emphasis placed on individualism (Lightsey, McQueen, & Anderson, 2005). As a consequence, an increased use of the language of SDH and health inequities in the United States is seen as much more recent than in countries like Canada, Great Britain, and other European countries; however, the ideas behind this language are not new in that country. When social medicine was developed as a division within academic medicine and the Yale Institute of Human Relations was set up in 1931, the expressed purpose of the institute was to "integrate medicine into research on social inequalities" (Porter, 2006, p. e39). The development of social medicine at Yale University was influenced by the need to introduce the social sciences into medicine (Viseltear, 1984). Social medicine in the United States did not have the widespread influence it had in Great Britain, mainly because of the overt political and ideological nature behind this movement; a challenge that continues to confront the adoption of the SDH as a link to or a means of reducing health inequities (Kelly, Bonnefoy, Morgan, & Florenzano, 2006). However, as Irvine et al. (2006) indicated, other developments in the United States in the 1970s such as beginning the "Healthy People" reports contributed to considering broader factors that influenced health even "act[ing] on the recommendations of the Lalonde Report and pioneer[ing] the introduction of national health targets" (p. 75).

More recently, the CDC (2010) advocated the use of an SDH approach for diseases such as HIV/AIDS, viral hepatitis, sexually transmitted diseases, and tuberculosis in order that together with individual factors, broader social and environmental factors are considered and inequities related to these diseases can be addressed. The CSDH (2008) framework on the SDH and health inequities was amended by CDC for use with "how determinants of health interact, influence inequalities, determines priorities, and target points for intervention" (p. 9). Within the American public health system there is an increased effort to advocate for the consideration of the SDH to address health inequities (Satcher, 2010). In the latest of the series on healthy people, "Healthy People 2020," the U.S. Department of Health and Human Services (2010) states a new addition is that the concepts of the SDH and health equity will be considered from a life course approach in meeting the specified goals.

There is certainly no lack of research evidence on health disparities in the United States (Braverman et al., 2011) and the need to rethink how to approach these disparities. Rethinking approaches to disparities was placed on the agenda for the 2012 summit *Nursing in 3D: Workforce Diversity, Health Disparities, and Social Determinants of Health* sponsored by Health Resources and Services Administration (HRSA). The proceedings of the summit were published in a special supplement to *Public Health Reports* in 2014. The purpose of the summit was to enable those attending to think about health equity in the United States through the three lenses of racial/ethnicity diversity in the nursing workforce, health diversities in specific populations in the country, and the SDH; suggesting the SDH framework would be a good approach to think about diversity in the workforce and health disparities in the population (Mahony & Jones, 2013). To achieve this change two important shifts are key: first, a move to a social determinant from an individual focus and second, a move to an equity model from one based on disparity (Srinivasan & Williams, 2014); shifts that had occurred in other countries at an earlier period. Nurses in the United States are seen as potential leaders to incorporate the SDH into their work to address many of the health problems and health inequities evident in that country (Lathrop, 2013).

THE SOCIAL DETERMINANTS IDENTIFIED

There have been various attempts, locally and globally, to identify the SDH. (See Table 28.2 for some examples of the SDH identified by different authors or by country.) Sometimes this has been by broad category (structural, environmental, behavioral, and individual factors) and sometimes by a particular material or social condition (poverty). One of the first instances of identification of the SDH was in the *Ottawa Charter for Health Promotion* (WHO, 1986) in which a list of prerequisites for health was identified. In most of the recent conceptualizations, generally agreed upon broad categories of the SDH are grouped by level or in a hierarchy (CSDH, 2008; Marmot, 2010). At the most distal or macrolevel, from the individual or population and sometimes referred to as upstream factors (Braverman et al., 2011), are general socioeconomic, cultural, and environmental conditions (Dahlgren & Whitehead, 2006) or the socioeconomic and political context (Solar & Irwin, 2010). Next are structural factors that include social and environmental conditions (Dahlgren & Whitehead, 2006) or socioeconomic position and other axes of social differentiation (e.g., gender, ethnicity; Kelly et al., 2006; Kelly, 2010; Solar & Irwin, 2010). More proximal to those affected are social and psychological

TABLE 28.2

Comparison of Social Determinants of Health or Determinants of Health Globally and by Country or Organization

	GLOBAL		
Source	WHO (1986)	WHO (Wilkinson & Marmot, 2003)	WHO (2011)
	Ottawa Charter for Health Promotion	*SDH: The Solid Facts*	*Rio Political Declaration on SDH*
Prerequisites for health:	1. Peace SDH 2. Shelter 3. Education 4. Food 5. Income 6. Stable ecosystem 7. Sustainable resources 8. Social justice and equity	1. Social gradient SDH 2. Stress 3. Early life 4. Social exclusion 5. Work 6. Unemployment 7. Social support 8. Addiction 9. Food 10. Transport	1. Early years' experiences 2. Education 3. Economic status 4. Employment and decent work 5. Housing and environment 6. Effective systems of preventing and treating ill health
Country	**Canada**	**Canada**	**United States**
Source	Raphael (2004)	Public Health Agency of Canada (PHAC; 2013)	Healthy People (U.S. Department of Health and Human Services, 2020)
Determinants	1. Early childhood development 2. Employment and working conditions 3. Food security 4. Health care services 5. Housing shortages 6. Income and its equitable distribution 7. Social exclusion 8. Social safety nets 9. Unemployment 10. Canadian women, aboriginal people, Canadians of color, and New Canadians	1. Income and social status 2. Social support networks 3. Education and literacy 4. Employments and working conditions 5. Social environments 6. Physical environments 7. Personal health practices and coping skills 8. Healthy child development 9. Biology and genetics endowment 10. Health services 11. Gender 12. Culture	1. Physical environment 2. Social environment 3. Individual behaviors 4. Biology and genetics 5. Health services

(continued)

TABLE 28.2

Comparison of Social Determinants of Health or Determinants of Health Globally and by Country or Organization (continued)

	New Zealand	Australia	Australia
Source	King (2000)	Turrell et al. (1999)	SDHA (2013)
	1. Knowledge and skills 2. Paid work 3. Economic standard of living 4. Civil and political rights 5. Social connectedness 6. Cultural identity 7. Leisure and recreation 8. Safety 9. Physical environment	1. Social, physical, and economic environment 2. Education 3. Employment 4. Occupation 5. Working conditions 6. Income 7. Housing and area of residence services	1. Social connectedness 2. Education 3. Gender 4. Physical environment 5. Ethnicity 6. Housing 7. Early childhood development 8. Health and social 9. Built environment 10. Employment and working conditions 11. Culture 12. Income
Organizations	**Canadian Nurses Association (2013)**		
SDH	1. Early childhood and access to education 2. Nature of employment and working conditions 3. Access to healthy food and adequate income 4. Social inclusion 5. Access to housing 6. Quality of built and natural environments 7. Ability to access and use health care		

systems (Dahlgren & Whitehead, 2006) or social cohesion and social capital as bridging factors from the structural determinants to the more downstream, meso or intermediary determinants of health (Solar & Irwin, 2010). Most proximal to individuals and populations, and if included are the micro, downstream (Braverman et al., 2011), or individual lifestyle factors (Dahlgren & Whitehead) or material circumstances, behavioral and biological factors and psychosocial factors (Solar & Irwin, 2010). In Table 28.2 is a comparison of the different factors included under various conceptualizations or models of the SDH. It would be expected that these specific factors would vary from country to country, and even globally and temporally, because of the importance of a particular social structure and its context at particular times when delineating the SDH for individuals and a population, region or country, as well as the dynamic nature of social structures (Kelly et al., 2007).

MODELS USED FOR SOCIAL DETERMINANTS OF HEALTH FRAMEWORK

A number of models have been developed that are used or adapted to illustrate an SDH framework, and these come from a variety of disciplines and are informed by varying theoretical perspectives (Dunn, Masyn, Yudron, Jones, & Subramanian, 2014). Most models are influenced by a social ecological design that is presented as a series of nested, multilevel, and interrelated factors (Brofenbrenner, 1977). Using a social ecological framework recognizes the embeddedness of humans (either as individuals or populations) within their environments and the social systems that characterize these environments. Perhaps the most widely used social ecological model, especially in the academic literature, is the "Rainbow" or Social Model of Health (Dahlgren & Whitehead, 2006). The Committee on the Social Determinants of Health conceptual framework (Solar & Irwin, 2010) is also a widely used model and could be considered a social ecological model. Other models can be found in the literature as well (Dolan et al., 2005).

Rainbow or Social Model of Health

This model, described as a social ecological model, was developed by Dahlgren and Whitehead (2006) and depicts the multiple levels of the SDH influences. Figure 28.1 illustrates this model. In the center of the model are individuals with their biological and demographic factors (age, sex, and genetics). The first level is identified as "individual lifestyle factors" and these are ones that can be modified through policy and programs that address lifestyle choices such as smoking and physical activity. Likewise, the second level "social and community networks" can be either conducive to health, if the networks are

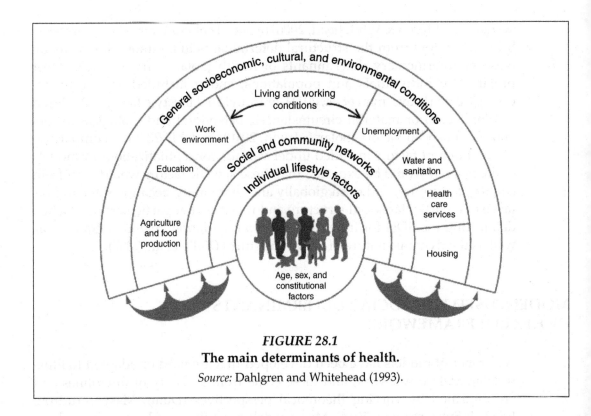

FIGURE 28.1
The main determinants of health.
Source: Dahlgren and Whitehead (1993).

present and functioning well, or not if the networks are poor or absent. The third level would be similar to what are often termed structural factors that affect health and in the model are: agriculture and food production, education, work environment, living and working conditions, unemployment, water and sanitation, health care services, and housing. The overarching level is the general socioeconomic, cultural and environmental conditions, also sometimes described as contextual factors. It is the various layers in interaction that are thought to influence human health. The Rainbow or Social Model of SDH is widely used in policy and research (Bambra et al., 2010).

CSDH Conceptual Framework

This model, described as the bringing together of "elements" identified as structural determinants and intermediate determinants, was developed through the work of the CSDH (2008) and is also a multilevel model as shown in Figure 28.2. It builds on the work of previous models in that it separates out the SDH from the social determinants of health inequities. The structural determinants are the social determinants of health inequities or the "causes of the cause" of poor health. At the left side of the model is the socioeconomic and political context and some of the structural mechanisms, such as governance, macroeconomic policies, social policies, public policies, and cultural

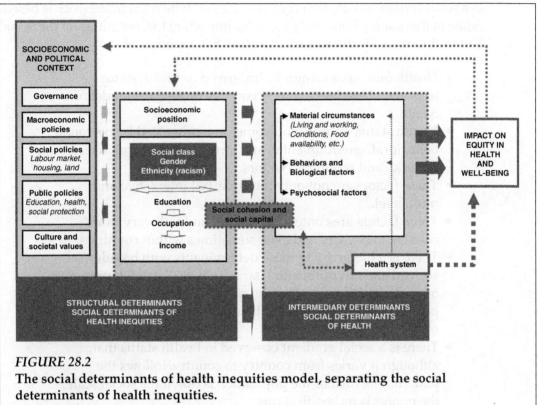

FIGURE 28.2
The social determinants of health inequities model, separating the social determinants of health inequities.

Source: Solar and Irwin (2010).

and societal values. These result in individuals being placed in a certain socioeconomic position determined by their social class, gender, and ethnicity through their education, occupation, and income within a particular socioeconomic and political context. The intermediate determinants are the SDH and they are categorized as material circumstances, behavioral and biological factors, psychosocial factors, and the health system. Social cohesion and social capital are seen as cutting across the structural and intermediate determinants. It is "underlying social determinants of health inequities operat[ing] through a set of intermediary determinants of health" that health outcomes are produced (Solar & Irwin, 2010, p. 6).

ASSUMPTIONS AND PRINCIPLES OF THE COMMITTEE ON THE SOCIAL DETERMINANTS OF HEALTH MODEL

Conceptual frameworks or models are important tools to present key concepts and the interrelationships between or among the concepts (Miles & Huberman, 1994; Ravitch & Riggan, 2012). Underlying any conceptual model is a set of certain assumptions or principles on which the framework is based. Some of the assumptions and principles important to Committee on the Social Determinants of Health Model and other SDH models are:

- Health outcomes cannot be improved or health status improved based on a purely curative or medical model of health.
- Health status or health outcomes are influenced by personal, behavioral, environmental, and structural (political, social, cultural, and economic) factors.
- These factors are not only multiple, but interactive and multilevel.
- These factors are context dependent and will vary from country to country and even sometimes within countries.
- There is a hierarchy to these determinants with broader societal and environmental (structural or distal determinants or upstream) factors often the cause or source of the more personal and behavioral (individual or proximal determinants or downstream) factors.
- There is a social gradient observed in health status that, although it varies from country to country, follows the pattern: The further the population is down the social scale, the poorer is its health status.
- Actions to address the SDH require an intersectoral (policy/ programs) and interdisciplinary (research) approach because several determinants lie outside the health sector.
- A community participatory approach that is contextually based is key.

In addition to these principles or assumptions, important assumptions or principles underpinning social determinants of health inequity are:

- Health is a human right and a matter of social justice.
- There is unequal and unjust access to the resources required for health, and these are the cause of health inequities.
- Adopting a social determinant of health equity lens is not value neutral; it is a political commitment.
- The goals for health equity and health care equity differ.
- Inequities in health are mainly determined by structural and not individual factors; therefore factors determining health inequities must be addressed at that level.
- If not addressed, the gap in health and health care will continue to widen and a consequent increase in health inequities will be observed.

EVIDENCE FOR SOCIAL DETERMINANTS OF HEALTH FRAMEWORK

The research evidence crucial to consider human health from an SDH framework, especially at a population level, is strong and continues to build (CSDH, 2008; Marmot, 2010). Much of this evidence, but not all, has come from commissioned reports that drew on population-based research (Acheson, 1998; Evans, Barer, & Marmor, 1994; National Forum on Health, 1996; Townsend et al., 1992; Wilkinson & Marmot, 2003). The WHO (2014) set up a series of nine knowledge networks to support the work of the CSDH and bring together evidence in a number of areas:

- Early child development (ECDKN)
- Employment conditions (ECKN)
- Globalization (GKN)
- Social exclusion (SEKN)
- Health systems (HSKN)
- Priority public health conditions (PPHKN)
- Urban settings (USKN)
- Women and gender equity (WGEKN)
- Measurement and evidence knowledge (MEKN)

The first eight knowledge networks addressed priority concerns under SDH and health equity, whereas the purpose of the MEKN was to provide guidance and stimulate discussion on issues of measurement and knowledge translation for practice and, in particular, design of policy (Bonnefoy, Morgan, Kelly, Butt, & Bergman, 2007).

RESEARCH AND THE SOCIAL DETERMINANTS OF HEALTH

Using an SDH framework for research presents a number of challenges. To identify some of the research issues associated with the SDH the CSDH (2008) established a network, MEKN, with the main objective "to collect, assess and synthesize global knowledge on existing methodologies to evaluate the effectiveness of policies, interventions and actions on social determinants of health which are aimed at improving health outcomes and health equity" (Bonnefoy et al., 2007, p. 8). Members of MEKN identified a number of conceptual and theoretical issues. These issues have been identified by others as well and remain challenges to the use of a SDH framework (Dunn et al., 2014; Kneipp & Drevdahl, 2003).

Conceptual or Definitional

As illustrated in the short historical overview of the development of the SDH, a number of different concepts and definitions have been used and these have changed over time with the resolution of some differences but not of others. A number of important questions are: (a) What are the differences between the concepts of SDH, health inequality, and health inequity? (b) What are the differences between health promotion, population health, and SDH? (c) How does the concept of social justice fit with the SDH?

Social Determinants of Health, Health Inequality, and of Health Inequities

A conceptual issue is that of clarifying the difference between the SDH, health inequality, and health inequities (Bonnefoy et al., 2007), an issue previously identified by Graham (2004). These three constructs are not the same even though they are highly interrelated. Recent work through the CSDH (2008) and the various networks of this commission has helped to make the distinction between the constructs, and this is reflected in the latest model. Although the SDH are descriptive of the "conditions in which people are born, grow, live, work, and age" (WHO, 2014, para. 1), the social determinants of health inequalities are "dimensional" and measure "the differences, variations, and disparities in the health achievements of individuals and groups" (Kawachi, Subramanian, & Almeida-Filho, 2002, p. 647). The same authors define health inequities as "normative" and refer to "those inequalities in health that are deemed to be unfair or stemming from some form of injustice" (p. 647). Health inequalities "arise" from the SDH and in as far as they are unfair or unjust, also give rise to health inequities (WHO, 2011).

As previously noted, many of the same factors have been conceptualized as differences, heterogeneities, disparities, inequalities, and inequities in health. Conceptualization and descriptive language are important "because they reflect different perspectives on the 'causes' of health outcomes and hence point to different solutions" (Reutter & Kushner, 2010, p. 270). In the United States, disparities was the language used and health disparities tended to be conceptualized as differences in disease patterns among particular groups or populations (Fink, 2009). Recently in the United States, there is a move to use the language of health inequities (Srinivasan & Williams, 2014) as well as an expanded definition of health disparities (Braverman, 2006). In Canada, "inequities" was the term used by Epp (1986); however, "heterogeneities" was the term used by Hertzman, Frank, and Evans (1994). They also focused on the determinants of health rather than the SDH; thus a move away from a more critical social science approach that had previously marked developments in Canada (Robertson, 1998). With the SDH framework, "health inequities" is the preferred term in that it is social structural factors, either directly or indirectly, that are being addressed because they are the "cause of the causes" for health outcomes.

A related conceptual issue is whether to consider and describe health inequities as disadvantages, gaps, or gradients (Kelly et al., 2006, 2007). Considering inequities as disadvantages implies a more neutral stance and could be equated with describing them as differences or heterogeneities. Differences or heterogeneities serve to acknowledge existence and even that some members of the population are disadvantaged, but carry no ethical or political implications and are inconsistent with an SDH approach that is based on a principle of equity (Kelly et al., 2006). Considering inequities as gaps leads to a focus on the sector of the population with the poorest outcome, and in select situations this may be required, but in the long run may not reduce relative changes that are required to reduce health inequities. The importance of thinking of inequities in terms of a gradient addresses both absolute and relative change and moving the whole population to achieve their highest potential for health. A particular framing of a problem has implications for what counts as evidence and how to best study or address the problem (Evans & Stoddart, 1994).

Social Determinants of Health, Health Promotion, and Population Health

Work on the SDH emerged from the concept of a "new health promotion" (Scriven, 2005). Much of the early histories on health promotion and SDH, therefore coincide. However, as Jackson et al. (2013) illustrated even though the SDH framework developed from early work on health promotion the two frameworks in many instances diverged with neither integrating the strength of the other and could benefit enormously from reintegration. One of the challenges in separating out differences is that health promotion in the broadest sense refers to "an holistic field of overlapping activity at primary, secondary and tertiary levels encompassing health education, lifestyle and preventative approaches alongside the policy, environment, legal and fiscal measures designed to advance health" (Scriven, 2005, p. 8). When the SDH are encompassed within health promotion the "policy and environment" activities are paramount especially if the goal is to address health inequities.

In Canada, the term that supplanted health promotion was "population health" (Federal/Provincial/Territorial Advisory Committee on Population Health, 1994) with a model of population health promotion incorporating the determinants of health and health promotion strategies (Hamilton & Bhatti, 1996). Understandably, the concepts and frameworks for population health and the SDH are sometimes used interchangeably. Some authors distinguish between the two and understand the SDH to be a subset of the population health framework, but contend that SDH do not encompass "inter- and intrapersonal determinants of health nor the intermediate processes that link these with the broader or 'social' or structural determinants of health" (MacDonald et al., 2013, p. 33). In contrast, the CSDH (2008) continued to describe the intermediary determinants of health as the SDH and the "structural determinants" as the social determinants of health inequities and integrated them within a single model (Solar & Irwin, 2010). Young (2005) examined the evolution of the term "population health," which originally was a substitute term for "health of populations" and later "as a field of study that focus on both health outcomes and health determinants, as well as the policies and interventions that link them" (p. 5). These constructs by Young's definition seem remarkably similar to the SDH. One of the distinguishing features between population health and the SDH is the level of analysis and the target of the interventions. Population health is aimed at a population or group level whereas the SDH could be used at the population level in which differential vulnerabilities and outcomes are observed as well as at an individual level where the differential consequences are experienced (Blas & Kurup, 2010).

Social Justice and SDH

Social justice is defined as

> the fair distribution of society's benefits, responsibilities and their consequences. It focuses on the relative position of one social grouping relationship to others in society as well as on the root cause of disparities and what can be done to eliminate them. (Canadian Nurses Association, 2010, p. 10)

Social justice is a concept that is increasingly found in nursing codes of ethics (Canadian Nurses Association, 2008; International Council of Nurses, 2012). The concept of social justice is tied to the SDH because of the role that the latter plays, particularly at the structural level, in producing health inequities. To assist nurses in applying the concept of social justice to programs, policies, or products, the Canadian Nurses Association (2010) has developed a social justice gauge. The gauge could be applied to nursing research using the SDH, especially at the proposal stage, to incorporate social justice.

Importance of Context

Understanding as fully as possible the context of the particular population to which an SDH framework is being applied is crucial because of the variation in social structure with country and over time (Kelly et al., 2006). The social structure must be inclusive of cultural, sociological, geographical, economic, and political influences particular to the population of concern. Care must be taken to distinguish between contextual knowledge and essentialized knowledge of the context; the former is knowledge "of" the context and the latter that "about" the context that is held by others (Anderson et al., 2009). Contextual knowledge allows for an understanding of how a particular place exerts influence and is influenced by selected factors, whereas essentialized knowledge may impose a worldview that does not adequately reflect the situation.

Findings based on the SDH ought to take into consideration "the unique particularities of each setting" best done through "extensive in-depth case studies" (Krumeich & Meershoek, 2014, p. 7).

Theory

An issue identified by MEKN is that of the dual responsibility of inferring causal pathways and agreeing on a theoretical explanation for the causation (Bonnefoy et al., 2007). The importance of theory to the SDH lies in the ability to put forward an explanation for the SDH as a cause in determining the health inequities observed between populations and countries or in the consequences they have for individuals and their health. The discussion of theoretical approaches to inequality began with the Black Report (Townsend et al., 1992, pp. 104–126) in which four possible explanations for the social gradient in health were explored. These explanations were grouped as: (a) artifact explanations; (b) theories of natural or social selection; (c) materialist or structural explanations; and (d) cultural/behavioral explanations. The authors concluded that the materialist or structural explanation held the most promise. Since those discussions, other authors have suggested other possible theoretical approaches or lens through which to view the research, such as critical theory or critical social theory (Stevens, 1989), feminist theory (Wuest et al., 2002), or critical social justice (Anderson et al., 2009). Although no one theoretical approach has been adopted, how the problem is theorized would have an important impact on practice and research activities or in how a research problem is framed.

Methodology

The origin of the evidence that supports an SDH approach has clearly arisen from a quantitative research paradigm. Epidemiological and social epidemiological studies were critical in the early development and will continue to play a role in monitoring any changes in the SDH and health inequities. A number of indicators have been used in measuring population health (Etches, Frank, Di Ruggiero, & Manuel, 2006) and would apply to quantitative research on the SDH. Types of data sets commonly used were census data and vital statistics records (births and deaths), health surveys, administrative data (health-related—health insurance, cancer, and other registries; and non-health-related—education, employment, and unemployment, and many others that address the SDH), and data from mapping (disease and resource distribution and climate changes); see Etches et al. (2006) and Harrison and Dean (2011). These sources are invaluable and techniques developed such as ability to link databases, perform multilevel analysis, and do statistical modeling make researching and monitoring the health of populations from an

SDH approach more feasible and powerful. Longitudinal studies are particularly important for assessing changes over time (Braverman et al., 2011). There are limitations as well to these approaches in that not all countries have well-developed databases, so other means for studying health status of populations need to be considered; neither might they have the resources to create these.

The use of the word "determinant" is strongly suggestive of causation. Part of establishing causation in research is to establish a causal link, in this instance a cause-and-effect interaction between variables with health status or health disparity, however, measured as the dependent variable. Key methodological questions (and related conceptual issues) are how best to measure health status and whether to use measures other than those of morbidity and mortality or self-reported health status. Key independent variables have been challenged as well, for example that of quantifying "social position," "socioeconomic status (SES)" and "social class" and what are the appropriate indicators (Kneipp & Drevdahl, 2003). SDH frameworks and models are multilevel, usually having three or more levels and thus present special challenges for measurement (Dunn et al., 2014). Challenges these authors identify are first, defining and conceptualizing the environment. It might seem evident in an SDH approach that these would be the determinants in the model; however, the researcher is still left with some quandaries. The first is of the environmental factors in a model how these variables can be operationalized or constructed so that they can be captured in measurement; for example, in Dahlgren and Whitehead's (2006) model in how to measure agriculture and food production or water and sanitation. The second is, in the particular context being studied, what determinants are *critical* to include, and at what level do these determinants operate. A second issue is what is the best source of the data. Related to the source of data is the "how" of data analysis and the capacity to test the multilevel influences. Even with advanced statistical techniques, overall conceptualization of the research is crucial as O'Campo and Urquia (2012) demonstrated in their comparison of studying a disease-specific model versus a generalized health impact model for adverse health outcomes related to pregnancy and birth. They concluded that the generalized health model was able to "detect stronger effects of social position on pregnancy related outcomes" (p. 1874) and thus would be more meaningful for research on the SDH.

Although quantitative studies predominated the early research on the SDH, that research landscape is changing as well. The consensus of participants in the MEKN was that all research approaches, whether quantitative, qualitative, or mixed methods, were equally valued for research into the SDH (Bonnefoy et al., 2007). It is important to understand causation, that is, how a particular determinant operates to contribute to health, interactions or what are the cumulative or intermediate effects of determinants, but equally important is to understand processes of what is happening and how. These processes will best be understood through a qualitative approach. For example, in a program designed to address a particular SDH, typically baseline measures are collected and later measures indicating the intervention worked or did not work will be collected at points along the way. However, it is equally important to understand how the program worked, under what conditions, and why some may have benefitted and others not; these are understandings that come from qualitative research (Bonnefoy et al., 2007). The basic principle on research methodology espoused by the MEKN is that the method must be the best one(s) for the problem(s) being studied (Bonnefoy et al., 2007).

Nursing scholars and others have used qualitative approaches in research with the SDH. A good example of the use of a qualitative approach was that by Wuest et al. (2002) who used grounded theory embedded in a participatory research design to identify how social, political, and economic structures and processes influenced marginalized groups of women's experiences. A second example is that by Gagnon, Carnevale, Mehta, Rousseau, and Stewart (2013) who used a focused ethnography with a group of migrant women to develop population-based interventions to address maternal–child health. They used a population health model and the SDH contained in that model to categorize the women's intervention needs. The interventions or modification to current interventions fit under income and social status, social support networks, education, personal health and practices and coping skills, healthy child development, and health services, which are well-defined SDH. A third example was an ethnographic study by Mao, Yang, Bottorff, and Sarbit (2014) in rural China to find out the personal and social determinants that influenced cigarette smoking. They used a nested, multilevel socioecological model consisting of individual, interpersonal, and environmental influences. Two of the environmental or structural factors that sustained the practice were economic (cigarettes as a payment and means to promote economic ties) and social (leisure activity and normalization of smoking despite a ban in certain settings).

Weight of Individual Studies

Another measurement and methodological issue is the weight of individual studies as evidence for the SDH. Large-scale population studies take up a great deal of resources and infrastructure to carry out the required research, but one means of overcoming this challenge is through reviews of smaller scale studies and/or the literature to provide further evidence for the SDH using different approaches. Even if a meta-synthesis is done it need not be limited to quantitative studies, because a number of models exist for gaining cumulative evidence from qualitative studies (Bonnefoy et al., 2007). Much of the work by nurse authors, sometimes in collaboration with other disciplines, on the SDH would fall into this category. Using the CSDH conceptual framework Williams-Brennan, Gastaldo, Cole, and Paszat (2012) did a scoping review to identify the SDH affecting access to cervical cancer screening. Their review was limited to 37 research articles on women in middle- and low-income countries. The SDH preventing screening were cultural (beliefs, values, and norms about cancer or women), lower education and income (affecting knowledge or access), and ethnicity. Alexander (2013) reviewed the literature on the social determinants of methadone use during pregnancy. She used a conceptual framework based on individual, social, and environmental determinants of drug use. Important determinants were mental health, intimate partner violence, racial disparities, and geography.

STRATEGIES FOR RESEARCH AND POLICY DEVELOPMENT ON THE SDH

A third methodological issue especially for policy development is what strategy or focus would best be adopted with an SDH approach. Dahlgren and Whitehead (2006) outline four different approaches; (a) integrated determinants of health strategy; (b) disease-specific strategy; (c) setting-based approach; and (d) group-specific strategy. Another approach could be added and that is determinant-specific, for example, built environment (DeGuzman & Kulbok, 2012) or food insecurity (Solberg, Canning, & Buehler, 2008). Research and policy and program development could fall within these approaches (Blas & Kurup, 2010). Although these approaches may be useful as a heuristic device, in reality a number of approaches, whereas not quite being fully integrated approaches, include two or more of the approaches, such as condition and group. As part of a scoping study and restricted to Canadian research on the SDH that included income, housing, food insecurity, and social inclusion, Muntaner et al. (2012) identified 109 studies. The majority were on income, followed by multiple determinants of health, social exclusion, housing, and food insecurity and with few exceptions supported the finding of inequalities in health. The most challenging, and most needed, of these approaches might be the integrated approach because of the comprehensive, participatory, interdisciplinary, and intersectoral nature of the approach (Barton, Miltin, Mulholland, Hardoy, & Stern, 2007).

Research by nurse researchers and in collaboration with colleagues that identified the inclusion of the SDH were categorized using Dahlgren and Whitehead's (2006) typology. An example of an integrated research approach is *Coasts Under Stress: Restructuring and Social-ecological Health* (Ommer with the Coasts Under Stress Research Project Team; Solberg, 2006). The research was based on a multilevel, multiscale (past, present, and future) socioecological model to understand the ecological and social determinants of health (on people, communities, and the environment). It was a 5-year, interdisciplinary, participatory (community-based) project that employed a variety of quantitative and qualitative methodologies focused on geographical areas in eastern (Newfoundland and Labrador) and western (British Columbia) areas of Canada. The end point was a number of policy implications for coastal communities struggling with the effects of social and environmental restructuring, a phenomenon threatening the health of these communities and the people living within them (Ommer, 2006).

A second approach or strategy is disease-specific (Dahlgren & Whitehead, 2006) and could be extended to include condition-specific. In this approach, policy or research is limited to a particular disease or condition and how it is related to the SDH. At a minimum the disease or condition must be linked to social and economic factors. This is one of the more commonly employed approaches or strategies and widely presented in the literature. A number of literature reviews on the SDH located within nursing were of this nature (Dysart-Gale, 2010—lesbian, gay, bisexual, transgendered, intersexed, and queer youth; Jackson, McGibbon, & Waldron, 2013—cardiovascular disease; Respress, Morris, Lewin, & Francis, 2013—adolescent depression; Williams et al., 2012—cervical cancer screening). A research example is that of Doornbos, Zandee, DeGroot, and De Maagd-Rodiguez (2013) who used SDH to study social determinants of women's mental health. Their work could also be grouped under group-specific because of their emphasis on vulnerable groups of women. The third approach or strategy is a setting-based approach. In this approach, a particular setting such as a workplace or educational setting is the target with the policy or research based on the SDH. No research based on a setting-based approach and that used the SDH was located in the nursing literature.

The fourth strategy or approach identified by Dahlgren and Whitehead (2006) is group-specific research and examples include but are not limited to women, children, older adults, and marginalized groups such as the homeless. In nursing research, women as a group-specific approach is fairly widely represented. Wuest et al.'s (2002) program of research using the SDH included groups of marginalized women such as single mothers and women leaving abusive relationships would fit this category as would the groups included by Gagnon et al. (2013) who focused on immigrant women and the categorization of their needs for maternal–child health interventions under the SDH categories. Some nurse researchers have focused on a single determinant of health as the main focus, such as Samuels-Denis (2006). Although her focus was on employment as a determinant of health in single mothers, she did integrate other SDH into her quantitative study. Employment status was important to this group of women, with those who were employed having fewer stressful events than those not employed. These stressful events were related to problems with housing, social isolation, and finances, which are other SDH. While some research has a primary focus and strategy using a particular SDH, findings often indicate the importance of a number of other

SDH and thus the research could be categorized as either group specific or an integrated approach.

SOCIAL DETERMINANTS OF HEALTH IN NURSING: POSSIBILITIES

The SDH are being integrated into the discipline of nursing and are influencing thinking and practice within the discipline. However, tracing the development, integration, and the influence of the SDH within nursing scholarship is very challenging. A search of bibliographic databases using the search terms "social determinants of health," "determinants of health," "health inequities," "health disparities," and "nursing" did identify a number of articles, reviews, and limited research utilizing this framework. One of the challenges of locating literature and research on the SDH in nursing is, as Wuest (2006) observed, that although nurses recognize how important this approach is, they do not always use it as an explicit framework or might use it as an explanation for findings rather than how the research or problem is framed. Additionally the SDH may be considered secondary in research and other works in the literature that are framed primarily in a health equity or a social justice framework or lens; even though the mechanism to achieve health equity and social justice in health is through the SDH, it may not turn up in a search on the SDH within nursing. For example, in Reutter and Krushner's (2010) discussion on how nurses could help reduce inequities in health, they suggest it is through "action on the social determinants of health" (p. 269). Another challenge is that by its very nature research using the SDH is often an interdisciplinary project, so the role of nursing may be invisible unless author affiliation makes this clear. In addition to these points, nursing would share with other disciplines some of the same conceptual and methodological issues that have been identified for research using the SDH that have been discussed in a previous section.

At least three nursing organizations have adopted position statements on the importance of integrating the SDH into nursing (Canadian Association of Nurses, 2013; New Zealand Nurses Organization, 2011; Royal College of Nursing, 2012). There is also some reference in the nursing education and practice literature for using the SDH. Using cardiovascular disease and taking a health-condition approach, Jackson et al. (2013) illustrated how strategies related to addressing racism and other SDH could be incorporated into practice, education, leadership and policy making, and research. In each of these areas it is critical to reflect on how the SDH have an impact on the individuals experiencing the health condition and how the nurses' understanding of SDH influences action. In keeping with an SDH and determinants of health inequalities advocacy and action on policies at a broader level are important strategies. A good example of the actual use of an education strategy, critical service learning, to improve a disadvantaged group's access to cardiac health screening is presented by Gillis and MacLellan (2013). Although their expressed purpose was to promote social justice and reduce health inequities, they acknowledge that an important aspect of their approach is the understanding of "root causes" of health inequities, completion of course work on "determinants of health," "recognition of the significant influences of the social determinants of health," and ability to analyze "the relationships among the determinants of health" (p. 66) were pre- or corequisites to the service learning proposed.

Despite the challenges, the SDH is a good conceptual framework for nursing; one to guide education, practice and research (Canadian Nurses Association, 2013; New Zealand Nurses Organization, 2011). First, health, and the environment in which it occurs, has long been considered important to nursing. The goal of nursing is to have a positive effect on health by protecting, promoting, restoring, and advocating for health at the individual, community, population, or even global level. To achieve this goal it is critical to know what factors determine that health, and as has been argued above, it requires an expanded view of the environment. Previously, the environment was conceptualized narrowly as the immediate physical environment of the client with little attention to the broader social structures or upstream factors that determine health. An SDH framework could provide nurses with the expanded view of the environment that is critical to their goals, social mandates, and ethical responsibilities.

An SDH framework offers a new and expanded view of achieving health, one that is interdisciplinary and collaborative across disciplines and sectors of our society. It is a way for nurses to practice to the full scope of practice that will be required to meet their professional, social, and moral mandates (Canadian Nurses Association, 2013; Mahony & Jones, 2013; Reutter & Kushner, 2010) and work collaboratively with others. As some nursing authors have suggested, a conceptual framework based on the SDH of health, and by implication social determinants of health inequities, offers much promise as an organizing framework for nursing education, practice, research, advocacy, and policy (Mahoney & Jones, 2013; McGibbon et al., 2008).

There is some movement toward integrating the SDH in nursing or at least advocating this integration (Canadian Nurses Association, 2013; Mahoney & Jones, 2013). The standards of the Community Health Nurses Association of Canada (2008) advocate health promotion by community health nurses from an SDH framework. More recently, the Registered Nurses' Association of Ontario (RNAO, 2013) building on the CSDH (2008) framework for SDH and health inequities in a paper *Fairer Societies for Better Health Equity* outlines actions to address the structural determinants of health inequities.

REFERENCES

Acheson, D. (1998). *Independent inquiry into inequalities in health.* Retrieved from http://web archive.nationalarchives.gov.uk/20130107105354/http://www.archive.official-documents .co.uk/document/doh/ih/contents.htm

Alexander, K. (2013). Social determinants of methadone in pregnancy: Violence, social capital, and mental health. *Issues in Mental Health Nursing, 34*, 747–751. doi:10.3109/01612840.2013 .813996

American Nurses Association. (2015). *Code of ethics for nurses with interpretative statements.* Retrieved from http://nursingworld.org/DocumentVault/Ethics-1/Code-of-Ethics-for-Nurses .html

Anderson, J., Rodney, P., Reimer-Kirkham, S., Browne, A. J., Basu Khan, K., & Lynam, J. (2009). Inequities in health and health care viewed through the ethical lens of critical justice theory: Contextual knowledge for the global priorities ahead. *Advances in Nursing Science, 32*, 282–294. doi:10.1097/ANS.0b013e3181bd6955

Bambra, C., Gibson, M., Sowden, A., Wright, K., Whitehead, M., & Petticrew, M. (2010). Tackling the wider social determinants of health and health inequalities: Evidence from a systematic review. *Journal of Epidemiology and Community Health, 64*, 284–291. doi:10.1136/jech.2008.082743

Barton, F., Miltin, D., Mulholland, C., Hardoy, A., & Stern, R. (2007). Integrated approaches to address the social determinants of health for reducing health inequity. *Journal of Urban Health, 84*(Suppl. 1), 164–173. doi:10.1007/s11524-007-9173-7

Blas, E., & Kurup, A. S. (2010). *Equity, social determinants and public health programmes.* Geneva, Switzerland: World Health Organization.

Bloch, J. R. (2011). Using geographical information systems to explore disparities in preterm birth rates among foreign-born and US-born Black Mothers. *Journal of Obstetric, Gynecological and Neonatal Nursing, 40*, 544–554. doi:10.1111/j.1552-6909.2011.01273.x

Bonnefoy, J., Morgan, A., Kelly, M. P., Butt, J., & Bergman, V. (2007). *Constructing the evidence base on the social determinants of health: A guide.* Retrieved from http://goo.gl/6EXWVC

Braverman, P. (2006). Health disparities and health equity: Concepts and measurement. *Annual Review of Public Health, 27*, 167–194.

Braverman, P., Egerter, S., & Williams, D. R. (2011). The social determinants of health: Coming of age. *Annual Review of Public Health, 32*, 381–398. doi:10.1146/annurev-publhealth-031210-101218

Brofenbrenner, U. (1977). Toward an experimental ecology of human development. *American Psychologist, 32*, 513–531.

Brunner, E., & Marmot, M. (2006). Social organization, stress, and health. In M. Marmot & R. G. Wilkinson (Eds.), *Social determinants of health* (2nd ed., pp. 6–29). Oxford, UK: Oxford University Press.

Butterfield, P. G. (1990). Thinking upstream: Nurturing a conceptual understanding of the social context of health behaviour. *Advances in Nursing Science, 12*, 1–8.

Canadian Nurses Association. (2005). *Social determinants of health and nursing: A summary of the issues. CNA backgrounder.* Retrieved from https://www.cna-aiic.ca/~/media/cna/page -content/pdf-en/social-determinants-of-health-and-nursing_a-summary-of-the-issues .pdf?la=en

Canadian Nurses Association. (2008). *Code of ethics for registered nurses*. Ottawa, ON, Canada: Author.

Canadian Nurses Association. (2010). *Social justice . . . a means to an end, an end in itself* (2nd ed.). Ottawa: Author.

Canadian Nurses Association. (2013). *Position statement: Social determinants of health*. Retrieved from http://www.cna-aiic.ca/~/media/cna/files/en/ps124_social_determinants_of_health_e.pdf

Centers for Disease Control and Prevention. (2010). *Establishing a holistic framework to reduce inequities in HIV, viral hepatitis, STDs, and tuberculosis in the United States*. Atlanta, GA: U.S. Department of Health and Human Services, Centers for Disease Control and Prevention. Retrieved from http://www.cdc.gov/socialdeterminants/docs/SDH-White-Paper-2010.pdf

Chang, W. C. (2002). The meaning and goals of equity in health. *Journal of Epidemiology and Community Health, 56*, 488–491. doi:10.1136/jeh.56.7.488

Chopoorian, T. J. (1986). Reconceptualizing the environment. In P. Moccia (Ed.), *New approaches to theory development in nursing* (pp. 39–54). New York, NY: National League for Nursing.

Cohen, B. E., & Gregory, D. (2009). Community health clinical education in Canada: Part 2—developing competencies to address social justice, equity, and the social determinants of health. *International Journal of Nursing Education Scholarship, 6*, 1–15. doi:10.2202/1548-923X.1638

Commission on the Social Determinants of Health. (2008). *Closing the gap in a generation: Health equity through action on the social determinants of health. Final Report of the Commission on Social Determinants of Health*. Geneva, Switzerland: World Health Organization. Retrieved from http://goo.gl/3x0ek9

Community Health Nurses Association of Canada. (2008). *Canadian community health nursing standards of practice*. Retrieved from http://goo.gl/s6laZz

Crighton, A., Robertson, A., Gordon, C., & Farrant, W. (1997). *Health care a community concern? Developments in the organization of Canadian health care services*. Calgary, AB, Canada: University of Calgary.

Dahlgren, G., & Whitehead, M. (1993). *Tackling inequalities in health: what can we learn from what has been tried?* (p. 19). Working paper prepared for the King's Fund International Seminar on Tackling Inequalities in Health, September 1993, Ditchley Park, Oxfordshire. London, King's Fund (mimeo). Retrieved from http://www.who.int/social_determinants/resources/leveling_up_part2.pdf

Dahlgren, G., & Whitehead, M. (2006). *Levelling up Part 2: European strategies for tackling social inequities in health*. Geneva, Switzerland: World Health Organization. Retrieved from http://goo.gl/fODFWN

DeGuzman, P. B., & Kulbok, P. A. (2012). Changing health outcomes of vulnerable populations through nursing's influence on neighbourhood built environment: A framework for nursing research. *The Journal of Nursing Scholarship, 44*, 341–348. doi:10.1111/j.1547-5069.2012.01470.x

Determinant. (2014). *Oxford dictionary online*. Retrieved from http://www.oxforddictionaries.com/us/definition/american_english/determinant

Dolan, A. H., Taylor, S. M., Neis, B., Eyles, J., Ommer, R. E, Schneider, D. C., & Montevecchi, W. A. (2005). Restructuring and health in Canadian coastal communities: A social-ecological framework of restructuring and health. *EcoHealth, 2*, 195–208. Retrieved from http://dx.doi.org/10.1007/s10393-005-6333-7

Doornbos, M. M., Zandee, G. L., DeGroot, J., & De Maagd-Rodriguez, M. (2013). Using community-based participatory research to explore social determinants of women's mental health and barriers to help-seeking in three urban, ethnically diverse, impoverished, and underserviced communities. *Archives of Psychiatric Nursing, 27*, 278–284. doi:htt://dx.doi.org/10.1016/j.apnu.2013.09.001

Dunn, E. C., Masyn, K. E., Yudron, M., Jones, S. M., & Subramanian, S. V. (2014). Translating multilevel theory into multilevel research. Challenges and opportunities for understanding the social determinants of psychiatric disorders. *Social Psychiatry and Psychiatric Epidemiology, 49*(6), 859–872. doi:10.1007/s00127-013-0809-5

Dysart-Gale, D. (2010). Social justice and social determinants of health: Lesbian, gay, bisexual, transgendered, intersexed and queer youth in Canada. *Journal of Child and Adolescent Psychiatric Nursing, 23*, 23–28. doi:10.1111/j.1744-6171.2009.0023.x

Edwards, N., & Cohen, E. (2012). Joining up action to address social determinants of health and health equities in Canada. *Healthcare Management Forum, 25*, 151–154. doi:.org/10.1016/j.hcmf.2012.07.002

Epp, J. (1986). *Achieving health for all: A framework for health promotion.* Ottawa: Minister of Supply and Services Canada.

Etches, V., Frank, J., Di Ruggiero, E., & Manuel, D. (2006). Measuring population health: A review of the indicators. *Annual Review of Public Health, 27*, 29–55. doi:10.1146/annurev.publhealth.27.021405.102141

Evans, R. G., Barer, M. L., & Marmor, T. R. (Eds.). (1994). *Why are some people healthy and others not? The determinants of health of populations.* New York, NY: Aldine de Gruyter.

Evans, R. G., & Stoddart, G. L. (1994). Producing health, consuming health care. In R. G. Evans, M. L. Barer, & T. R. Marmor (Eds.), *Why are some people healthy and others not? The determinants of health of populations* (pp. 27–64). New York, NY: Aldine de Gruyter.

Federal/Provincial/Territorial Advisory Committee on Population Health. (1994). *Strategies for population health: Investing in the health of populations.* Ottawa: Minister of Supplies and Services. Retrieved from http://goo.gl/ZyRgMJ

Fink, A. M. (2009). Toward a definition of health disparity: A concept analysis. *Journal of Transcultural Nursing, 20*, 349–357. doi:10.1177/1043659609340802

Flaskerud, J. H., & Nyamathi, A. M. (2002). Guest editorial: New paradigm for health disparities needed. *Nursing Research, 51*, 139.

Frank, J. W., & Mustard, J. F. (1994). The determinants of health from a historical perspective. *Daedalus, 123*, 1–19. Retrieved from http://www.jstor.org/stable/20027264

Gagnon, A. J., Carnevale, F., Mehta, P., Rousseau, H., & Stewart, D. E. (2013). Developing population intervention with migrant women for maternal-child health: A focused ethnography. *BMC Public Health, 13*, 471–484. doi:10.1186/1471-2458-13-471.

Gillis, A., & MacLellan, M. A. (2013). Critical service learning in community health nursing: Enhancing access to cardiac screening. *International Journal of Nursing Education Scholarship, 10*, 63–71. doi:10.1515/ijnes-2012-0031

Graham, H. (2004). Social determinants and their unequal distribution: Clarifying policy understandings. *The Milbank Quarterly, 82*, 101–124.

Hamilton, N., & Bhatti, T. (1996). *Population health promotion: An integrated model of population health and health promotion*. Retrieved from http://www.phac-aspc.gc.ca/ph-sp/php-psp/index-eng.php#toc

Harrison, K. M., & Dean, H. D. (2011). Use of data systems to address social determinants of health: A need to do more. *Public Health Reports, 53*, 1–5. Retrieved from http://www.jstor.org/stable/41639296

Hertzman, C., Frank, J., & Evans, R. G. (1994). In R. G. Evans, M. L. Barer, & T. R. Marmor (Eds.), *Why are some people healthy and others not? The determinants of health of populations* (pp. 67–92). New York, NY: Aldine de Gruyter.

Honjo, K. (2004). Social epidemiology: definition, history and research examples. *Environmental Health and Preventive Medicine, 9*, 193–199. doi:http://dx.doi.org/10.1265/ehpm.9.193

Institute for Population and Public Health. (2014). *Canadian Institutes for Health Research*. Retrieved from http://www.cihr-irsc.gc.ca/e/13777.html

International Council of Nurses. (2012). *The ICN code of ethics for nurses*. Geneva, Switzerland: Author. Retrieved from http://goo.gl/zvX3Lk

Irvine, L., Elliott, L., Wallace, H., & Crombie, I. K. (2006). A review of major influences on current public health policy in developed countries in the second half of the 20th century. *The Journal of the Royal Society for Health promotion, 126*, 73–78. doi:10.1177/146642006063182

Irwin, A., & Scali, E. (2007). Action on the social determinants of health: A historical perspective. *Global Public Health, 2*, 235–256. doi:10.1080/17441690601106304

Irwin, A., & Scali, E. (2010). *Actions on the social determinants of health: Learning from previous experiences*. Social Determinants of Health Discussion Paper 1. Retrieved from http://goo.gl/Y9wA5e

Jackson, S. F., Birn, A.-E., Fawcett, S. B., Poland, B., & Schultz, J. A. (2013). Synergy for health equity: Integrating health promotion and social determinants of health approaches in and beyond the Americas. *Revista Panamericana de Salud Pública, 34*, 473–480.

Jackson, J., McGibbon, E., & Waldon, I. (2013). Racism and cardiovascular disease: Implications for nursing. *Canadian Journal of Cardiovascular Nursing, 23*(4), 12–18.

Kawachi, I., Subramanian, S. V., & Almeida-Filho, N. (2002). A glossary for health inequalities. *Journal of Epidemiology and Community Health, 56*, 647–652. Retrieved from http://jech.bmj.com/content/56/9/647.full

Kelly, M. P. (2010). The axes of social differentiation and the evidence base on health equity. *Journal of the Royal Society of Medicine, 103*, 266–272. doi:10.1258/jrsm.2010.100005

Kelly, M. P., Bonnefoy, J., Morgan, A., & Florenzano, F. (2006). *The development of the evidence base about the social determinants of health*. Geneva, Switzerland: World Health Organization. Retrieved from http://goo.gl/7UktQw

Kelly, M. P., Morgan, A., Bonnefoy, J., Butt, J., Bergman, V., and the Measurement and Evidence Knowledge Network. (2007). *The social determinants of health: Developing and evidence base for political action. Final Report to World Health Organization commission on the social determinants of health from the measurement and evidence knowledge network*. Retrieved from http://goo.gl/6TbnDR

King, A. (2000). *The New Zealand health strategy: Discussion document*. Wellington, NZ: Ministry of Health. Retrieved from http://www.moh.govt.nz/notebook/nbbooks.nsf/0/f6c8df90d2020c814c2568fc0011d53a/$FILE/nzhsdisc.pdf

Kneipp. S. M., & Drevdahl, D. J. (2003). Problems with parsimony on research on social determinants of health. *Advances in Nursing Science, 26,* 162–172.

Krumeich, A., & Meershoek, A. (2014). Health in global context: Beyond the social determinants of health? *Global Health Action, 7,* 23506. doi:10.3402/gha.v7.23506

Lalonde, M. (1974). *A new perspective on the health of Canadians: A working document.* Ottawa, ON, Canada: Government of Canada.

Lathrop, B. (2013). Nursing leadership in addressing the social determinants of health. *Policy, Politics, and Nursing Practice, 14,* 41–47. doi:10.1177/1527154413489887

Lightsey, D., McQueen, D., & Anderson, L. (2005). Health promotion in the USA: Building a science-based health promotion policy. In A. Scriven & S. Garman (Eds.), *Promoting health: Global perspectives* (pp. 266–278). New York, NY: Palgrave MacMillan.

MacDonald, S., Newburn-Cook, C., Allen, M., & Reutter, L. (2013). Embracing the population health framework. *Nursing Inquiry, 20,* 30–41. doi:10.1111/nin.12017

Mahony, D., & Jones, E. J. (2013). Social determinants of health in nursing education, research and health policy. *Nursing Science Quarterly, 26,* 280–284. doi:10.1177/08943/84/3489186

Mao, A., Yang, T., Bottorff, J. L., & Sarbit, G. (2014). Personal and social determinants sustaining smoking practices in rural China: A qualitative study. *International Journal for Equity in Health, 13,* 12. Retrieved from http://www.equity.healthj.com/content/13/1/12

Marmot, M., & Wilkinson, R. G (Eds.). (2006). *Social determinants of health* (2nd ed.). Oxford, UK: Oxford University Press.

Marmot, M. (2001). From Black to Acheson: Two decades of concern with inequalities in health. A celebration of the 90th birthday of Professor Jerry Morris. *International Journal of Epidemiology, 30,* 1165–1171. doi:10.1093/ije/30.5.1165

Marmot, M. (2010). *'Fair societyhealthy lives'.* UCL Institute of Health Equity. Retrieved from http://www.instituteofhealthequity.org/projects/fair-society-healthy-lives-the-marmot-review

McGibbon, E., Etowa, J., & McPherson, C. (2008). Health care access as a social determinant of health. *The Canadian Nurse, 104*(7), 23–27.

McKeown, T. (1976). *The modern rise of population.* New York, NY: Academic Press.

McKeown, T. (1979). *The role of medicine: Dream, mirage, or nemesis?* (2nd ed.). Oxford, UK: Basil Blackwell.

Meleis, A. I. (2012). *Theoretical nursing: development and progress* (5th ed.). Philadelphia, PA: Wolters Kleiver Health/Lippincott Williams & Wilkins.

Miles, M. B., & Huberman, A. M. (1994). *Qualitative data analysis* (2nd ed.). Thousand Oaks, CA: Sage.

Muntaner, C., Ng, E., & Chung, H. (2012). *Better health: An analysis of public policy and programming focusing on the determinants of health and health outcomes that are effective in achieving the healthiest populations.* Canadian Health Services Research Foundation. Retrieved from http://archives.enap.ca/bibliotheques/2013/06/030429303.pdf

National Forum on Health. (1996). *What determines health?* Ottawa, ON, Canada: Minister of Public Works and Government Services Canada.

New Zealand Nurses Organization. (2011). *Closing the gap: How nurses can help achieve health access and equality.* [Position statement]. Retrieved from http://www.nzno.org.nz

Irvine, L., Elliott. L., Wallace, H., & Crombie, I. K. (2006). A review of major influences on current public health policy in developed countries in the second half of the 20th century. *The Journal of the Royal Society for Health promotion, 126,* 73–78. doi:10.1177/1466424006063182

O'Campo, P., & Urquia, M. (2012). Aligning method with theory: A comparison of two approaches to modelling the social determinants of health. *Maternal and Child Health Journal, 16,* 1870–1878. doi:10.1007/s10995-011-0935-1

Ommer, R. E with the Coasts Under Stress Research Project Team. (2007). *Coasts under stress: Restructuring and social-ecological health.* Montreal and Kingston, Canada: McGill Queen's University Press.

Ommer, R. E. (2006). *Coasts under stress: Restructuring and social-ecological health, policy reflections.* St. John's, NL, Canada: ISER Books.

Pauly, B. M. (2013). Challenging health inequities: Enacting social justice in nursing practice. In J. L. Storch, P. Rodney, & R. Starzomski (Eds.), *Towards a moral horizon: Nursing ethics for leadership and practice* (pp. 430–447). Toronto, ON, Canada: Pearson.

Pederson, A., Rootman, I., & O'Neill, M. (2005). Health promotion in Canada: Back to the past or towards a promising future? In A. Scriven & S. Garman (Eds.), *Promoting health: Global perspectives* (pp. 255–278). New York, NY: Palgrave MacMillan.

Porter, D. (2006). How did social medicine evolve, and where is it heading? *PLoS Medicine, 3*(e399), 1667–1672. doi:10:1371/journal.pmed.00

Public Health Agency of Canada. (2013). *What makes Canadians Healthy or unhealthy?* Retrieved from http://www.phac-aspc.gc.ca/ph-sp/determinants/determinants-eng.php

Raphael, D. (Ed.). (2004). *Social determinants of health: Canadian perspectives.* Toronto, ON, Canada: Canadian Scholars' Press Inc.

Raphael, D. (2010). *About Canada: Health and illness.* Halifax, NS, Canada: Fernwood Publishing.

Raphael, D. (2011). A discourse analysis of the social determinants of health. *Critical Public Health, 2,* 221–236. doi:10.1080/09581596.2010.485606

Ravitch, S. M., & Riggan, M. (2012). *Reason and rigour: How conceptual frameworks guide research.* Thousand Oaks, CA: Sage.

Registered Nurses Association of Ontario. (2013). *Fairer societies for better health equity.* Retrieved from http://goo.gl/KBDPfg

Respress, B. N., Morris, D. L., Lewin, L. C., & Francis, S. A. (2013). Social determinants of adolescent depression: An examination of racial differences. *Issues in mental Health Nursing, 34,* 539–549. doi:10.3109/01612840.2012.758206

Reutter, L., & Kushner, K. E. (2010). 'Health equity through action on the social determinants of health': Taking up the challenge in nursing. *Nursing Inquiry, 17,* 269–280.

Risjord, M. (2010). *Nursing knowledge: Science, practice, and philosophy.* Oxford, UK: Wiley-Blackwell.

Robertson, A. (1998). Shifting discourse on health in Canada: From health promotion to population health. *Health Promotion International, 13,* 155–166. doi:10.1093/heapro/13.2.155

Royal College of Nursing. (2012). *Health inequalities and the social determinants of health.* [Position Statement]. Retrieved from https://www2.rcn.org.uk/__data/assets/pdf_file/0007/438838/01.12_Health_inequalities_and_the_social_determinants_of_health.pdf

Samuels-Denis, J. (2006). Relationship among employment status, stressful life events, and depression in single mothers. *Canadian Journal of Nursing Research, 38,* 59–80.

Satcher, D. (2010). Commentary: Include a social determinants of health approach to reduce health inequities. *Public Health Reports, 125*(Suppl. 4), 6–7. Retrieved from http://www.jstor.org/stable/41434913

Scriven, A. (2005). Promoting health: A global context and rationale. In A. Scriven & S. Garman (Eds.), *Promoting health: Global perspectives* (pp. 1–13). New York, NY: Palgrave MacMillan.

Scriven, A., & Garmin, S. (Eds.), (2005). *Promoting health: Global perspectives.* New York, NY: Palgrave MacMillan.

Segall, A., & Fries, C. J. (2011). *Pursuing health and wellness.* Oxford, UK: Oxford University Press.

Social Determinants of Health Alliance (SDHA). (2013). Retrieved from socialdeterminants.org.au

Solar, O., & Irwin, A. (2010). *A conceptual framework for action on the social determinants of Health. Social determinants of health discussion.* Paper 2 (Policy and Practice). Retrieved from http://goo.gl/xkq6Cv

Solberg, S. M., (2006). Researching the social determinants of women's health. *Canadian Journal of Nursing Research, 38,* 169–174.

Solberg, S. M., Canning, P., & Buehler, S. (2008). Changing patterns of household food consumption in rural communities of Atlantic Canada. In C. C. Parish, N. J. Turner, & S. M. Solberg (Eds.), *Resetting the kitchen table: Food security, culture, health, and resilience in coastal communities* (pp. 161–175). New York, NY: Nova Science Publishers Inc.

Srinivasan, S., & Williams, S. D. (2014). Transitioning from health disparities to a health equity research agenda: The time is now. *Public Health Reports, 129*(Suppl. 2), 71–76.

Stevens, P. E. (1989). A critical social reconceptualization of environment in nursing: Implications for methodology. *Advances in Nursing Science, 11*(4), 56–68.

Townsend, P., Davidson, N., & Whitehead, M (Eds.). (1992). *Inequalities in health: The Black Report and the Health Divide.* New York, NY: Penguin.

Turrell, G., Oldenburg, B., McGuffog, I., & Dent, R. (1999). *Socioeconomic determinants of health: Towards a national research program and a policy and intervention agenda.* Canberra, Australia: Queensland University of Technology, School of Public Health/Ausinfo. Retrieved from http://eprints.qut.edu.au/585/1/turrell_health_inequalities.pdf

U.S. Department of Health and Human Services. (2010). *Healthy people 2020 framework.* Retrieved from https://www.healthypeople.gov/sites/default/files/HP2020Framework.pdf

Villarruel, A. M., Bigelow, A., & Alvarez, C. (2014). Integrating the 3Ds: A nursing perspective. *Public Health Reports, 129,* 37–44. Retrieved from http://goo.gl/84kpJU

Viseltear, A. J. (1984). Milton C. Winternitz and the Yale Institute of Human Relations: A brief chapter in the history of social medicine. *The Yale Journal of Biology and Medicine, 57,* 869–889. Retrieved from http://goo.gl/ufwzlU

Whitehead, M. (1987). *The Health Divide: Inequalities in health in the 1980s.* London, UK: Health Education Council.

Whitehead, M., & Dahlgren, G. (2006). *Levelling up (Part 1): A discussion paper on concepts and principles for talking about social inequities in health.* Retrieved from http://goo.gl/2HfdcE

Wilkinson, R. G., & Marmot, M. (Eds.). (2003). *Social determinants of health: The solid facts* (2nd ed.). Copenhagen, Denmark: The Regional Office for the World Health Organization. Retrieved from http://goo.gl/ehmm20

Williams, G. H. (2003). The determinants of health: Structure, context and agency. *Sociology of Health and Illness, 25,* 131–154. doi:10.1111/1467-9566.00344

Williams-Brennan, L., Gastaldo, D., Cole, D. C., & Paszat, L. (2012). Social determinants of health associated with cervical cancer screening among women living in developing countries. *Archives of Gynecology and Obstetrics, 286,* 1487–1505. doi:10.1007/s00404-012-2575-0

World Health Organization. (1978). *Declaration of Alma-Ata International Conference on Primary Health Care, Alma-Ata, USSR.* Retrieved from http://www.who.int/publications/almaata_declaration_en.pdf

World Health Organization. (1986). *The Ottawa charter for health promotion.* Retrieved from http://www.who.int/healthpromotion/conferences/previous/ottawa/en

World Health Organization. (2011). *Rio political declaration on social determinants of health.* Retrieved from http://www.who.int/sdhconference/declaration/Rio_political_declaration.pdf

World Health Organization. (2014). *What are the social determinants of health?* Retrieved from http://www.who.int/social_determinants/sdh_definition/en/

Wuest, J. (2006). Guest editorial: Towards understanding women's health through a social determinants lens. *Canadian Journal of Nursing Research, 38,* 3–5.

Wuest, J., Merritt-Gray, M., Berman, H., & Ford-Gilboe, M. (2002). Illuminating social determinants of women's health using grounded theory. *Health Care for Women International, 23,* 794–808. doi:10.1080/073993302901123226.

Young, T. K. (2005). *Population health: Concepts and methods* (2nd ed.). New York, NY: Oxford University Press.

SECTION VIII

TOWARD CERTAINTY: BUILDING A MATURE THEORETICAL BASE

In this section, we move toward agreement through techniques of meta-synthesis. Qualitative meta-synthesis is an initial move toward certainty, by "combining" the findings of several similar studies, conducted in different contexts and settings, by different investigators. The outcome is a theory of the same level of abstraction.

TOWARD CERTAINTY: BUILDING A MATURE THEORETICAL BASE

Janice M. Morse

TOWARD CERTAINTY: QUALITATIVE META-SYNTHESIS

"The truth *is not a thing of fact or reason," he chortles.*
"The truth *is just what* everyone agrees *on."*
—David Côté (2005, p. 167)

Meta-synthesis includes various techniques for integrating the findings of studies addressing a similar topic, into a more "general" theory. The technique is used in both qualitative as well as quantitative research, so we have to be careful not to confuse *qualitative* meta-synthesis with *quantitative* meta-synthesis techniques. Quantitative meta-synthesis and meta-analysis use statistical techniques, usually for combining trials and comparing effect sizes to determine efficacy (Cumming, 2012). These statistical methods are well developed, commonly used, and various software packages have been developed to facilitate these analyses. They are also a component of the Cochrane systematic reviews (Noyes, Popay, Pearson, Hannes, & Booth, 2008).

On the other hand, qualitative meta-synthesis is still in the developmental phase. There are several types of "metas": Noblitt and Hare introduced meta-ethnography in 1988; Patterson, Thorne, Canam, and Jillings describe a "meta-study" in three analytic phases (meta-data, meta-method, and meta-theory); and Sandelowski (2006) worries about "meta-jeopardy." Thorne (2008) defines meta-synthesis as: "research approaches that integrate the collective products of extant bodies of qualitative research findings using systematic, formal processes for the purpose of generating overarching inductively derived claims about phenomenon of interest." These claims "extend beyond the scope of what would have been achievable within the temporal, spatial, or epistemological confines of individual studies."

But when attempting synthesis, there is a problem for qualitative researchers. While replication is an important part of validation for quantitative researchers, qualitative research does not intentionally replicate. That is, if someone has "done "a qualitative study on a particular topic, in a particular group, in a particular context, unless there is a reason to suspect that study is lacking something, then qualitative researchers usually accept that study as "done," and select an allied topic or explore the topic in a different population or context. The primary reason is that reading the findings—about the theoretical structure of a study—interferes with the inductive processes of the second project, and therefore is a threat to validity. Processes of verification within the conduct of qualitative research are designed to ensure rigor during construction. In fact, "not having any new findings" is a criteria for rejection from the journal *Qualitative Health Research.*

Data for a meta-synthesis are obtained from several similar theories that address the same phenomenon. Qualitative researchers do not intentionally replicate, so that studies will be "similar," but not precisely the same as each other. Perhaps researchers have not seen the first study when they conducted the second, or they used a slightly different theoretical perspective, or method or sample, or they worked at a different level of analysis.[1] Researchers may have used different labels for categories and themes in their studies, or created a different type of model, so that the studies appear to be different. In fact, if you ask five researchers to study the same phenomenon (or even used the same data), you would not be very likely to get similar results (but not the *same* results). Each investigator may have examined these data from his or her own perspective, thereby producing different results. Very occasionally in his or her struggle to understand all aspects of the concept, the other studies may have been conducted by the same researcher, and the meta-synthesis is the combination of all of these studies. An example of this is Beck's research program exploring postpartum depression (Beck, 2013, 2015, 2016) and the meta-synthesis of postpartum depression (2002, 2007, 2013).

One of the most important tasks in meta-synthesis is locating relevant and pertinent studies about the same topic.[2] These are then analytically "merged," and the resulting conceptualization or theory is usually more significant than any of the original studies. As such, qualitative synthesis is the "rigorous study of qualitative findings (versus raw data), and results in the reconceptualization of the original conclusion" (Finfgeld, 2003) and may suggest new directions for practice (Paterson, 2013, p. 331), or even used as evidence base for practice (Beck, 2009).

---

[1] For example, see Wertz et al. (2011), in which each method is described as a lens.

[2] For hints about literature searching, see Finfgeld-Connett and Johnson (2012). Literature search strategies for conducting knowledge-building and theory-generating qualitative systematic reviews.

THE DEVELOPMENT OF META-SYNTHESIS

In the past two decades there has been a number of "styles" of meta-syntheses developed according to methods of the original study and goals of the research outcomes. Some of the researchers have used studies that follow the same method (for instance, grounded theory or ethnography). In fact, the first text for combining qualitative studies was Nobit and Hare's (1988) for meta-ethnography. In nursing, Paterson, Thorne, Canam, and Jillings (2001) published a text outlining criteria for method study, followed by Sandelowski and Barroso's text in 2007, and Hanes and Lockwood (2012). Meanwhile the methods were refined in the literature by a number of authors (Finfgeld, 2003; Thorne, Jenson, Kerney, Noblit, & Sandelowski, 2004; Paterson, Canam, Joachin, & Thorne, 2001).

Purposes of Meta-Synthesis

Meta-synthesis may be used for a variety of purposes, either descriptive or interpretative. Descriptively, Popay et al. (2006) describe the synthesis of narratives for the effects of the evidence and factors shaping the implementation of the intervention. For instance, their example of "Interventions for promoting smoke alarm ownership and function" includes the preference for studies with predefined categories, and integration of the quantitative results as well as the qualitative narrative. They have a preference for developing a "common rubric" (p. 28), to evaluate the quantitative data.

How to Conduct a Meta-Synthesis

Your task however, will be greatly simplified if the studies selected all use the same method, such as, all grounded theory studies, for the *form* of the theories in the first-level analysis will be more comparable with one another.

When conducting meta-synthesis, the goal is to develop a *representative* solution, one contributed by all (or at least most) of the studies identified. Think of it as creating a *mean*—the most average, most typical, solution. As data are derived from different studies representing similar experiences, think of your task as finding a mathematical average from textual sources. There will be the equivalent of outliers; do not ignore them—address them in your text—but focus on the *most frequent*, "middle" data.

Take a large sheet of paper (of course), and open each theory by placing the concepts and attributes in cells across the paper, one author's theory per row. This enables you to then compare each author's trajectory with other authors' theories.

Each common piece of the process forms a part of your new theory, the outcome of your study. As you proceed, you are reducing the random noise or variation and moving toward theoretical clarity. You may or may not choose to use the labels from the original theories in the resulting theory. You may choose to create new labels or select the "best" label from all of the theories, as you merge and condense the descriptions.

One researcher may have a more detailed description than the others. There are no rules about how much you use from each theory, or if one theory forms the "backbone" of the new theory or not. Throughout the process, keep the main ideas associated with each of the original sources, so that appropriate credits may be given.[3]

Interpretatively, researchers have used meta-synthesis to move findings toward formal grounded theory, as in Kearney's (2001) study on domestic violence. The assumptions underlying the literature on fatigue were examined by Paterson et al. (2001). More recently, Beck (2011) developed a model of "causal looping" of the experience of new mothers. Four of the experiences were considered positive, and "balancing" or negative. She describes the "domino effect" of traumatic childbirth experiences.

In Chapter 30, Finfgeld-Connett demonstrates the development of the concept of *nursing presence*. She synthesizes 4 linguistic analyses of presence and 14 qualitative studies. The goal is to develop the concept of nursing presence, which is then presented with all the conceptual components and a model showing the antecedents, the attributes, and outcomes of the concept—moving toward a low-level theory. You will note that in order to conduct such a study, the studies that comprise these data must be reasonably focused within a similar context—in this case patient care.

The second example (Chapter 31, also contributed by Finfgeld-Connett) is a synthesis of homelessness literature. Finfgeld-Connett demonstrates the development of homeless women, and their "distorted perceptions of competency," receptiveness to assistance," and "therapeutic strategies" about how care for these women may be framed. She makes an argument for care that has a "personalized structure" and provides autonomy when working with homeless women with substance abuse. You will note in this study that the context is much broader, and therefore, to compensate for the increase in scope, the sample is much larger. The database consists of 60 reports and 45 studies, using grounded theory methods to organize these data. The large sample used in Finfgeld-Connett's study facilitates the movement toward recommendations for practice.

---

[3] Q: If the outcome resembles the original theories, why bother doing this?
ANS: By seeking "theoretical agreement" between the authors of independent studies, we create a theory with more certainty and more generalizability, even if it remains at the same level of abstraction.

REFERENCES

Beck, C. T. (2002). Postpartum depression: A metasynthesis. *Qualitative Health Research, 12*(4), 453–472.

Beck, C. T. (2007). Exemplar: Teetering on the edge: A continually emerging theory of postpartum depression. In P. L. Munhall (Ed.), *Nursing research: A qualitative perspective* (pp. 273–292). Burlington, MA: Jones &Bartlett.

Beck, C. T. (2009). Metasynthesis: A goldmine for evidence-based practice. *Association of peri-Operative Registered Nurses Journal, 90*(5), 701–710.

Beck, C. T. (2011). A metaethnography of traumatic childbirth and its aftermath: Amplifying causal looping. *Qualitative Health Research, 21*(3), 301–311.

Beck, C. T. (2015). Middle range theory of traumatic childbirth: The ever-widening ripple effect. *Global Qualitative Nursing Research, 2*. doi:10.1177/2333393615575313

Beck, C. T. (2016). *Developing a program of research*. New York, NY: Springer Publishing.

Côté, D. (2005). *Wicked the grimmerie*. New York, NY: Hyperion.

Cumming, G. (2012). *Understanding the new statistics: Effect sizes, confidence intervals, and meta-analysis*. New York, NY: Routledge.

Finfegld-Connett, D., & Johnson, E. D. (2012). Literature search strategies for conducting knowledge-building and theory-generating qualitative systematic reviews. *Journal of Advanced Nursing, 69*, 194–204. doi:10.1111/j.1365-2648.2012.06037.x

Finfgeld, D. L. (2003). Metasynthesis: The state of the art—So far. *Qualitative Health Research, 13*(7), 893–904.

Hannes, K., & Lockwook, C. (2012). *Synthesizing qualitative research: Choosing the right approach*. Chichester, England: Wiley-Blackwell.

Kearney, M. H. (2001). Enduring love: A grounded formal theory of women's experience of domestic violence. *Research in Nursing & Health, 24*(4), 270–282.

Noblit, G. W., & Hare, R. (1988). *Meta-ethnography: Systematizing qualitative studies*. Newbury Park, CA: Sage.

Noyes, J., Popay, J., Pearson, A., Hannes, K., & Booth, A. (2008). Qualitative research and Cochrane reviews. In J. Higgins & S. Green (Eds.), *Cochrane handbook for systematic reviews of interventions* (pp. 571–592). Chichester, West Sussex, England: John Wiley & Sons.

Paterson, B. (2013). Metasynthesis. In C. T. Beck (Ed.), *Routledge international handbook of qualitative research* (pp. 331–346). New York, NY: Routledge.

Paterson, B. L., Canam, C., Joachim, G., & Thorne, S. E. (2001). Embedded assumptions in qualitative studies of fatigue. *Western Journal of Nursing Research, 25*, 119–133.

Paterson, B. L., Thorne, S. E., Canam, C., & Jillings, C. (2001). *Meta-study of qualitative health research: A practical guide to meta-analysis and meta-synthesis* (Methods in Nursing Research, Vol. 3). Thousand Oaks, CA: Sage.

Popay, J., Roberts, H., Sowden, A., Petticrew, M., Arai, L., Rodgers, M., . . . Duffy, S. (2006). *Guidance on the conduct of narrative synthesis in systematic reviews*. ESRC Methods Programme. Retrieved from http://goo.gl/CqxmXT

Sandelowski, M. (2006). "Meta-jeopardy": The crisis of representation in qualitative metasynthesis. *Nursing Outlook, 54*(1), 10–16.

Sandelowski, M., & Barroso, J. (2003). Classifying the findings in qualitative studies. *Qualitative Health Research, 13,* 905–923.

Thorne, S. E. (2008). Meta-synthesis. In L. Givens (Ed.), *The SAGE encyclopedia of qualitative research methods.* Los Angeles, CA: Sage.

Thorne, S., Jensen, L., Kearney, M. H., Noblit, G., & Sandelowski, M. (2004). Qualitative metasynthesis: Reflections on methodological orientation and ideological agenda. *Qualitative Health Research, 14*(10), 1342–1365.

Wertz, F. J., Charmaz, K., McMullen, L. M., Josselson, R., Andersen, R., & McSpaldden, E. (2011). *Five ways of doing qualitative analysis: Phenomenological psychology, grounded theory, discourse analysis, narrative research, and intuitive inquiry.* New York, NY: Guilford.

30

META-SYNTHESIS OF
NURSING PRESENCE[1]

META-SYNTHESIS OF NURSING PRESENCE

Due, in part, to its spiritual and philosophical underpinnings, nursing presence is a complex concept that is vague and difficult to delineate (Smith, 2001). It is often confused with other concepts such as caring, empathy, therapeutic use of self, support, and nurturance (Gardner, 1992). Adding to this confusion is the finding that presence has been fragmented into numerous types (e.g., Easter, 2000; Osterman & Schwartz-Barcott, 1996), used indiscriminately (Smith, 2001), and combined with other concepts such as caring (e.g., Covington, 2003; Engebretson, 2000; Nelms, 1996). Currently, the concept of presence has unclear boundaries and is poorly defined (Doona, Haggerty, & Chase, 1997; Osterman, 2002).

Despite this lack of clarity, presence is a component of several nursing frameworks (e.g., Humanistic Nursing [Paterson & Zderad, 1988]; Human Science and Human Care [Watson, 1988]; Science of Unitary Human Beings [Rogers, 1990]; Human Becoming [Parse, 1998]), and its significance to nursing has been extolled by numerous scholars (e.g., Chase, 2001; Doona et al., 1997; Engebretson, 2000; Gardner, 1992; Hines, 1992; Osterman, 2002; Osterman & Schwartz-Barcott, 1996). For these reasons and in order to ensure the ongoing emergence of nursing theory and knowledge, it is important that the concept of presence be further clarified.

To accomplish this goal, it has been recommended that substantive findings related to the concept of presence be synthesized (Smith, 2001). Although findings from one synthesis (Fredriksson, 1999) already existed, studies related to the phrase *caring presence* were included in the data analysis.

---

[1] Reprinted with permission from Finfgeld-Connett (2006).

In addition, several recent works related to presence were not available at the time it was carried out. Thus, a meta-synthesis of qualitative findings related to nursing presence was conducted. These findings are reported in this chapter.

METHODOLOGY

Meta-synthesis methods for this investigation were adapted from Finfgeld (2003). Meta-synthesis is a research method that is used to rigorously study qualitative findings (versus raw data) and results in reconceptualizations of original conclusions (Finfgeld, 2003). Meta-synthesis is restricted to the analysis of qualitative findings; thus, quantitative results were not included in this study.

Based on familiarity with the existing literature related to presence, it was surmised from the outset that coding categories could be saturated based on findings extracted from the nursing literature; thus, data from other disciplines were not included in this investigation. It was also deemed important to limit the sample to findings within nursing because the ultimate goal of this concept development study was to move toward the formulation of nursing-specific theory. This perspective is in keeping with Penrod and Hupcey's (2005) contention that use of multidisciplinary literature may result in overgeneralization of findings.

The nursing literature was searched using the electronic version of Cumulative Index to Nursing and Allied Health Literature (CINAHL). All available years were reviewed (1982–2005) using the key words presence, concept analysis, qualitative studies, grounded theory, phenomenology, and ethnography. The results were limited to English language publications. *Dissertation Abstracts* (1861–2005) was searched online using the combined key terms presence and nursing. Books related to nursing presence were located using the Missouri Bibliographic Information User System (MOBIUS), a search engine that links multiple academic libraries throughout the state. In combination, these electronic searches resulted in over 1,300 references, which were individually reviewed for possible inclusion in this study. Reference lists of articles, dissertations, and book chapters were also scanned for relevant documents.

Criteria for inclusion in this study consisted of results from concept analyses and qualitative studies of presence that used established data analysis methods. Use of findings from differing epistemological perspectives (e.g., concept analysis, phenomenology, grounded theory) was deemed as a strength due to their complementary nature (Finfgeld, 2003). Anecdotal discussions of the concept along with qualitative analyses that labeled the concept post hoc were excluded.

Analyses and studies of the phrase *caring presence* were excluded, because caring has not been fully conceptualized (Brilowski & Wendler, 2005; Smith, 2001), caring and presence are easily confused (Gardner, 1992), and the two constructs require differentiation (Covington, 2002, 2003; Gilje, 1993). It is anticipated that results from this meta-synthesis will help to delineate presence so that it can be better differentiated from concepts such as caring, empathy, therapeutic use of self, support, and nurturance.

Four linguistic concept analyses and 14 qualitative studies of presence were included in this study (see Table 30.1). Investigations were not excluded based on quality, since universally accepted and empirically reliable criteria for evaluating qualitative studies for use in meta-syntheses do not exist (Sandelowski & Barroso, 2003). In addition, valuable data can be inadvertently excluded based on unnecessary restrictions (Sandelowski, Docherty, & Emden, 1997). The qualitative studies included in this

TABLE 30.1
Publications Included in Meta-Synthesis

AUTHOR(S)/YEAR	TYPE OF INVESTIGATION	DATA SOURCES
Benner (1984)	Qualitative	Nurses
Cavendish et al. (2003)	Qualitative	Nurses
Doona, Haggerty, and Chase (1997)	Qualitative	Nurses
Duis-Nittsche (2002)	Qualitative	Nurses, patients
Easter (2000)	Concept analysis	Literature
Fuller (1991)	Qualitative	Nurses
Gilje (1992)	Concept analysis	Literature
Gilje (1993)	Qualitative	Patients
Hemsley and Glass (1999)	Qualitative	Nurses
Hines (1992)	Concept analysis	Literature
MacKinnon, McIntyre, and Quance (2005)	Qualitative	Patients
McKivergin and Daubenmire (1994)	Concept analysis	Literature
Miller and Douglas (1998)	Qualitative	Nurses
Mohnkern (1992)	Qualitative	Nurses
Osterman (2002)	Qualitative	Nurses, patients
Pettigrew (1988)	Qualitative	Family
Savenstedt, Zingmark, and Sandman (2004)	Qualitative	RNs, nursing staff
Wilson (1986)	Qualitative	Staff, documents, film

investigation reflect the perspectives of staff (primarily nursing staff), patients, and significant others.

Identical data analysis methods were used for findings from all studies, regardless of their epistemological origins (e.g., concept analysis, phenomenology, grounded theory, etc.). Each reference was carefully studied and findings were highlighted. After reading only a few documents, in vivo and metaphorical codes emerged, which provided a beginning structure for data analysis. In keeping with methods suggested by Finfgeld (2003) and grounded theory strategies (Strauss & Corbin, 1998), the initial coding structure was shaped by Walker and Avant's (2005) broad process categories (i.e., antecedents, attributes, and consequences). Outside of offering a structure for coding, Walker and Avant's (2005) methods were not used to conduct this investigation.

Ongoing analysis of the findings was accomplished using an electronic matrix; codes and categories were added, combined, and deleted. Substantive categories and codes that were saturated were subsequently synthesized and translated to create a model. Links among constructs were explicated with the assistance of written memos and diagrams, and a new interpretation of nursing presence was formulated.

FINDINGS

Nursing presence is an interpersonal process that is characterized by sensitivity, holism, intimacy, vulnerability, and adaptation to unique circumstances. Potential recipients demonstrate a need for and openness to presence, and nurses are willing to enact it. To engage in presence, nurses must possess personal and professional maturity, and their nursing care must be based on moral principles of commitment and respect for individual differences. They must also practice within an environment that is conducive to presence.

Presence results in enhanced mental well-being for nurses and patients and improved physical well-being for recipients. In keeping with the nature of a process, the outcomes of nursing presence go on to influence its enactment in the future. These findings are illustrated in Figure 30.1 and are discussed in detail throughout the remainder of this article.

Attributes

Presence consists of a process that is enacted in moments or over days, weeks, and years (Fuller, 1991; Gilje, 1993; Hines, 1992; Mohnkern, 1992; Miller & Douglas, 1998; Wilson, 1986). Given extended periods of time, a rhythmic pattern of presencing develops between the nurse and patient (Easter, 2000; Gilje, 1993; Miller & Douglas, 1998; Osterman, 2002). This process is characterized by interpersonal sensitivity (Doona, Chase, & Haggerty, 1999; Duis-Nittsche,

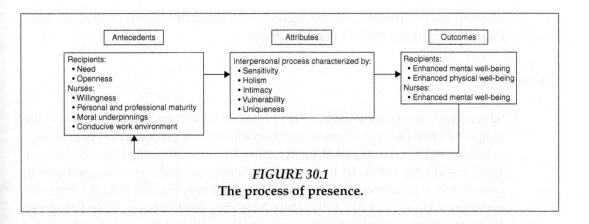

FIGURE 30.1
The process of presence.

2002; Gilje, 1993; Hemsley & Glass, 1999; MacKinnon, McIntyre, & Quance, 2005; Pettigrew, 1988) and is holistically focused on each individual's physical, psychological, and spiritual well-being (Doona et al., 1999; Duis-Nittsche, 2002; McKivergin & Daubenmire, 1994).

Presence involves being with another in an intimate way (Duis-Nittsche, 2002; Fuller, 1991; Wilson, 1986). Close physical proximity is the norm and includes engaged availability, affectionate touching, and attending to personal needs (Easter, 2000; MacKinnon et al., 2005; Mohnkern, 1992). Sensitive verbal communication (Duis-Nittsche, 2002; Hines, 1992; MacKinnon et al., 2005; Pettigrew, 1988) may be used to manage psychological and spiritual concerns; however, these issues may also be addressed nonverbally by listening or making knowing eye contact (MacKinnon et al., 2005; Pettigrew, 1988).

Nurses enact presence not only with patients but also with their significant others (Cavendish et al., 2003; Duis-Nittsche, 2002; MacKinnon et al., 2005; Pettigrew, 1988). Within these relationships, trust must be established (Easter, 2000; Gilje, 1993; Hines, 1992; MacKinnon et al., 2005; Pettigrew, 1988; Savenstedt, Zingmark, & Sandman, 2004) so that risk taking is possible. Each individual is compelled to become personally vulnerable (Gilje, 1993; Hemsley & Glass, 1999; Miller & Douglas, 1998; Osterman, 2002; Pettigrew, 1988) and reciprocally share in physical, spiritual, and psychological ways (Duis-Nittsche, 2002; Mohnkern, 1992; Savenstedt et al., 2004). For all parties involved, this means lowering defenses (Duis-Nittsche, 2002; Fuller, 1991; Gilje, 1993; Hemsley & Glass, 1999) and mutually experiencing feelings such as attachment (Gilje, 1993), sacredness (Hemsley & Glass, 1999), suffering (Fuller, 1991), and neediness (Mohnkern, 1992).

Presence occurs within a context of dynamic adaptation to unique circumstances (Doona et al., 1999; Gilje, 1993; MacKinnon et al., 2005). Depending on the situation, nurses may be present in various ways and on a variety of levels (Duis-Nittsche, 2002; Fuller, 1991; Mohnkern, 1992; Osterman, 2002). To enable this type of flexibility, each individual is viewed through a lens of unconditional positive regard and acceptance (Cavendish et al., 2003; Gilje, 1993; Hines, 1992; Pettigrew, 1988).

Antecedents

Several precursors are necessary for presence to be carried out. The first is the recipient's need for presence, which is evidenced by physical and psychological distress (Doona et al., 1999; Easter, 2000; Fuller, 1991; Gilje, 1993; Mohnkern, 1992; Pettigrew, 1988). In the context of need, an individual's openness to presence is also necessary, and the nurse is actively invited into the patient's experience (Doona et al., 1999; Duis-Nittsche, 2002; Easter, 2000; Pettigrew, 1988). In reciprocal fashion, the nurse must be willing to engage in intentional presence (Doona et al., 1999; Duis-Nittsche, 2002; Fuller, 1991; Pettigrew, 1988). There must be intent to spend time (Doona et al., 1999; Duis-Nittsche, 2002), internalize another's struggles (Doona et al., 1999; Fuller, 1991; Pettigrew, 1988), and share personal energy (Duis-Nittsche, 2002; Fuller, 1991; Gilje, 1992; Mohnkern, 1992) to diminish distress.

Due to its complex nature, nurses who enact presence must be personally and professionally mature. From a personal standpoint, nurses must know (Easter, 2000; Fuller, 1991; Gilje, 1993) and accept themselves (Benner, 1984; Duis-Nittsche, 2002; Mohnkern, 1992) such that they are well-balanced and centered individuals (Doona et al., 1999; Gilje, 1992, 1993; Mohnkern, 1992). They must also possess clinical competence and expertise in the physical and psychosocial domains of nursing practice (Duis-Nittsche, 2002; Easter, 2000; Fuller, 1991; Hines, 1992; Mohnkern, 1992). From a moral perspective, presence is underpinned by a commitment to help (Easter, 2000; Miller & Douglas, 1998; Mohnkern, 1992; Pettigrew, 1988) and a respect for individual differences (Cavendish et al., 2003; Duis-Nittsche, 2002; Gilje, 1993; Hines, 1992; Pettigrew, 1988; Wilson, 1986).

Presence takes shape within the milieu at hand (MacKinnon et al., 2005; Osterman, 2002); thus, a final precursor to the enactment of presence is a conducive work environment. Favorable elements include supportive colleagues (Miller & Douglas, 1998; Pettigrew, 1988; Wilson, 1986), adequate time (Duis-Nittsche, 2002; Pettigrew, 1988) and staffing (Pettigrew, 1988; Wilson, 1986), and judicious emphasis on technology and tasks (Fuller, 1991; MacKinnon et al., 2005; Pettigrew, 1988) versus psychological and spiritual concerns.

Outcomes

Recipients of nursing presence report enhanced mental well-being. There are feelings of safety and security (Gilje, 1993; Pettigrew, 1988), decreased stress (Fuller, 1991; Gilje, 1993), increased coping (Easter, 2000; Pettigrew, 1988; Wilson, 1986), and elevated self-esteem (Easter, 2000; Gilje, 1993; Pettigrew,

1988). Revitalization occurs (Duis-Nittsche, 2002; Easter, 2000; Gilje, 1992, 1993), and patients feel as if they grow in the experience through new understandings (Doona et al., 1999; Easter, 2000; Gilje, 1992, 1993). In keeping with a process orientation, presence has a sustained therapeutic effect that may last long after the actual event (Gilje, 1992, 1993; Hines, 1992; Pettigrew, 1988).

Nursing presence is also associated with enhanced physical well-being. Investigators allude to general improvements in physiological status using terms such as "recovery," "remission," and "healing" (Duis-Nittsche, 2002; Fuller, 1991; Hemsley & Glass, 1999). In addition, they report specific changes in physical health such as decreased pain (Easter, 2000; Fuller, 1991). When loss of life is inevitable, there is the sense of a better death experience (Mohnkern, 1992; Pettigrew, 1988).

Findings suggest that nurses also experience improved mental well-being resulting from presence (Duis-Nittsche, 2002; Easter, 2000). Improvements are evidenced by satisfaction (Duis-Nittsche, 2002; Easter, 2000; Miller & Douglas, 1998), learning and maturation (Doona et al., 1999; Easter, 2000; Hemsley & Glass, 1999; Miller & Douglas, 1998), revitalization (Duis-Nittsche, 2002; Easter, 2000; Miller & Douglas, 1998; Mohnkern, 1992), and self-confidence (Doona et al., 1999; Easter, 2000; Duis-Nittsche, 2002; Mohnkern, 1992). Providing personal and professional maturity does not antecedently exist (Doona et al., 1999; Gilje, 1992, 1993; Mohnkern, 1992), there is the possibility of energy depletion and fatigue (Duis-Nittsche, 2002; Miller & Douglas, 1998; Mohnkern, 1992). This potentiality points to the important role that personal and professional maturity plays in tempering the demands of nursing presence.

In keeping with the premise that nursing presence consists of a process, outcomes will influence antecedents. As such, recipients have less need for presence; however, based on previous experience, they are more open to it in the future. Nurses are enabled to engage in presence based on enhanced satisfaction (Duis-Nittsche, 2002; Easter, 2000; Miller & Douglas, 1998), learning and maturation (Doona et al., 1999; Easter, 2000; Hemsley & Glass, 1999; Miller & Douglas, 1998), revitalization (Duis-Nittsche, 2002; Easter, 2000; Miller & Douglas, 1998; Mohnkern, 1992), and self-confidence (Doona et al., 1999; Duis-Nittsche, 2002; Easter, 2000; Mohnkern, 1992). It is also inferred that managers and administrators will continue to gain an appreciation for the benefits of nursing presence and, thus, strive to maintain a working environment that encourages it.

DISCUSSION

Findings from this meta-synthesis offer a more thorough and comprehensive understanding of the concept of nursing presence. Nursing presence is an interpersonal process that is characterized by sensitivity, holism, intimacy, vulnerability, and adaptation to unique circumstances. Presence results in positive outcomes for nurses and recipients, which go on to encourage the enactment of presence in the future. In order for presence to emerge, patients must possess a need for and openness to it. Nurses must be willing, personally and professionally mature, and act on prescribed moral principles. They must also work within an environment that is conducive to nursing presence.

In keeping with meta-synthesis methods (Finfgeld, 2003), refutational findings were sought throughout the data analysis process. Despite openness to refutational results and active attempts to saturate and synthesize these types of findings, none emerged. This includes a lack of evidence that presence results in negative outcomes. Ergo, presence appears to be an inherently positive experience, and negative outcomes are the result of another process.

Findings from this work suggest that antecedents (e.g., personal and professional maturity, conducive work environment) are necessary in order for presence to be enacted. That said, it is hypothesized that incidental presence is possible in situations in which antecedents are nascent or lacking. For example, it may be possible for a novice nurse to enact presence, given the support and guidance of a mentor (e.g., Engebretson, 2000). Alternately, a mature nurse may be able to employ presence within a nonconducive environment. These scenarios are in keeping with Morse's (1995) probabilistic view of nursing concepts and her assertion that they are organized around properties or clusters of connected elements rather than rigid criteria. The probabilistic view allows for concept commonality and cohesion coupled with contextual fluidity and variation.

Based on findings from this investigation and Sherwood's (1997) meta-synthesis of caring, it is clear that nursing presence and caring have many overlapping components. Both concepts appear to be processes that are composed of interpersonal sensitivity, expert nursing practice, and an intimate reciprocal relationship between nurse and patient. Researchers are encouraged to use advanced concept development methods such as, concept correction and comparison (Morse, 1995), to further delineate and differentiate presence from nursing phenomena such as caring and empathy.

In the past, researchers have delineated types of nursing presence (e.g., Easter, 2000; Osterman & Schwartz-Barcott, 1996). For the short term, this may be an important exercise in understanding the nuances of the phenomenon. In the long run, however, it may inhibit comprehension of the whole. Many psychosocial phenomena within nursing (e.g., caring, courage, empowerment) can be classified on continua, but appreciating the essence of the whole is necessary in order to make concepts functional components of the discipline's lexicon.

Another practice that inhibits useful analysis and understanding of the concept of presence is the tendency to combine the term with constructs such as caring (e.g., Covington, 2003; Engebretson, 2000; Nelms, 1996). Although the phrase *caring presence* has a nice ring, neither term holds it boundaries;

similarities and differences between the two concepts need to be explicated. Until this is accomplished, scholars are cautioned against such practices.

Although close physical proximity is the norm when enacting presence, telehealth technology (e.g., telephone, videoconferencing, Internet) is forcing nurses to explore the possibility that presence can be executed when nurses and patients are not in the same location (Sandelowski, 2002). Savenstedt et al. (2004) brought this issue to the foreground in their study of synchronous videoconferencing with older adults. Their initial findings suggest that tele-communicated presence is possible using some of the same techniques that are employed in face-to-face settings.

Placing presence within the context of a process begs a discussion of the practicality of this phenomenon within a time-sensitive health care system. An analysis of the process elements suggests that selective antecedents, such as development of personal and professional maturity are, by nature, time intensive. Once these antecedents are in place, however, it seems possible that presence may require very little time to unfold, which should allay some anxiety about the practicality and cost-effectiveness of nursing presence within the current health care milieu.

Nurses are encouraged to note that many of the findings used in this investigation can only be found in dissertation format. Although dissertations offer a rich source of data, they are not always readily available and may be costly to access. For this reason, scholars are urged to publish their work in more easily accessible peer-reviewed journals.

SUMMARY

Given the visibility of presence within numerous nursing frameworks (e.g., Parse, 1998; Paterson & Zderad, 1988; Rogers, 1990; Watson, 1988), nurses are compelled to do a better job of delineating the concept. To this end, findings from this meta-synthesis add to the overall understanding of the construct. In the future, researchers are encouraged to use advanced concept development methods to further delineate and differentiate presence from other nursing phenomena such as caring. In addition, nurses are cautioned against parsing the term and combining it with other vaguely defined constructs. Finally, researchers are urged to consider how nursing presence can be preserved using telehealth technology and in time-sensitive health care settings.

REFERENCES

Benner, P. (1984). *From novice to expert: Excellence and power in clinical nursing practice*. Menlo Park, CA: Addison Wesley.

Brilowski, G. A., & Wendler, M. C. (2005). An evolutionary concept analysis of caring. *Journal of Advanced Nursing, 50,* 641–650.

Cavendish, R., Konecny, L., Mitzeliotis, C., Russo, D., Luise, B. K., Lanza, M., . . . Bajo, M. A. M. (2003). Spiritual care activities of nurses using nursing interventions classification (NIC) labels. *International Journal of Nursing Terminologies and Classifications, 14,* 113–124.

Chase, S. K. (2001). Response to "The concept of nursing presence: State of the science." *Scholarly Inquiry for Nursing Practice: An International Journal, 15,* 323–327.

Covington, H. (2002). *Caring presence: Journey toward a mutual goal* (Unpublished doctoral dissertation). University of Colorado Health Sciences Center, Denver, CO.

Covington, H. (2003). Caring presence: Delineation of a concept for holistic nursing. *Journal of Holistic Nursing, 21,* 301–317.

Doona, M. E., Chase, S. K., & Haggerty, L. A. (1999). Nursing presence: As real as a Milky Way bar. *Journal of Holistic Nursing, 17,* 54–70.

Doona, M. E., Haggerty, L. A., & Chase, S. K. (1997). Nursing presence: An existential exploration of the concept. *Scholarly Inquiry for Nursing Practice: An International Journal, 11,* 3–16.

Duis-Nittsche, E. R. (2002). *A study of nursing presence* (Unpublished doctoral dissertation). University of Texas Medical Branch, Galveston, TX.

Easter, A. (2000). Construct analysis of four modes of being present. *Journal of Holistic Nursing, 18,* 362–377.

Engebretson, J. (2000). Caring presence: A case study. *International Journal for Human Caring, 4*(2), 33–39.

Finfgeld, D. L. (2003). Metasynthesis: The state of the art—So far. *Qualitative Health Research, 13*(7), 893–904.

Finfgeld-Connett, D. (2006). Meta-synthesis of presence in nursing. *Journal of Advanced Nursing, 55,* 708–714. doi:10.1111/j.1365-2648.2006.03961.x

Fredriksson, L. (1999). Modes of relating in a caring conversation: A research synthesis on presence, touch and listening. *Journal of Advanced Nursing, 30,* 1167–1176.

Fuller, J. G. (1991). *A conceptualization of presence as a nursing phenomenon* (Unpublished doctoral dissertation). University of Utah, Salt Lake City, UT.

Gardner, D. L. (1992). Presence. In G. M. Bulechek & J. C. McCloskey (Eds.), *Nursing interventions: Essential nursing treatments* (pp. 191–200). Philadelphia, PA: W. B. Saunders.

Gilje, F. (1992). Being there: An analysis of the concept of presence. In D. A. Gaut (Ed.), *In the presence of caring in nursing* (pp. 53–67). New York, NY: National League for Nursing.

Gilje, F. L. (1993). *A phenomenological study of patients' experiences of the nurse's presence* (Unpublished doctoral dissertation). University of Colorado Health Science Center, Denver, CO.

Hemsley, M., & Glass, N. (1999). "Super" presencing nurse healers' stories of healing. *The Australian Journal of Holistic Nursing, 6,* 25–31.

Hines, D. R. (1992). Presence: Discovering the artistry in relating. *Journal of Holistic Nursing, 10,* 294–305.

MacKinnon, K., McIntyre, M., & Quance, M. (2005). The meaning of the nurse's presence during childbirth. *Journal of Obstetric, Gynecologic and Neonatal Nursing, 34,* 28–36.

McKivergin, M. J., & Daubenmire, M. J. (1994). The healing process of presence. *Journal of Holistic Nursing, 12,* 65–81.

Miller, M. A., & Douglas, M. R. (1998). Presencing: Nurses commitment to caring for dying persons. *International Journal for Human Caring, 2*(3), 24–31.

Mohnkern, S. M. (1992). *Presence in nursing: Its antecedents, defining attributes and consequences* (Unpublished doctoral dissertation). University of Texas, Austin, TX.

Morse, J. M. (1995). Exploring the theoretical basis of nursing using advanced techniques of concept analysis. *Advances in Nursing Science, 17*(3), 31–46.

Nelms, T. (1996). Living a caring presence in nursing: A heideggerian hermeneutical analysis. *Journal of Advanced Nursing, 24,* 368–374.

Osterman, P. A. (2002). *A participant observation study of experienced nurses' presence in daily care* (Unpublished doctoral dissertation). University of Rhode Island, Kingstown, Rhode RI.

Osterman, P., & Schwartz-Barcott, D. (1996). Presence: Four ways of being there. *Nursing Forum, 31*(2), 23–30.

Parse, R. R. (1998). *The human becoming school of thought: A perspective for nurses and other health professionals.* Thousand Oaks, CA: Sage.

Paterson, J. G., & Zderad, L. T. (1988). *Humanistic nursing.* New York, NY: John Wiley & Sons.

Penrod, J., & Hupcey, J. E. (2005). Concept advancement: Extending science through concept-driven research. *Research and Theory in Nursing Practice, 19*(3), 231–241.

Pettigrew, J. M. (1988). *A phenomenological study of the nurse's presence with persons experiencing suffering* (Unpublished doctoral dissertation). Texas Woman's University, Denton, TX.

Rogers, M. E. (1990). Nursing: Science of unitary, irreducible, human beings: Update 1990. In E. A. M. Barrett (Ed.), *Visions of Rogers' science-based nursing* (pp. 5–11). New York, NY: National League for Nursing.

Sandelowski, M. (2002). Visible humans, vanishing bodies, and virtual nursing: Complications of life, presence, place, and identity. *Advances in Nursing Science, 24*(3), 58–70.

Sandelowski, M., & Barroso, J. (2003). Classifying the findings in qualitative studies. *Qualitative Health Research, 13,* 905–923.

Sandelowski, M., Docherty, S., & Emden, C. (1997). Qualitative metasynthesis: Issues and techniques. *Research in Nursing & Health, 20,* 365–371.

Savenstedt, S., Zingmark, K., & Sandman, P. O. (2004). Being present in a distant room: Aspects of teleconsultations with older people in a nursing home. *Qualitative Health Research, 14,* 1046–1057.

Sherwood, G. D. (1997). Meta-synthesis of qualitative analyses of caring: Defining a therapeutic model of nursing. *Advanced Practice Nursing Quarterly, 3,* 32–42.

Smith, T. D. (2001). The concept of nursing presence: State of the science. *Scholarly Inquiry for Nursing Practice: An International Journal, 15,* 299–322.

Strauss, A., & Corbin, J. (1998). *Basics of qualitative research: Techniques and procedures for developing grounded theory.* Thousand Oaks, CA: Sage.

Walker, L. O., & Avant, K. C. (2005). *Strategies for theory construction in nursing* (4th ed.). Upper Saddle River, NJ: Pearson.

Watson, J. (1988). *Nursing: Human science and human care: A theory of nursing.* New York, NY: National League for Nursing.

Wilson, H. S. (1986). Presencing–social control of schizophrenics in an antipsychiatric community: Doing grounded theory. In P. L. Munhall & C. J. Oilerss (Eds.), *Nursing research: A qualitative perspective* (pp. 131–144). Norwalk, CT: Appleton-Century-Crofts.

Deborah Finfgeld-Connett, Tina L. Bloom, and E. Diane Johnson

31

PERCEIVED COMPETENCY AND RESOLUTION OF HOMELESSNESS AMONG WOMEN WITH SUBSTANCE ABUSE PROBLEMS[1]

> *We are approaching a new age of synthesis. Knowledge cannot be merely a degree or a skill . . . it demands a broader vision, capabilities in critical thinking and logical deduction without which we cannot have constructive progress.*
>
> —Li Ka-shing

Despite evidence of relative prosperity in some places, homelessness remains a problem in many locales. Homelessness in Canada is estimated to range from 150,000 to 300,000 (Intraspec.ca, 2010), and in Australia the numbers are thought to hover around 105,000 (Australian Bureau of Statistics, 2008). Over the course of a year, it is estimated that 1,593,150 individuals in the United States experience homelessness. Of that number, approximately 605,397 (38%) are women residing in shelters (Substance Abuse and Mental Health Services Administration [SAMHSA], 2011). Reasons for homelessness among women include a lack of jobs and public assistance funds and a coinciding increase in poverty and home foreclosures. Other exacerbating problems among women include domestic violence, mental illness, substance abuse, and a commensurate lack of affordable treatment programs (Human Resources and Skills Development Canada [HRSDC], 2010; National Coalition for the Homeless [NCH], 2009).

Moving homeless women into stable housing can be challenging when substances of abuse such as alcohol, cocaine, and heroin are involved.

---

[1] Reprinted with permission from Finfgeld-Connett, Bloom, and Johnson (2012).

Among a sample of homeless women from three Canadian cities, 82% (n = 193) were found to have at least one type of substance abuse disorder (Torchalla, Strehlau, Li, & Krausz, 2011). In the United States, it is estimated that women comprise one-fifth of the homeless who are admitted to substance abuse treatment facilities. About half of these individuals report between one and four prior treatment episodes, and 20% report five or more treatment experiences (SAMHSA, 2004). Given these recidivism rates, efforts to systematically examine and fine-tune assistance programs for homeless women with substance abuse problems are needed (O'Campo et al., 2009).

We conducted the current meta-synthesis following a prior investigation in which the process of becoming homeless, being homeless, and resolving homelessness among persistently homeless women was investigated (Finfgeld-Connett, 2010a). Based on findings from that study, it appears that becoming and being homeless are likely to involve maladaptive experiences of interpersonal abuse, neglect, and/or abandonment, all of which may be fueled by the psychic instability and/or immoral proclivities of close associates. Other contextually permeating factors include circumstantial poverty and transience, and social service system barriers. These barriers appear to extend beyond mere problems of availability and accessibility. Of particular note are more intangible impediments pertaining to trust and overall integrity of the system.

Based on findings from this same meta-synthesis (Finfgeld-Connett, 2010a), it was also concluded that resolving homelessness among a heterogeneous group of persistently homeless women involves cyclic stages. These women tend to seek assistance when crises occur, but they remain vulnerable to homelessness. It is not unusual for persistently homeless women to repeatedly engage–disengage–engage with the social service system prior to making sustained efforts to become stably housed. The cyclic nature of this process prolongs the resolution of homelessness and is attributable, at least in part, to substance abuse problems (Burlingham, Andrasik, Larimer, Marlatt, & Spigner, 2010; Finfgeld-Connett, 2010a). The specific purpose of this investigation was to articulate new insights relating to the cyclic process of resolving homelessness among adult women with substance abuse problems.

METHODOLOGY

Qualitative Meta-Synthesis

Qualitative meta-synthesis, as outlined by Finfgeld-Connett (e.g., 2009a, 2009b, 2010a), was used to conduct this investigation. This method was inspired by the work of Noblit and Hare (1988), Miles and Huberman (1994), and the grounded theory approaches of Corbin and Strauss (2008) and Strauss and Corbin (1990). Qualitative meta-synthesis does not involve data aggregation or any other quantitative method. It is not a secondary analysis of raw qualitative data, nor is it a type of meta-analysis. Meta-synthesis is a methodology in which qualitative findings from existing research reports are systematically acquired and qualitatively analyzed and synthesized (Finfgeld-Connett, 2010b). Qualitative meta-syntheses result in novel interpretations of qualitative findings that cannot be identified in original research reports (Thorne, Jensen, Kearney, Noblit, & Sandelowski, 2004).

Within the context of meta-synthesis work, validity is not dependent on the logic of replication (Thorne et al., 2004); rather, it is based on trustworthiness (Lincoln & Guba, 1985). One way that trustworthiness is established is through transparent data extraction and analysis processes. To this end, these iterative processes are described next.

Sample

There is some overlap ($n = 23$) between the reports that comprise the database for this study ($N = 60$) and a prior investigation ($N = 45$; Finfgeld-Connett, 2010a); however, with the help of an expert reference librarian (third author), the pool of potential research reports was greatly expanded for this study. In addition, unlike the prior investigation, research reports were excluded if substance abuse issues were not addressed.

Electronic databases that were searched included Cumulative Index to Nursing and Allied Health Literature (CINAHL), ETOH Archival Database, GenderWatch, Google Books, Ovid MedLine, ProQuest Dissertations, PsycINFO, Scopus, and Social Work Abstracts. Customized search strategies, were used to maximize the potential of each unique database and to exclude reports such as those that pertained solely to children, adolescents, and men, or those that were not conducted using qualitative methods. These tailored search strategies resulted in over 5,500 English language citations, with unavoidable duplication across databases.

A cursory review of each citation title and abstract was conducted to further eliminate publications that were clearly not reports of qualitative research relating to homeless women. This resulted in the identification of 90 promising reports that were subsequently secured for further evaluation. Thirty of these were eliminated for one or more reasons. For example, findings relating to substance abuse could not be identified, or findings relating to women could not be separated from those pertaining to men, or findings relating strictly to homeless women could not be isolated from those associated with low-income women. In total, 60 reports of qualitative research, dating from 1990 to mid-2010, comprised the sample for this investigation. This number consisted of 30 published peer-reviewed articles, 7 books, and 23 theses/dissertations.

Data Extraction, Analysis, and Synthesis

To avoid potential theoretical bias, grounded theory process concepts (e.g., antecedents, attributes, outcomes, and interrelationships among constructs; Corbin & Strauss, 2008; Strauss & Corbin, 1990) were the only theoretical foundations that were used for data analysis. Coding structures from a prior investigation (Finfgeld-Connett, 2010a) were not used to guide data analysis since the foci of this study and that one differed.

A data collection form that was adapted from Finfgeld-Connett (2010a) was used to gather information pertaining to each study such as aim/purpose, theoretical framework, methods, and sample. This information was used throughout the data analysis process to provide context. When available, information relating to substance abuse treatment strategies was also gathered; however, the utility of these data was limited because they were inconsistently reported across studies.

Each research report was carefully read, and the findings were highlighted. In keeping with meta-synthesis methods, findings were limited to researcher interpretations rather than raw data such as quotations (Finfgeld, 2003; Finfgeld-Connett, 2010a). To avoid bias, all interpreted findings, regardless of how they compared with the researchers' preconceived ideas, were extracted from the original research reports and placed into data analysis matrices for coding and categorizing. Concrete and in vivo codes were initially used to ensure a firm grounding in the data. To further ensure well-grounded results, metaphorical coding was carried out in small iterative and reflexive steps. Subsequently, memos were iteratively and reflexively composed and revised to clearly articulate singular codes, explicate abstract categories, and delineate links among concepts (Finfgeld-Connett, 2010a). Memos were gradually translated into provisional lines of argument and continually evaluated against the original data to assess for truthfulness and fittingness with associated findings. This reflexive and iterative process continued until conceptual clarity was achieved and the core concept of perceived competency was fully articulated (Corbin & Strauss, 2008; Finfgeld-Connett, 2010a; Noblit & Hare, 1988).

Trustworthiness

In addition to the data collection and analysis methods that have already been outlined, the following steps were taken to enhance trustworthiness. First, instead of vetting research reports in their entirety for quality, each finding was evaluated based on its credibility and fittingness within the emergent findings (Pawson, 2006). Based on this strategy, only those findings that lacked support within the context of the current investigation were omitted. This is in contrast to potentially rejecting all findings from an entire research report based on the way that a study is presented or written. The approach used to conduct this investigation is consistent with the fact that no known valid method currently exists for judging the overall quality of qualitative research based on written reports (Centre for Reviews and Dissemination, 2009). In the end, only those findings that lacked support within the context of the current investigation were excluded from further consideration. This is in contrast to rejecting all findings from an entire research report based on the way a study is presented or written. For example, because research reports as old as 20 years were included in the database, each finding was carefully vetted for currency. In large part, data relating to the topic under investigation transcended time. Those that did not were excluded from further analysis. These included time-sensitive findings pertaining to treatment funding and public policy initiatives.

It is notable that because findings from multiple qualitative investigations comprise a meta-synthesis database, several forms of triangulation are inherent to the methodology. These types of triangulation include a variety of research frameworks (i.e., phenomenology, ethnography, grounded theory, etc.), sampling methods, data analysis methods, and researchers (Finfgeld, 2003; Finfgeld-Connett, 2010b).

In the case of this meta-synthesis, the second author independently reviewed codes and memos at critical junctures in the data analysis process and provided feedback to the first author. Her feedback was used to reflexively review coding, categorizing, and memoing, and to make adjustments that were congruent with the data.

FINDINGS

Overview

The reports included in this investigation represent studies that were carried out in the United States ($n = 51$), Canada ($n = 3$), and Australia ($n = 1$). One was a multisite study (Canada and Scotland), and in four instances, the data collection locations were undisclosed. In light of contextual information, these four studies appear to have been carried out in the United States and Canada.

The findings that comprised the sample for this meta-synthesis represent data from 1,871 homeless women. This includes data from 674 Black women, 346 White women, 252 Hispanic women, 100 women who were classified as other, and 499 individuals whose race/ethnicity remain unknown. The study database also included findings generated from 251 staff and 74 members of the public. These numbers do not account for countless others who were included in the research process through observation and participant observation.

Findings from the meta-synthesis portion of this investigation are presented next. This meta-synthesis is not comprehensive; instead, it is intended to orient the reader and to provide an overview of the findings. Based on the results of this meta-synthesis, distorted perceptions of competency, which are shaped by dysfunctional relationships and mental health problems, appear to make it challenging for women with substance abuse problems to resolve homelessness. Women with low and high levels of perceived competency grapple with challenges related to structure and control, trust, and hopelessness. Therapeutic strategies for approaching women with distorted perceptions of competency include careful assessment, caring, personalized structure and control, development of interpersonal trust, and instillation of hope. Targeted efforts to manage substance abuse and other exacerbating mental health problems are also consistent with optimal care.

Perceived Competency

Perceived competency is a concept that is inferred based on the findings of this meta-synthesis. It is the personally interpreted ability to make decisions, take action, and execute positive change in one's life. Perceived competency exists on a continuum and is based on individual insights and interpretations. Given the enduring personal and interpersonal challenges that many homeless women face (Marcus, 2001; Padgett, Hawkins, Abrams, & Davis, 2006), they tend to present with varying levels of perceived competency. Some homeless women project a high level of perceived competency whereas others project very little. Still others lie somewhere in the middle. Supporting references are used to explicate these ideas in the following paragraphs.

Low Perceived Competency

Women with low levels of perceived competency are likely to present as chronically homeless owing to a sense of personal paralysis (Lineberger, 2009). They are apt to psychologically distance themselves from the reality of their situations (Acquaviva, 2000) and to disassociate from their mental and physical health care needs (Enriquez, 2005; Liebow, 1993). These women tend to see themselves as unable to effect positive change, and they attribute their gridlocked status to forces beyond their control such as the economy or the bureaucratic system (Williams, 2003). Using this mindset, fatalism tends to become a consoling way to explain a powerful and unjust world, and blame and loathing may be projected elsewhere (Acquaviva, 2000; Brink, 2001; Carroll & Trull, 2002; Lineberger, 2009; Williams, 2003). Although adaptive in some ways, this nihilistic worldview is apt to inhibit change by obfuscating links between personal behavior and negative consequences. It may also lead to acquiescence and behavioral inertia on the part of the individual (Acquaviva, 2000; Gelberg, Browner, Lejano, & Arangua, 2004).

High Perceived Competency

Women with high levels of perceived competency also tend to present as intransigently homeless; however, their affect may be notably different than those individuals with low levels of perceived competency. Freedom and the liberty to abide by one's own value system and rules are likely to take priority over getting help in a structured setting that functions based on conventional mores and regulations (Fogel, 1997; Patterson, 2003). These women may see the treatment environment as alien, and expectations of social service providers may exceed their willingness or ability to adapt. Instead of feeling more stable and secure in a structured environment (Fogel, 1997), they tend to feel out of control, and their behavior may be disruptive (Fogel, 1997; Grella, 1994).

Homeless women with high levels of perceived competency appear to overestimate their ability to independently execute change and improve their lives outside of therapeutic environments. Based on this vantage point, they may repress or deny injustices and assume personae of strength, toughness, and autonomy (Huey & Quirouette, 2010). These women have been known to go so far as to believe that they are exceptionally lucky, skillful, strong, or manipulative. At this polarity of the continuum, homeless women may perceive that societal rules do not apply to them, which can lead to aggressive, antisocial, or criminal activities (Carroll & Trull, 2002; Gentry, 2003; Luhrmann, 2008). Consequently, they may habitually gravitate toward illegal and unsustainable activities such as drug sales and sex work (Geter, 1993; Greene, Ball, Belcher, & McAlpine, 2003; Marcus, 2001; Wheeler, 2006).

Perceived Competency at Mid-Continuum

It is inferred that homeless women in the middle of the perceived competency continuum appear to have a relatively good grasp of their personal assets and limitations, and they tend to possess skills that are needed to effectively make decisions and resolve problems. These women are better equipped than those on the margins of the continuum to assertively approach social service providers, gain knowledge, build healthy supportive relationships, establish conventional daily routines, and pursue job and housing leads (Banyard, 1995; Gillette, 2001; Haydon, 2005; Sysko, 2002). They tend to be more adept at instituting creative coping strategies, and they are not as likely to rely on social services for extended periods of time (Grella, 1994). These women are not the focus of this investigation.

Factors That Shape Perceived Competency

Dysfunctional Relationships

High and low perceptions of competency tend to emerge in the context of dysfunctional relationships. Homeless women are likely to have been raised in unstable homes where there was a history of multigenerational dysfunction and loss (Trickett & Chung, 2007). It is not unusual for their parents to have been divorced, deceased, and/or substance abusers. As youth, many homeless women endured some form of neglect and physical and emotional abuse, and they may have been raised by relatives or placed in foster care at an early age (Acquaviva, 2000; Carroll & Trull, 1999, 2002; Haydon, 2005; Marcus, 2001).

As adults, homeless women frequently report that they have experienced familial abuse and/or alienation (Carroll & Trull, 2002; Lineberger, 2009; Trickett & Chung, 2007; Wheeler, 2006). Although they may seek refuge with sympathetic acquaintances and family members, these relationships are tenuous, tensions escalate over time, and eventually the women feel compelled to leave (Belcher, Greene, McAlpine, & Ball, 2001; Brink, 2001; Montgomery, McCauley, & Bailey, 2009; Williams, 2003). As a result of these types of experiences, many homeless women do not have the opportunity to develop healthy interpersonal relationships (Belcher et al., 2001), and their social support systems are, at best, fragile (Brink, 2001; Gillette, 2001; Williams, 2003).

Among individuals with low levels of perceived competency, it is inferred that innate needs to stay interpersonally connected may sometimes override needs to ensure one's own well-being and safety (D'Amico, Barnes, Gilbert, Ryan, & Wenzel, 2009; Urbanoski, 2001). In an attempt to create mutually fulfilling relationships, these women are apt to endure a number of different types of interpersonal abuse for the short term in hopes of satisfying their need for fulfilling relationships in the long run (Haydon, 2005; Liebow, 1993; Lineberger, 2009).

Among homeless women with high levels of perceived competency, it appears that they are also likely to engage in maladaptive interpersonal relationships, but they are apt to take a different form. These women may be less likely to become closely linked with men who will abuse them, but they remain highly vulnerable to ubiquitous violence and the negative consequences of activities such as serial monogamy and drug use with strangers (e.g., exposure to HIV; Bourgois et al., 2004; Luhrmann, 2008).

Substance Abuse and Mental Health Problems

In some instances it is difficult to determine which comes first, substance abuse or homelessness. Many times there is a family history of substance abuse or, at the very least, it can be documented at an early age (Carroll & Trull, 1999, 2002; Lineberger, 2009; Schretzman, 1999). Foregoing that, it is not unusual for substance abuse to emerge once a woman becomes homeless. Homeless women may resort to using drugs and alcohol in order to belong, please a sexual partner, and/or to escape from painful realities (Brink, 2001; Enriquez, 2005; Padgett et al., 2006). No matter its inception, a self-perpetuating cycle of substance abuse and homelessness may take shape (Belcher et al., 2001). In addition, this problem may be fueled by other acute and chronic mental health conditions such as anxiety and personality, mood, and psychotic disorders (Hatton, Kleffel, Bennett, & Gaffrey, 2001; Magee & Huriaux, 2008; Sysko, 2002; Trickett & Chung, 2007).

It is inferred that substance abuse and/or mental health problems may exacerbate the misperceptions that women on each end of the perceived competency continuum experience. In severe cases, individuals may suffer from delusions of grandeur, which could significantly escalate problems related to high perceived competency. Conversely, delusional thinking could reduce a woman's already diminished sense of perceived competency and make it difficult for her to initiate positive changes (Acquaviva, 2000; Carroll & Trull, 1999, 2002; Gillette, 2001; Haydon, 2005; Marcus, 2001; Padgett et al., 2006; Trickett & Chung, 2007; Sysko, 2002; Williams, 2003; Woods-Brown, 2001).

Perceived Competency and Receptiveness to Assistance

Structure and Control Issues

The notion that many homeless women do not have well-developed adaptive skills that are needed to make long-term positive changes in their lives is supported by qualitative research findings (Carroll & Trull, 2002; Greene et al., 2003; Lineberger, 2009; Wheeler, 2006). In different ways, homeless women on each end of the perceived competency continuum appear to struggle with structure and control issues. Homeless women with low perceived competency tend to flounder and acquiesce when they are left to their own coping devices. They prefer to abdicate decision making to others, and they are apt to flourish within supportive environments that are highly controlling and structured (Hill, 1991; Lindsey, 1997). At times, they may unobtrusively adhere to unwarranted rules and regulations simply because they fear denial of services if they do not comply (Liebow, 1993; Luhrmann, 2008; Williams, 2003).

In contrast, the same structure and control that is comforting to women with low levels of perceived competency may be interpreted as oppressive to those on the opposite end of the competency continuum. Women with high levels of perceived competency tend to deeply resent structured and controlling environments. They dislike that activities such as eating, sleeping, and parenting are subject to focused scrutiny and regulation (Fogel, 1997; Flores, 2006; Geter, 1993; Gillette, 2001; Haydon, 2005; Marcus, 2001; Wheeler, 2006; Urbanoski, 2001). They are also highly critical of the fact that, due to restrictive rules and procedures, they are unable to make personal decisions (Connolly, 2000; Urbanoski, 2001; Wheeler, 2006). Consequently, women with elevated levels of perceived competency find it difficult to benefit from highly structured programs of assistance, and they are apt to leave prior to fully benefitting from the services that are available (Fogel, 1997; Patterson, 2003).

Trust Versus Mistrust

Due, at least in part, to a history of non-normative developmental experiences such as abuse and neglect, persistently homeless women appear to have difficulty making adaptive decisions and functioning with their own best interests in mind (Cook, 1995). One long-term repercussion includes difficulty forming adaptive interpersonal relationships with peers, significant others, and family members (Acquaviva, 2000; Carroll & Trull, 1999, 2002; Haydon, 2005; Lineberger, 2009; Marcus, 2001; Wheeler, 2006).

In an effort to protect themselves from additional victimization and trauma, homeless women may have difficulty forming adaptive interpersonal connections with beneficent social service personnel (Haydon, 2005). Homeless women do not always trust that the social service system works with their best interests in mind, and they do not necessarily take advantage of the help that is available to them (Sysko, 2002). For example, homeless women do not always believe that social service providers tell them the truth (Acquaviva, 2000; Connolly, 2000) or that the justice system will protect them (Brink, 2001). They may also fear that information they share with social service providers will be used against them when child custody decisions are at stake (Hatton, Kleffel, Bennett, & Gaffrey, 2001; Woods-Brown, 2001).

Due to a lack of trust, homeless women on each end of the perceived competency continuum may find it difficult to benefit from the services that are available (Sysko, 2002). Individuals with low perceived competency may not feel confident disclosing and asserting themselves, and they are likely to behave in servile and obsequious ways. These women may shape their needs to fit the services that are available rather than forthrightly seeking out assistance that is designed to specifically meet their needs (Liebow, 1993; Luhrmann, 2008; Williams, 2003). For instance, to meet their need for food and shelter, women with substance abuse problems have been known to feign domestic abuse in order to receive assistance at a facility that specializes in intimate partner violence. This type of behavior tends to obfuscate their real problems and hinders rehabilitation efforts (Geter, 1993; Gillette, 2001).

Alternatively, women with high levels of perceived competency who lack trust may be reluctant to enter or remain in the system unless a crisis occurs. Compassionate outreach efforts may be needed to recruit them into helping environments (Apfel, 2007; Gelberg et al., 2004), and once enrolled, they may be reluctant to disclose personal information (Liebow, 1993; Gillette, 2001; Marcus, 2001). To retain them in the system, considerable effort may be needed to establish and maintain trusting relationships.

Hopelessness

Creating a new life can be challenging, even under ideal circumstances. These challenges tend to be magnified when individuals are prone to distorted perceptions of competency, and the system they must work within is rife with imperfections. For instance, complex bureaucracy is a widespread problem that can make it difficult for women with relatively few interpersonal skills to benefit from the services that are available (Brink, 2001; Hatton, 2001; Marcus, 2001; Wheeler, 2006). It is these types of problems that may heighten frustration and lead to a sense of hopelessness among women with both low and high levels of perceived competency.

Given their proclivity to develop a sense of powerlessness and to assume an inactive stance (Acquaviva, 2000; Carroll & Trull, 2002; Lineberger, 2009; Williams, 2003), it is reasonable to infer that women with low levels of perceived competency may experience a sense of hopelessness. At first, they may attach this feeling strictly to themselves. Later, they may extend this same feeling to a system that they perceive to be inefficient and ineffective. Alternatively, women with high levels of perceived competency are thought to feel hopeless when they are forced to operate within a system that they view as overly restrictive and punitive (Fogel, 1997; Liebow, 1993; Marcus, 2001; Patterson, 2003; Williams, 2003). A key difference between these two groups of women is that in the case of the latter, their sense of hopelessness tends to transcend the personal and be projected onto the bureaucratic system. In effect, this defense mechanism may help women with high levels of perceived competency preserve their distorted perception of competency.

PROVISION OF SERVICES IN THE CONTEXT OF DISTORTED PERCEPTIONS OF COMPETENCY

Careful Assessment

For different reasons, women on each end of the perceived competency continuum may find it difficult to optimally benefit from social services. For this reason, careful assessment is recommended (Apfel, 2007; Bridgman, 2003; Flores, 2006; Lindsey, 1997; Magee & Huriaux, 2008; Urbanoski, 2001; Williams, 2003; Woods-Brown, 2001). Having a sense of each woman's position on the perceived competency continuum is anticipated to help social service providers create and implement the most effective and efficacious assistance possible.

Supplied with accurate assessment information, social service providers are better able to foresee how homeless women may present themselves, request assistance, and respond when assistance is offered. For instance, homeless women with high levels of perceived competency would be expected to present themselves as being more capable and less in need than those with low levels of perceived competency. In addition, substance abuse problems would be anticipated to further complicate attempts to resolve homelessness (Apfel, 2007; Bridgman, 2003; Flores, 2006; Lindsey, 1997; Magee & Huriaux, 2008; Urbanoski, 2001; Williams, 2003; Woods-Brown, 2001).

Caring

Based on the available evidence, it cannot be assumed that social service providers will routinely provide assistance in a caring manner. This is despite the fact that caring is perceived to be an important attribute of therapeutic assistance (Gillette, 2001; Gelberg et al., 2004; Liebow, 1993). In particular, homeless women comment on the therapeutic benefits of compassion, kindness, empathy, support, and respect. Patient, nonjudgmental communication and collaboration are valued, and the women emphasize how noncaring approaches obfuscate attempts to assist (Apfel, 2007; Gelberg et al., 2004; Gillette, 2001; Magee & Huriaux, 2008; Urbanoski, 2001; Wenzel, D'Amico, Barnes, & Gilbert, 2009). Caring is perceived to be particularly important given that many homeless women are survivors of various forms of interpersonal trauma. It is also inferred that caring may help to diminish treatment barriers related to trust.

Development of Interpersonal Trust

Regardless of their position on the perceived competency continuum, distrust of the social service system may result in treatment barriers. Distrust is thought to stem from previous experiences in which homeless women put their trust in individuals who ultimately disappointed or failed them (Acquaviva, 2000; Carroll & Trull, 1999, 2002; Haydon, 2005; Marcus, 2001). Homeless women may also lose trust in the social service system because they were stigmatized, shamed, or blatantly mistreated by helping professionals (Acquaviva, 2000; Brink, 2001; Connolly, 2000; Gillette, 2001).

In addition to building trust through caring, a holistic approach is recommended (D'Amico et al., 2009; Gelberg et al., 2004; Williams, 2003; Woods-Brown, 2001). This is not meant to imply that all services are needed or appropriate for every individual. On the contrary, each woman enters the system with her own unique needs and requires customized care and assistance (Apfel, 2007; Bridgman, 2003; Flores, 2006; Magee & Huriaux, 2008; Urbanoski, 2001; Williams, 2003; Woods-Brown, 2001). Assistance programs that are not well-tailored to individual needs are inferred to promote distrust and alienation because women may perceive that their problems are not being addressed or taken seriously.

Although homeless women build supportive relationships with social service personnel (Haydon, 2005), they cannot rely solely on these individuals for nurturance and support. For this reason, they may require assistance establishing trusting relationships with individuals outside of the helping professions. Prior to doing this, however, homeless women may need support to relinquish nonadaptive relationships (Sysko, 2002) that are characterized by interpersonal abuse and substance use (Greene et al., 2003; Schretzman, 1999; Sysko, 2002).

Care providers are encouraged to foster adaptive relationships among homeless women. Researchers indicate that homeless women can build healthy supportive relationships with other homeless women that cross race, ethnicity, and sexual orientation (Haydon, 2005; Gillette, 2001). Bonding occurs based on the fact that the women share similar backgrounds and challenges, and they do not judge each other (Urbanoski, 2001). These types of supportive relationships may be helpful in terms of maintaining abstinence from alcohol and drugs (Sysko, 2002), providing comfort, and enhancing financial stability (Acquaviva, 2000).

Personalized Structure and Control

In different ways, homeless women on each end of the perceived competency continuum struggle with structure and control issues. Women with low levels of perceived competency tend to thrive in more controlled and structured environments (Liebow, 1993; Luhrmann, 2008; Williams, 2003). Conversely, women with high levels of perceived competency are likely to resent these same types of milieus (Fogel, 1997; Geter, 1993; Gillette, 2001; Haydon, 2005; Marcus, 2001; Wheeler, 2006; Urbanoski, 2001). For these reasons, social service providers are encouraged to optimize assistance efforts by providing personalized structure and control (Apfel, 2007; Bridgman, 2003; Flores, 2006; Haydon, 2005; Magee & Huriaux, 2008; Urbanoski, 2001; Williams, 2003; Woods-Brown, 2001).

Most homeless women appear to understand the need for at least some structure and control in order to live safely and amicably among others. They may even express a sense of appreciation and relief when they know that beneficent staff are present to ensure that behavioral expectations are clear and rules are judiciously applied (Bridgman, 2003; Sysko, 2002). For these individuals, fully explaining the ground rules and offering clear rationale if objections are raised may be enough to create a therapeutic milieu (Apfel, 2007).

There may also be times when personalized structure and control means letting women know what type of help is available and allowing them to decide whether they will accept and actively use the services that are offered (Bridgman, 2003). This also means allowing the women to deal with the consequences of their decisions, despite the fact that they may be painful (Connolly, 2000). There are, of course, instances when this type of laissez-faire approach would not be appropriate, and priorities such as safety would take precedence.

Instillation of Hope

Homeless women on both ends of the perceived competency continuum may have difficulty formulating a realistic vision of what their lives could be like. As homeless individuals, they may not see their options as plentiful, and/or they may not see one option as being significantly better than another (Grella, 1994;

Montgomery, McCauley, & Bailey, 2009). When making choices, they may feel as if they face the classic dilemma of choosing the lesser of two or more evils (Lineberger, 2009). For these reasons, it is important for those who work with homeless women to instill the belief that they are worthy of a better life and to help them envision what their lives might realistically look like (Gillette, 2001; Haydon, 2005; Montgomery et al., 2009; Sysko, 2002). To avoid perpetual disappointment and lapses into hopelessness, care providers are urged to acknowledge challenges and help homeless women envision small incremental improvements rather than the ideal (Apfel, 2007; D'Amico et al., 2009; Haydon, 2005; Liebow, 1993; Magee & Huriaux, 2008; Schretzman, 1999; Sysko, 2002).

To instill and sustain hopefulness, providers are urged to help homeless women on both ends of the perceived competency continuum develop new skill sets. Armed with new skills, individuals in each group have the potential to use them to suit their unique needs. For instance, newly acquired communication skills have the potential to enable individuals with low and high levels of perceived competency to interact more assertively rather than passively or aggressively (Banyard, 1995; Hatton et al., 2001). Other skill sets that could be honed include the art of compromise, collaborative goal setting, and decision making (Apfel, 2007; Barkley, 1996; Connolly, 2000; D'Amico et al., 2009; Flores, 2006; Gentry, 2003; Haydon, 2005; Magee & Huriaux, 2008). Homeless women could also benefit from learning basic living skills such as how to apply for benefits, manage money, and get and maintain a job (Marcus, 2001; Wheeler, 2006; Williams, 2003). Each of these is action-oriented and has the potential to lead to immediate positive results and reinforcement, which may be desperately needed when individuals are experiencing hopelessness.

Another strategy that is recommended for dealing with hopelessness is spirituality. Spirituality is thought to provide homeless women with hope that their lives will improve and the supplemental nurturance that they need to see them through the process (Greene, Ball, Belcher, & McAlpine, 2003; Gillette, 2001; Sysko, 2002; Urbanoski, 2001). Spiritual sustenance is also associated with the intrapsychic and interpersonal support that they may require to overcome substance abuse problems (Greene et al., 2003).

Management of Substance Abuse and Mental Health Problems

It may be difficult for persistently homeless women to take steps in a positive direction given substance abuse and mental health problems (Banyard, 1995; Grella, 1994) that may exacerbate distorted perceptions of competency. The use of psychotherapeutic agents may be in order to treat some acute and chronic problems (Apfel, 2007). In addition, individual, substance abuse, and trauma-informed therapy are frequently recommended (Apfel, 2007; Kissman, 1999; Williams, 2003; Woods-Brown, 2001). Careful assessment is needed to know when and what type of counseling is most appropriate. For instance, counseling may be eagerly accepted in crisis situations, but individuals may be less receptive as presenting problems are resolved. This may be particularly true for individuals with high levels of perceived competency, and flexibility may be required to capture therapeutic opportunities and effectively meet the targeted needs of recipients (Urbanoski, 2001).

DISCUSSION

Perceived Competency and Related Concepts

Many factors contribute to persistent homelessness among women. They include substance abuse, economics, and mental illness (HRSDC, 2010; NCH, 2009). Results from this investigation also point to the role that long-term dysfunctional interpersonal relationships play in the emergence of distorted perceptions of competency and homelessness among women.

It has been suggested that differences such as comorbid mental health problems, culture and ethnicity, domestic abuse, motherhood, and even transgender issues should be accommodated to provide optimum care to homeless women (Apfel, 2007; Bridgman, 2003; Flores, 2006; Magee & Huriaux, 2008; Urbanoski, 2001; Williams, 2003; Woods-Brown, 2001). Although this may be true, evidence from this investigation supports the notion that perceived competency could potentially transcend these differences. As such, service providers are urged to carefully determine where homeless women lie on the perceived competency continuum and accommodate their care accordingly.

Self-Efficacy

Outside of grounded theory, which was used to guide the research methods, no other theoretical or conceptual frameworks were employed to carry out this investigation. To examine the findings further, a systematic comparison is recommended to evaluate the similarities and differences between concepts such as self-efficacy and perceived competency. A comprehensive comparison of these two concepts is beyond the scope of this report; however, a cursory review is offered.

Like perceived competency, self-efficacy is thought to exist on a continuum ranging from low to high, and individuals on the low end of the continuum are anticipated to require considerable assistance to make adaptive changes in their lives. Aside from this similarity, differences between the two concepts abound. Unlike perceived competency, it is proffered that the more self-efficacy that individuals possess the more likely it is that they will be able to make adaptive changes in their lives (Bandura, 2004). This is counter to findings from this investigation in which homeless women who lie in the middle of the perceived competency continuum are seen as better prepared to improve their living situations than those on the high end of the continuum.

It is noteworthy that the theorized correlation between high levels of self-efficacy and adaptive change among homeless women and women who have endured long-term abuse and trauma is not robust (Benight & Bandura, 2004; Epel, Bandura, & Zimbardo, 1999). For this reason, researchers are urged to further examine the value of concepts such as perceived competency to more fully explain the process of resolving homelessness among women.

Empowerment

Qualitative researchers do not begin research investigations devoid of information relating to their topic of interest. To manage this potential threat to trustworthiness, data analysis is conducted in a reflexive manner (Finlay, 2002). In the case of this investigation, it was tentatively hypothesized at the start that empowerment would emerge as an important strategy for helping homeless women with substance abuse problems become stably housed. In fact, empowerment was a working code well into the latter stages of data categorizing and memoing. As data analysis and synthesis progressed, however, it became clear that empowerment does not fully capture the complexity involved in such things as personalizing structure and control, making collaborative decisions, and instilling hope among women with vastly different levels of perceived competency.

Autonomy

A similar conclusion can be inferred about autonomy, a concept that was identified by O'Campo et al. (2009) in their systematic review of homeless adults with substance abuse problems. It is averred that undifferentiated promotion of autonomy among women with high levels of competency may exacerbate existing distortions. Conversely, women with low levels of perceived competency, who prefer structure, may find unbridled autonomy to be overwhelming. For these reasons, it is recommended that careful assessment and tailored promotion of autonomy be instituted to meet the unique needs of each woman.

Limitations

All meta-syntheses involve inherent limitations. Among the most serious is the researcher's distance from the original research participants. This limitation was minimized by conducting expansive sampling and carrying out careful and comprehensive data extraction. This potential limitation was also minimized by staying close to the data and using in vivo codes and transparent metaphors throughout the data analysis and synthesis processes.

In keeping with O'Campo et al. (2009) results from a qualitative synthesis related to homeless adults, clear guidelines for improving substance abuse outcomes could not be inferred from the data that were available for this investigation. In the case of this study, it has already been noted that data related to specific substance abuse treatment strategies were inconsistently reported across studies. In addition, although researchers were interested in substance abuse problems, immediate needs such as housing seemed to take precedence followed closely by a keen interest in the women's overall well-being rather than merely her status as a substance abuser. The latter most likely relates to the complexities involved in becoming and being homeless and resolving homelessness versus the more limited role that substance abuse may play as a coping mechanism (Burlingham et al., 2010).

SUMMARY

Framing care for persistently homeless women within the context of perceived competency offers a new way of understanding the plight of these women and shaping interventions to assist them to establish healthier and more stable lives. Social service providers are encouraged to carefully assess homeless women's receptiveness to assistance based on their level of perceived competency and to intervene accordingly. Suggested therapeutic strategies include development of trust, personalized structure and control, instillation of hope, and careful management of mental health problems that may exacerbate distorted perceptions of competency.

Based on the results of this investigation, social service providers are asked to reconsider blanket admonitions to enhance self-efficacy and promote empowerment and autonomy among homeless women with substance abuse problems. In addition, research is recommended to explore the similarities and differences between perceived competency and self-efficacy. Researchers are also urged to carefully examine the effectiveness of personalized structure and control versus undifferentiated efforts to promote empowerment and autonomy when working with homeless women who are on the margins of the perceived competency continuum.

FUNDING

The authors disclosed receipt of the following financial support for the research and/or authorship of this article: The project described was supported by Grant Number R21DA024749 from the National Institute on Drug Abuse. The content is solely the responsibility of the authors and does not necessarily represent the official views of the National Institutes of Health.

REFERENCES

Acquaviva, K. D. (2000). *A qualitative study of the sexuality of women living in a homeless shelter* (Unpublished doctoral dissertation). University of Pennsylvania, Philadelphia, PA.

Apfel, J. (2007). *Creating surviving the streets: A trauma-informed treatment guide for homeless women* (Unpublished doctoral dissertation). Alliant International University, San Francisco, CA.

Australian Bureau of Statistics. (2008). *Homelessness in Australia.* Retrieved from http://goo .gl/bbNEqz

Bandura, A. (2004). Health promotion by social cognitive means. *Health Education & Behavior, 31,* 143–164.

Banyard, V. L. (1995). "Taking another route": Daily survival narratives from mothers who are homeless. *American Journal of Community Psychology, 23,* 871–891.

Barkley, K. M. (1996). *Social change and social service: A case study of a feminist battered women's shelter* (Unpublished doctoral dissertation). Eugene, OR: University of Oregon.

Belcher, J. R., Greene, J. A., McAlpine, C., & Ball, K. (2001). Considering pathways into homelessness: Mothers, addictions, and trauma. *Journal of Addictions Nursing, 13,* 199–208.

Benight, C. C., & Bandura, A. (2004). Social cognitive theory of post-traumatic recovery: The role of perceived self-efficacy. *Behaviour Research and Therapy, 42,* 1129–1148.

Bourgois, P., Prince, B., & Moss, A. (2004). The everyday violence of hepatitis C among young women who inject drugs in San Francisco. *Human Organization, 63,* 253–264.

Bridgman, R. (2003). *Safe haven: The story of a shelter for homeless women.* Toronto, ON, Canada: University of Toronto.

Brink, L. A. (2001). *"My guardian angel is working overtime:" The health issues and life stories of six homeless women* (Unpublished master's thesis). Gonzaga University, Spokane, WA.

Burlingham, B., Andrasik, M. P., Larimer, M., Marlatt, G. A., & Spigner, C. (2010). A house is not a home: A qualitative assessment of the life experiences of alcoholic homeless women. *Journal of Social Work Practice in the Addictions, 10,* 158–179.

Carroll, J. J., & Trull, L. A. (1999). Homeless African American women's interpretations of child abuse as an antecedent of chemical dependence. *Early Child Development and Care, 155,* 1–16.

Carroll, J. J., & Trull, L. A. (2002). Drug-dependent homeless African-American women's perspectives of life on the streets. *Journal of Ethnicity in Substance Abuse, 1,* 27–45.

Centre for Reviews and Dissemination. (2009). *Systematic reviews: CRD's guidance for undertaking reviews in health care.* Retrieved May 4, 2011, from http://www.york.ac.uk/inst/crd/pdf/ Systematic_Reviews.pdf

Connolly, D. R. (2000). *Homeless mothers: Face to face with women and poverty.* Minneapolis, MN: University of Minnesota.

Cook, M. A. (1995). Substance-abusing homeless mothers in treatment programs: A question of knowing. *Contemporary Drug Problems, 22,* 291–316.

Corbin, J., & Strauss, A. (2008). *Basics of qualitative research: Techniques and procedures for developing grounded theory.* Los Angeles, CA: Sage.

D'Amico, E. J., Barnes, D., Gilbert, M. L., Ryan, G., & Wenzel, S. L. (2009). Developing a tripartite prevention program for impoverished young women transitioning to young adulthood: Addressing substance use, HIV risk, and victimization by intimate partners. *Journal of Prevention & Intervention in the Community, 37,* 112–128.

Enriquez, M. P. (2005). *Health care accessibility for homeless women in Long Beach, California* (Unpublished master's thesis). California State University, Long Beach, CA.

Epel, E. S., Bandura, A., & Zimbardo, P. G. (1999). Escaping homelessness: The influences of self-efficacy and time perspective on coping with homelessness. *Journal of Applied Social Psychology, 29,* 575–596.

Finfgeld, D. L. (2003). Metasynthesis: The state of the art—So far. *Qualitative Health Research, 13*(7), 893–904.

Finfgeld-Connett, D. (2009a). Model of therapeutic and non-therapeutic responses to patient aggression. *Issues in Mental Health Nursing, 30,* 530–537.

Finfgeld-Connett, D. (2009b). Management of aggression among demented or brain-injured patients: A process of entering the patient's world. *Clinical Nursing Research, 18,* 272–287.

Finfgeld-Connett, D. (2010a). Becoming homeless, being homeless, and resolving homelessness among women. *Issues in Mental Health Nursing, 31,* 461–469.

Finfgeld-Connett, D. (2010b). Generalizability and transferability of meta-synthesis research findings. *Journal of Advanced Nursing, 66,* 246–254.

Finfgeld-Connett, D., Bloom, T. L., & Johnson, E. D. (2012). Perceived competency and resolution of homelessness among women with substance abuse problems. *Qualitative Health Research, 22,* 416–427. doi:10.1177/1049732311421493

Finlay, L. (2002). "Outing" the researcher: The provenance, process, and practice of reflexivity. *Qualitative Health Research, 12,* 531–545. doi:10.1177/104973202129120052

Flores, C. (2006). *Domestic violence shelters: Changes and challenges* (Unpublished master's thesis). Southern Illinois University, Carbondale, IL.

Fogel, S. J. (1997). Moving along: An exploratory study of homeless women with children using a transitional housing program. *Journal of Sociology and Social Welfare, 24,* 113–133.

Gelberg, L., Browner, C. H., Lejano, E., & Arangua, L. (2004). Access to women's health care: A qualitative study of barriers perceived by homeless women. *Women & Health, 40,* 87–100.

Gentry, Q. M. (2003). *Risk in the rough: An ethnographic inquiry of how poor African-American women who smoke crack reduce their risks for HIV-infection* (Unpublished doctoral dissertation). Georgia State University, Atlanta, GA.

Geter, R. S. (1993). *Crack prostitution in Philadelphia: A career model* (Unpublished doctoral dissertation). University of Pennsylvania, Philadelphia, PA.

Gillette, S. C. (2001). *"Listen to their conversation very carefully:" Homeless women talk about their health and AIDS prevention* (Unpublished doctoral dissertation). University of Washington, Seattle, WA.

Greene, J. A., Ball, K., Belcher, J. R., & McAlpine, C. (2003). Substance abuse, homelessness, developmental decision-making and spirituality: A women's health issue. *Journal of Social Work Practice in the Addictions, 3,* 39–56.

Grella, C. (1994). Contrasting a shelter and day center for homeless mentally ill women: Four patterns of service use. *Community Mental Health Journal, 30,* 3–16.

Hatton, D. C. (2001). Homeless women's access to health services: A study of social networks and managed care in the US. *Women & Health, 33,* 167–181.

Hatton, D. C., Kleffel, D., Bennett, S., & Gaffrey, E. A. N. (2001). Homeless women and children's access to health care: A paradox. *Journal of Community Health Nursing, 18,* 25–34.

Haydon, E. (2005). *Homemaking/making home: The domestic lives of women living in poverty and using illicit drugs* (Unpublished master's thesis). University of Toronto, Toronto.

Hill, R. P. (1991). Homeless women, special possessions, and the meaning of "home:" An ethnographic case study. *Journal of Consumer Research, 18,* 298–310.

Huey, L., & Quirouette, M. (2010). "Any girl can call the cops, no problem": The influence of gender on support for the decision to report criminal victimization within homeless communities. *British Journal of Criminology, 50,* 278–295.

Human Resources and Skills Development Canada. (2010). *The homeless partnering strategy.* Retrieved September 2, 2010, from http://goo.gl/94Nk5x

Intraspec.ca. (2010). *Homeless in Canada.* Retrieved September 18, 2010, from http://goo.gl/Y9wA5e

Kissman, K. (1999). Time out from stress: Camp program and parenting groups for homeless mothers. *Contemporary Family Therapy, 21,* 373–384.

Liebow, E. (1993). *Tell them who I am: The lives of homeless women.* New York, NY: Free Press.

Lincoln, Y. S., & Guba, E. G. (1985). *Naturalistic inquiry.* Newbury Park, CA: Sage.

Lindsey, E. W. (1997). The process of restabilization for mother-headed homeless families: How social workers can help. *Journal of Family Social Work, 2,* 49–72.

Lineberger, K. A. (2009). *Unfortunate choices: "Risk in the lives of street-level sex workers and non-sex working streetwise women* (Unpublished doctoral dissertation). University of Colorado, Denver, CO.

Luhrmann, T. M. (2008). "The street will drive you crazy": Why homeless psychotic women in the institutional circuit in the United States often say no to offers of help. *American Journal of Psychiatry, 165,* 15–20.

Magee, C., & Huriaux, E. (2008). Ladies' night: Evaluating a drop-in programme for homeless marginally housed women in San Francisco's mission district. *International Journal of Drug Policy, 19,* 113–121.

Marcus, W. S. (2001). *Tracing bitter roots of personal violation and social displacement: A comparative phenomenological study of the life histories of homeless mothers and their dependent children* (Unpublished doctoral dissertation). State University of New York, Buffalo, NY.

Miles, M. B., & Huberman, A. M. (1994). *Qualitative data analysis* (2nd ed.). Thousand Oaks, CA: Sage.

Montgomery, P., McCauley, K., & Bailey, P. H. (2009). Homelessness, a state of mind? A discourse analysis. *Issues in Mental Health Nursing, 30,* 624–630.

National Coalition for the Homeless. (2009). *Why are people homeless?* Retrieved from http://www.nationalhomeless.org/factsheets/why.html

Noblit, G. W., & Hare, R. (1988). *Meta-ethnography: Systematizing qualitative studies.* Newbury Park, CA: Sage.

O'Campo, P., Kirst, M., Schaefer-McDaniel, N., Firestone, M., Scott, A., & McShane. (2009). Community-based services for homeless adults experiencing concurrent mental health and substance use disorders: A realist approach to synthesizing evidence. *Journal of Urban Health: Bulletin of the New York Academy of Medicine, 86,* 965–989.

Padgett, D. K., Hawkins, R. L., Abrams, C., & Davis, A. (2006). In their own words: Trauma and substance abuse in the lives of formerly homeless women with serious mental illness. *Psychological Assessment, 76,* 461–467.

Patterson, W. A. (2003). *Substance abuse treatment profiling: A case study of the St. Jude Women's Recovery Center* (Unpublished doctoral dissertation). University of Louisville, Louisville, KY.

Pawson, R. (2006). Digging for nuggets: How "bad" research can yield "good" evidence. *International Journal of Social Research Methodology, 9,* 127–142. doi:10.1080/13645570600595314

Schretzman, M. K. (1999). *Voices of successful women: Graduates of a residential treatment program for homeless addicted women with their children* (Unpublished doctoral dissertation). The City University of New York, New York, NY.

Strauss, A., & Corbin, J. (1990). *Basics of qualitative research: Grounded theory procedures and techniques.* Newbury Park, CA: Sage.

Substance Abuse and Mental Health Services Administration. (2004). Characteristics of homeless female admissions to substance abuse treatment: 2002. *The DASIS Report.* Retrieved from http://media.samhsa.gov/data/2k4/FemHomeless/FemHomeless.pdf

Substance Abuse and Mental Health Services Administration. (2011). *Current statistics on the prevalence and characteristics of people experiencing homelessness in the United States. Department of Health and Human Services.* Retrieved from http://www.samhsa.gov/sites/default/files/programs_campaigns/homelessness_programs_resources/hrc-factsheet-current-statistics-prevalence-characteristics-homelessness.pdf

Sysko, H. B. (2002). *A study of homeless mothers in transition from shelter to stable housing* (Unpublished doctoral dissertation). University of Pittsburgh, Pittsburgh, PA.

Thorne, S., Jensen, L., Kearney, M. H., Noblit, G., & Sandelowski, M. (2004). Qualitative metasynthesis: Reflections on methodological orientation and ideological agenda. *Qualitative Health Research, 14*(10), 1342–1365.

Torchalla, I., Strehlau, V., Li, K., & Krausz, M. (2011). Substance use and predictors of substance dependence in homeless women. *Drug and Alcohol Dependence, 118*(2–3), 173–179. doi:10.1016/j.drugalcdep.2011.03.016

Trickett, E. M., & Chung, D. (2007). Brickbats and bouquets: Health services, community and police attitudes and the homeless experiences of women 45 years and over living in rural South Australia. *Rural Social Work and Community Practice, 12,* 5–15.

Urbanoski, K. H. (2001). *Counselling in shelters for Aboriginal women* (Unpublished master's thesis). University of Calgary, Calgary, Canada.

Wenzel, S. L., D'Amico, E. J., Barnes, D., & Gilbert, M. L. (2009). A pilot of a tripartite prevention program for homeless young women in the transition to adulthood. *Women's Health Issues, 19,* 193–201.

Wheeler, C. A. (2006). *The needs and challenges of homeless families with children as perceived by homeless-service agencies* (Unpublished doctoral dissertation). Indiana University, Indianapolis, IN.

Williams, J. C. (2003). *"A roof over my head:" Homeless women and the shelter industry.* Boulder, CO: University Press of Colorado.

Woods-Brown, L. Y. (2001). *Ethnographic study of homeless mentally ill persons: Single adult homeless and homeless families* (Unpublished doctoral dissertation). University of South Florida, Tampa, FL.

DEVELOPING THEORY
USING META-ANALYSIS

> *"I am paying for this microphone!"*
> —Ronald Regan (when the moderator threated
> to cut off his mike at a debate he paid for)

Brainstorming: Sorting Out Meta-Analysis

Morse: *But studies overlap in different ways. They overlap
            because they are about the same phenomenon or the
            same concept, or they overlap because they are
            about the same disease entity, or they overlap
            because they are about something else. And you
            have to make your decision about what it is you are
            collecting studies on. And people go around collect-
            ing studies about illness. Now when Joy [Johnson]
            and I put together all of those studies on illness, we
            were criticized because people said that Norris's
            study was about abortion, and "abortion wasn't ill-
            ness." This is ridiculous. And when I told Judy
            [Norris], she said, "My study wasn't about abor-
            tion; it wasn't about illness— it was about soul
            ache."*
            *So what our theory is about is human responses to a
            threat to the self, or whatever. And if you look at it
            that way, then Judy's study fits perfectly. If we*

create these artificial boundaries and don't let these studies, as Glaser says, "earn their way into data," then you get into a whole lot of trouble, and you have a tremendous threat to validity—if you want to use that bad V word.
So that's why I think you have to start with the most abstract concept and work down.

May: *That's a nice bit of intellectual footwork! But 99% of folks, who attempt to do that, can't do that. Even in my field if you took all the quantitative work on at-risk childbearing—there are not very many, but you could pile them up on the table. But then to push through and find out what the study really was about. And to think: this one is about "techno- logical management of conditions." And this one is about "suffering and anticipatory grief." Do you see it's a level problem? You've got apples and Tues- days. And the source data don't necessarily tell you [what it's about]. Jan [Morse] had to get inside those studies and then say, "But what did they really do?"*

Morse: *But it is false for us to go and collect studies on heart attacks and strokes.*

Sandelowski: *But it's the way you start. In order to get to the point where you are—that's something that's invented by the analysis. And in order to get there, you have to go through this process. A naturally occurring way to start is, "Gee, I am interested in people's responses to heart attack," and then to say the essence of this thing is not the heart attack, per se. The main part of the analytic work is getting there—you don't get there first.*

Morse: *You are totally right. But I don't know if you have to do the coding, or if you have to be theory- smart—the problem is, if you start off with the data, you get bogged down. You get into not seeing the forest for the trees thing—you can't get there. To do a meta-analysis, you have to decide on your goal before you start. So you are doing this ana- lytic stuff and working almost deductively, orga- nizing your theory.*

—Wuest and Merritt-Gray (1997)

META-ANALYSIS

Throughout this book we have discussed various ways to develop solid, clear, and appropriate concepts. In this chapter we will discuss how to create a mid-range theory from multiple interrelated studies that resulted in lower level theories. *Qualitative meta-analysis* has a different purpose, and therefore a different outcome, than qualitative meta-synthesis techniques. Recall that meta-synthesis "smoothes" categories across attributes, looking for commonalities, for the "most similar," for common agreement, to make the original concepts or theory stronger. When doing meta-synthesis, researchers use studies that address a similar area or processes, and the final labels used in the theory may or may not be the same as (or similar to) those used in the original study. It makes for a stronger theory about a certain topic.

On the other hand, qualitative meta-analysis is a technique that develops a higher level theory from a cluster of studies from different contexts and different populations, but studies that address the same concept and the same phenomenon. Rather than meta-synthesis that produces a concept about the same topic, meta-analysis produces a *higher level concept*. For instance, in Chapter 33 we use grounded theories that address all sorts of illness problems to develop a meta-analysis of the experience of illness.

Qualitative meta-analysis uses data and analyzes the internal structures of mid-range theories to create new, higher level, formal theory (Estabrooks, Field, & Morse, 1994; Schreiber, Crooks, & Stern, 1997). This formal theory is different and more insightful than the studies from which it has been derived; it is at a higher level of abstraction, and the study represents the domain of the higher level concept. By conducting a meta-analysis, the researchers are working with a different level of data and manipulating it differently, than when using the meta-synthesis. Researchers are working with the concepts and theories developed from other studies.

For instance, in this example, grounded theory studies that have developed theory about women adjusting to heart attacks, having a hysterectomy, discharge from a psychiatric hospital, mothers involved in their daughters' abortions, and husbands' experiences during their wives' chemotherapy are used to create a higher level theory of illness. The theory of illness is much broader in scope than any of the single theories from which it is composed, and most importantly, is applicable to conditions that were not included in the original study—and to the experience of people who are yet to experience illness. It is a way to make the resulting theory more generalizable, more useful. If done well, the theory should be applicable to future instances of the phenomenon. That is, the theory developed in Chapter 33 should be also applicable to cases or illnesses that are not included in the original analysis. The level of abstraction is not particular to any specific illness.

In the literature there is some crossover with the terms "meta-synthesis" and "meta-ethnography" (Sandelowski, 2003). Therefore meta-analysis may be found as meta-ethnography (Noblit & Hare, 1988) or qualitative meta-data-analysis (Paterson, Thorne, Canam, & Jillings, 2001). Note that this process of meta-analysis and the outcomes are quite different from meta-synthesis.

DOING META-ANALYSIS

Data for meta-analysis are derived from a number of studies that address the same concept, but in different topics. Does that make sense?

To Select Your Studies

Supposing you are interested in a concept, such as posttraumatic stress disorder (PTSD); you may identify studies describing returned soldiers, people who have had serious accidents, or even women who experienced difficult childbirth. All of these studies do not have a context in common; they do not have a population in common, but they address the same concept. And as with meta-synthesis, your task will be easier if they all use the same methods that will produce the same theoretical form. In the Chapter 33, the studies are all about various aspects of different health crises, using Glaserian grounded theory (Glaser, 1978).

What is meant by "theoretical form?" Theory developed from ethnography does not have the same theoretical form as grounded theory. Ethnographic theory is usually explanatory; it may contain one or many concepts that are linked. But this theory does not usually describe a process. In grounded theory there are usually stages and transitions, and a core variable, so that when you place the theories on a large chart and "open the concepts" there is usually a structure that makes the theories comparable.

The goal of phenomenology or of narrative inquiry may not be to produce theory, or even a "theoretical scheme," and the themes developed in each study may not be comparable. Is it easy to do a meta-analysis with perhaps a group of studies that have each used a different method? No. I don't think so. When studies have used different methods, the results are usually at a different level of abstraction and *link,* rather than when developed theoretically by integration. Therefore, in such a case, I would keep each study intact and consider using *theoretical coalescence* (as described in Chapter 34).

Meta-Analysis Method

Read the studies carefully and "open" the studies, copying the concepts and the attributes onto a large chart. Kept each study confined to one row across the page, so that it is easy to compare columns when you are seeking common processes between theories.

How to Think: How to Synthesize When Doing Meta-Analysis

First, combining the studies may appear an impossible jumbled mess, because authors will not have used common labels, or even followed an apparent common path. Now think about each stage in the process in the studies. *Think above the data*; this means generally looking for commonalities more abstractly than it is presently described. *Float above the data.* You may have to merge categories or separate categories; merge processes or split cells in some cases. Your thinking should also use your theoretical knowledge of theories already developed. Ask yourself: What is new here? Unique here? What is similar? Are there concepts that will encompass two or more of the described processes? Think until your head aches. Then think some more.

By thinking generally at first, think beyond the particular. In doing so, you are moving beyond the individual categories. Keep thinking about what each central theme *implies.* Think how you can smooth out these categories. Then build the concepts, recreating a new theoretical scheme. Having the raw data available is a plus, for you may be able to go back to the original interviews to seek, confirm, or to check out new ideas. But remember if you are using the raw data, you will need institutional review board (IRB) approval.

DEVELOPING THE ILLNESS-CONSTELLATION MODEL

In the *Illness-Constellation Model* (Morse & Johnson, 1991; Chapter 33), we report on the perspective of the ill person as well as the perspectives of significant others. Do the experiences of the significant other follow, or otherwise resemble, those of the patient. Do they lag or are they ahead of the patient? (For instance, is the family given information that the patient does not know, or vice versa?) How does this work, when the family member is less mature (as in Norris's study of the mothers whose daughters were having an abortion), or in cases when for instance the elderly family member is cognitively confused?

The next step is to prepare the new, more abstract encompassing theory. As with meta- synthesis, take care to provide appropriate credit to the original authors' work.

The new theory will have a greater level of abstraction, greater scope, and be more generalizable that the original theories. It will have new labels, and it will be applicable to other illnesses not included in the first set of theories. It will be able to predict outcomes for patients and their families.

Introducing the Illness-Constellation Model

Although published in 1991, the *Illness-Constellation Model* (Morse & Johnson, 1991) is still relevant to the illness process. In addition to its clinical application, the model has formed the basis of the curricula in undergraduate nursing programs in the Netherlands and is still used as the physical therapy curriculum in the United States.

This meta-analysis is developed from five grounded theories, all of which used Glaserian grounded theory.

Learning to Live Again: The Process of Adjustment Following A Heart Attack
(Johnson, 1990; Johnson & Morse, 1991)

Feeling unwell? At what point do you consider yourself sick? And when you are sick, at what point do you call the ambulance? The process of waiting to see if the symptoms dissipate, the testing to find out what makes the symptoms worse or better can continue for several days. To admit that one requires help is to admit that the symptoms are beyond one's control. The signs and symptoms of a heart attack often begin insidiously and escalate over a period of hours. Heart attacks have a paradoxical nature. Although potentially fatal, the early signs of a heart attack mimic minor complaints. Unless the heart attack is extensive, the early symptoms may be interpreted as indigestion, the flu, a pulled muscle, or food poisoning. For example, in the following study, one participant delayed seeking medical attention for 3 days.

The irony of delaying treatment is caused in part by the mixed messages given to the public. On one hand, the signs and symptoms of a heart attack are well publicized because it is assumed that people who recognize the combination of symptoms will seek help early. On the other hand, people are reluctant to go to hospital emergency rooms or "bother" their physicians with seemingly minor complaints. Media accounts of the health care system often give the impression that there is a major concern with an overutilization of health care facilities and with the cost of nonurgent consultations. Furthermore, health care professionals are frequently annoyed by nonurgent consultations and become condescending toward patients with "minor" complaints. In turn, these attitudes manage to embarrass patients and ensure that they learn not to "misuse" emergency services.

The process of assessing the severity and meaning of symptoms and somatic experiences continues for patients through the acute and rehabilitative phases. It is almost as if they are constantly holding their breath, hoping that each twinge is not another heart attack. This process is not only internal, but it also includes carefully monitoring the response of others, especially the responses of health care professionals. Spoken or unspoken, implicit or explicit indications of their progress are used by heart attack patients to gauge their recovery. Seemingly minor signs of progress, such as looks of relief from health care professionals, and successfully achieving milestones, such as walking a flight of stairs, provide concrete evidence of progress for heart attack patients. But is this enough? Unfortunately it is not enough because the mixed messages continue: "You are well enough to do without a cardiac monitor, but it must be attached when you exercise." "You are recovering well, but keep taking your medication." Heart attack victims' lives are plagued by uncertainties. They must continue to test their abilities until they once again trust their bodies.

The Experience of Women Having a Hysterectomy
(Marie Andreé Chassé, 1991)

One of the strengths of using qualitative methods is that these methods allow the researcher to consider the context of the phenomenon as well as the phenomenon itself. Respecting the context of a phenomenon involves allowing the informants to tell the stories and share the experiences that they believe are relevant. Although Chassé was initially interested in the process of recovery following a hysterectomy, she soon discovered that her informants could not simply discuss their recoveries; rather, they had to discuss all of the events surrounding the hysterectomy beginning with the exacerbation of symptoms and their first hunches that something was wrong. The informants could not separate their recoveries from the initial stages of the hysterectomy decision-making process because part of the recovery process involved resolving the issue of whether they had made the right decision when they consented for surgery. Chassé was sensitive to this fact and incorporated the rich data regarding pre-surgery decision making into her analysis.

Becoming Ordinary: Leaving a Psychiatric Hospital
(Beverley Lorencz, 1991)

A significant problem in qualitative research is trying to understand the patient's perspective when the patient is unable to speak or to express himself or herself. If the patient is unable to speak (as in the case of preverbal infants or aphasic adults) the researcher is forced to use observational techniques such as participant observation or ethology. Both of these techniques involve a certain amount of researcher inference when the research question pertains to patient feelings. If the patient is able to speak but is confused, glimpses of the patient's reality may be obtained through interviews if the researcher has extraordinary skill and patience, especially when the researcher is competing with the multiple voices and realities with which the delusional patient must contend. The value of this latter approach is evident in this chapter.

Lorencz's thesis committee recognized the problems associated with using a verbal technique with patients who may not be able to express themselves, and she was strongly recommended not to undertake her study on the experiences of adults with schizophrenia who are about to be discharged. Despite this recommendation, she continued with this onerous study to the amazement and awe of her thesis committee members. One of the most crucial qualities of an excellent researcher (along with creativity, sensitivity, and wisdom) is perseverance. Perseverance is the most essential quality of a researcher in that it ensures completion of a difficult project and enables the researcher to prove that certain data are obtainable despite overwhelming odds. When conducting the interviews for this study Lorencz often waited for more than a minute for responses to her questions. When the responses came they often were responses to another voice—an internal voice—and as a result the interview often seemed nonsensical, slow, and convoluted. Throughout data collection these apparently irrelevant glimpses into the experiences of these patients were interpreted not as nonsensical delusions, but as the informant's own reality. As a result a creative and powerful grounded theory emerged from this study.

Mothers' Involvement in Their Adolescent Daughters' Abortions (*Norris, 1991*)

In the case of this study, Norris observed mothers waiting for their daughters' return from the operating room where they had gone for a therapeutic abortion. The lack of support for these women, either from professionals or from friends and/or family members, was striking because the mothers seemed to be more distressed than their daughters. Wondering about how she could best help these women Norris searched for material in the library and to her amazement found very little. It is these gaps in the literature that indicate the dire need for qualitative research.

The timing of in-depth, interactive interviews raises many ethical questions. In this study, Norris did not consider her role to be that of a counselor and she felt she should not be involved in the abortion decision-making process; therefore, her first contact with the mothers was after the procedure had commenced and her interviews were conducted by telephone 1 week later. During the interviews, however, she found it was easy to obtain retrospective accounts of the decision-making process as the mothers needed to tell their stories at the beginning.

Although it was not Norris's intention, the process of telling the story was therapeutic for these women. Mothers began their stories tentatively but as they relaxed the words poured forth rapidly. As accounts progressed the informants seemed to experience a release of pent-up emotions. All interviews seemed to end on a light note, for example, with humorous banter about "why mothers of adolescent daughters go grey." Once or twice, when

Norris attempted a second interview, she discovered that the mothers were not interested in talking about their experiences a second time. It was as if there had been a grand catharsis in the first interview, and having told the story the informants considered the issue closed. Many of these women had not had the opportunity to tell their stories to a compassionate listener. Some husbands, if told about the abortion, were not a source of support because they considered abortion to be a woman's matter for their wife "to take care of" and mothers were often reluctant to confide in their relatives and friends. For these reasons telephone counseling services would provide women with the opportunity to talk out the abortion experiences anonymously with a neutral listener.

The Unrelenting Nightmare: Husbands' Experiences During Their Wives' Chemotherapy
(Sharon Wilson, 1991; Wilson & Morse, 1991)

One of the greatest changes to have occurred in the past 30 years in health care is the recognition of patient rights and the rights of the relatives involved in the patient's experience. Whereas in obstetrics the husband has been incorporated into the childbirth experience, in oncology the spouse is paradoxically included and excluded. At one time the spouse was the only person given information regarding the diagnosis, and he or she was urged to keep this information from the patient. More recently, although some information is still kept "behind the scenes" and only given to the spouse, physicians have become more open with patients. Although the spouse's role in supporting the patient is now acknowledged, often the spouse is still made to feel like "the third wheel" in the treatment setting; even so, spouses often suffer during the patients' illness experience. The value of this study is the exploration and explication of the experience of the person closest to a patient undergoing chemotherapy.

One of the hazards of repeated, in-depth, interactive interviews is that the researcher may also become embedded in the informant's nightmare. How does the researcher listen to such suffering and remain detached? How does the researcher "get inside the mind" of the informant and remain unscathed?

REFERENCES

Chassé, M. A. (1991). The experience of women having a hysterectomy. In J. Morse & J. Johnson (Eds.), *The illness experience: Dimensions of suffering* (pp. 89–139). Newbury Park, CA: Sage.

Estabrooks, C. A., Field, P. A., & Morse, J. M. (1994). Aggregating qualitative studies: An approach to theory development. *Qualitative Health Research, 4,* 503–511.

Glaser, B. G. (1978). *Theoretical sensitivity.* Mill Creek, CA: Sociology Press.

Johnson, J. (1991). Learning to live again: The process of adjustment following a heart attack. In J. M. Morse & J. L. Johnson (Eds.), *The illness experience: Dimensions of suffering*. Newbury Park, CA: Sage.

Johnson, J. J., & Morse J. M. (1991). Preserving the self: Women having cardiac surgery. *Heart & Lung: The Journal of Critical Care, 23*(2), 99–105.

Lorencz, B. (1991). Becoming ordinary: Leaving a psychiatric hospital. In J. Morse & J. Johnson (Eds.), *The illness experience: Dimensions of suffering* (pp. 140–200). Newbury Park, CA: Sage. Retrieved from http://content.lib.utah.edu/u?/ir-main

Morse, J. M., & Johnson, J. (1991). *The illness experience: Dimensions of suffering*. Newbury Park, CA: Sage Publications.

Noblit, G. W., & Hare, R. (1988). *Meta-ethnography: Systematizing qualitative studies*. Newbury Park, CA: Sage.

Norris, J. (1991). Mothers' involvement in their adolescent daughters abortions. In J. Morse & J. Johnson (Eds.), *The illness experience: Dimensions of suffering* (pp. 201–236). Newbury Park, CA: Sage.

Paterson, B. L., Thorne, S. E., Canam, C., & Jillings, C. (2001). *Meta-study of qualitative health research: A practical guide to meta-analysis and meta-synthesis* (Methods in Nursing Research, Vol. 3). Thousand Oaks, CA: Sage.

Sandelowski, M. (2003). Qualitative meta-analysis. In M. Lewis-Beck, A. Bryman, & T. Liao (Eds.), *The Sage encyclopedia of social science research methods* (pp. 893–894). Thousand Oaks, CA: Sage.

Schreiber, R., Crooks, D., & Stern, P. N. (1997). Qualitative meta-analysis. In J. Morse (Ed.), *Completing a qualitative project: Details and dialogue* (pp. 311–326). Thousand Oaks, CA: Sage.

Wilson, S. (1991). The unrelenting nightmare: Husbands' experiences during their wives' chemotherapy. In J. Morse & J. Johnson (Eds.), *The illness experience: Dimensions of suffering* (pp. 237–313). Newbury Park, CA: Sage.

Wilson, S., & Morse, J. M. (1991). Living with a wife undergoing chemotherapy: Perceptions of the husband. *Image: Journal of Nursing Scholarship, 23*(2), 78–84.

Wuest, J., & Merritt-Gray, M. (1997). Participatory action research: Practical dilemmas and emancipatory possibilities. In J. Morse (Ed.), *Completing a qualitative project: Details and dialogue* (pp. 283–309). Thousand Oaks, CA: Sage.

TOWARD A THEORY OF ILLNESS: THE ILLNESS-CONSTELLATION MODEL[1]

> *Get the habit of analysis—analysis will in time enable*
> *synthesis to become your habit of mind.*
> —Frank Lloyd Wright

Wellness is a state of optimal comfort that is disrupted by the occurrence of an illness episode. Although illness physiologically generally affects *one* individual, the experience of illness can affect and involve the entire family and other significant people in the experience of suffering, pain, and threats to life. Consequently, illness may be viewed as a distressing and disruptive period during which the minimization of suffering and the attainment of comfort become paramount. Because the ramifications of illness extend suffering beyond the individual to the family and others, *attaining comfort* takes the form of any number of strategies used by the ill individual, by those who are close to the ill individual and who share the suffering, or as an interactive process negotiated by any number of individuals involved in the illness experience. The goal of those involved in the illness experience is to decrease the suffering of the ill person or the shared suffering, thereby increasing well-being.

In the literature there are two major conceptualizations of the illness experience. First, illness has been conceptualized as the individual's experience of symptoms, which has been extensively described as the *medical model* (Figure 33.1). From this perspective the practitioner focuses on the individual and is *primarily* interested in the patient's report of physical symptoms as cues to underlying disease processes. A second view focuses on the *person* and considers illness behavior as the ability of the ill person to cope with or to respond to the disease process. For example, Lazarus (1966) viewed illness

---

[1] Reprinted with permission from Morse, J. M., & Johnson, J. L. (Eds.). (1991). *The illness experience: Dimensions of suffering*. Newbury Park, CA: Sage. Retrieved from http://content.lib.utah.edu/cdm/singleitem/collection/uspace/id/10102/rec/149

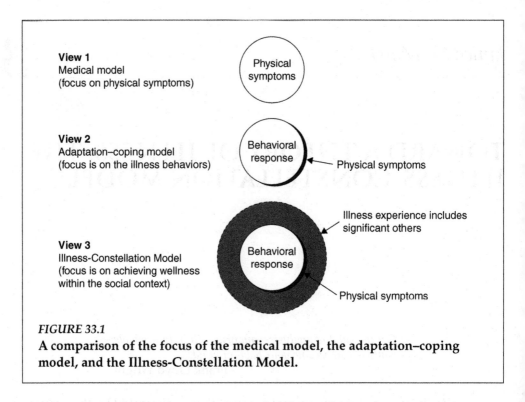

FIGURE 33.1

A comparison of the focus of the medical model, the adaptation–coping model, and the Illness-Constellation Model.

as a cultural, mental, and somatic stressor that threatens bodily harm and disrupts motivational behavior. More recently, researchers who use the phenomenological method have viewed illness from this perspective (e.g., see Kaufman, 1988). Thus this second conceptualization of the illness experience is more complex because it incorporates not only the physical symptoms, but it also incorporates the human responses to these symptoms.

A more comprehensive view of illness, called the *Illness-Constellation Model*, was developed. This model viewed illness as an experience that affects the sick person *and* his or her significant others. From this perspective, the ramifications of the individual's illness experience cause profound changes in the interactions, roles, and relationships of those involved in the illness experience and result in a loss of normalcy. Particularly in the case of serious illness there is interplay of compensatory relationships between the sick person and his or her family and friends. The task of *regaining normalcy*, of regaining former roles and relationships with others, is a legitimate task that must be resolved before the person regains a high level of wellness.

In the Illness-Constellation Model, the illness experience is defined as a four-stage process. *Stage I* is the *Stage of Uncertainty*, and in this stage the individual detects or suspects signs of illness and attempts to make sense of these symptoms by determining their severity and meaning. Those closest to the ill person (usually family members and friends) observe that the sick person is unwell, but these observations may lag behind the experience of the ill person—or alternatively the ill person may have to inform others of the illness, for example in the case of a woman discovering a breast lump.

Stage II, the *Stage of Disruption,* begins when the individual makes a decision that the illness is real, is serious, and decides to seek help. This stage may also be initiated by the confirmation of a medical diagnosis or by the person suddenly becoming so ill that the decision to seek help is taken out of his or her hands by another person, for example taking the ill person to the doctor or calling an ambulance. This is a stage of crisis, a stage in which the individual relinquishes control and withdraws by *distancing* him or herself from the situation. At this point the individual becomes totally dependent on health care professionals and family members. Significant others become aware of the illness and the threat it poses, and they may hover, be vigilant, and, as concerned friends or relatives, *suffer* with the individual. In the case of serious illness, relatives and friends assume the day-to-day responsibilities of the ill person, such as taking care of the ill person's children.

Stage III is the *Stage of Striving to Regain Self,* and in this stage the ill person *strives to make sense* of the illness. During this stage the ill person examines the past for reasons that explain the illness, and he or she tries to predict the future ramifications of the illness. Significant others find themselves *committing to the fight,* working and assisting with treatments and day-to-day tasks, and supporting and encouraging the individual. *Preserving self,* which involves conserving and focusing energy, becomes a priority for the sick person, while significant others engage in *buffering* behaviors; that is, behaviors that reduce stimuli and protect the sick person from undue stressors. As the ill person is placed in a passive role, he or she must constantly negotiate and renegotiate with others in order to preserve his or her self-identity, control, and roles, and as he or she regains wellness, he or she must negotiate and prove to him or herself and to others that he or she is well enough to resume tasks and responsibilities that have been assumed by others. Significant others who permit the ill person to be dependent and provide assistance with day-to-day tasks are hesitant to force the ill person to resume activities, yet they realize that although it is necessary for the sick person to relinquish some of his or her responsibilities and become dependent, total relinquishment on occasion may be harmful. The skill is to attain a balance or a reciprocal relationship in which the needs of both individuals are respected.

Frequently, this balance is attained by the sick person *setting goals,* and the attainment of these goals may indicate physiological improvement or a return to social functioning. While setting these goals, family and friends endure the illness process, policing and modifying the ill person's goals to ensure that they are realistic and attainable and providing necessary, realistic support and encouragement.

The last stage, *Stage IV,* the *Stage of Regaining Wellness,* is the stage in which the ill person *attains mastery* by regaining former relationships and the control of self. During this stage, the ill person determines when he or she is "better" or adjusts to and accepts a changed level of functioning. Family and friends assist the ill person in *making it through,* providing support and allowing the ill person to gradually regain control of his or her life. The ill person focuses on *taking charge,* learning to trust his or her body, to recognize and monitor symptoms closely, and to live within the new limits set by the illness.

Table 33.1 summarizes the five studies included in this text and identifies the major strategies that were used by families and individuals in the various

---

TABLE 33.1
The Stages of Illness as Described in Five Grounded Theories

TOPIC (AUTHOR)

Women's adjustment following health attack (Johnson)	Women having hysterectomy (Chasse)	Leaving the psychiatric hospital (Lorencz)	Mothers' involvement with daughters' abortions (Norris)	Husbands' experience during their wives' chemotherapy (Wilson)
Defending Oneself	**Experiencing and Disruption**	**Being a Failure**	**Suspecting Pregnancy**	**Identifying the Threat**
Normalizing Symptoms	Experiencing Symptoms	Not Making It Being Overwhelmed	Informing Assessing Sexual	Suspecting Finding Out
Struggling to Maintain the Status Quo	Learning to Read the Body	Getting Admitted	Activity Monitoring	↓
Distancing Oneself	Negotiating Medical	↓	Being Vigilant	**Engaging in the Fight**
↓	Management	**Being in Boot Camp**	↓	Resolving Inducting
Coming to Terms	↓	Planning for	**Taking Responsibility**	Enduring
Facing One's Mortality	**Struggling to Preserve**	Goal Attainment	Considering Alternatives	Finalizing ↓
Making Sense	**Wholeness**	Assessing	Consenting	**Becoming a**
Facing Limitations	Observing the Changes	Readiness	Waiting	**Veteran**
Looking to the Future	Managing the	Getting Out	↓	Making it
↓	Separation	↓	**Reconciling the Abortion**	Through
Learning to Live	Becoming a	**Anticipating Mastery**	Grieving	Recognizing Changes
Preserving Self Minimizing	Patient ↓	Becoming Ordinary	Seeking Closure Assessing the	Making Time
Uncertainty Establishing	**Recovering**		Outcome ↓	
Guidelines for Living	Adjusting to Changes		**Recovering**	
↓	Coming to		Putting it Behind	
Living Again	Terms			
Accepting Limitations Refocusing Attaining Mastery				

stages of illness. From the stages and strategies of the Illness-Constellation Model (see Table 33.2), developed by synthesizing the findings of these five studies, we elicited the commonalities of each stage and compared the main characteristics of each of the models.

In the following sections, the Illness-Constellation Model is discussed in detail in order to show how it affects both individuals and their significant others. As each strategy describes the ill person's response, the equivalent strategy that describes the response of the family or friends is also discussed. For example, in the Stage of Uncertainty, both the ill person and the significant others engage in suspecting, and this is listed as "Suspecting ↔ Suspecting." Next, the ill individual engages in Reading the Body, and the significant others engage in Monitoring. These strategies are listed in tandem as "Reading the Body ↔ Monitoring."

TABLE 33.2

The Stages of Illness and Focus of the **Illness-Constellation**
Model *as Described in Five Grounded Theories*

ILLNESS-CONSTELLATION MODEL

SELF	OTHERS

Stage 1: The Stage of Uncertainty

• Suspecting	• Suspecting
• Reading the Body	• Monitoring
• Being Overwhelmed	• Being Overwhelmed

Stage 2: The Stage of Disruption

• Relinquishing Control	• Accepting Responsibility
• Distancing Oneself	• Being Vigilant

Stage 3: Striving to Regain Self

• Making Sense	• Committing to the Struggle
• Preserving Self	• Buffering
• Renegotiating Roles	• Renegotiating Roles
• Setting Goals	• Monitoring Activities
• Seeking Reassurance	• Supporting

Stage 4: Regaining Wellness

• Taking Charge	• Relinquishing Control
• Attaining Mastery	• Making It Through
• Seeking Closure	• Seeking Closure

STAGE I: THE STAGE OF UNCERTAINTY

Suspecting ↔ Suspecting

The illness experience commences as the individual begins to *suspect* that something is wrong. They note that things are not quite right—their periods are irregular, they seem more stressed, a "funny feeling" of nausea overtakes them, they lose their appetite, or they find a lump in their breast—and confronted with these symptoms, the individual begins to suspect that something is wrong:

> I thought, "Gee, should I stop for lunch or shouldn't I?. . . I
> didn't have any breakfast today, maybe I'm feeling a bit hun-
> gry." So 1 made myself a half a sandwich. I normally make a
> whole sandwich, and I thought, "I wonder why."

Family and friends may also note behavioral changes in the ill individual or they may be directly told by the ill individual about suspicious symptoms. In turn, family and friends also are drawn into the process of suspecting. Doubts begin to creep into the minds of the individual and family members as they grapple with the idea that something serious may be happening.

Reading the Body ↔ Monitoring

The symptoms experienced by the ill individual may begin insidiously and slowly, and the question the person asks about each subtle change is: *Is this normal?* For example, in Chasse's hysterectomy study, women tolerated increasingly severe dysmenorrhea, watching their periods to see if this one would be heavier than the last, to see if the pain was increasing in severity, or if the menstrual flow was normal or heavy. People begin *reading their body* by using their own past experiences to evaluate the present symptoms and, when the uncertainty continues, by comparing their own symptoms with their friends' experiences with menstruation. Chasse referred to this process as *establishing the boundaries of normalcy.* Similarly, in Johnson's study of women heart attack victims, although the illness onset was necessarily more acute, all of the informants tried to evaluate the seriousness of the symptoms and to place the symptoms within the boundaries of known, familiar, and more common but less serious illnesses. At the onset of the heart attack these individuals tried to explain their symptoms as "the flu" or "something they ate." One informant, who had the classical signs of heart attack listed on a bookmark, still did not interpret his symptoms correctly. Yet all of Johnson's informants were surprised at the fuss, speed, and sense of urgency their symptoms created when they finally consulted a doctor or reported to the emergency room. Were these people expecting heart attack symptoms to be more painful or more dramatic? Or did they not seek help, as Johnson suggests, because they preferred to remain in control and to regard their symptoms as trivial? The flu or the upset stomach was considered such a trivial complaint that these individuals would rather avoid the embarrassment of "troubling the doctor" than have their fears alleviated:

> *I only had a slight idea what might be happening, but I thought the standard, "Hey it can't be me." So I got up and threw up once. I was getting weaker all the time. But I stayed at work for the day.*

In order to accurately read their bodies, ill individuals begin to identify *triggers* or situations that stimulate an attack or worsen or alleviate the symptoms. Again, in Chasse's study, this occurred frequently and over a long period of time before the women accepted the fact that their periods were abnormal and that they should seek medical help.

This process of normalizing symptoms is not limited to physical symptoms; emotional states are evaluated as well. For example, in Lorencz's study, the informants in the psychiatric hospital complained about increasing loneliness, problems with interpersonal relationships, and problems remaining employed, but again, one thing was clear: they saw themselves as "not making it" and needing some help.

It is important to note that others also observed the sick person: *monitoring* the ill person for symptoms or assessing their level of wellness. In Norris's study, the mothers did this as soon as they suspected their daughters were involved in sexual relations, observing their daughters for signs of pregnancy:

> I've kept this to myself, but being a mother who washes her
> daughters' clothes, I do know when they have their monthlies.
> And I noticed that [daughter!] didn't have anything on her
> clothes. It flashed through my mind (that she was pregnant) . . .
> I certainly didn't want to believe it.

Similarly, Wilson reported that husbands of women undergoing chemotherapy monitored their wives over an extended period of time in order to determine what was happening to them.

Being Overwhelmed ↔ Becoming Overwhelmed

Eventually, the symptoms develop to a point where the individual is *overwhelmed*, both physically and emotionally, by a sense of uncertainty. Perhaps the process of deciding when you are sick *enough* to need a doctor is easiest when the symptoms are so severe that there is no question that medical help should be obtained immediately or when the situation is taken "out of the sick person's hands." The state of limbo, of the patient not feeling well and yet not being sick, may be so stressful that receiving an actual diagnosis, the confirmation of being sick and the respite from an intolerably ambiguous situation, may be almost a relief:

> It's the unknown, the not knowing, which is the most stressful.
> It's fear of the unknown; fear of your mind starting to go off in
> all directions. You imagine all kinds of things.

On the other hand, the confirmation of malignancy (e.g., finding a breast lump) may be devastating. The way the diagnosis is received by the patient depends on the severity of symptoms, the type of disease and prognosis, and the course of the illness.

If physicians dismiss the reported symptoms and do not provide the expected care or if they suggest unacceptable treatments or surgery the patient begins to "doctor hop," consulting one doctor after another. Chasse notes that her informants said many physicians did not give them information when requested, and in many encounters her informants were not treated with empathy and respect. Despite the fact that they were reporting severe and quite disabling symptoms they felt the physicians treated their complaints as "all in their head," and because they felt that they were not being taken seriously they were not in a position to negotiate treatments. If the patient's spouse is supportive during this time, this support adds weight or credence to the suspicion that something is *really* wrong, and the process of seeking medical help is eased considerably for the individual.

As family and friends witness the ill individual seeking medical assistance the fact that their relative or friend is ill becomes a reality. Often the friends and relatives *become overwhelmed* by worry and concern, particularly if they detect that the individual concerned is worried. Apprehension begins to grow during this waiting period, particularly if it is necessary for the ill person to undergo tests to rule out serious complaints. They vacillate, one moment considering the possibility of a devastating disease and the next moment reassuring themselves that such bad news is unlikely:

> Waiting for results from the lab was really a torture situation. It
> was extremely stressful when you suspected very strongly, and
> yet nobody [will] come out and [say] this is what it is. When
> you're waiting for the phone to ring, you're wondering. It was
> very stressful waiting to hear. You felt so damn helpless.
> Phoning didn't seem to help. Nothing seemed to help.

STAGE II: STAGE OF DISRUPTION

The Stage of Disruption begins when the individuals realize that medical intervention is required and they no longer have a choice about whether or not they can manage their symptoms alone: either the symptoms are too severe or the uncertainty is unbearable. A critical point is reached whereby either the person (or if they are unable, their relatives) transfers the responsibility for decision making to the physician.

Relinquishing Control ↔ Accepting Responsibility

Once the sick person enters the medical system, he or she no longer *really* makes decisions: choices become a medical prerogative. Rather than presenting alternatives for the patient to select or allowing the patient to decide whether or not treatment will even be instigated, the physician presents the selected course of treatment. Several factors contribute to the *relinquishing of control* on the part of the patient. First, in the physician–patient relationship the physician is often viewed as the expert and the patient as the follower of expert advice. Second, urgent situations often necessitate the relinquishment of control, either because immediate action on the part of the physician is necessary or because the patient is not considered competent enough to make an informed decision. This lack of competence is exacerbated because of symptoms such as pain and the patient is not considered knowledgeable enough to make an informed decision, and perhaps because the patient is seen as a "case" rather than as a *person*.

This sense of lack of control is also felt by family members. For example, although the mothers and daughters in Norris's study had received permission from the Therapeutic Abortion Committee to have an abortion, they had difficulty grasping the fact that the abortions were *actually going* to take place, that the nightmare would soon be over. Similarly, Wilson notes that following the diagnosis for cancer her informants "were overwhelmed by the speed with which things happened." Once told about the diagnosis, these informants were pushed "from the frying pan to the fire, pretty quick," and they felt the necessity to receive immediate treatment. They felt *thrust* into a new situation, and there was "nothing they could do about it." This sense of immediacy was accelerated because they had an image of the cancer cells multiplying exponentially on a daily basis. Patients in this situation feel they have no choice but to trust the decisions of the physician. When a suspected heart attack victim experiences emergency care, the speedy response of health professionals is legendary. The patients are not active participants in their treatments; rather, they are viewed as objects that "have things done to them." Perhaps the most extraordinary description of this phase is from the psychiatric patients in Lorencz's study:

> And the, all of a sudden, wham, I'm stuck in the hospital, and I
> was changed . . . and then the doctors got at me, and I was
> changed. I was—I didn't—I didn't give a damn for a while, eh?
> And the, and then, it got harder, even harder. And then the

> doctors got at me, and that's where I'm at. The doctors are
> talking about me, eh? What they think I am, and what they think,
> feel I want, and what I—do, and what I think, and stuff like that.

Seeing the vulnerability of the ill person and his or her inability to make decisions or to take control, the family and friends feel compelled to *accept responsibility* for them. Family members feel that they must "keep it together," not giving in to their own feelings of being out of control because they feel a sense of responsibility to act for their family member:

> It reinforced for me that I'm here because I want to be here. She
> still is my daughter and my little girl. I wouldn't want to be
> anywhere else but here, and I am taking responsibility for her
> and for her error.

The family and friends' sense of responsibility is derived in part from the fact that they are healthy and their friend or family member is sick. Family members feel obliged to help in any way. They complete small tasks such as notifying others by phone and fetching basic articles for the sick person even though they are exceedingly worried and concerned. These small tasks keep them busy and help to relieve their anxiety. Consequently, helping is a comforting strategy. As one informant in Wilson's husband study indicated, "If you want to survive the situation, you really have to turn yourself into something that can be helpful to the person that's sick."

Distancing Oneself ↔ Being Vigilant

The loss of control requires total relinquishment of self on the part of the patient. In order to cope with the situation, they begin to *distance themselves*. Patients describe this as feeling as though they are automated; once begun, it seems that treatments cannot be stopped. As recipients of treatment, ill individuals have little input into the decision-making process, and often they do not even know what is happening to them or who their doctor is. Often patients complain that things seem foggy, unreal, and that they have trouble grasping what is happening to them:

> Afterwards, it didn't seem like I had a heart attack. It didn't
> seem real. I thought, "Somebody else had it." It was funny. And
> it was kind of interesting. I thought about the fact that I had a
> heart attack, and it seemed almost impossible. It was like my
> brain didn't want to accept it.

During this time, relatives are *vigilant*, and although recognizing that their ill relative is unable or unwilling to take full control, they wait in the periphery in case they are needed or wanted. They struggle to get information, to understand what is happening, and to learn about the ramifications and outcome of the illness. Being vigilant often involves long periods of waiting and these waiting periods seem endless to the relatives. The family and friends feel that they must become the ill person's eyes and ears, trying to pick up whatever information they can in order to protect the sick person:

> You had to change your life-style a whole bunch. On those
> days, you obviously couldn't plan on going out. You had to be
> around to take *care* of your wife.

The patient in turn realizes the seriousness of the situation by the fact that the family is watching over him or her. The drain of knowing their family is waiting affects the sick patient, and this waiting increases their concern: "I was tense, she was tense. She got tenser from me, and I got tenser from her. We just kind of went around in a circle for a while." A patient in the intensive care unit (ICU) reported seeing her children "come off" the elevator while "they [the staff] were working over [her]." Although her children could not get close enough to communicate with her, she saw fear on their faces. Thus it is clear that the concept of *being vigilant* adds credence to the fact that the illness experience is a shared experience, occurring within reciprocal, dynamic relationships.

The Stage of Disruption ends as the individual begins to gain a sense of what is happening to him or her. They no longer feel that everything is in a fog and they are able to regain a sense of reality and engage more actively in the treatment process. For some individuals this stage is terminated by an acceptance of the terrifying fact that something has gone terribly wrong. No longer is it necessary for the individual to relinquish all control to physicians and family. Realizing that they must take some responsibility for themselves, they move into the Stage of Striving to Regain Self.

STAGE III: STRIVING TO REGAIN SELF

Making Sense ↔ Committing to the Struggle

The Stage of Striving to Regain Self begins when the individual comes to grips with the illness and the future ramifications of the illness. They attempt to *make sense* of what has happened by asking friends and relatives who are present for details about their admission, resuscitation procedures, how they behaved while in pain, and other incidents that they can barely remember. They may also seek information from staff members or ambulance drivers. They examine events leading up to the crisis, they replay the story in their minds, and they tell and retell events to visitors and others as a part of making sense and accepting their present situation.

Inherent in this stage is the well-documented process of soul searching for the "real" reason that *they* were stricken with this illness. Some find "just" cause, for example cancer of the uterus caused by a long past illicit abortion or a heart attack caused by living too well. Others are unable to answer the question "why me?":

> I kept thinking about it for the first month after I got home . . .
> Just going over in my mind "Why did this have to happen?"
> And then I'd sit and ponder over it.

Family members go through a similar process, asking why, blaming themselves, and taking responsibility for the illness. This was evident in Norris's study where mothers accepted responsibility for their daughters' pregnancy, feeling somehow they should have been able to prevent this disaster. They wondered if this could have been avoided if they had been more strict, educated their daughters more completely, or somehow ensured that their daughters were properly using birth control.

Ill individuals are also confronted with the fact that their lives have been irrevocably altered. Although they might regain former functioning, because of the illness experience they see themselves in a new light. The suffering inherent in the illness experience forces the individual and the families to re-examine their lives, appreciating the things they had often taken for granted. They confront their mortality and re-examine their values. For some this is a positive experience encouraging them to redirect their life goals; for example, by making their relationships with their families a new priority. For others, however, the crisis of illness is so devastating that the implications are beyond comprehension. The sense of devastation that results from this may lead to depression, marital conflict, and withdrawal. The fact that life is irrevocably altered by the illness experience is clearly evident in all of the studies. For example, Lorencz's informants recognized that they would not only have to deal with the trauma of hospitalization but also the stigma attached to being sent to a place for "crazies." Mothers consenting to their daughters' abortions realized that their perceptions of who their daughters were would never be the same. Women who had experienced a hysterectomy faced the fact that they would never be able to bear children again. Husbands faced the threat that cancer would eventually recur in their wives. The fact that lives were permanently changed by the experience was clear when Wilson's informants discussed their wives' struggles even though their wives had died years ago.

Often any attempt by the relatives to make sense of the crisis is short-lived as they believe they should not focus on themselves but should commit all of their efforts toward helping their ill family member. For example, Wilson described how husbands had to "get it together" so that they could *commit* to the care of their wives. Thus while the individual is trying to make sense of what has occurred, the family and friends are beginning to look to the future and are committing to the struggle that remains ahead.

Preserving Self ↔ Buffering

The immediate need of the person who is ill is the desire to regain control and preserve self. This is particularly difficult in the hospital environment as decision making is often out of the control of the perons. Sometimes the person may not even choose when and how to breathe. For example, they have to cough on command (even if it hurts) and they cannot go to the bathroom when they wish, choose their own meals, or eat whenever they want. Being unable to make even the simplest, most basic decision is demeaning and threatens the person's self-identity. Furthermore, removal from the home environment and the workplace removes the cues that make one a unique individual and that give life purpose. The statement "Don't worry I've taken care of it" does not placate; instead, it increases the feelings of alienation and uselessness.

In order to *preserve a sense of self,* the ill person begins to assert him or herself and to reclaim control. They question treatment ("What's this pill for?"), and they seek information about their diagnosis, test results, and prognosis. They attempt to alleviate the signs of distress in their relatives' faces by trying to appear cheerful ("much better") and making light of their illness in order to minimize the concern demonstrated by their visitors:

> So they're [the informant's children] watching [the cardiac monitor]. They think they're going to get me excited, and I'm going to drop dead or something. So one day I looked up at it, and as I'm twisting to look up, I noticed it all went funny, and then I twisted a little more, and it went really funny . . . So next time [my children came], I started wiggling around, and I said, "Hey, now watch that IV . . . The older one said, "You're going to kill yourself. You can't do that." I said, "Oh yes I can. Watch this. Isn't it neat!" But you gotta have some fun or else you'd drop dead in there.

The relatives recognize that they must *buffer* and protect the ill person. They hover, attempting to shelter the ill individual from concern and worry:

> You do whatever you have to do for someone you love to make it as easy as possible. Everything I did was strictly for my wife. I had to do everything to make it easier.

The paradoxical nature of buffering is that it is done to protect the patient and allow the patient the time and energy needed to get well. If the buffering is excessive and too complete, however, they increase the sick person's stress as they sever the person from the outside world and deny the ill person a sense of purpose. This extreme buffering may become so protective that it retards recuperation and may even become disabling.

Renegotiating Roles ↔ Renegotiating Roles

Both individuals and their families must *renegotiate roles* and responsibilities as the ill person recovers. Responsibilities are essential to the patient's sense of self and reclaiming former roles is the major strategy used as the individual strives to regain self. Often ill individuals attempt to regain a sense of control over their home and work environments, even while still in hospital, by giving instructions, orders, and making decisions. Continuing to have input in their "other lives" outside the hospital helps them to feel like human beings rather than anonymous patients.

Once they return home ill individuals will often attempt to regain a sense of sameness in the home so that the disruption of illness is minimized. This was particularly true in Wilson's study when the families contained children or in Norris's study where it was important to maintain secrecy, when it was essential that the facade of normalcy was maintained. At this point patients are attempting to minimize the seriousness of their conditions by being cheerful and reassuring their families, while the family members, on the other hand, are attempting to coddle and reassure the patient. For the sick person, maintaining normalcy by reclaiming roles minimizes the impact of the illness and maintains the illusion that they are closer to recovery than they are in reality. Although these people are sick, somewhat dependent, and in need of help, the relatives must realize that they need to allow the sick person, within limits, to give to them. As one informant in Johnson's study said, "I think everybody needs to be useful. If you have a feeling of being useless, I think you feel what's the use of living sort of thing." Thus the relationship becomes one of intricate interplay with the sick person, to some extent concealing symptoms and negotiating in order to be treated as "normal" while others observe for cues that suggest the sick person is able to cope. Much like a dance, the sick person and the well person accept and relinquish tasks. Recovery is not a linear process but rather it depends on the resources of the sick person at any particular point in time.

Setting Goals ↔ Monitoring Activities

It is important for ill individuals to believe that they will not remain ill forever. In order to feel that they are making progress, they often set goals for themselves. Accomplishing small goals such as walking a block or managing a stressful situation helps the individual feel that he or she is regaining control and is making progress in the struggle. In the case of the psychiatric patients in Lorencz's study, the schizophrenic patients worked to retain positive self-regard and planned for specific goal attainment. Because these individuals were not "making it" prior to their admissions they did not want to go back to the past but rather they were future-oriented, fantasizing about a normal life upon discharge:

> I'm gonna make a promise to myself that I'm gonna get out of that group home in_____and get an apartment. And earn a . . . wage and eventually, eventually get back on my own and eventually earn my own keep, you know.

Meanwhile, family members are concerned that their relative might "overdo it," and they monitor the activities of the ill person, trying to ensure that they do not "push themselves" too hard. They chaperone, hover, and observe all the activities of the ill person, sometimes from a distance and are always prepared to intervene if needed.

Seeking Reassurance ↔ Supporting

Throughout the Stage of Striving to Regain Self, a sense of uncertainty prevails, and the individual is forced to constantly seek reassurance from health care professionals as they strive for a sense of control. Seemingly trivial decisions, such as how much activity to engage in, when to regain sexual activity, or whether to lift a heavy object, are overwhelming as individuals attempt to manage their recovery. It is only through a process of trial and error that daily routines are constructed to accommodate ongoing symptoms and fears:

> I'm still going through it, and I think, "Oh, I'm sure I can do this myself," and "Why can't I do it?" I'm scared of overdoing it. I'm worried whether I should have a fear like that. I'm scared to do too much. And what is frustrating is I think, "Well, should I do it, or shouldn't I do it? Why do I have a fear of doing anything until I ask somebody if I can do it?"

Recognizing the uncertainty of their ill relative, family members engage in supporting the ill individual, giving them praise and encouragement and trying to instill in them a sense of hope. Family members offer support to the individual who is ill by making lifestyle changes, second-guessing his or her needs, reading about the illness, trying to remain positive (even if they do not feel positive), and by trying not to notice or comment upon the devastating effects of the illness.

STAGE IV: REGAINING WELLNESS

When the patients have once more regained a sense of self, they enter into the rehabilitative Stage of Regaining Wellness. This stage does not necessarily coincide with the patient's discharge from the hospital. The major tasks of this stage are regaining former relationships without the dependency of illness and once more asserting control over their own lives, learning to trust their bodies, putting the illness behind them, and attaining mastery.

Taking Charge ↔ Relinquishing Control

Relationships with friends and family members gradually return to resemble former patterns without the imbalance caused by the dependency that accompanies relationships when one of the partners is ill. Frequently the initiation of these changes comes from the rehabilitating person who is anxious to once again take charge. Often the recovering individuals feel that this is necessary in order to demonstrate their health and their competencies. For example, in Lorencz's study, patients felt they had to prove to themselves and to others that they were capable of surviving on their own after discharge. For other patients, this process of taking charge involved unwise actions:

> I changed my living room around two weeks ago. My husband
> came home and just about shot me. . . . He said, "Good Christ,
> it's been that way for four years, it can stay that way." But I
> think it looks much nicer now, there's more room in it.

Often, dependent persons are anxious to take charge as they find the oversolicitousness of friends and family members to be both inappropriate and inhibiting:

> Well, there was a little anger building up in me because she's
> the oldest one, and she was the most protective. Like, I would
> get up out of my chair, and "No, no Mom, don't. Where are you
> going? What are you going to do?" "I want to go to the
> bathroom." "Well, okay." And if I'd get up to do something,
> "No, no mom, no, no. You can't do that. No, no. Let me do it.
> Don't go upstairs again, oh no." And she'd be walking behind
> me and follow me up the stairs. I said, "I can go up and down
> the stairs twice; 1 day, and that's all I do." I'd go to take a spoon
> out of the cupboard drawer, "No, no mom, sit down. I'll do that
> for you." Well, it just finally got to me. . . .So I just had to yell at
> her. And I yelled at her really good.

At other times the ill individual is forced into an independent role because of the demands of everyday living:

> Like the other day, he hit the corner of the heat register there
> and cut his little head open, and I mean, people say don't lift
> him up. But I think that was half my problem 'cause I lifted my
> son way too early, but they don't understand, like, how can you
> say no to a two year old?

As the ill individual begins to take charge, family and friends begin to relinquish control. This is possible because they see tremendous signs of improvement in the ill individual and are beginning once again to trust the ill individual's abilities and judgments. Seeing the ill individual return to activities such as lifting, driving a car, or returning to work reinforces the perception that the individual is once again able to care for him or herself. Although some degree of monitoring may be maintained, it is usually done on a covert basis. If family or friends are unwilling to relinquish their control, ill individuals will increase their efforts to assert control over their own lives.

Attaining Mastery ↔ Making It Through

Throughout this final stage, ill individuals gradually learn to trust their abilities, and they work toward *attaining mastery*. They learn what their limitations are and how to extend their previous limits until they consider themselves well. Tentative trials of new physical tasks gradually give way to confident efforts:

> I'll tell you one of my happiest times was the summer after
> I had my heart attack . . . We went to Banff, to Johnson
> Canyon . . . and we walked up the mountain there for hours.
> But I walked careful. I walked easy because I hadn't had my
> heart attack all that long ago. And I get to about four miles up
> there, hey, I felt great, and I thought, "God, I'm not cripple."
> The last thing you want to be is a cripple. Nobody wants to be.
> A blind person doesn't want to be blind, and a deaf person
> doesn't want to be deaf, and a heart attack doesn't want to be
> a couch potato.

As small goals are reached and progress becomes evident, the overwhelming idea of rehabilitation becomes more manageable. Furthermore, "promotions" such as day passes and increased privileges for psychiatric patients facilitate the testing of the ill person's ability to make it in the "real world":

> By going through, going through the ropes, to use a cliché,
> I feel more comfortable having the approval of somebody
> professional saying, "When l started working in the snack bar, I
> felt more confident about being around more other people and
> being—putting myself in a social situation where the noise level
> and the conversation level was quite high—the potential for
> getting strained."

At this time the individual has to relearn the cues for reading the body, to learn when to become concerned over symptoms and the meaning of these symptoms. Perhaps because of the potentially serious ramifications of mis-reading symptoms and signs, this task requires a lot of energy and awareness. Constant comparisons are made with others or with one's previous state in order to determine if one is progressing and if symptoms should be a source of concern:

> I still got my same temper and everything, but something really
> has to happen to get me in a bad mood. Like before, it didn't
> take nothing. I just switched from one mood to the other with
> no reasoning, no nothing behind it, so that plays on your mind,
> too. You think you're going crazy.

The process of attaining mastery can continue for a prolonged period of time. Eventually, as confidence and a sense of control are regained, the individual is able to put the illness behind him or her and focus on other aspects of his or her life. A sense that he or she has regained wellness occurs gradually and becomes evident only when he or she realizes that he or she is no longer spending long periods of time being consumed by worry and concerns. Tasks are eventually completed without thinking twice about them, and the individual is able to put the illness experience behind.

As the individual works toward regaining mastery, family and friends focus on making it through. Although they rejoice in the victories of the ill person, they continue to be concerned about the future, unwilling to be convinced that the end of the illness is in sight. Often the family is concerned about reoccurrences. They do not want to become too enthusiastic about progress in case a setback is experienced.

Seeking Closure ↔ Seeking Closure

In this final stage, a major task that ill individuals and their family members engage in is that of seeking closure. Individuals cannot "get on with their lives" until they have satisfactorily resolved what has happened to them. For example, Chasse's informants said they could not move to a state of wellness until they resolved the question of whether they had made a correct decision when they had a hysterectomy. Those who were unable to affirm their decision to have a hysterectomy were unable to regain a feeling that their lives were back to normal:

> I feel so sad. I feel so empty inside, you know . . . Towards my
> younger baby, I feel like I have to stick with her all the time. It's
> just an unbelievable feeling. I never felt that way before.

The family members also attempt to put the illness behind them. Although it is no longer a central concern, the poignancy of this experience, particularly the vulnerability of their partner, relative, or friend, remains with them. Having lived through the nightmare of an acute illness the family has a need to bring closure to the event. This desperate need for closure is expressed by a mother whose daughter had an abortion:

> I feel some kind of need to write closure to this, and I don't
> know how to do that. I should feel some sense of relief that it's
> over with, but there is so much pressure and tension and stress
> there that I have not been able to bleed it off effectively . . .
> I am at a loss to know what it is that I need help with. I haven't
> identified that for myself yet. Like I know what it's not . . . I can
> tell you what it's not, but I cannot yet tell you what it is. I am
> going to have to work this through.

Full closure, however, is never attained for the individual or for the family members. Heart attack victims continue to work hard to prevent another occurrence. Mothers continue to monitor their daughters' sexual activity to ensure that an unwanted pregnancy does not occur, and husbands vigilantly monitor their wives' health for signs of recurrence of cancer or metastasis.

Some individuals may be unable to return to a state of wellness following the illness experience. Failure to resolve the experience, the continuation of symptoms, and disability may all contribute to an inability to successfully put closure to the experience. Finally, it should be noted that the illness experience is not a simple linear process. Individuals experience "highs" and "lows" in this process, and some may return to previously completed stages several times. What does seem clear is that an individual will be unable to move on to a progressive stage until the previous one is complete.

Minimizing Suffering

In the Illness-Constellation Model, the core variable that underlies the entire process for both patients and their family and friends is *minimizing suffering*. The process of minimizing suffering consists of a variety of strategies directed at reducing the physical and psychological discomfort of illness, the social distress extending from changed roles and responsibilities, and the uncertainty of the unknown future. Suffering was therefore conceived to be a comprehensive concept incorporating the experience of both acute and chronic pain, the strain of trying to endure, the alienation of forced exclusion from everyday life, the shock of institutionalization, and the uncertainly of anticipating the ramifications of the illness:

> When you're thrown down into a pool, and you can't swim,
> and you don't have a life preserver, that's the way 1 felt for a
> long time. In other words, struggling. It was hard to get up in
> the morning knowing that you were going to have another one
> of those days which was unpredictable.

There is no doubt that the nature of the suffering experience has not been clearly described, and there is much work to do in the exploration of individuals' experiences as they cope and struggle with suffering in the illness experience. Furthermore, individuals do not suffer alone. The experience of suffering has ramifications for all those who are associated with the ill person:

> The pain of watching somebody that you love going through
> pain, going through agony, that is the hardest part. That is the
> hardest part of the whole thing to deal with that. That was my
> hardest part—it wasn't the caring or the cleaning up or the
> helping her to the washroom or getting the pills.

Because the nature of suffering incorporates physiological as well as psychological and social dimensions, *minimizing suffering* may be considered a *Basic Social, Psychological, Physiological Process (BSPPP)* in the Illness-Constellation Model.

DISCUSSION

Here, we have attempted to arrive at some general understanding of the illness experience. Clearly there is much research left to do before this complex process is fully understood. Although recent years have witnessed an increased interest in the experiences of those who are ill (Conrad, 1990), investigations have tended to examine illness by examining the individual's response to diseases. The biomedical model is frequently used as a structure for understanding individuals' responses to specific diagnoses such as epilepsy (Scambler & Hopkins, 1990), Parkinson's disease (Pinder, 1988), or postpartum depression (Harkness, 1987). Alternatively, researchers have focused on responses to specific symptoms, such as hypoglycemia (Hunt,

Browner, & Jordon, 1990; Singer, et al., 1987) or pain (Zborowski, 1969). Clearly, these investigations have offered valuable, *albeit* fragmented insights. It is ironic, however, to note that the medical model continues to be used to sample for behavioral theory. Perhaps the current fragmentation of illness theory is because of the a priori classification of behaviors based on medical diagnosis. Indeed, even the chapters of this book have been derived using this perspective of patients with medical problems. Attempts to move away from the medical model in illness theory need to be made, however. It is clear that there are commonalities in the illness experience that bridge the boundaries created by the disease taxonomy. These can be elicited just as Selye (1976) observed the physiological syndrome of "just being sick" many years ago.

Clearly, it is time to move on and develop a broader understanding of the illness experience using human behavior as a basis for developing theory. As the five studies included in this book have demonstrated, there are remarkable similarities in the ways individuals and their families and friends live through and cope with the illness experience, and from these similarities the strength of the Illness-Constellation Model is derived. Although the Illness-Constellation Model overcomes some of the limitations of current illness theory in that it incorporates the experiences of individuals and their families and friends and is not limited to a single diagnosis, there is still much work to be done in this area. Instead of investigating illness as a series of discrete categories or isolated responses we need to further develop this model and continue to investigate the illness experience comprehensively.

In particular, the role of the family needs to remain at the forefront of illness research. Too often the illness experience has been conceptualized as individualistic rather than reciprocal. Because of emotional ties, family and friends are intimately involved in and affected by the life of the ill individual and the impact that illness has on these individuals needs to be included. Another area that also needs to be considered is how individuals isolated from friends and family manage with their illness, particularly in Stage II of the Illness-Constellation Model, the Stage of Disruption; in particular, older adults are often without the support of family. How do these individual experiences differ from those with support systems? This area needs to be carefully investigated.

Another aspect of illness requiring careful consideration is the experience of those who do not recover from what is considered by medical personnel to be a recoverable disease. The plight of the "cardiac cripple" who is determined by a physician to be physically well, yet is only able to function at a minimal level is a typical example of this phenomenon (Cassem & Hackett, 1977). There are countless examples of individuals who have suffered from a variety of diseases and are unable to regain wellness despite the fact that they have officially recovered from their disease. Conversely, there are individuals who remain physically disabled but reach a high level of wellness (Trieschmann, 1980). Both of these examples illustrate the inappropriateness of using medical diagnoses as the basis for examining illness behavior. Thus perhaps it is time to ignore the medical diagnosis and to use behavioral indicators when sampling for studies that are exploring behavior.

Suffering is inherent in the illness experience, particularly as these studies show in more serious illnesses. The experience of suffering may be short and intense or it may be a prolonged and insidious strain that "does not go away." The nature of suffering reflects the variable and often erratic course of illness. Yet despite the pervasive nature of suffering and the integral relationship of suffering and illness, this concept has been largely ignored in the research literature. There is a need for intensive investigation in this area.

In recent years, the focus of many qualitative studies has been on chronic illness. It is not clear to us, however, how chronic illness is differentiated from acute illness. Authors do not state if they use medical criteria or the criterion of duration to define "chronic," although we suspect it is the former. Nevertheless, when these chronic illnesses are examined from an experiential perspective their course is not dissimilar from that of acute illnesses. Perhaps the differentiation between acute and chronic illness represents a false dichotomy. There are similarities between the experiences of those who suffer an acute illness, those who suffer chronic illness, and those who may technically suffer from a nonillness, such as those who are undergoing abortions (see Norris, 1982). Certainly, the Illness-Constellation Model appears to fit acute and chronic patterns of illness. It appears that the "flare-ups" or exacerbations that occur in chronic illness are similar to episodes of acute illnesses. Furthermore, although a disease such as a myocardial infarction is officially classified as acute, the recuperative period is prolonged and the impact of this disease on the individual's life is permanent. At this point there is a need for further research to examine these chronic illnesses with a view to exploring further the acute–chronic differentiations.

Although the Illness-Constellation Model is not intended to explicate a "standard" response to the illness experience, it does provide important insights into how the ill individual and significant others respond to their situations. Clearly, variation in these experiences is expected and future investigation will enrich and explicate this model. Furthermore, this model is not intended to describe a linear process; rather, it is a process that may involve regression as well as progression. For example, individuals may progress to Stage III and later deteriorate to Stage II. Or as indicated in Wilson's study cancer patients in Stage IV return to the Stage of Uncertainty (Stage I) as the individual suspects that the disease is recurring.

In 1984, Armstrong noted that the explication of the patients' view is not a recent innovation. Patients have always been expressive about their experiences. What is new is that we are beginning to listen more attentively and to give credence to the patient's perspective. We are hearing the same stories but with new ears and with new research methods and we are gaining new insights. Our changing attitudes toward patient care places new value on the illness experience as an important area of investigation. This refocusing of health care ensures that the patient is treated as a person, that the family is included in the care, and that the care is humane.

OTHER EXAMPLES OF QUALITATIVE META-ANALYSIS

(Beck 2011)

Developed from six studies on birth trauma, and the resulting posttraumatic stress disorder (PTSD), Beck developed a theory of Amplified Causal Loops (Beck, 2011). In four studies, original triggers of amplifying feedback loops reinforced the experience (in a positive direction) and two studies balanced (in a negative direction) the experience. The experiences were birth trauma, breastfeeding, mother–infant interaction, anniversary of the birth, and subsequent childbirth, with the negative experiences balancing or breaking the positive experiences that reinforce the PTSD birth experience.

A theory of Uncertain Motherhood (Marck, Field, & Bergum, 1994) developed from six grounded theories, relating to different stages and conditions around pregnancy and birth. Conditions were infertility, unexpected pregnancy, "guarding" the mother–unborn child relationship, live birth following still birth, having a preterm baby, and when a child has a birth defect. Themes relating to Uncertain Motherhood were:

- Everything has changed: a journey into vulnerability

  - Anything can happen

- An inner dialogue with uncertainty

  - A possible mother: trust and vulnerability
  - Negotiating the risk
  - Uncertain motherhood as a hidden conversation
  - Mothering pains: Responding to the call of a child

- The search for care: relationship between caregivers and women

  - Divergent knowledge

- Living through mothering experiences when the outcome is uncertain

  - Identifying a threat
  - Appraising the threat (low threat/high threat)

- Protecting the self
- Blaming self/blaming others
- Connecting/disconnecting
- Telling others/not telling others
- Seeking information/blocking information (pp. 269–291)

The authors write:

> . . . not every woman took home a child to nurture and raise. It was not every woman's goal to do so, and for many women, it was an impossible goal. What every woman took out of this experience of uncertain motherhood was not a living child, but the experience of having responded to the notion of mothering a child.
>
> For each woman, responding to the possibility of motherhood was a unique and deeply personal struggle, one that brought pain and a need to make sense of her experience. Understanding came as each woman experienced her pain and as she found others who would witness and share it honestly (Marck, Field, & Bergum, 1994).

REFERENCES

Beck, C. T. (2011). A metaethnography of traumatic childbirth and its aftermath: Amplifying causal looping. *Qualitative Health Research, 21*(3), 310–311. doi:10.1177/1049732310390698

Cassem, N. H., & Hackett, T. P. (1977). Psychological aspects of myocardial infarction. *Medical Clinics of North America, 61,* 711–721.

Conrad, P. (1990). Qualitative research on chronic illness: A commentary on method and conceptual development. *Social Science & Medicine, 30,* 1257–1263.

Harkness, S. (1987). The cultural medication of postpartum depression. *Medical Anthropology Quarterly, 1,* 194–209.

Hunt, L., Browner, C. H., & Jordon, B. (1990). Hypoglycemia: Portrait of an illness construct in everyday use. *Medical Anthropology Quarterly, 4,* 191–210.

Kaufman, S. R. (1988). Towards a phenomenology of boundaries in medicine: Chronic illness experience in the case of stroke. *Medical Anthropology Quarterly, 2,* 338–354.

Lazarus, R. A. (1966). *Psychological stress and the coping process.* New York, NY: McGraw-Hill.

Marck, P. B., Field, P. A., & Bergum, V. (1994). A search for understanding. In P. A. Field & P. B. Marck (Eds.), *Uncertain motherhood: Negotiating the risks of the childbearing years* (pp. 268–298). Thousand Oaks, CA: Sage.

Morse, J. M., & Johnson, J. L. (Eds.). (1991). *The illness experience: Dimensions of suffering.* Newbury Park, CA: Sage. Retrieved from http://content.lib.utah.edu/cdm/singleitem /collection/uspace/id/10102/rec/149

Norris, C. (1982). *Concept clarification in nursing.* Rockville, MD: Aspen.

Norris, J. (1991). Mothers' involvement in their adolescent daughters abortions. In J. Morse & J. Johnson (Eds.), *The illness experience: Dimensions of suffering* (pp. 201–236). Newbury Park, CA: Sage. Retrieved from http://content.lib.utah.edu/u?/ir-main,2008

Pinder, R. (1988). Striking balances: Living with Parkinson's disease. In R. Anderson & M. Bury (Eds.), *Understanding health and social care* (pp. 67–88). Boston, MA: Unwin Hyman.

Scambler, G., & Hopkins, A. (1990). Generating a model of epileptic stigma: The role of qualitative analysis. *Social Science & Medicine, 30,* 1187–1194.

Selye, H. (1976). *The stress of life.* Boston, MA: Butterworths.

Singer, M., Fitzgerald, M. H., Madden, M. J., Voight von Legat, C., & Arnold, C. D. (1987). The sufferer's experience of hypoglycemia. In J. A. Roth & P. Conrad (Eds.), *Research in the sociology of health care: The experience and management of chronic illness* (Vol. 6, pp. 147–176). Greenwich, CT: JAI Press.

Trieschmann, R. (1980). *Spinal cord injuries: Psychological, social and vocational adjustment.* Elmsford, NY: Pergamon.

Zborowski, M. (1969). *People in pain.* San Franciso, CA: Jossey-Bass.

SECTION IX

TOWARD THEORY-BASED INTERVENTIONS

As noted in Chapter 27, applying quantitative criteria to qualitative inquiry, researchers erroneously write that their findings are not generalizable because of the limitations in the sample size and ethnic composition and so forth. However, these quantitative criteria have developed because quantitative researchers are attempting to match certain sociological demographic indicators between their study sample and the population to which they are generalizing. These indicators have no relevance for qualitative generalization. Qualitative researchers abstract their findings and are moving the theory across to another situation. If certain features pertaining to the situation are the same in both settings, then the theory may be used in the new setting.

Earlier we spoke about conducting a series of qualitative studies about the same topic, involving different patient groups, from different perspectives, or using different levels of analysis from macro- to microscopic. Theoretical coalescence allows you to link studies addressing a general substantive area, studies that address the scale of high-level concept, but in different contexts and patient populations experiencing different problems, which are linked by some overall high-level concept. All of the studies have something to do with the overall concept. Then instead of conducting a meta-analysis looking for commonalities between studies, we look to more abstract commonalities that have to do with a central conceptual process. In this way, we link attributes, decontextualizing from each study, and combine these features to build to an abstract higher level mid-range theory. This theory may then ultimately be recontextualized and applied to multiple settings.

The goal is to produce an abstract theory consisting of principles that may be applicable to any situation, that may be subsequently tested, that will provide a frame for, and understanding of, practice, and be applied in myriad settings whenever a need for comfort is manifest.

TOWARD THEORY-BASED
INTERVENTIONS

34

THEORETICAL COALESCENCE

> *We are proposing a theory of theories that sees theory as a conceptual*
> *system invented to some purpose—when seen in its full*
> *consequences—has revolutionary possibilities.*
> —Dickoff & James (1968, p. 203)

Theoretical coalescence is a method of combining a series of studies into a whole, to create a higher level theory. The advantages of theoretical coalescence are obvious. It gives new meaning to mid-range theory, enabling it to be moved "up a notch" to a higher level; it enables a theory with *increasing scope* to be developed, and it encompasses increasing complexity. In this way it counters many of the problems we have been discussing with qualitatively derived theory, while at the same time retaining the connection of the theory with the data and the applicability of theory with praxis.

Since the 1990s, researchers have been encouraged to obtain increasing depths of understanding around a research topic. Rather than conducting one small research study after another in a scattered area, they have been encouraged to conduct multiple research projects in a general area, connected laterally or horizontally, to increase knowledge and generalizability of the project. In qualitative inquiry, this is to create a larger theory; in quantitative research this is to develop certainty.

THE LIMITED SCOPE OF MID-RANGE THEORY

Qualitative inquiry is always limited in scope. Qualitative theories are usually small and developed from a small sample within a restricted group and a delimited context. Further, because of the nature of saturation and because the researcher is usually working alone, qualitative studies are often narrow and delimited. However, at the same time there is great confusion about the ability of these mid-range theories to generalize. As each of these "small" studies is published, so does the researcher's "evidence base" and compiled understanding of the whole—of the mid-range theory—become revealed, piece by piece, to build a comprehensive understanding. Theoretical coalescence is a method that formalized these processes of theoretical integration.

Developing Theory From Multiple Qualitative Projects

How do you plan and select these studies? All of the studies are complete projects in themselves and published separately. Investigators are generally interested in a topic and keep conducting studies around that topic. Previously this was called a *research program*, but a more interesting term, *multiple methods*, is now used. Importantly, multiple-method designs are conducted so that the projects will be deliberately synthesized at some point. Research programs were "looser," less well integrated. Previous studies were used to justify the next study (or series of studies) as the investigator worked toward solving some particular problem. With qualitative studies used for theoretical coalescence, the researcher is still seeking understanding, Some of the studies may be partly synthesized and minor models developed, but the end results are very different than a quantitative "solution"—and the application of the research, as a theory, bears no comparison—yet it is equally important for practice.

Developing a Theory of Increasing Scope

Because research is conducting studies according to a certain topic, these studies may be conducted in different areas, with different age groups, cultural groups, illnesses, and at different times in the illness process. Some of the studies may be of different levels of analysis—microanalytic or macroanalytic. Some may even involve quantitative analysis or different methods of qualitative inquiry, producing a different type of data and different types of findings. Some studies may be conducted at a particular point in time; others may be longitudinal. In this way the scope of the overall theory expands in ways that a single study cannot. Conducting a collection of such studies provides differing perspectives, until the research has "3D" vision of the topic, and can answer broad and significant analytic questions. These "data" form the basis for the emerging theory.

Developing Theory of Increasing Complexity

The differing contexts, patient groups, perspectives of those involved (patients, caregivers, families), points in time, levels of analyses, and types of results produce a mirage that resembles the complexity of reality. But the researcher has control. The researcher has a unique perspective that is both within and removed from the patient, and can view the problem from many angles and directions so that inquiry does not stop with a pile of publications. The most exciting part of the inquiry is about to begin. The researcher can then answer the "so what?", and start to bring forth the most interesting and significant ramifications of the previous years of effort.

Can theoretical coalescence be conducted with a collection of studies carried out by others and pieced together as a meta-analysis? Perhaps. It is much easier if the researcher has access to the data and knows it intimately. In this way, *cognitive sliding* is less likely to occur. Researchers will not be guessing about meanings and bending interpretations unconsciously nor deliberately as they fit their findings.

Can theoretical coalescence be conducted by a research team? Certainly—but ideally the team will share the same lab so that constant communications will be the norm. The team should not "fit and force" findings, but work together as they conduct each project, knowing intimately the nuances of each, asking questions of each other's data and emerging analyses. Such research is expensive, but the rewards are paradigm-molding.

Theoretical Coalescence: Developing a High-Level Mid-Range Theory

Theoretical coalescence is a process of:

1. *Identifying significant concepts.*
2. *Evaluating the development of the concepts common to each study:* This will have probably been conducted as each study was conducted, but, for instance in quantitative studies, this may be so. Do these core concepts need to be present in each study? No—other studies may contribute to other types of knowledge. At this point do not exclude any study that you may think may be useful.
3. *Diagramming the concepts, and their position overall*: Locate each concept for each theory, its level of abstraction, and position on the trajectory (noting the target population and so on). Map the concept in position according to the primary contribution it makes to the overall theory.
4. *Identifying the attributes common to each example of the concepts.* Open each of the concepts and seek common attributes between the concepts. This will provide some indication about how the concepts interlock and share attributes or characteristics across conceptual boundaries. Link them laterally or horizontally by connecting them according to shared attributes.

5. *Developing analytic questions about the nature of the overarching concept, identifying the answers in each study, and the attributes/characteristics of each study.*
6. *Diagramming and writing the mid-range theory.*

Figure 34.1 is an example of how a collection of studies may link together. Notice there is no deliberate replication—they do not overlap. Such replication is unnecessary, for we have attended to rigor in the process of inquiry when developing each study. But these studies are theoretically connected, sharing characteristics that contribute to the theoretical development. These characteristics may be deliberately obvious, as in a naturalistic experiment, or they may not be immediately evident, and only by exploring characteristics across studies be understood as useful to the developing theory. Taken as a set, these studies overcome the criticism of the limitations of qualitative inquiry (*small scale, insignificant*), and provide a mid-range theory that is clinically useful and applicable.

The different shapes of the studies represent scope, different populations, age groups, and contexts of the studies. In Figure 34.1, *a* represents a hole—a gap in the research program revealing missing information—or a study planned in the future.

The previous list of five steps makes it appear easy to conduct the last synthesizing procedure to develop the theory. Again the key is developing appropriate analytic questions that are pertinent to the emerging theory. Remember that comfort and discomfort are emotions that are manifest behaviorally. They are signified by expressions and actions and vocalizations. Comforting is an action sometimes initiated by empathetic and compathetic and emotions, and resulting in actions, and sometimes reflective responses. In this case, it is from this perspective, that the analytic questions are developed.

When using theoretical coalescence, each theory is decontextualized to the basic processes and attributes that need to be involved in comforting emotions, actions, processes, and outcomes. Analytic questions first take the form of looking for commonalities between the studies, considering in part

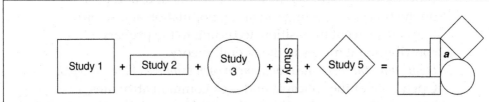

FIGURE 34.1
Placing studies laterally using *theoretical coalescence*, to create a mid-range theory of broader scope than any single study.

a, gap, new data needed.

the different stages of the process of comforting and identifying the major components. Later the questions may even be yes/no, presence or absence questions confirming the axioms of the theory.

Chapters 34 and 35 are examples of theoretical coalescence. The first is a theory of comfort and comforting; the second the *Praxis Theory of Suffering.* This is our goal: a comprehensive theory of nursing, developed from sound and pertinent concepts—one that guides nursing, one that is relevant and patient-centered, but developed rigorously from data. In the 48 years since Dickoff and James expressed their desire for such nursing theory—have we achieved it? Perhaps this is the time: We now have the tools, the methods, the means—and we know what we need. Although we may not reach Dickoff and James's (1968) goal of developing a "conceptual scheme," that will revolutionize nursing, at least we are trying to begin.

REFERENCE

Dickoff, J., & James, P. (1968). A theory of theories: A position paper. *Nursing Research, 17*(3), 197–203.

THE EVOLUTION OF OUR UNDERSTANDING OF SUFFERING: *THE PRAXIS THEORY OF SUFFERING*

The primary role of nursing is to care for those who are ill or are undergoing a physical or psychological health crisis. As a profession, we have developed an extensive base of rote and standardized procedures for caring for the physiological body; as well as some knowledge of suffering in general and the subconcepts, such as grief, and care of the patient and the family when suffering. But our understanding about the *behaviors* of those who are ill and are suffering remains sorely inadequate. Medicine, as a profession, over the past two centuries has developed a compendium of signs and symptoms, mostly developed from informal observations by practicing physicians. These collectively became an encyclopedic knowledge of behaviors that largely became classified as symptoms providing diagnostic cues. Nursing sorely lags in its comprehension of patient behaviors. Most of our therapeutic inter-actions are based on "intuition" (a concept that is poorly described and con-sequently difficult to teach), using trial and error, and implicit, informal learning in the clinical setting.

Yet, human behavior is patterned. In everyday life, we classify and develop lay concepts, and these lay concepts themselves may serve as gate-ways for researchers to use as metaphors and mirrors to develop the human understanding and the knowledge that nursing is seeking. In addition, quali-tative research methods have developed rapidly over the past two decades; these methods themselves provide access, which allows interpretation of implicit and explicit behaviors, and are used as a means to access empathetic insight into the experiences of others. But, with a charge of attending to suffer-ing, nursing has another professional demand: nurses must respond to the needs of the patients within the microseconds that interactions are paced: Nurses do not always have the privilege of knowing what is causing the distress, nor the circumstances that underlie the problem. They must act instantly and based only upon what they see. I call this "reading behavior." In the clinical setting, nurses must respond rapidly to behavioral cues. Sometimes, as Benner and Tanner (1987) noted, these observed cues have physiological bases ("Mrs. Smith—are you all right?"), but often these behaviors result from emotional distress, and the nurse is required to *respond* to the distressed patient without knowing or understanding the cause. Yet, even though the nurse may not know the cause, distress is a complex emotion manifest in many ways with many emotional displays that demand different responses from the nurse so he or she may respond appropriately and therapeutically.

In this chapter, I:

A. Discuss the *background* to the *Praxis Theory of Suffering*
B. Discuss *the physiology of the Praxis Theory of Suffering*, describing how people move through suffering, and provide an overview of how the model "works"
C. Provide an in-depth *description of the major concepts* of *enduring* and *emotional suffering* and the *transition* between the two states, and finally
D. Discuss *suffering as Praxis*.

BACKGROUND

I have been studying these behavioral manifestations of distress for almost three decades, primarily by conducting various types of qualitative inquiry. Patient participants with a number of different illnesses or injuries (both sudden and chronic), as well as the bereaved, have shared their stories and agreed to be observed. From these data, I have been able to delineate behavioral modes of suffering. When one asks those who are suffering to "tell their story," in the process of narration, the emotions they felt at the time re-emerge. I call this *emotional re-enactment* (Morse, 2002), and it lends validity and credence to the research. I collected narrative interviews with those who were recovering from major accidents, illnesses, or bereavement; I also conducted observational research in the trauma room, emergency departments (EDs), and in hospital units. I observed videos of birthing (Bergstrom et al., 2009; Bergstrom, Richards, Morse, & Roberts, 2010), and conducted interviews with patients, relatives, and nursing staff. In the past three decades this has resulted in approximately 27 studies of suffering behaviors.

Despite the emerging patterns from which states of suffering have been identified, behaviors of suffering are neither constant nor stable; the different causes of the suffering, and the different meanings this has for individuals that the suffering signified, result in differences in responses in intensity and duration of suffering. I labeled the first major behavioral state as *enduring*, and the second, *emotional suffering*. My goal was to develop behavioral indices of these behaviors, so that nurses may recognize these states clinically, that they may be taught, and so that strategies that ease and relieve suffering (that is, comforting) may be identified (see Chapter 36). I explored how people "exited" the state of enduring *if* the cause of their distress was removed; and the behaviors that those who were enduring used to release the energy that was contained, without moving into emotional suffering. I observed how people responded to the behavioral cues of those who were enduring, and expanded these databases by using photographs from newspapers and those appearing on the Internet. Finally, I conducted microanalysis of the behavioral transition between enduring and suffering (Morse, Beres, Spiers, Mayan, & Olson, 2003).

Throughout, I noted that, despite the fact that enduring was extraordinarily common, and was even evident in movies,[1] it was not clearly described in the literature.[2] Of importance is the fact that enduring was a concept that may be observed as participants told their stories during interviews. Because enduring behaviors are so internalized, those who are enduring do not have insight into their own behaviors. They will tell you that they are "managing well," or are coping "fine," rather than "bearing it" (whatever *it* may be) and this suppression inhibits or blocks our ability as researchers to understand their experience.

I explored the second state, *emotional suffering*, the same way. Those who were emotionally suffering were so focused on their own sorrow that they were sometimes even unable to articulate without sobbing. One student who was studying the experience of fathers of sons who had died of AIDS found fathers too distressed to tell their stories, despite the fact that they wanted to be a part of the study. She gave the father a lapel microphone and took him for a walk on his farm; only then was he able to speak of his suffering.

When narrating their stories, participants transitioned from enduring to emotional suffering, and the patterns of the transitioning behaviors were, in retrospect, evident, even during interviews. Then, in 2003, we constructed and deliberately analyzed these transitional behaviors inherent by collecting videotaped interviews of those who were suffering from various illnesses, accidents, or the relatives of those who experienced the death of a loved one. This enabled us to synchronize the emotional state (as manifest in facial expression [Ekman & Friesen, 2003]) with the content of monologue as their stories unfolded (Morse et al., 2003).

---

[1] An excellent depiction of enduring behavior is by William Hurt in *The Accidental Tourist* (1988, Warner Bros. Inc.).

[2] Some authors write of "enduring suffering," but if the concepts of enduring and emotional suffering are used as they are defined and described here, enduring suffering (see, for instance, Duggleby, 2000) is not possible: One cannot simultaneously suppress and release emotions.

The most extraordinary observation from this research program was that the behaviors were similar between participants regardless of what was being suffered. In hindsight, this should not have been unexpected: If we enter a room where everyone is laughing, we do not need to hear the joke to understand that these people were enjoying something funny. Of course, there was individual variation in the expression—as well as contextual and cultural variation, and variation by age and gender—but the important point is that now we have achieved our interpretative goal: We can now describe the dominant indicators of enduring and emotional suffering, so that nurses may quickly identify and meet the needs of the emotional states of patients who are suffering.

Early Conceptualizations of Suffering

Before 1991, I had a number of master's students conducting grounded theory studies on a number of topics, but primarily illnesses. In 1991, six of these grounded theories were published in a single volume, *The Illness Experience: Dimensions of Suffering* (Morse & Johnson, 1991). The title was suggested by the publisher—until that time I was more interested in comfort and comforting, and had not considered that the "umbrella" of this research program was under the rubric of suffering. However, Chapter 33 of this book was the meta-analysis, developing the *Illness-Constellation Model*, which clearly showed the significance of suffering and provided the initial groundwork for the development of the *Praxis Theory of Suffering* and the initial descriptions of enduring and emotional suffering behavior. As we began to research comfort and comforting, it was evident that until we understood *suffering* and were able to interpret states of suffering, we would not be able to understand comforting. This research was also essential to be able to interpret the changing nature of suffering during comforting interactions.

In 1993, I worked with a postdoctoral fellow, Barbara Carter, and she brought her theory of the *reformulated self* to my attention. In light of this, we analyzed secondary data and developed the enduring further, identified strategies of enduring as ways of *preserving self* (Morse & O'Brien, 1995), and developed the preliminary model of the *Praxis Theory of Suffering* (Morse & Carter, 1995). This work continued to be developed, with new versions published in 2001, 2011, and 2015.

Theoretical Cohesion: Targeted Data Collection to Understand States of Suffering

Our insight into the *Praxis Theory of Suffering* did not come all at once, and the studies described in Figure 35.1 were neither conducted systematically nor

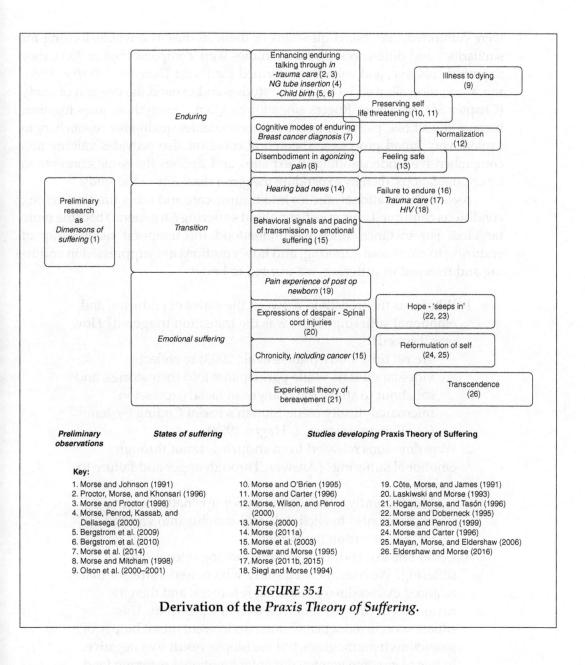

| Preliminary observations | States of suffering | Studies developing Praxis Theory of Suffering |

FIGURE 35.1

Derivation of the *Praxis Theory of Suffering.*

Key contained in figure:

Key:

1. Morse and Johnson (1991)
2. Proctor, Morse, and Khonsari (1996)
3. Morse and Proctor (1998)
4. Morse, Penrod, Kassab, and Dellasega (2000)
5. Bergstrom et al. (2009)
6. Bergstrom et al. (2010)
7. Morse et al. (2014)
8. Morse and Mitcham (1998)
9. Olson et al. (2000–2001)

10. Morse and O'Brien (1995)
11. Morse and Carter (1996)
12. Morse, Wilson, and Penrod (2000)
13. Morse (2000)
14. Morse (2011a)
15. Morse et al. (2003)
16. Dewar and Morse (1995)
17. Morse (2011b, 2015)
18. Siegl and Morse (1994)

19. Côte, Morse, and James (1991)
20. Laskiwski and Morse (1993)
21. Hogan, Morse, and Tasón (1996)
22. Morse and Doberneck (1995)
23. Morse and Penrod (1999)
24. Morse and Carter (1996)
25. Mayan, Morse, and Eldershaw (2006)
26. Eldershaw and Morse (2016)

sequentially. The conceptualization of suffering occurred over time as the studies were conducted, and, in retrospect, by thinking about the collective whole—"fit" occurred later. The studies contributing to the theory accrued as we first conducted research into the illness experience. These data collected for the "comfort grant" commenced in the ED and trauma centers; video and interview data collected on comforting also contained important data describing states of suffering, as well as descriptions of the ways in which suffering diminished as patients were comforted.[3] We asked questions of these studies as a whole, looking for similarities and differences. As these studies were compiled (Figure 35.1), they appeared cohesive, and collectively formed the *Praxis Theory of Suffering*. Theoretical cohesion allowed us to link the studies and expand the domain of study (Chapter 34). As Mister Rogers sings for children, "Everything goes together, because it's all one piece," internal cohesion enables qualitative researchers to explore very broad processes. Theoretical cohesion also provides validity and comprehensive understanding; it explores and applies the same concepts to other populations, thereby expanding the generalizability of the study.

As our observational studies into trauma care and other life-threatening conditions continued, our questions about suffering (in general) became more targeted. For instance, once we understood the temporal relationship of enduring to emotional suffering, and how emotions are suppressed in enduring and released in suffering, we wanted to know:

1. What was the transition between the states of enduring and emotional suffering? How was the transition triggered? How was it paced?

   We set up a study (Morse et al., 2003) to collect videotaped data while participants told their stories, and set about to study the changes in facial expression microanalytically using Ekman's Facial Coding System (see Ekman, Friesen, & Hager, 1978).

2. Were emotions released from enduring, if not through emotional suffering? (Answer: Through anger and failure to endure).

   Most recently, we deliberately set up "naturalistic experiments" to elicit data and insights into various processes within the model.

3. Could one exit enduring without moving into emotional suffering? We constructed a study, which used a stressor that required extraordinary enduring resources, and then the reason to endure was removed form the particant. This situation occurred when women underwent breast biopsy of a suspicious mammogram, but the biopsy result was negative. In this case, some women did enter emotional suffering (and cried tears of relief); others became "high" and giggly. Yet others continued to suffer, fully believing they did have cancer (the doctor simply had not found it yet; Morse et al., 2014).

These findings were then incorporated into the *Praxis Theory of Suffering*.

---

[3] This work was supported with federal grants: In 1994, I received a 5-year renewal from the National Institute of Nursing Research (NINR), National Institutes of Health (NIH), specifically to explore suffering in comforting; in 1998 I received a grant from the Canadian Institutes of Health Research (CIHR) to identify patterns of suffering; and in 2001 I received a grant from the Alberta Cancer Foundation.

THE PHYSIOLOGY OF THE MODEL

The model of the *Praxis Theory of Suffering* is shown in Figure 35.2. It is not a linear model, although all enter the model when they learn of a distressful event. However, within the model, individuals may take a number of pathways; they may remain in a particular state for as long as they need to, move from enduring to emotional suffering, and find that their emotions are too intense, and again retreat to enduring.

For earlier versions of this model, see Morse (2001, 2011b, 2015) and Morse and Carter (1996).

Entering Enduring

All persons enter the model when they hear of or experience a distressful event. The event may be hearing bad news about their own diagnosis, or their loved one, or they (or their loved one) may have a sudden serious accident or died. These events may begin suddenly, or the persons may go through a period suspecting that something is wrong.

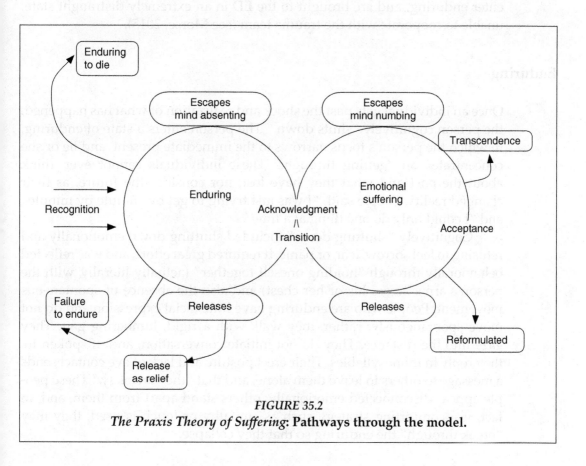

FIGURE 35.2
The Praxis Theory of Suffering: **Pathways through the model.**

Inevitably, persons pass through a period of shock, horror, and unreality. But as soon as they recognize what has happened, they enter into the state of enduring. Enduring is important; it enables the persons to keep functioning. I argue that the most important function during enduring is the suppression of emotions. They deliberately suppress feelings of panic, terror, or horror, so that the persons may protect themselves or those for whom they are responsible. If there has been a car accident, the persons will "check themselves out" to determine the extent of their own injuries. They ask people standing by (lay first-aiders) "not to move them," and may even direct rescue persons.

Failure to Endure

"Failing to endure" became an important component of the theory. In retrospect, we saw these behaviors in Laskiwski's ethnography of spinal cord injured patients (Laskiwski & Morse, 1993)—who had "tantrums," and "swore"—and later reports of relatives in the trauma center when their loved ones were receiving emergency care (Morse & Pooler, 2002).

Enduring mechanisms may fail if the person is inebriated, has taken drugs, or is in excruciating pain or severely injured. These people may not enter enduring, and are brought to the ED in an extremely distraught state, unable to cooperate with the trauma team (see Morse, 2015).

Enduring

Once an individual gets past the shock and realization of what has happened, the person cognitively "shuts down." The person enters a state of enduring, in which the person's focus narrows to the immediate present, and he or she concentrates on "getting through." These individuals cannot even think about the past and what they have lost, nor consider the future, as their changed reality. People said, "I was just trying to get by, minute by minute" and "I could only do one thing at a time."

Cognitively "shutting down" included shutting down emotionally and refusing to feel sorrow, fear, or panic. It required great effort, and was reflected behaviorally through "holding oneself together" (actually literally, with the person's arms across his or her chest) and also the absence of spontaneous movement. People who are enduring have little facial expression and do not move spontaneously; rather, they walk with a rigid, lumbering gait. They gaze into the distance. They do not initiate conversation, and, if spoken to, they reply in monosyllables. Their erect posture and lack of eye contact sends a message to others to leave them alone, and that "they are okay." These people appear disconnected emotionally; others stand apart from them, and, in fact, if a comforting strategy such as empathy or touch is used, they may "break through" the enduring so that they collapse.

Enduring enables people to continue with their daily lives and responsibilities, albeit mechanically. A study of fathers whose wives were undergoing chemotherapy (Wilson & Morse, 1993) described how fathers managed their work roles as well as family responsibilities (cooking and caring for the children) by "blocking" (enduring) emotions.

People who are seriously ill or injured appear in a state of enduring. The lack of emotional expression conserves their energy. We labeled this state as "preserving self" (Morse & O'Brien, 1995)—a concept that has expanded to refer to strategies that people use to retain their identity in such debilitation illnesses as Parkinson's disease (Vann-Ward, 2016) or dementia (Surr, 2006). As the person becomes closer to dying, he or she may quietly move from this state, "slipping away" as he or she dies (Olson et al., 2000–2001).

Cognitive mechanisms are in place during enduring to reduce suffering. In the case of agonizing pain, it was clear from the interviews that the person disembodied the painful parts of their body; for instance, referring to one's own hand as "it" (Morse & Mitcham, 1998). Using this signal in the interviews, we could trace the phase in rehabilitation when these individuals re-embodied once the pain was controlled and "took their bodies back."

The Attributes of Enduring

From this descriptive research we identified four conceptual attributes of enduring. These are:

1. Maintaining control of self
2. Living in the present moment
3. Removing oneself from the situation
4. Being aware of the danger or consequences of emotional disintegration (Morse, 2011b, 2015).

Maintaining Control of Self

Self-control is a process in which the emotions of despair are deliberately suppressed. For example, when learning of a diagnosis, the extent of one's injuries, or that someone has died, panic threatens to overwhelm the person. He or she grapples with the news, trying to understand, but at the same time the person is trying to disbelieve what he or she is actually hearing. These individuals do not know and cannot grasp the ramifications of the situation, and it takes deliberate effort to maintain self-control.

At the moment of receiving bad news, the body shuts down. People report hearing a buzz in their ears, or may not be able to hear at all, but just see the physician's mouth move.

> It's like I wasn't there; It was happening to someone else; My legs just absolutely collapsed underneath me; I was in shock for days, you know, physical, its physical shock. (Hogan, Morse, & Tasón, 1996, p. 52)

Often the response is physical, with individuals reporting that their legs gave way and that they fell on the floor. Others respond with a howl.

> I started howling, and howling, crying from some place that is almost animal, absolutely beyond a kind of mental thing at all. Its just animal...I just fell apart, fell on the couch and howled for about fifteen minutes because, I guess, I thought he was gonna be here when I got back (from a trip), and he wasn't. And I just howled. (Hogan, Morse, & Tasón, 1996, p. 53)

Once the immediate news is received, these individuals refuse to let the sorrow or shock "show on their face" for fear of upsetting others. Cognitively, they block tears from forming, refuse to complain, and deliberately refuse to think about the ramifications of whatever is being suffered. They strive to maintain a normal schedule, do not tell others, and are aware that displays of crying or sorrow are distressing to others and conceal whatever they may be suffering.

> I think it's an unconscious thing you do. You have to guard yourself—it's a measure of self control you have. You have to guard yourself against allowing [breaking down]. I suppose it's a form of emotional distance, that you are disciplined emotion- ally. Now you don't ever allow yourself to cry. You don't do it especially in their presence. I did that [crying] in the car, coming and going, running around. (Morse & Carter, 1996, p. 54)

This suppression of emotions is so extreme that it is manifested behav- iorally. People who are enduring do not display facial expressions of sorrow but appear to gaze off into the distance. They stand erect with a dignified expression, and may appear to walk stiffly without spontaneous movement. Family members and caregivers stand apart without touching them.

Living in the Present Moment

Individuals who are enduring reduce the distress by limiting their immediate focus to whatever they are doing at the moment. They refuse to consider the future ramifications of the event by focusing intensely on the present. This enables them not to feel overwhelmed, to focus on one task at a time so they may get through the next moment, hour, or day. At the extreme end, trauma patients control the situation by focusing on breathing in and breathing out. In the intensive care unit, burn patients in extreme pain watch the clock move minute by minute, and count numbers of treatments. Those in bereavement get through the day one step at a time. All of these people tell us that they cannot see the big picture—it causes too much anxiety or sorrow—they focus on getting through the next minute, next hour, or next day.

Removing Oneself From the Situation

Those who are enduring avoid contact with others who may express sympathy, or publicly acknowledge whatever is being suffered. Such condolences for the bereaved "make the death real." Therefore, these bereaved avoid going to church or to stores where they are known and may meet their neighbors. Those who are injured avoid the glances and looks of others, preferring to remain at home until they are ready to handle the emotions that such interactions evoke.

Aware of the Consequences of Emotional Disintegration

All of the aforementioned strategies are temporary. Continual effort is required to reduce the effects of the calamity, injuries, or deaths overwhelming these individuals. Resisting crying becomes an ever-present goal and these people are afraid that "if they begin to cry they will not be able to stop." They are metaphorically afraid they will "break down," and if they move into emotional suffering, they will not be available to help others, to care for their children, and that their own distress will distress others. Enduring is a stoic state.

Enduring was often deliberate, requiring effort to "refuse to cry." In interviews, people often paused, blinding and fighting back tears, willing themselves not to cry, and re-entering enduring. At other times, in particular when a sympathetic comment was unexpected and it broke through the seal of enduring, people may "break down" in emotional suffering.

Of importance, those who are enduring do not tolerate sympathy, empathy, or even acknowledgment of what they are experiencing. The condolences offered by others is an additional "think" to endure. Those in the bereavement study spoke of the importance of sympathy cards: "You could read them, when you were *ready*." Therefore, the nursing interactions with the person who is enduring, described in Chapter 26, are to stand apart, not to use comforting touch, not to overwhelm the person with information, and not to use comforting strategies that one uses with a person in emotional suffering.

We conducted an ethnography of children who were normally nursed at home, but on respirators, who were invited to summer camp (Morse, Wilson, & Penrod, 2000). There, the cognitive strategies of enduring took a different form, as children compared tracheostomy tubing ("like mine") and entered into physical abilities that were usually the purview of more active children, such as horse riding, swimming in a pool, and even parading in a Mardi Gras.

What do patients endure? First, they endure the physical discomforts and pain of illness, injury, or childbirth. As with the trauma patient, this enduring often requires coaching in the form of "talking through" using the Comfort Talk Register (Proctor et al., 1996) behavioral assistance with behavioral control, as midwives who are expert at talking through demonstrate

(Bergstrom et al., 2009, 2010). Nurses use the register to talk patients through painful procedures, such as nasogastric (NG) tube insertion (Morse et al., 2000) in which patient behaviors must be coordinated with the nursing action in order for safe completion of the task.

Patients also endure fears of a poor prognosis, of surgery and other treatments, of loss of a physical ability, or even loss of a body part. They lose relationships, home, and family, and suffer financially and spiritually. They have day-to-day irritants and loss of control, as they wait and wait. These processes also are reflected as enduring behaviors, and are managed cognitively as they try to make sense of their predicament. Hearing bad news is a common situation that patients experience, yet there is little information about what patients can actually hear when they are given bad news. Processes of enduring override comprehension, so that little of what is reported to the patient may be actually later recalled (Morse, 2011a).

What is failure to endure? If a patient is overwhelmed with pain, fear, or terror, or the illness is unbearable and the person can no longer "take it," the person loses control.

> Participant: Then they sent me to the hospital for a right—you know—catheterization. And they told me I had a heart condition that my brother and my father had died from. So I just—
> Int: Tell me what you did—
> Partic: I threw magazines around; kicked chairs; and threw a regular fit. (Dewar & Morse, 1995, p. 961)

In trauma care, nurses describe patients who are *terrified* or *lose control*. Patients who are terrified may be seriously injured, and often inebriated. They shout, loudly protest, and resist care (calling "Nooooooo!!! There is nothing wrong with it!! STOP!"). They may struggle and try to get up from the gurney.

Those who are *out of control* display screaming, hysterical, and bellowing behavior. They do not speak in coherent sentences, but use single words that are often unintelligible, guttural sounds. They yell at maximum volume and do not respond to staff commands. Staff no longer interact with these patients; they simply go ahead administering essential care.

If removing oneself from the situation is not possible, as previously noted, the persons may fight care (Morse, 2015). If the failure to endure occurs in a nonthreatening situation, and the person has the ability, the emotions of enduring may be expulsed as anger or rage. The persons in the ED waiting room may kick the soda machine when losing a quarter—an action that he or she would not normally do. The emotions appear as shouting, and often a lack of control. In a study of the spinal cord unit, the patients often lost control and swore, which was interpreted as an expression of grief due to their lost abilities (Laskiwski & Morse, 1993). More commonly, however, is that the person moves into emotional suffering.

I am often asked: "How long do people endure?" People endure apparently for as long as they need to; they transition into emotional suffering, but if the emotions are too powerful and they fear they cannot be controlled, they immediately move back into enduring.

But enduring was not a continuous state: When these fathers needed to emotionally suffer, they did so in private by, for instance, stopping the car on the way home from work to cry. Other participants reported similar behaviors of hiding their emotional suffering: A wife of a seriously burnt linesman would retreat to the bathroom, crying in the shower. But the "switch" between enduring and emotional suffering is clearly delineated, and we called the state between enduring and emotional suffering *transition*. Individuals can move between enduring, in which emotions are suppressed, and emotional suffering, in which emotions are released. When transition is triggered, emotion overwhelms these individuals, and if they choose not to display sorrow, they may fight to regain control of enduring.

Mind Absenting Escapes for Enduring

Cognitively, these patients remove themselves from the situation by focusing intensely on tasks. In the rehabilitation unit, these patients focus on puzzles (especially jigsaw puzzles) or television. Women may knit. All appreciate nurses' small talk and jokes, repeating them endlessly as a distraction. These strategies remove these people from their situation, although temporarily. Patients tell us that they keep busy and focus.

Enduring to Die

While many studies have been conducted on dying in oncology, few have connected the illness trajectory with dying. In this study, as the patients began physical deterioration and entered a stage of progressive withdrawal, we termed it enduring to die. Emotions were "buried" beneath the surface, and families reduced their distractions and boundaries. Visitors were reduced to a minimum, and patients lived moment by moment, a process we labeled *cocooning*. These patients were resigned to dying, and simply "faded away."

Relief as Release

In the previously described study of women undergoing diagnosis for breast cancer (Morse et al., 2014), we examined data for reports of women exiting the state of enduring without releasing as in emotional suffering. Some did release by displaying tears (the physician reported "we get more tears from those who are negative"), but some did respond with joy, laughter, and giggles.

Transition: Moving Between Enduring and Emotional Suffering

At this time, we realized that people who transitioned from enduring to emotional suffering are transitioned for the purpose of releasing the pent-up emotions of enduring, when they could no longer be contained, or they no longer needed to endure. It occurs when the individual acknowledges that the loss has actually occurred.

> I was letting it in little by little, because, even when he passed
> away, I know I had this feeling that if I really let myself feel the
> way I really feel, If I let myself out of control, that my heart
> would break. That's what I felt. (Morse & Carter, 1996, p. 52)

Some participants would try to keep talking to maintain control, and if they were able to return to the neutral expression of enduring, they were able to return to the actual state of enduring. However, most became agitated and would reach for a tissue or start rocking back and forth; their eyes would then tear up as they moved into emotional suffering.

A microanalysis of the facial expressions that occur in the transition between enduring and suffering is extraordinarily patterned. The first indicator of the transition from enduring to emotional suffering was frequent, rapid, undirected movement of the eye. Participants' eyes darted around the room but remained unseeing and unfocused (Morse et al., 2003). As emotions broke through the neutral facial expression, participants would cease speaking, frown, their lips began to quiver, and they often raised their hands to their mouths, pressing their fingers against their lips. About this time, their eyes would tear up. Speech was marked with swallowing and cracking of the voice, and with long pauses. Their eyes would blink rapidly as they tried to regain control. The mean time for these transitions from enduring to emotional suffering was 18.9 seconds (a range of 7.5 to 35 seconds); see Figure 35.3(a).

Transitioning into emotional suffering may be uncontrolled or may be deliberate and controlled. If controlled, persons feel that they are "ready"; if it is uncontrolled and unexpected, persons may be "sideswiped," the barriers of enduring break down, and they may even collapse on the floor.

Emotional Suffering

What Is Emotional Suffering?

Emotional suffering is a state of distress in which emotions are released and expressed (Morse, 2001, p. 51). The emotional resources can no longer be controlled or contained within persons and overwhelm them as despair, grief, and sorrow. They mourn the lost past and the irretrievably altered future. They weep, cry, and sob, often publicly; their facial expression is one of sorrow, lined and "drooped." Their posture is stooped; they sigh and talk incessantly in a sorrowful voice about whatever it is they are suffering. When persons are emotionally suffering, they accept the event in the past and recognize the ramifications of their loss that has resulted in their present predicament.

Emotional suffering is physically exhausting. Those who are suffering demand to be held and comforted; they want to be held and they appreciate a listening ear. Their body posture sends a message to others: Comfort me. However, emotional suffering is not a consistent state; emotions may come in waves, varying in intensity, as persons recall their plight. At this time, they are psychologically working through, mourning their lost past and their altered perception of the future.

With Nancy Hogan, I studied the emotional suffering of bereavement, interviewing those who were at least 6 months from the death of their loved one. As survivors told their stories of the course of their bereavements, the intensity of the emotions changed according to the nature of the ongoing narrative (Hogan et al., 1996). We interviewed those with relatives whose death was expected (those with chronic illness or the aged) and those whose death was unexpected (from suicide, accident, or acute illness); we interviewed those whose loss they considered timely (i.e., older adults) or untimely (too young).

This *experiential theory of suffering* revealed that the emotional responses varied according to the nature of the death of the loved one, and that the context determined the course of the bereavement itself. The relatives of those who were expecting the death endured during the illness, and then moved into emotional suffering relatively quickly and experienced intense grief. The emotional suffering was not one that was "resolved," but rather one that was adapted "to the reality of the loss," and that the "deaths changed the survivors in permanent ways" (Hogan et al., 1996, p. 62).

Mind Numbing Escapes for Emotional Suffering
Mind numbing escapes are those activities that remove the person from the situation. For those who are emotionally suffering, these are watching TV excessively, drinking, using drugs, or excessive sleeping.

Releases for Emotional Suffering
Releases are activities that distract the person from the emotional suffering. People who are emotionally suffering do not like to be alone. Activities, such as talking on the phone, going to the movies, staying with friends, and eating, are important.

Acceptance: "Coming Out of Emotional Suffering?"
Once a person accepts that which is being suffered and comes to terms with the altered life, he or she may begin to move out of suffering. Hope seeps in and the individual views life with a new perspective. These people reorder

their values and priorities about life and living, recognizing that they are different people from having suffered. They feel privileged and able to help others who are in the midst of enduring and emotional suffering. They often work to serve others through advocacy activities, lean to support groups, volunteer at hospitals, and so forth. It is clear that one emotionally suffers as long as one needs to suffer. In our study of bereavement, suffering was continuing at 32 years (Hogan et al., 1996). But others reported lives that were richer and fuller following the experience of emotional suffering. We recall Carter's (1993) concept of "reformulated self" and the literature describing transcendence (see Chapter 20, Eldershaw & Morse, this volume).

Reformulated Self

Those who leave emotional suffering come to see their lives with a new perspective, and reorder their own values and priorities about how they want to live their life. They have an urge to give back, especially to others who are suffering. For instance, one burn patient reported that she took a course in camouflage makeup so that she could help other burn patients. They feel in a special position to help others, and helping others fills them with joy.

These victims reformulate and consider themselves better for the experience of suffering:

> I'm sort of caught between the person I was, and—I'm not the
> person I was. And I'm kind of growing—but I'm not quite sure
> where I'm growing. I guess you can't see the end of the road. I
> have a new path to follow, but exactly where I am going, I don't
> know. I trust in the Lord and go, like I say, slowly. But I do get
> very impatient. I look at life differently. I have a constant battle
> back and forth. A part of me wants the way I was before, so that
> I still get depressed and frustrated when I go shopping because I
> feel limited in what I can wear, with the long-sleeve aspect of
> things. I'm still not ready to wear sleeveless things . . . some days
> I'm ready and some days I'm not. (Morse & Carter, 1996, p. 55)

Suffering as Praxis

The Importance of Learning to "Read" the Patient's State
Teaching/Learning Suffering
Nurses can usually recognize the states of suffering from the descriptions of the behaviors: They have seen suffering in their personal lives, as well as in the clinical setting. They recognize the posturing, the facial expressions, and patterns of speech with those who are enduring and suffering.

Figure 35.3 is a comparison of facial expressions of those who are enduring, in transition, and emotional suffering. In enduring, the face is relatively blank, except for the brow, which may be furrowed. In transition, the face looks as if the persons have "shut down": They look away, hold their hand to their lips, close their eyes—which start to tear. If persons continue into emotional suffering (and they do not always do this—some may move back into enduring), their eyes may tear and close, they look away, their mouth is pulled back, and their head is down.

Differences in posture between those who are enduring and those who are emotionally suffering are great. Those who are enduring stand erect, with their head up, in a dignified stance. They do *not* give signals that they would welcome to be touched, hugged, or comforted. Quite the opposite—the cue

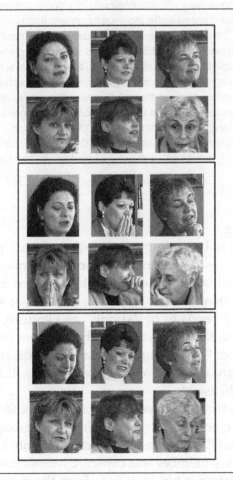

(A) Enduring: Face lacks spontaneous expression; eyes gaze into the distance; brow is furrowed.

(B) Transition: Eyes close or look away, and may start to tear; speech hesitates; mouth pulls back; hand may come up to the face, with fingers over the mouth.

(C) Emotional suffering: Eyes tear, or lids are closed; brow furrowed; mouth pulled back; head down.

FIGURE 35.3

Faces of suffering: (A) enduring, (B) transition, and (C) emotional suffering.

Source: Morse et al. (2003). Reprinted with permission from Sage Publications.

they send is that they want to be left alone, and people do step back. Those who are suffering are "crumbled" and have the appearance of needing to be held. They accept touch and a listening ear.

Nursing interactions for patients in each of these states differ according to the patient state, as the patient's degree of comprehension and ability to hear and respond differs with each state. Of importance, patient states may rapidly change as the patient's condition changes, levels of pain vary, and emotions are triggered, such as fear.

TO DO 35.1. LEARN TO IDENTIFY STATES OF ENDURING FROM EMOTIONAL SUFFERING

1. Search the web for groups of people who are suffering. You will notice that if you use "suffering" as the search term, you will retrieve great works of art, depicting emotional suffering. But if you search for current events that have caused suffering—earthquakes, floods, fires, accidents, and so forth—you will get very interesting pictures from which you can easily identify states of enduring or emotional suffering. Examine both the person that the photographer has targeted and the states of the people in the background. Often the target person is emotionally suffering and those in the background are enduring. Why do photographers target those who are emotionally suffering rather than enduring? Examine the proximal relationships of groups of people. Who are the supporters and who are releasing emotions? Who are the comforters? Note the states (enduring or emotional suffering) of each person.
2. Examine photographs of formal ceremonies, such as funerals. Do you think conventions and ceremonies support enduring or emotional suffering behaviors in the bereaved? How? Why?

The Synchrony of Suffering

Within families, there appears to be an implicit code that during periods of crisis, family members take care of one another. Family members tend to "monitor" each other to ensure that the others are "okay." When one person is emotionally suffering, another will tend to assume the role of supporter; one person in the family group tends to be "strong" and endure, watching over the others and assuming tasks. However, later they may switch roles so that the strong enduring member "takes a turn" and suffers. If the mother has particular responsibilities toward children or other tasks, she will move into enduring to manage them, if she is able.

We were able to explore patterns of interactions between those who were enduring and those who were emotionally suffering in family groups as they entered the trauma room to visit their injured or ill family member (Morse & Pooler, 2002). If the injured family member was conscious, those family members who were emotionally suffering hid their face from the patient. Those who were enduring often took their lead from the nurse and repeated her instructions: "You are doing fine"; "Brave girl"; "We're proud of you, you're so strong" (Morse & Pooler, 2002, p. 247).

Patient States in Trauma Care

The next phase of the research was to simultaneously explore states of suffering and comforting. I considered the optimal setting for exploring states of suffering to be in the trauma center, so I videotaped 178 resuscitations in three medical centers, as well as collected many targeted interviews with patients, staff, and relatives. These observational video data were particularly significant, as the actions may be replayed, slowed, and zoomed; interrater reliability established; and the dialogue recorded. The styles of interactions for the trauma patient are described elsewhere (Morse, 2015, pp. 557–585).

From these data we developed a compendium of states of the trauma patient. While it is clear that some of these states may be classified as "enduring"—for instance, "scared"—and some as emotional suffering (e.g., frightened), others were a "failure to endure" ("terrified" and "out of control"). The behaviors were on a continuum, from scared, to anxious, to frightened, to terrified, to out of control, and those at the extreme end (very dangerous states [Morse, 2015]). When "terrified" and "out of control," the person fights essential care, forcing the caregivers to restrain the patient with physical restraints or use pharmaceutical medications. (If with physical restraints or being held by assistants, the patient will continue to resist, which may cause further injury to the patient.)

Patient States May Be Modified by the Caregiver; Such Actions Are a Component of Care

Interactions with patients who are suffering must be provided within the patient's state (Morse, 2000). Patients who are enduring must be interacted with and provided with care that supports their state of enduring. They should not be touched; empathic statements should not be used, as such statements are resisted by the persons and break through enduring. Often significant others, recognizing the pent-up emotions, feel that "if she would cry, she would be all right" and use approaches intending to move the person to emotional suffering. However, interactions must follow the cues of the individual who is suffering; the person will transition into emotional suffering once he or she is ready.

On the other hand, patients who are emotionally suffering must be provided with comforting strategies that support the emotional suffering. These are described in the *Praxis Theory of Comfort and Comforting* (Chapter 36).

TO DO 35.2. CONSIDER THE EMOTIONAL CONTAGION OF SUFFERING

Enduring and emotional suffering trigger emotions in us as observers. How do these emotions differ? What kinds of responses in the observer do they elicit?

REFERENCES

Benner, P., & Tanner, C. (1987). How expert nurses use intuition. *The American Journal of Nursing, 87*(1), 23–34.

Bergstrom, L., Richards, L., Morse, J., & Roberts, J. (2010). How caregivers manage pain and distress in second stage labor. *Journal of Midwifery and Women's Health, 55*(1), 38–45.

Bergstrom, L., Richards, L., Proctor, A., Bohrer-Avila, L., Morse, J., & Roberts, J. (2009). Birth talk in second stage labor. *Qualitative Health Research, 19,* 954–964.

Carter, B. J. (1993). Long-term survivors of breast cancer: A qualitative descriptive study. *Cancer Nursing, 16*(5), 354–361.

Côté, J. J., Morse, J. M., & James, S. G. (1991). The pain experience of the post-operative newborn. *Journal of Advanced Nursing, 16,* 378–387.

Dewar, A., & Morse, J. M. (1995). Unbearable incidents: Failure to endure the experience of illness. *Journal of Advanced Nursing, 22*(5), 957–964.

Duggleby, W. (2000). Enduring suffering: A grounded theory analysis of the pain experience of elderly hospice patients with cancer. *Oncology Nursing Forum, 27*(5), 825–831.

Ekman, P., & Friesen, W. V. (2003). *Unmasking the face: A guide to recognizing emotions from facial clues.* Los Altos, CA: ISHK.

Ekman, P., Friesen, W. V., & Hager, J. (1978). *The Facial Action Coding System (FACS): A technique for the measurement of facial action. Palo Alto.* Palo Alto, CA: Consulting Psychologists Press.

Eldershaw, P. L., & Morse, J. M. (2016). Self-transcendence and self-reformulation: one concept or two? In J. M. Morse (Ed.), *Analyzing and conceptualizing the theoretical foundations of nursing* (pp. 357–386). New York, NY: Springer Publication Company.

Hogan, N., Morse, J. M., & Tasón, M. C. (1996). Toward an experiential theory of bereavement. *Omega, 33*(1), 43–65.

Laskiwski, S., & Morse, J. M. (1993). The spinal cord injured patient: The modification of hope and expressions of despair. *Canadian Journal of Rehabilitation, 6*(3), 143–153.

Mayan, M., Morse, J. M., & Eldershaw, L. P. (2006). Developing the concept of self-reformulation. *International Journal of Qualitative Studies on Health and Well-Being, 1*(1), 20–26.

Morse, J. M. (2000). On comfort and comforting. *American Journal of Nursing, 100*(9), 34–38.

Morse, J. M. (2001). Toward a *Praxis Theory of Suffering. Advances in Nursing Science, 24*(1), 4759.

Morse, J. M. (2002). Emotional re-enactment [Editorial]. *Qualitative Health Research, 12*(2), 147.

Morse, J. M. (2011a). Hearing bad news. *Journal of Humanistic Medicine, 32,* 187–211. doi:10.1007/s10912-011-9138-4

Morse, J. M. (2011b). The *Praxis Theory of Suffering.* In J. B. Butts & K. L. Rich (Eds.), *Philosophies and theories in advanced nursing practice* (pp. 569–602). Sudbury, MA: Jones & Bartlett.

Morse, J. M. (2015). The *Praxis Theory of Suffering.* In J. B. Butts & K. L. Rich (Eds.), *Philosophies and theories in advanced nursing practice* (pp. 559–586). Sudbury, MA: Jones & Bartlett.

Morse, J. M., Beres, M., Spiers, J., Mayan, M., & Olson, K. (2003). Identifying signals of suffering by linking verbal and facial cues. *Qualitative Health Research, 13*(8), 1063–1077.

Morse, J. M., & Carter, B. J. (1995). Strategies of enduring and the suffering of loss: Modes of comfort used by a resilient survivor. *Holistic Nursing Practice, 9*(3), 33–58.

Morse, J. M., & Carter, B. (1996). The essence of enduring and the expression of suffering: The reformulation of self. *Scholarly Inquiry for Nursing Practice, 10*(1), 43–60.

Morse, J. M., & Doberneck, B. M. (1995). Delineating the concept of hope. *Image: Journal of Nursing Scholarship, 27*(4), 277–285.

Morse, J. M., & Johnson, J. L. (Eds.). (1991). *The illness experience: Dimensions of suffering.* Newbury Park, CA: Sage.

Morse, J. M., & Mitcham, C. (1998). The experience of agonizing pain and signals of disembodiment. *Journal of Psychosomatic Research, 44*(6), 667–680.

Morse, J. M., & O'Brien, B. (1995). Preserving self: From victim, to patient, to disabled person. *Journal of Advanced Nursing, 21*, 886–896. doi:10.1046/j.1365-2648.1995.21050886.x

Morse, J. M., & Penrod, J. (1999). Linking concepts of enduring, suffering, and hope. *Image: Journal of Nursing Scholarship, 31*(2), 145–150.

Morse, J. M., Penrod, J., Kassab, C., & Dellasega, C. (2000). Evaluating the efficiency and effectiveness of approaches to nasogastric tube insertion during trauma care. *American Journal of Critical Care, 9*(5), 325–333.

Morse, J. M., & Pooler, C. (2002). Patient-family-nurse interactions in the trauma-resuscitation room. *American Journal of Critical Care, 11*(3), 240–249.

Morse, J. M., Pooler, C., van Ward, T., Maddox, L., Olausson, J. M., Roche-Dean, M., . . . Martz, K. (2014). Awaiting the diagnosis of breast cancer: Strategies of enduring for preserving self. *Oncology Nursing Forum, 41*(4), 350–359. doi:10.1188/14.ONF.350-359

Morse, J. M., & Proctor, A. (1998). Maintaining patient endurance: The comfort work of trauma nurses. *Clinical Nursing Research, 7*(3), 250–274.

Morse, J. M., Wilson, S., & Penrod, J. (2000). Mothers and their disabled children: Refining the concept of normalization. *Health Care for Women International, 21*(8), 659–676.

Olson, K., Morse, J. M., Smith, J., Mayan, M., & Hammond, D. (2000–2001). Linking trajectories of illness and dying. *Omega, 42*(4), 293–308.

Proctor, A., Morse, J. M., & Khonsari, E. S. (1996). Sounds of comfort in the trauma center: How nurses talk to patients in pain. *Social Sciences & Medicine, 42*, 1669–1680.

Siegl, D., & Morse, J. M. (1994). Tolerating reality: The experiences of parents with HIV+ sons. *Social Science & Medicine, 38*, 959–971.

Surr, C. A. (2006). Preservation of self in people with dementia living in residential care: A socio-biographical approach. *Social Science & Medicine, 62*(7), 1720–1730.

Vann-Ward, T. (2016). *Preserving the core self: The challenging and strategic processes for people with Parkinsonism* (Doctoral dissertation). University of Utah, Salt Lake City, UT.

Wilson, S., & Morse, J. M. (1993). Living with a wife undergoing chemotherapy: Perceptions of the husband. *Image: Journal of Nursing Scholarship, 23*(2), 78–84.

36

TOWARD UNDERSTANDING COMFORT AND COMFORTING

Nurses who work in the hospital, work with patients who have ongoing irreversible, irretrievable suffering. Physical suffering, emotional suffering, mental suffering—anguish beyond belief . . .
—Morse, Whitaker, and Tasón (1996, p. 91)

I have been interested in comfort as long as I have been a researcher. In my doctoral program I was uneasy with the concept of caring as the "essence of nursing" (Leininger, 1978) as caring did not encompass the *tasks* of nursing, and appeared to be focused on the nurse, rather than the patient. I argued that such a perspective on caring frequently led to the outcome of caring as the *nurse* feeling better; such a perspective on caring was not always a patient-centered concept (Morse, 1992).

My understanding of comfort and comforting came from conducting many studies, starting with masters' and PhD students' dissertation's and later supported by post doctoral students. The early studies were based on patients' experiences, mainly using grounded theory methods; all were published, but it took the preparation of the *Illness-Constellation Model* to recognize the relationship between suffering and comforting.

My first federally funded grant from the National Center for Nursing Research (NCNR; now the National Institute of Nursing Research) was to delineate the concept of comfort. We did that, but only partway through the subsequent 5-year extension grant did we recognize that we had to focus on suffering first. Until we understood suffering (that is, what was being comforted), we could not understand comfort.

The problem was that the state of suffering itself interferes with the expression of suffering, so that conducting interviews to understand suffering (which everyone seems to do) is the most ineffective way to understand the suffering experience. People who are enduring suppress the emotions that you are trying to understand, to the extent that your interviews sound like police reports—short sentences devoid of emotion. If the person is in the state of emotional suffering, the emotions themselves often make the interviews unintelligible. And perhaps, some would argue, interviewing that causes such distress is unethical. At best, interviews conducted *during the active part of suffering* provide only a part of the story. Once the person comes out of suffering he or she gains new insights into the experience. These later interviews are not invalid, as some argue: People do not forget those experiences, as psychologists suggest. In fact, returning to those memories evokes the same emotional responses during interviews, but with less intensity, a phenomenon which I call "emotional re-enactment" (Morse, 2002).

Later in the research program, observational studies of trauma care provided the most useful insights into the mutual interaction between comforting and suffering. Once I understood what the states of suffering were, I could see suffering in my interviews, both enduring and emotional suffering, as well as the transitions between the two. It was present in the statements and descriptions and also in the intonations, expressions, and behaviors of those being interviewed. Most of all, in the videos, I could see the responsiveness of caregivers to suffering, that is, comforting.

Thus, the studies that form a part of this analysis of comfort were also a part of the analysis of suffering (Chapter 36), for comforting is the "flip side" of suffering. These two concepts always occur together, often simultaneously. Comforting rarely occurs unless there is suffering (i.e., a need for comfort) at some level.

With my coinvestigators and graduate students, for more than two decades we analyzed comforting in palliative care, bereavement, major accidental injuries (in emergency departments, including trauma resuscitation), intensive care unit (ICU), spinal cord injury units, transplant units, with postoperative infants in the neonatal intensive care unit (NICU), in oncology units, in rehabilitation, and even a summer camp for children on ventilators who were normally nursed at home. We explored comfort and comforting from the perspective of the patient, the relatives, and the nurses, and we explored techniques of comforting. We used interview research, linguistic analysis, observational methods, video ethnography, grounded theory, phenomenology, and, of course, various types of concept analysis to determine the exact nature of the comforting strategies. We explored self-comforting, nurse comforting, and other comforting, including lay and professional strategies. We studied patients at various levels of discomfort, from minimal to chronic to acute, intolerable agony; states of discomfort and fear, and the emotional pain of losing a loved one and even one's own dying.

ASSUMPTIONS ABOUT COMFORT AND COMFORTING

1. We know a tremendous amount the individuals' experience of infirmary, illness, injury, rehabilitation, dying, disability, abnormality, and health seeking and health maintenance behaviors—under the rubric of emotional, physical, and spiritual responses (see, for example, Kolcaba, 2003).

2. We know that if we alleviate symptoms the individual is more *physically* comfortable, but that the meaning of the symptoms, that is, *what the symptom represents*, remains.

Therefore:

    a. The physical easing is important, but in itself, is not enough (e.g., consider palliative care and dying; physical easing does not remove the prognosis, disability, etc.).

    b. Most illness impairs, scars, changes body image, and changes the self. (These are rehabilitation and chronicity models; also models of adjustment, adaptation and normalization.)

    c. Even *curing* (removal of symptoms and restoration of self) changes people forever—and results in changes to self. While curing is a significant goal, it is incomplete.

3. *Suffering is a social event.* I maintain that the most basic response to infirmary, illness, injury, rehabilitation, dying, disability, abnormality, and mental disability, is one of suffering—*enduring and emotionally suffering.* The response extends beyond the individual affected, and also affects the family, friends, caregivers and, in fact, those who come in contact or who know of (or even hear about) the affected individual.

4. *Enduring and emotional suffering vary in intensity and form,* depending on the nature of the individual's needs. For example, so far we have identified three types of enduring (enduring to live, enduring to survive, and enduring to die), a trajectory of enduring to emotional suffering, to the reformulated self, and the intersection of some other concepts involved in the process (Morse, 2001, 2011; see also Chapter 5).

5. *How enduring and emotionally suffering are manifest* is culturally and contextually prescribed, within the most basic parameters of *preserving self* (Morse, 2012).

6. *Medical treatment is necessary, is usually selected and is morally right.* Technically competent care is a necessary right.

Similarly, comforting is a necessary right, as are the obligation of health care professionals and the moral obligation of family, and society.

7. *Comfort is a relative state, an optimal state achieved by each individual.* Comforting is an effort expended by the individual and by others to assist the individual to reach that goal. Comfort may also be a state attained by a family, group, community, or nation.

8. *Comforting consists of curing.* Comfort consists of symptom relief. Comforting consists of providing technically competent care. Comforting consists of supporting the individual to endure, easing the individual through the process of suffering. Comforting is aiding the individual to attain a state free of distress/discomfort. Comfort is healthy living; a comfortable life is a healthy life.

9. *For nursing, the primary responsibility for providing comfort* is targeted toward monitoring and alleviation of symptoms, supportive and restorative functions, including psychosocial and spiritual support, moving the individual toward health.

10. For nursing, the act of comforting consists of caring, which motivates the provision of comfort and keeps the technical aspects of care humanistic, and providing comforting actions/procedure(s). The procedure may be a routine intervention (such as giving an injection in a way that causes minimal distress), providing a comforting strategy, which uses the nurses' self (such as touch being there or verbal interaction), or supporting a comforting environment.

DOING THEORETICAL COALESCENCE

Building a Database

In order to conduct *theoretical coalescence* (Chapter 34), one needs a comprehensive database. Recall that these studies, as a set, must contain studies at different levels of analysis, from different perspectives and at different times of the process. These studies need to be comprehensive and derived from different methods. Thus, these studies enable the phenomenon of interest to be viewed from different perspectives, from micro to macro, and focus on different aspects of the process.

Box 36.1 shows these studies sorted into categories according to the areas that they cover. Some of these studies have been introduced earlier in the book. For all of these studies I have these data and also additional

BOX 36.1. STUDIES CONTRIBUTING TO THE VARIOUS DIMENSIONS OF COMFORT AND COMFORTING

A. COMFORT

Three studies contributed to the development of insight into the nature of comfort and the concept of comfort:

1. Morse, J. M. (1983). An ethnoscientific analysis of comfort: A preliminary investigation. *Nursing Papers/Perspectives in Nursing, 15*(1), 6–19.
2. Morse, J. M., Bottorff, J. L., & Hutchinson, S. (1994). The phenomenology of comfort. *Journal of Advanced Nursing, 20,* 189–195.
3. Morse, J. M., Bottorff, J. L., & Hutchinson, S. (1995). The paradox of comfort. *Nursing Research, 44*(1), 14–19.

B. THE NEED FOR COMFORTING

1. Côté, J. J., Morse, J. M., & James, S. G. (1991). The pain experience of the post-operative newborn. *Journal of Advanced Nursing, 16,* 378–387.
2. Dewar, A., & Morse J. M. (1995). Unbearable incidents: Failure to endure the experience of illness. *Journal of Advanced Nursing, 22*(5), 957–964.
3. Morse, J. M., & Carter, B. (1996). The essence of enduring and the expression of suffering: The reformulation of self. *Scholarly Inquiry for Nursing Practice, 10*(1), 43–60.
4. Hogan, N., Morse, J. M., & Tasón, M. C. (1996). Toward an experiential theory of bereavement. *Omega, 33*(1), 43–65.
5. Morse, J. M., & Carter, B. J. (1995). Strategies of enduring and the suffering of loss: Modes of comfort used by a resilient survivor. *Holistic Nursing Practice, 9*(3), 33–58. [Reprinted in Danish: Ed. Nete Gress Klinisk Sygrpleje, bd 1,11, og 111, 2000]
6. Morse, J. M. (1989). Cultural responses to parturition: Childbirth in Fiji. *Medical Anthropology, 12*(1), 35–44.

C. RESPONSES TO SIGNS OF DISTRESS

1. Solberg, S., & Morse, J. M. (1991). The comforting behaviors of caregivers toward distressed post-operative neonates. *Issues in Comprehensive Pediatric Nursing, 14*(2), 77–92.
2. Wilson, S., & Morse, J. M. (1991). Living with a wife undergoing chemotherapy: Perceptions of the husband. *Image: Journal of Nursing Scholarship, 23*(2), 78–84.
3. Morse, J. M., Miles, M. W., Clark, D. A., & Doberneck, B. M. (1994). Sensing patient needs: Exploring concepts of nursing insight and receptivity used in nursing assessment. *Scholarly Inquiry for Nursing Practice, 8*(3), 233–254.
4. Siegl, D., & Morse, J. M. (1994). Tolerating reality: The experiences of parents with HIV[+] sons. *Social Science & Medicine, 38,* 959–971.
5. Morse, J. M., Mitcham, C., & van der Steen, V. (1998). Compathy or physical empathy: Implications for the caregiver relationship. *Journal of Medical Humanities, 19*(1), 51–65.
6. Penrod, J., Morse, J. M., & Wilson, S. (1999). Comforting strategies used during nasogastric tube insertion. *Journal of Clinical Nursing, 8,* 31–38.
7. Olson, K., Morse, J. M., Smith, J., Mayan, M., & Hammond, D. (2000–2001). Linking trajectories of illness and dying. *Omega, 42*(4), 293–308.

D. SELF-COMFORTING

1. Johnson, J. L., & Morse, J. M. (1990). Regaining control: The process of adjustment following myocardial infarction. *Heart and Lung, 19*(2), 126–135.
2. Flaming, D., & Morse, J. M. (1992). Minimizing embarrassment: Boys experiencing pubertal changes. *Issues in Comprehensive Pediatric Nursing, 14,* 211–231.
3. Laskiwski, S., & Morse, J. M. (1993). The spinal cord injured patient: The modification of hope and expressions of despair. *Canadian Journal of Rehabilitation, 6*(3), 143–153.
4. Morse, J. M., & Carter, B. J. (1995). Strategies of enduring and the suffering of loss: Modes of comfort used by a resilient survivor. *Holistic Nursing Practice, 9*(3), 33–58.
5. Morse, J. M., & O'Brien, B. (1995). Preserving self: From victim, to patient, to disabled person. *Journal of Advanced Nursing, 21,* 886–896. doi:10.1046/j.1365-2648.1995.21050886.x
6. Penrod, J., & Morse, J. M. (1997) Strategies for assessing and fostering hope: The hope assessment guide. *Oncology Nurses Forum, 24*(6), 1055–1063.
7. Morse, J. M. (1997). Responding to threats to integrity of self. *Advances in Nursing Science, 19*(4), 21–36.
8. Morse, J. M., & Mitcham, C. (1998). The experience of agonizing pain and signals of disembodiment. *Journal of Psychosomatic Research, 44*(6), 667–680.
9. Morse, J. M., Wilson, S., & Penrod, J. (2000). Mothers and their disabled children: Refining the concept of normalization. *Health Care for Women International, 21*(8), 659–676.
10. Morse, J. M., Pooler, C., Vann-Ward, T., Maddox, L., Olausson, J. M., Roche-Dean, M., . . . Martz, K. (2014). Awaiting the diagnosis of breast cancer: Strategies of enduring for preserving self. *Oncology Nursing Forum, 41*(4), 350–359.

E. ATTRIBUTES OF COMFORT

1. Morse, J. M., Solberg, S. M., Neander, W. L., Bottorff, J. L., & Johnson, J. L. (1990). Concepts of caring and caring as a concept. *Advances in Nursing Science, 13,* 1–14.
2. Morse, J. M., Bottorff, J., Neander, W., & Solberg, S. (1991). Comparative analysis of the conceptualizations and theories of caring. *Image: Journal of Nursing Scholarship, 23*(2), 119–126.
3. Hupcey, J., Penrod, J., Morse, J., & Mitcham, C. (2001). An exploration and advancement of the concept of trust. *Journal of Advanced Nursing, 36*(2), 282–293.
4. Morse, J. M., Bottorff, J., Anderson, G., O'Brien, B., & Solberg, S. (1992). Beyond empathy. Expanding expressions of caring. *Journal of Advanced Nursing, 17,* 809–821.
5. Morse, J. M., Anderson, G., Bottorff, J., Yonge, O., O'Brien, B., Solberg, S., & McIlveen, K. (1992). Exploring empathy: A conceptual fit for nursing practice? *Image: Journal of Nursing Scholarship, 24*(4), 274–280.
6. Estabrooks, C., & Morse, J. M. (1992). Toward a theory of touch: The touching process and acquiring a touching style. *Journal of Advanced Nursing, 17,* 448–456.
7. Morse, J. M., & Doberneck, B. M. (1995). Delineating the concept of hope. *Image: Journal of Nursing Scholarship, 27*(4), 277–285.

F. THE COMFORTING RELATIONSHIP

1. Morse, J. M. (1991). Negotiating commitment and involvement in the patient-nurse relationship. *Journal of Advanced Nursing, 16,* 455–468.
2. Bottorff, J. L., & Morse, J. M. (1994). Identifying types of attending: Patterns of nurses' work. *Image: Journal of Nursing Scholarship, 26*(1), 53–60.

3. Hupcey, J. E., & Morse, J. M. (1995). Family and social support: Application to the critically ill patient. *Journal of Family Nursing, 1*(3), 257–280
4. Morse, J. M., & Mitcham, C. (1997). Compathy: The contagion of physical distress. *Journal of Advanced Nursing, 26*, 649–657.
5. Morse, J. M., & Intrieri, R. (1997). Patient-patient communication in a long-term care facility. *Journal of Psychosocial Nursing & Mental Health Services, 35*(5), 34–39. [Abstracted in *American Journal of Nursing, 97*(7), 9–10]
6. Morse, J. M., Havens, G., DeLuca, A., & Wilson, S. (1997). The comforting interaction: Developing a model of nurse-patient relationship. *Scholarly Inquiry for Nursing Practice, 11*(4), 321–343.
7. Wilson, S., Morse, J. M., & Penrod, J. (1998). Developing reciprocal trust in the caregiving relationship. *Qualitative Health Research, 8*, 446–465.
8. Wilson, S., Morse, J. M., & Penrod, J. (1998). Absolute involvement: The experience of mothers of ventilator-dependent children. *Health & Social Care, 6*(4), 224–233.

G. THEORETICAL EXPANSION USING OTHER MODELS; OTHER POPULATIONS

1. Hupcey, J. E., Penrod, J., & Morse, J. M. (2000). Establishing and maintaining trust during acute care hospitalizations. *Scholarly Inquiry for Nursing Practice: An International Journal, 14*(3), 227–242.
2. Morse, J. M., & Pooler, C. (2002) Patient-family-nurse interactions in the trauma-resuscitation room. *American Journal of Critical Care, 11*(3), 240–249.
3. Bergstrom, L., Richards, L., Proctor, A., Bohrer-Avila, L. Morse, J., & Roberts, J. (2009). Birth talk in second stage labor. *Qualitative Health Research, 19*, 954–964.
4. Bergstrom, L., Richards, L., Morse, J., & Roberts, J. (2010). How caregivers manage pain and distress in second stage labor. *Journal of Midwifery and Women's Health, 55*(1), 38–45.
5. Morse, J. M. (2011). Hearing bad news. *Journal of Humanistic Medicine. 32,* 187–211. doi:10.1007/s10912-011-9138-4

H. UNDERSTANDING THE MICROANALYTIC MECHANISMS OF COMFORTING

1. Solberg, S., & Morse, J. M. (1991). The comforting behaviors of caregivers toward distressed post-operative neonates. *Issues in Comprehensive Pediatric Nursing, 14*(2), 77–92.
2. Morse, J. M., Solberg, S., & Edwards, J. (1993). Caregiver-infant interaction: Comforting the postoperative infant. *Scandinavian Journal of Caring Sciences, 7,* 105–111.
3. Solberg, S., & Morse, J. M. (1991). The comforting behaviors of caregivers toward distressed post-operative neonates. *Issues in Comprehensive Pediatric Nursing, 14*(2), 77–92.
4. Bottorff, J. L., & Morse, J. M. (1994). Identifying types of attending: Patterns of nurses' work. *Image: Journal of Nursing Scholarship, 26*(1), 53–60.
5. Morse, J. M., Miles, M. W., Clark, D. A., & Doberneck, B. M. (1994). Sensing patient needs: Exploring concepts of nursing insight and receptivity used in nursing assessment. *Scholarly Inquiry for Nursing Practice, 8*(3), 233–254.
6. Proctor, A., Morse, J. M., & Khonsari, E. S. (1996). Sounds of comfort in the trauma center: How nurses talk to patients in pain. *Social Sciences & Medicine, 42,* 1669–1680.
7. Morse, J. M., & Mitcham, C. (1997). Compathy: The contagion of physical distress. *Journal of Advanced Nursing, 26,* 649–657.
8. Morse, J. M., & Proctor, A. (1998). Maintaining patient endurance: The comfort work of trauma nurses. *Clinical Nursing Research, 7*(3), 250–274.

9. Morse, J. M. (2000). Responding to the cues of suffering. *Health Care for Women International, 21,* 1–9.
10. Morse, J. M., Beres, M., Spiers, J., Mayan, M., & Olson, K. (2003). Identifying signals of suffering by linking verbal and facial cues. *Qualitative Health Research, 13*(8), 1063–1077.

I. THE COMFORTING ENVIRONMENT

Comforting role of funeral directors:
1. Hyland, L., & Morse, J. M. (1995). Orchestrating comfort: The role of funeral directors. *Death Studies, 19,* 453–474.

J. THEORETICAL

1. Morse, J. M. (1992). Comfort: The refocusing of nursing care. *Clinical Nursing Research, 1,* 91–11.
2. Morse, J. M. (1996). The science of comforting. *Reflections, 22*(4), 6–8.
3. Morse, J. M. (1997). Conceptualizing a theory of comfort. *Health SA Gesondheid, 2*(2), 3–9. [Reprinted in Afrikaans: Konseptualisering van 'n Gemaksteorie. *Health SA Gesondheid, 4*(4), 3–10]
4. Morse, J. M., & Penrod, J. (1999). Linking concepts of enduring, suffering, and hope. *Image: Journal of Nursing Scholarship, 31*(2), 145–150.
5. Morse, J. M. (2000). On comfort and comforting. *American Journal of Nursing, 100*(9), 34–38.

unpublished data in interviews and videotapes. I first discuss the evidence derived from each area and number the references to the key in Box 36.1 to expedite reading. Then, later in this chapter, I put the theory together as a whole.

As early as 1983, I knew that comforting consisted of types of talking, patterns of touch, and styles of listening. Importantly, I realized that we did not have the language to describe the combinations and types of touch-talk-listening, and without that terminology it sounded so *dumb*; so basic; so obvious. I now understand why the language is not developed: most of these comforting interactions are beyond awareness. They are reflexive and automatic, and a natural component of interactions, which is implicit. But I now realize they can be described, should be described, and even be taught.

When thinking about discomfort, slight, constant or overwhelming, one realizes that it is a state in the body and the mind. Therefore with Hutchinson and Bottorff, I conducted two phenomenological studies to determine what a state of comfort was like experientially (cited in Box 36.1 as A.2 and A.3).

Comfort was a state that had a myriad of meanings, depending on the nature of the discomfort(s). Discomfort was a state that was largely beyond the control of the person, so that with the loss of control the body does not obey its will (is "*dis*obedient"). Pain makes the person feel vulnerable and fragile; pain threatens, and one feels violated. *Dis*-ease deceives, occurring silently, shattering the person on diagnosis; *dis*-ease betrays, as the person tries to conceal symptoms and continue living day to day. Chronic and intractable pain must be endured, with the body resigned to becoming a changed body. Comfort was a state or relief, even temporary ease, and one that is not usually achieved alone, but in the relationship with another, often a nurse. Illness and injury place the patients' awareness of their bodies in the foreground, dominating their consciousness and disrupting their movements, ability to speak, and their "orientation to the world." Enduring pain and discomfort disrupts time, presence, orientation to the world, and interrupts taken-for-granted bodily experiences.

Nightingale (1860/1969) was correct: "When the patient is comfortable, they have no need for a nurse." When comfortable, the body loses its dominance and is beyond awareness. However, comfort is not something that is achieved quickly and easily, but something that is attained as a process, in small incremental steps. Often, it is an interactive act, achieved with the assistance of others. And that "other" is frequently the professional charge of a nurse.

Ask Analytic Questions of the Studies

To move the analysis forward, I use the technique of asking analytic questions (described in Chapter 17). Rather than asking the questions of *data* (i.e., interviews and observations notes), in the period of analysis, we asked analytic questions of the studies themselves.

This we know:

Comforting occurs in an interaction.

QUESTION: What conditions, events, *signals*, start the comforting action?

The Infant Pain Study

A graduate student, Judy Côté, conducted an ethological study of infant pain in the NICU (Côté, Morse, & James, 1991). Videotaped data enabled us to see microanalytically, moment-by-moment, infant pain responses to painful stimuli, as well as postoperative pain. Later, with Shirley Solberg (Morse, Solberg, & Edwards, 1993; Solberg & Morse, 1991), we realized we could use these videotapes to observe the infants' *signals* and the nurses' hands comforting the infant—and listened to the nurses' vocalizations of comforting. But we could do more. We would observe the infants' responses to the comforting actions. We could describe it, time it, and look for changes in the pattern of comforting when it stopped, and describe the infants' level of comfort at the time the comforting action ceased.

The pattern of comforting was fascinating. Touch was rhythmic, structured, and cycled as pat-pat-pat-pat-pat, rub-rub-rub-rub, stroke-stroke-stroke-stoke, rock-rock-rock-rock. Often the infant was crying hard, and the crying did not ease. In fact, with the rocking, the intensity of the infant's distress increased. One type of rocking was to hold the infant's hands and move his or her arms from side to side, so that when lying, the infant was moved from side to die.

Look at Figure 36.1, for what our data looked like.

TO DO 36.1. ANALYSIS OF INFANT'S DISTRESS PATTERNS

Examine these data presented in Figure 36.1.

1. Examine the timelines, and the incidences of verbal (v) and touching(*).
2. Why do you think comforting touch is so sporadic?
3. Was comforting always given in response to a cue of distress?
4. Why do you think the verbal comforting is so sparse?

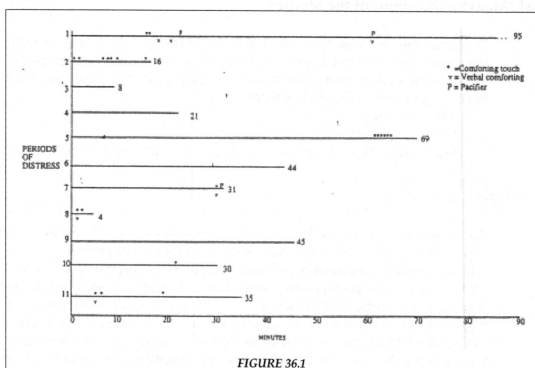

FIGURE 36.1
One infant's periods of distress, during comforting.
Source: Solberg and Morse (1991).

Help Me Think

Is comforting always given in response to a cue or signal of distress? What happens if the cue or signal is ignored by caregivers?

Let us count how many times the infant was given comforting touch during the period of distress. Why was it so infrequent?

Now, when we looked on the tape, the infant was not given comforting touch when he or she was not distressed. Why?

Why was verbal comforting so seldom used?

Here is a "rule"

In behavioral research, anything that is 100% clear (accepted), is usually so obvious that it is no longer interesting, so we will expect a few exceptions (or negative cases). And, when we look at those instances in the tape, we see that, at that time, the nurse apparently had nothing to do, and was touching (absentmindedly "fiddling with") the sleeping infant.

Perhaps the verbal comforting was used so infrequently because comforting occurs in response to the infant's cues, and in this case, with intubated infants, the cry was silent? Nurses did NOT need to say, "There, there," or "Shhhh," or sing, or "coo" to these babies. Rather, they were seen carrying on conversations with the nurses caring for the infant in the next crib.

This conjecture could be confirmed within the data set by examining all instances of comforting with and without verbal comforting. Actually, we did this analysis, and it was confirmed as statistically significant (Morse, Solberg, & Edwards, 1993).

Comforting is given in response to patient's cues, and if these cues are absent (in this case the babies had a silent cry), the matching comforting strategy is not given (i.e., verbal comforting).

Question: Are Comforting Actions Patterned and Routinized?

We examined patterns of comforting from instance to instance (the same nurse and the same infant), or from different nurses and the same infant, or between infants (differing nurses and different infants). The same rhythm and pattern of comforting touch remained. The cycle of touch was the same (pat-pat-pat-pat-pat, rib-rub-rub-rub, stroke-stroke-stroke-stroke-stoke, rock-rock-rock-rock); but whereas the number of pats or the order of the pats or strokes was different, the patterns were strikingly similar.

Question: How Long Does Comforting "Last?"

Touch: A comforting touch intervention will be tried for 10 to 20 sec (rarely longer). If the intervention is not "working" (i.e., produce a reduction in discomfort) it is changed and another type of comforting touch tried. With intubated infants, after approximately 20 min, if the infant had not settled, the nurse would turn away to other tasks. Therefore, comforting interventions are time-limited.

Therefore, from this study we know that:

- Comforting occurs in response to a signal or cue from the patients *AND* rarely occurs when the signal or discomfort is not present.
- Cues of discomfort must be evident, and the need for comforting signaled to the caregiver. If this is missing, or the nurse "misses" the signal, the patient is unlikely to receive comfort.
- This means that comfort is patient-led.
- Patterns of comforting (touch) are very similar, and are learned or initiated in the clinical setting.
- Comforting interventions are time-limited.

The Next Step Is to Confirm These Findings With Another Data Set: Trauma Studies

Data used in the trauma studies consisted of continuous videotapes of patients as they were admitted for trauma resuscitation. Video cameras were mounted on the wall; 178 recordings were made in 3 trauma centers. The purpose was to record nurse-comforting strategies used for extremely distressed patients as they were brought into the trauma department.[1]

The Comfort Talk Register

When patients were brought into the trauma room extremely distressed, we observed extraordinary nurse-comforting techniques that helped the patient maintain control (Morse & Proctor, 1998; Proctor, Morse, & Khonari, 1996). They bent over, above the patient's face, so their own face was about 10 inches from the patient (see Figure 36.2). If the patients had their eyes open, they held their gaze, and spoke in a very loud voice, instantly responding to their cries or utterances.

---

[1] Institutional review board (IRB) consents were obtained from all caregivers (nurses, physicians, consultants; relatives). Notifications and reminders to technicians, ambulance staff, cleaners, and orderlies were given. *Patients*: Taping was commenced as soon as the patient entered the room, and these tapes were placed in the Quality Assurance data set until the patient's consent was obtained. Patients were informed about the study as soon as they were able to comprehend; consent was obtained as soon as they were able to give consent. If the patient did not agree to participate, the tape was erased. If the patient consented, all identifiers (patient's face and names) were removed from the tape. Children's consents were obtained from the parent or guardian; older children provided assent.

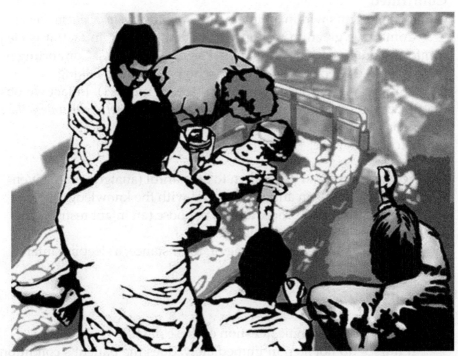

FIGURE 36.2
Posturing in "talking through" using the comfort talk register. The nurse's head is approximately 15 inches above the patient's face.
Courtesy of Nicky Pearson.

Nurses spoke, using special intonations, which we called the *comfort talk register*. They spoke in short sentences. Content analysis showed that they met four functions: (a) helping patients hold on (endure), (b) obtaining information, (c) gaining information about procedures, and (d) giving information about procedures. Intonation referred to pitch changes over an entire phrase. The intonation contours were rising and falling of pitch, which gave additional meaning over and above the meaning communicated by the speech. Sometimes the nurse was communicating to calm the patient "You're O.K., you're O.K., honey"; to warn the patient "You will feel a little prick in your arm"; to assess the patient "Does it still hurt?" and to get them to endure, "You can do this" (Proctor, Morse, & Khonari, 1996). Comforting touch was with a firm palmer touch. Nurses rarely stroked or patted distraught adults, but patients often would grab and clutch the nurse's hand, when it was offered.

Interpretation
The nurse always interrupted patients' cries, and rarely "disturbed" the patients when they were lying quietly.

Confirmed

Comforting occurs within an interaction, *in response to a patient cue.*

Comfort is given in response to patient signals. In fact, it is clear that comforting interventions *interrupt* the signal of distress. Comforting is given quickly. Nurses step in immediately, with holding and talking.

This is a very strong relationship (see Figure 36.1). In fact we observed that, except in some circumstances, *comforting does not occur unless the patient signals for, or requires comforting, or the nurse observes a cue.*

Exceptions were:

1. Procedures that are known to be painful (analgesics are given ahead of time in anticipation and with the knowledge that this is a painful procedure). A papoose (an infant restraint) may be placed on an infant.
2. The absentminded stroking of, for instance, a sleeping infant

Analytic Questions

Next, we asked an analytic question of these data:

If nurses do not step in immediately, does the patient's condition escalate, diminish, or stay the same?

Findings

Examination of the videotapes showed that if the signals were not attended to, the patient's condition escalated. They moved rapidly through the stages of scared, anxious, frightened, to terrified, and then, out of control. They became increasingly vocal, and fought caregivers. When providing care under such circumstances became dangerous for the patients, they were restrained by others (nurses held their hands to prevent flailing or placed their arms over the patients' thighs), and the analgesics were quickly provided as soon as possible.

Therefore, externally, the comforting person(s) countered the distress and assisted the persons to regain control.[2] In this context, comforting is therapeutic, minimizing injury by preventing the person from fighting essential care, and enabling them to cooperate with care. It reduces harm from the injuries, and it expedites care.

---

[2] This is a logical conjecture, for we cannot determine *how* therapeutic comforting is experimentally, but only by using logic. For instance, if the patient had a head injury, the increased intercranial pressure from fighting caregivers will exacerbate the intercranial bleed, and patients with fractured limbs often try to move those limbs.

Analytic Questions

Are the comforting strategies provided for each patient state distinct? Or are the same strategies used for any type of distress signal?

In Chapter 35, we classified the states of trauma patients "into scared," "anxious," "frightened," "terrified," and "out of control." The answer to this analytic question is that a different type of comforting strategy must be used for patients in each state.

Comforting Strategies if the Patient is Scared

Recall from Chapter 35 that scared patients lie very still, listening intently and trying to piece information together. Talk that is comforting for them is continuous. The nurse gives a "running commentary" about everything that she is doing: "I'm just behind you Mr. Smith, and I am hanging a new IV. You are doing real well. Now, I am over here charting the IV fluid. Great. Now, I just want to look at . . ." The nurse talk in this case does not have the intonation of the Comfort Talk Register, but is rather in the tone of normal conversation. These patients need someone with them constantly; *nurse presence* is a vital comforting strategy for scared patients.

Comforting Strategies if the Patient Is Anxious

Anxious patients watch the nurse closely, following his or her every movement, and often talking very fast and continuously. If the nurse looks concerned, they will ask: "What's wrong! What's wrong!" If the nurse wants to give them information, it is difficult to know if they really heard what she said, for they interrupt whatever she is saying, asking even more questions. Nurses must listen, and follow the patients' tone. Some of these patients may conceal their anxiety. If your anxious patient is joking, reciprocate and follow his or her lead. If important instructions are to be given to these patients, make certain he or she repeats everything back. These patients will accept light comforting touch, and they should not be left alone.

Comforting Strategies if the Patient Is Frightened

Patients who are *frightened* are restless, verbal, and defensive. If they do not receive comforting strategies, their condition may escalate very quickly into *terrified*. Remain with the patient. They need constant reassurance, and may even respond to *talking though*. Protect the patient by keeping the number of caregivers close to the patient at a minimum. The patient is given warning of procedures and is assured that only one procedure will be conducted at a time, and with the patient's acknowledged permission.

Comforting Strategies if the Patient Is Terrified

Terrified patients are very restless, verbally loud, and respond only sometimes when spoken to. They must be addressed loudly and clearly, for they may be hearing the nurse's voice, although their eyes may be closed. If overtly distressed, *talking through* is very effective in helping them to maintain control, to permit essential care, and preventing their emotional state from escalating to out of control. With skilled care, they may cooperate with treatments, and remain in control. The person who is providing the comfort talk should not leave the patient's side, use firm touch, and respond to any vocalizations using the comfort talk register.

Comforting Strategies if the Patient Is Out of Control

When patients are out of control, they are restless and vocalizing very loudly. They do not respond to commands and appear to be almost unaware of the caregivers. This is a very dangerous state, and these patients must be sedated so that urgent emergency care may proceed.

From these data we conclude that the type of comforting offered to patients in different states is substantially different. The patterns and type of nurses' talk, touch, listening and presence are different for each patient's state, and if the "wrong" type is used, then the patient's condition will escalate. If the right pattern of comforting is used, the patient's state will remain as such, or the patient's *comfort level* will be lowered to the next state.[3] Comforting interactions intercept the vocalizations and behaviors that signal distress, and comforting behaviors are immediately effective. If a comforting action does not have the expected effect, nurses will immediately change it.

Now, the next analytic question is as follows.

Are comforting strategies distinct for each patient state?

From the above descriptions, we learned that comforting strategies must "match" the patient's condition.

For instance, if a scared patient is treated as anxious, with strategies appropri- ate for anxious, they rapidly deteriorate and become anxious. If the nurse missed a patient signal or patient cue, then the patient's behaviors deteriorate. Fortunately, most of the comforting actions are learned in everyday conversation, and mistakes on the part of the nurse are easily corrected. However, if a nurse begins using a comforting strategy, one that is "working," and it is suddenly stopped, or she or he leaves the patient, the patient's condition immediately escalates.

Confirmed

Comforting strategies are tailored to the patient's state.

Inappropriate comforting actions are correctable and are "forgiven."

---

[3] The patient's *comfort level* is a term used by nurses to refer to the patient's state of comfort. Nurses use the six states of comfort level described here.

To date, nurses have not been taught about microanalytic comforting strategies. How did they learn them? We asked the nurses: "Well," they said, "when you are new to trauma care, you watch the experienced nurses *like a hawk* for at least a year." We surmised that such levels of intense comforting are a combination of intuitive compassion, a willingness to ease the distress, learned by modeling, and by making and correcting mistakes.

Now, the next analytic question is as follows:

What if the Strategy for the Wrong Patient State Was Used?

We saw mistakes—when the wrong comforting strategy was used. Examples were touch that caused pain, a statement that aroused the patient, scared patients who were left alone, and so forth. When nurses saw that what they were doing was not appropriate, and caused the patient to react, or exacerbated their distress, they immediately apologized, withdrew, and changed the comforting strategy used.

Confirmed

Comforting caregiver comforting mistakes were instantly corrected.

The second part of the *malleability of comforting* is that comforting mistakes are forgiven if the nurse instantly apologizes and changes her comforting strategy to a more appropriate one. As comforting strategies benefit the patient, the strategies must change as the patient's state changes:

Comforting processes were malleable: Comforting strategies changed as the patient's condition changes and becomes more comfortable.

Eventually, when the patient relaxes, the nurse is able to leave the patient, letting him or her to rest.

Question:

Is comfort always "patient-led"?

Nurses know if a procedure is known to be painful, and in these cases analgesics are given proactively. Otherwise, all comforting procedures are given in response to patient cues. That is, all comforting strategies are patient-led and must be "demanded" by the patient.

Mitigating the Distress of Nasogastric Tube Insertion

The videotapes of trauma care provided an opportunity for observing *how* nurses talked patients though painful procedures, such as nasogastric (NG) tube insertion. Although nursing texts provide detailed instruction on the mechanical techniques of NG tube insertion, these texts remind nurses only to "explain procedure to the patient," but do not tell them *how* they should explain or *what* they should say, and *how to say it*.

Our microanalysis of videotapes of 32 NG tube insertions revealed that there were three styles of talking to the patient: affective, technical, and a blend of technical and comforting (Morse, Penrod, Kassob, & Dellesega, 2000). The fourth style, *mixed,* described more than one caregiver, each using a different style.

With the *affective (comforting)* style the nurse is concerned about causing discomfort and withdraws the tube quickly; she also uses terms of endearment, and consoling talk:

". . . . *Big swallow; swallow it down, big swallow. Swallow, honey, swallow. That's a boy.* [patient gags and the tube is withdrawn] . . . *Take it easy now . . .*" (p. 328).

With the *technical* style, the nurse's explanation centers on the patient instructions ("*Swallow—swallow—swallow* [Pause]. *Tell me your name.*" [p. 328]).

With the *blended* style, nurse's talk combines features of the two styles:

> Ok. We're going to do this. If you help me, it makes it a little easier,
> Okay? But it's still going to be unpleasant. The big thing is when I
> ask you to swallow, try and swallow. It's not going to be easy though,
> okay? (p. 328)

When we examined the efficacy of the trials, surprisingly the blended type was more effective, resulting in fewer trials to insert the tube and was therefore more successful. The technical style was next in effectiveness, and the affective style was least effective. This study is important, showing that the style of the verbal coaching of patient during NG tube insertion affects the success rate.

Who Provides Comfort?

In all of these studies, if the nurse was providing a procedure, comforting was provided by the person assisting the nurse. Usually this was because the person conducting the procedure was necessarily trying to maintain a sterile field or manipulating equipment, but having a second nurse there "for the patient" allows the nurse providing the treatment to focus on the actual procedure. Care is safer.

When we first published the results of the comfort talk register, I presented often to hospitals and nurse administrators the advantages of having a nurse available for the patient to assist with *talking through*, in areas in which patients are acutely distressed, such as trauma care, or labor and delivery. But budgetary concerns have always overridden patient safely, even with this evidence.

Were Comforting Strategies Always the Responsibility of the Caregiver?

Gradually, we recognized that comforting strategies were also the responsibility of the individual who was suffering. The concept of *enduring* was significant, and described as *taking it* or *bearing it,* in Chapter 35, the *Praxis Theory of Suffering.*

Analytic Question: What Is Self-Comforting?

Self-comforting was apparent in two forms: Physical and cognitive.

The physical discomfort *signals* the nurse and provides cues into the source of distress. For example, if patients are in pain, they will *posture,* and *protect the painful part of their body.* They will hold and protect that painful area if they have a migraine, they will squint and move away from light and noise, and they will lie very still. They may or may not vocalize. With severe pain, they may be pale, perspire, and grimace. *Self-comforting* strategies are posturing and protecting, as mentioned earlier.

If the patient has chronic pain, or is emotionally distressed, they will move into a state of enduring. As described in Chapter 29, emotions are suppressed, along with spontaneous movements and spontaneous speech. As identified in our study of women undergoing diagnosis for breast cancer (Chapter 24; Morse et al., 2014), women used deliberate cognitive strategies to reduce distress, putting thoughts of cancer "at the back of their minds."

Some Strategies Were Not Deliberate

Analysis of interviews with burn patients revealed that they disembodied the part of the body in which the pain was excruciating (Morse & Mitcham, 1998). They disembodied the painful parts of their bodies, using *it, the, this,* rather than *my, mine* to refer to their own body parts. This appears to be a special human capacity to maintain the integrity of the self during prolonged and agonizing experiences. For instance, a lineman who received an electric shock reported:

> . . . . *And* the *right leg was burnt quite badly, and the whole outside of* the *leg was burnt down to* the *bone—you could see bones and sinews in there, and at the very bottom—it also exited—not on the bottom of* the *foot at the bottom of* the *leg, like right at the side of* the foot was really burnt bad, too. (Morse & Mitcham, 1998, p. 669)

What Comforting Behaviors Are Conducted by the Other, in Consideration for the Sufferer?

Both patients and relatives try to conceal their distress from each other, so as not to "upset" the other. Patients will minimize, not report pain, not disclose symptoms, and try to normalize, even to the extent of telling jokes and maintaining a happy face.

Patients and relatives know that emotional suffering is contagious—it signals to others exactly how serious the illness is, and the need for comfort. Distress sends a message, "hug me, hold me, listen to me, stay with me, I am afraid." But the same fear that patients feel will somehow be transmitted to the relatives, and increase their distress. So patients conceal.

The pain response is also transmitted and shared with others. The compathetic response has been described in Chapter 13, and in serious injuries, the vicariously shared pain may be so strong as to cause caregivers to faint or to vomit, and therefore interrupt caregiving.

TO DO 36.2. IS COMFORTING A ONE-TO-ONE ACTIVITY?

At times of disaster, our president comforts the nation. Think of 9/11, and if and how "comforting a nation" was accomplished. How is bad news delivered on the television?

Comforting Interventions Are Time-Limited

The comforting strategies discussed here are time-limited. A comforting touch or a verbal response may have an "efficacy" for only a few seconds. For this reason, the strategy should be offered until the patient settles and no longer needs the comforting. Yet in our videos, comforting touch intervention may be tried for 10 to 20 sec (rarely longer), and if there was no change in the infant's condition, if the intervention was not "working" (i.e., produce a reduction in discomfort) then the comforting strategy was changed and another type tried. If that did not work after some minutes, then the nurse would stop trying to comfort. If the infant had not settled, the nurse would turn away to do other tasks. In the trauma room, a patient with a head injury asked the nurse repetitively: "How's my wife?" The nurse answered 32 times. Then, she turned the lights down and left the room.

Can an Environment Be Comforting?

Most people have a special place to be when in need of solace. They may find a church, a garden, the beach, or a mountain top comforting. The places are usually private, so they may cry, and those places are often beautiful and associated with happier memories.

Hyland and Morse (1995) studied the comforting interactions of funeral directors. This study was interesting because the funeral directors had a professional responsibility to comfort. The funeral home itself provides atmosphere that is intended to comfort: subdued lighting, soft music, flowers, comfortable chairs, and a muted color scheme (Hyland & Morse, 1995).[4] Examine the front stage/backstage organization of the funeral home, with the places for care of the body and office work, segmented from the public mourning areas. When you attend a funeral, watch how funeral directors monitor the bereaved by hovering silently in the background, and stepping forward when needed. The public face of funeral directors is one of grave solemnity. If they are alone and in the public view, such as driving the hearse, they may be talking, cracking jokes, but all with a straight face and barely moving their lips.

My friend attended a funeral for a 12-year-old girl who died in a riding accident. When she returned, she said "all the girl's friends were there in their riding gear, and the horse was outside the church. At the reception, the father was quiet, politely shaking guests' hands—he could not take it, and left—but the mother comforted the room." I was stunned . "How do you comfort a *room*?," I asked.

My friend said, "The girl's mother moved around the room quietly hugging and thanking her daughter's friends for coming. She said "It's all right. It will be alright."

AXIOMS

Next, we examined the analysis of all of the studies to identify common characteristics according to context (see Table 36.1). Patient cues and signals of distress were present in all of the studies, so that this formed a very strong characteristic. Other characteristics were not present in all of the studies, but as a whole provided a comprehensive picture of comforting.

From these data and interpretive insights we have some very strong axioms:[5]

---

[4] In America we have separated death from the hospital, removing the bodies as discretely as possible. The hospital in Seoul, Korea, that I visited had the morgue and funeral parlors as a part of the hospital. Families could move seamlessly from dying in palliative care to the services needed by the family immediately following death.

[5] An axiom is a premise that is self-evident, and may be accepted "as true" without discussion.

TABLE 36.1
Characteristics of Comforting Across Studies

CHARACTERISTICS OF COMFORTING	STUDY								
	Enduring and suffering	Patient states	Trauma studies	Disembodiment	Enduring to die	Infant pain study	Vent camp	Commitment and involvement	Diagnosis for breast cancer
Self-comforting strategies	✓	✓	✓	✓	✓		✓	✓	✓
Patient cues/signals	✓	✓	✓	✓	✓	✓	✓	✓	✓
Patient-led	✓	✓	✓		✓	✓	✓	✓	✓
Nurse responsiveness to cues of distress			✓			✓	✓		✓
Nurse comforting interrupts signals of distress	✓	✓	✓			✓			
Comforting strategies are particular to patient's state of discomfort	✓	✓	✓						
Intuitive recognition of discomfort	✓	✓	✓			✓	✓	✓	
Nurse has a compendium of comforting strategies	✓		✓				✓	✓	
Malleability of comforting strategies	✓		✓			✓			
Comforting strategies match patient state	✓		✓				✓	✓	
Sequential application of comforting strategies	✓		✓			✓			
Nurse's style of care	✓		✓				✓	✓	✓
Evolving comforting relationship	✓	✓						✓	
Comfort Level	✓	✓	✓	✓	✓	✓	✓	✓	

- The type of comforting provided is dependent on the context, circumstance, type and intensity of suffering.
- Comforting strategies must match each state of suffering: If the wrong comforting strategy is used, the suffering intensifies.
- The alleviation of suffering, comfort, is achieved incrementally, through the application of multiple comforting actions.
- Comforting interactions intercept the vocalizations and behaviors signaling distress.
- Comforting interventions are time-limited. If started they should be continued until the person's condition changes.
- Comforting strategies are patterned and routinized.
- Comforting is a malleable action: It may be modified to meet immediate needs as signaled by the patient, corrected if the strategy is unhelpful, and continued as long as it is needed.
- Cues of discomfort must be evident, and the need for comforting signaled to the caregiver. If this is missing, the patient is unlikely to receive comfort.
- Caregiver comforting actions are "forgiving" and immediately correctable.
- If self-comforting is evident, these efforts should be supported by the caregiver.

These are general and abstract statements. Remember them. Remember how suffering and comforting interface.

SUMMARY

The process of developing mid-range theory using theoretical coalescence is a long-term endeavor, but one that compensates for the criticisms of qualitative research—that it is small sample research and is limited in scope. Theoretical coalescence increases the generalizability, the application, and the significance of the theory.

TO DO 36.3. TRACE THE DEVELOPMENT OF A MID-RANGE THEORY

Mid-range theories do not usually arise from a single project (but they may do). More often, the theories arise out of thinking that takes place over many years and with the conduct of many projects. This is true for both qualitative and quantitative mid-range theory. Select and read one of the theories listed in Box 23.1 using the reference list for that article, gather all of the previous articles written by the author about the theory, and examine the development of the theory.

REFERENCES

Côté, J. J., Morse, J. M., & James, S. G. (1991). The pain response of the postoperative newborn. *Journal of Advanced Nursing, 16*(4), 378–387.

Hyland, L., & Morse, J. M. (1995). Orchestrating comfort: The role of funeral directors. *Death Studies, 19*, 453–474.

Kolcaba, K. (2003). *Comfort theory and practice: A vision for holistic health care.* New York, NY: Springer Publishing.

Leininger, M. M. (1978). *Transcultural nursing: Concepts, theories and practices.* New York, NY: John Wiley & Sons.

Morse, J. M. (1992). Comfort: The refocusing of nursing care. *Clinical Nursing Research, 1,* 91–113.

Morse, J. M. (2001). Toward a praxis theory of suffering. *Advances in Nursing Science, 24*(1), 47–59.

Morse, J. M. (2002). Emotional re-enactment [Editorial]. *Qualitative Health Research, 12*(2), 147.

Morse, J. M. (2011). The Praxis Theory of Suffering. In J. B. Butts & K. L. Rich (Eds.), *Philosophies and theories in advanced nursing practice* (pp. 569–602). Burlington, MA: Jones & Bartlett.

Morse, J. M. (2012). *Qualitative health research: Creating a new discipline.* Walnut Creek, CA: Left Coast Press.

Morse, J. M., & Mitcham, C. (1998). The experience of agonizing pain and signals of disembodiment. *Journal of Psychosomatic Research, 44*(6), 667–680

Morse, J. M., & Proctor, A. (1998). Maintaining patient endurance: The comfort work of trauma nurses. *Clinical Nursing Research, 7*(3), 250–274.

Morse, J. M., Penrod, J., Kassab, C., & Dellasega, C. (2000). Evaluating the efficiency and effectiveness of approaches to nasogastric tube insertion during trauma care. *American Journal of Critical Care, 9*(5), 325–333.

Morse, J. M., Pooler, C., Vann-Ward, T., Maddox, L., Olausson, J. M., Roche-Dean, M., . . . Martz, K. (2014). Awaiting the diagnosis of breast cancer: Strategies of enduring for preserving self. *Oncology Nursing Forum, 41*(4), 350–359.

Morse, J. M., Solberg, S., & Edwards, J. (1993). Caregiver-infant interaction: Comforting the postoperative infant. *Scandinavian Journal of Caring Sciences, 7*, 105–111.

Morse, J. M., Whitaker, H., & Tasón, M. (1996). The caretakers of suffering. In J. Chesworth (Ed.), *Transpersonal healing: Essays on the ecology of health* (pp. 91–104). Newbury Park, CA: Sage.

Nightingale, F. (1860/1969). *Notes on nursing: What it is and what it is not.* New York, NY: Dover.

Proctor, A., Morse, J. M., & Khonsari, E. S. (1996). Sounds of comfort in the trauma center: How nurses talk to patients in pain. *Social Science & Medicine, 42*(12), 1669–1680. doi:10.1016/0277-9536(95)00298-7

Solberg, S., & Morse, J. M. (1991). The comforting behaviors of caregivers toward distressed post-operative neonates. *Issues in Comprehensive Pediatric Nursing, 14*(2), 77–92.

THE PRAXIS THEORY OF COMFORT AND COMFORTING[1]

> *Asked by elderly woman:*
> *"What do you call a group of nurses?"*
> *Answer: "A comfort!"*

What, then, is *comfort*? At the broadest level in Chapter 36, we developed axioms for the Theory of Comfort and Comforting. These were derived from research, from multiple projects. They are assumptions that I held to be reasonable, all things considered, and provided a context for the macro- and microanalytic processes inherent in the theory.

CONTEXTUAL FACTORS INFLUENCING COMFORT AND COMFORTING

There is one more series of factors before we put all of these components together—and that is the context in which comforting (and nursing) occurs. In addition to the overly narrow focus of interaction or the superficial focus of relationship studies, research has ignored many fundamental facts inherent in the nurse–patient situation. These characteristics are as follows.

The Patient Is Usually Cared for by Many Nurses in the Course of a Single Day

Although one nurse may be responsible for the development and implementation of a patient's care plan, due to the demands of 24-hour care, shift work,

---

[1] This chapter has been published in part from Morse, J. M., DeLuca-Havens, G. A., & Wilson, S. (1997). The comforting interaction: Developing a model of nurse-patient relationship. *Scholarly Inquiry for Nursing Practice, 11*(4), 321–343.

the demands of days off and for meal and coffee breaks, care is actually provided by many nurses with different levels of preparation, and holding different relationships with the patient. These nurses may have a "relationship" established with this particular patient or be unfamiliar, presenting a new face to the patient. Furthermore, nursing care is not equally distributed between patients. Some nurses interact with some patients more frequently and for greater periods of time than others.

Surprisingly, despite differences in nursing education, experience, and relationships, these teams of nurses are presumed by administration to being able to provide adequate, and roughly equivalent, care. In short, it is assumed that once these nurses have read the patient's chart, they are considered, from the administration's perspective, as interchangeable (Morse et al., 1992). Of course, this attitude—the "warm body" style of nursing administration—acknowledges only entry-level clinical competency. It does not acknowledge the significance of the *relationship* component of the nurse–patient relationship. In fact, nursing administration intentionally organizes staff to prevent such relationships from developing, and to protect nurses from becoming "involved" with patients. The result is that patients rarely refer to nurses (and even more rarely to one particular nurse), and if they do, they speak of "the nurses" as a collective. It is interesting that nurses, unlike physicians, are almost never referred to by name.

Nursing Care is Often Provided by Groups of Caregivers Working Simultaneously

The second characteristic of the nurse–patient relationship occurs when major procedures are being performed, when the patient requires assistance (such as lifting and, we know, comforting), when urgent care is being provided, or when complex tasks are being performed. In these instances, several nurses may be simultaneously involved in the care, with one nurse directing the team. If the care is painful or the patient is a child and his or her parents are visiting, the nurse may second the parent or a non-nurse (such as an aide or an orderly) to assist. The nurse usually directs, coordinates, and accepts responsibility for the procedure.

The Nurse Does Not Serve as an Independent Therapist, but Rather as an Agent of the Physician or the Institution

Because the individual nurse is considered interchangeable and part of a team, any confidential information given to a particular nurse is recorded in the patient's chart or passed on informally in the patient's report. This indicates that the nurses themselves consider such information to belong, albeit for the patient's good, to the greater arena of pertinent "patient information" to which the team of nursing and medical staff has access. Despite the recording and reporting of such information, the nurse still considers him or herself to have retained patient confidentiality. This action also indicates that nurses consider themselves to be agents of the institution and the physician, something that Wolgast (1992) has labeled an "artificial person." Nurses are not in an autonomous position in regard to making decisions for patient treatment, and they demonstrate greater allegiance to the medical staff and the institution than to the patient. Such a clinical reality is not explicitly stated to patients, and when disclosure of a confidence occurs, it may result in the loss of trust and profound changes in the nurse–patient relationship.

THE PRAXIS THEORY OF COMFORT AND COMFORTING

Components of Comforting

Comforting consists of caring (as a motivator for the nurse to provide comfort and to monitor the patient condition throughout the process) and a comforting action, or interaction, provided as a process, until the patient reaches an endurable *comfort level*.

Comfort Encompasses Caring

Comfort is a concept that incorporates the caring focus of nursing—which enables us to see the cues and signals of suffering and motivates us to comfort—and a comforting action or task (Morse, 2000b). Note that when comfort is the central concept for nursing, nursing care is focused on the patient (in contrast to caring, which is focused on the nurse). Within this framework, nurses' use of touch and talk are **not** indicators of caring per se; rather, they are comforting strategies that are responses to *signals of suffering*. They are *strategies for alleviating suffering* (Morse, 1992). Comforting therefore cannot be separated from suffering.

What Is a Patient's Comfort Level?

The patient's *comfort level* is the degree of *dis*comfort that is tolerable or bearable, and the goal of nursing is always to minimize the patient's discomfort and to maximize the patient's comfort state. The comfort level may thus be perceived as a continuum ranging from complete comfort to extreme agony, and the patient's comfort level is dynamic, continuously fluctuating on this continuum. Comfort level is used between nurses as a means of quickly communicating the patient's state of comfort and determining their comfort needs.

The comfort level is **not** *a measure of pain, but rather how well a patient is tolerating or enduring the pain.*

Comforting Is a Process

Nurse-comforting interventions are not a "one-shot" intervention, but a process that occurs in many iterative steps at the microanalytic level (as a therapy) and within the interaction and the developing relationship (as a psychosocial intervention). These processes form the *comforting-interaction loop* in which a need for comfort is observed or requested, the comforting action occurs, the patient is re-evaluated, and another comforting action is provided, and so forth.

Examples of the comforting-interaction loop may be:

- Observing that the patient appears in pain (noting the *cues of distress* or *signals of suffering*), verifying the pain with the patient (action), administering an analgesic action (comforting action), and observing signs that the pain was subsequently alleviated
- Observing the patient appears cold and is shivering (noting the *behavioral cue*), fetching a warm blanket (comforting action), and observing the patient appears more relaxed and warmer

As nursing tasks increase in complexity, so do the comforting actions:

- During childbirth the nurse observes the patient is becoming distressed (a signal of suffering), and uses her voice (comforting interaction, such as "talking through" or an expression of empathy) to assist in synchronizing the second-stage labor until the woman regains control (see Bergstrom et al., 2009).
- In the trauma room during resuscitation, a patient is scared but lying still (caring observation). The nurse provides presence, and a "running commentary," talking constantly, describing everything that she and the trauma team are doing (Chapter 35). Later, the patient said that she "just listened to that nurse's voice and held on."
- During trauma resuscitation, the nurse observes that the patient is terrified (a *signal* of suffering), and she uses the *Comfort Talk Register* to enable the patient to hold on, and hold still (a comforting action) until the analgesics take effect (see Morse & Proctor, 1998; Proctor, Morse, & Khonsari, 1996).

The *comforting-interaction loop* continues until comfort is no longer needed and is no longer demanded by the patient. From this perspective, comforting is a major component of every nursing action, minor or major, transitory or prolonged, including the provision of the technical aspects of care as well as direct and indirect comforting strategies. *Making the patient comfortable is the goal of nursing* (Morse, 1992).

Comfort is attained as an immediate, short-term goal (i.e., comforting), which is to ease and relieve or to assist the patient to endure and to last through a procedure. This is congruent with the dictionary definition of comfort: to ease, relieve, or to "make strong." When patients are comfortable, that is, when comfort is attained, they have no need for a nurse (Nightingale, 1860/1969). The long-term goal of comfort is the achievement of relief or optimal health.

Definition

Comfort is a *relative and optimal state of well-being that may occur during any stage of the illness–health continuum* (Morse, 1992).

Providing Comfort

I suggest that the comforting process consists of the nurse recognizing a *patient cue* or *signal of distress* (indicating a patient need), assessing, and intervening with a comforting strategy or procedure. The outcome or patient response cues or signals are then assessed or evaluated by the nurse, another strategy implemented, and so forth. It sounds very simple, but it is extraordinarily difficult to research and to document the efficacy of comforting strategies.

What Is a Patient *Cue*?

A patient cue may be in the form of a pain response, restlessness, an utterance, expression, or even a request. Patient cues indicate discomfort, and by responding to such cues, nurses provide comfort. For example, nurses may adjust the patient's position, offer or administer pain medications, and so forth. In other words, patient cues motivate the nurse to provide comforting strategies, even if the patient has not requested such care.

What Is a *Signal of Distress*?

Signals of distress are larger groupings of patient cues that clearly indicate a patient problem—usually, acute distress. The behavioral signals of distress may be accompanied and reinforced by physiological signs of distress—increased pulse, falling blood pressure, and so forth. A signal of distress may even be a verbal request or complaint.

What Is a Comfort Strategy?

Comforting strategies are methods or techniques of comforting the distressed person. While not unique to nursing, it is nursing's role, and privilege, to use comfort strategies when caring for the distressed person. Comfort strategies may be as follows.

Direct

These are strategies administered directly to the patient. *Direct strategies* are universal patterns of touch, talking, and listening, which may be used to keep the patient in control by eye contact, voice, such as in *talking the patient through* painful procedures, and the responsive use of touch. Recall, while comforting strategies are patterned, they are also particular to the patient's state. They also include providing appropriate explanations, as well as providing competent care; they include providing gender, age, and culturally appropriate care.

It is crucial that the comfort strategies match the patient's *comfort level* because using comfort strategies that are intended for a different state will result in the escalation of discomfort. Comfort strategies are variable. An experienced nurse has a large repertoire and changes the strategies in accordance with the patient's state. Thus, while the comfort strategies used are nurse-controlled, they are patient-led.

Indirect

These are strategies that control the actions of others or manipulate the environment. *Indirect strategies* include such actions as providing warmth, quiet, or darkness and are used for protecting the patient, to pace and sequence care to minimize distress, and to manipulate the environment to maximize patient rest and prevent fatigue. They also include monitoring, the administration of an analgesic, and to minimize distress, and to perform the therapies and plan of care for the patient.

The Context of Comforting

Comfort strategies vary in complexity. They may be as simple as placing a hand on the patient's shoulder; it may be as technical as responding to a code with efficiency, speed, and competence. A comfort strategy may be keeping vigilance while the patient "sleeps," or it may be forcefully getting the patient out of bed, despite protests of, "It hurts!," "Not today!," and "Wait—I'm not ready."

Nurse-comforting strategies buffer the injury/illness experience and alleviate the intensity of symptoms for the patient. Because comfort strategies are *variable* and *context-dependent*, they cannot be formulated. Rather, the expert nurse has an enormous repertoire of comforting strategies and is versatile in their application. An expert nurse "reads the patient" by reassessing situational *clues* or *signals of distress*, patient *cues*, and responds to triggers in the situation. The expert nurse instantly recognizes *patient cues* or *signals of distress*. The expert nurse is *versatile*, so that if a comforting strategy does not work, is ineffective, or causes discomfort, then another comforting strategy is used. Expert nurses have a large *compendium of comforting strategies* that they provide sequentially according to the patient's state and perceived need. Assessment of the attainment of the optimal comfort level is ongoing.

What About Self-Comforting? The Patient's Approach

Recall from the *Praxis Theory of Suffering*, (Chapter 35) that when encountering loss or an illness that must be endured, individuals try to maintain control and not panic. This is the first step in self-comforting. Individuals tend to "shut down," and put whatever they are suffering about at the back of their minds (Morse et al., 2014). They suppress emotions of panic, horror, and fear, and in the process, move into a state of enduring. They reassure themselves, and try to maintain normality in their lives, concealing their worry or symptoms. A patient may deny or refuse to acknowledge the illness or the symptom; consider this as another form of self-comforting, which may not be in the patient's best interest.

TO DO 37.1. WATCH PATIENTS BEFORE VISITING AND THEN WATCH THEM GREET VISITORS

Describe their changes in behaviors. Describe their "before visitor" and "during visit" behaviors. Do they report their "complaints" and pains to their visitors as they do to you?

Self-comforting also takes the form of behaviors: We recognize posturing to minimize pain; we see patients moving with an altered gait to minimize pain; we see toddlers rocking or patients lying very still and refusing to move because "it hurts." All of these behaviors are self-comforting strategies.

Patient Actions in Assessing the Nurse

Behaviors that are unique to the patients as recipients of care are those that evaluate the nurse, decide whether or not to trust the nurse's care, that is, to *relinquish for care*, and form patterns of relating. These patient actions influence the relationship and provide the patient with the control that influences the nurse's response and the nurse's actions. Each independent contact or interaction results an implicit negotiation from which the nurse–patient relationship evolves.

Patients use strategies to evaluate their nurse. First, the patient determines whether or not the nurse is a "good person." For example, the patient questions the nurse about her personal life disguised as social conversations such as, "Are you from around here?" and "Do you have children?" Second, the patient determines if the nurse is a "good" nurse. For example, the patient checks whether or not the nurse "likes her job," where she went to nursing school, and how long she has been nursing. Patients also "get references" from other patients ("Is she a good nurse?") and evaluate if the nurse has "good hands." If the nurse rates adequately, and the patient decides to trust the nurse, the patient then makes overtures by being a "good patient" and being friendly. Patients may give gifts (such as chocolates) and compliments either directly to the nurse or deliberately to other patients or visitors within the nurse's hearing. On the other hand, if the patient does not trust the nurse, the patient uses strategies to prevent the nurse from "knowing" him or her by refusing to make eye contact, focusing dialogue on symptoms and treatments, and may become demanding, coercive, uncooperative, and/or manipulative (Morse, 1991b).

The level of trust developed results in *patient-led patterns of relating* with the nurse. As stated earlier, if the patient does not trust the nurse, the patient may use behaviors that nurses have labeled as "difficult." These patients, depending on their needs, condition, and behaviors, control the type of relationship that eventually develops. In this sense, the type of relationship is *patient-controlled*, and the nurse responds to these patient cues. For instance, if the patient chooses to enter a joking relationship, the patient manifests joking behaviors that, in turn, elicit teasing behavior and responses from the nurse. If the patient is in pain, the responses elicited from the nurse are those behaviors appropriate for a patient in pain. With each nurse–patient contact, the relationship develops and eventually evolves to become one that meets the needs of both the nurse and the patient.

NURSING APPROACH

A *nursing approach* supports the patient's self-comforting strategies. The nursing approach is a patterned, normative, and professional behavior granted to a nurse by society because of her professional role, education, and responsibilities. They include role behaviors that typify a nurse and provide her with access to the patient and to the patient's body for particular expected, necessary tasks of greeting, assessment, confidences, surveillance, treatments, care of bodily functions and hygiene, and so forth. The nursing approach includes all of the "scripted" questions and tasks of assessment, treatment, and caregiving.

Styles of Care

A style of care is the nurse's manner of approaching individual patients. Nurses unconsciously adapt their style of care to match the patient's perceived needs. Nurses' styles of care vary according to the patient's affect, age, gender, culture, and condition. Nurses may greet an elderly patient in pain with quiet respect, or a child with distraction, and an upbeat tone. Or nurses may counter a patient's affect, cajoling a depressed patient or being stern with a noncompliant. The nurse's interaction with each patient is different.

A nurse's posturing and approach is often dictated by, and matches, the style of care. And often, microanalytic comforting strategies accompany the style of care: Consider whether or not the nurse touches or hugs a patient. Embedded in the style of care is the nurse's personality. Some nurses are quiet and consoling; others are lighthearted and funny. Some nurses find it easy to talk to a patient and "draw" him or her out. Others keep to the nursing "script."

TO DO 37.2. IDENTIFYING STYLES OF CARE

Observe a situation in which nurses are moving from one patient to another, such as an intermediate level care, the medical-surgical unit in the emergency department. Notice how the nurse talks softly to the patient in pain, with her head inches from the patient's ear; teases the responsive, anxious patients to normalize the situation; approaches children very cautiously and waits until they respond, permitting her to come close.

Record these approaches and the patient's responses.

Within these various approaches used by nurses, or "styles of care," are embedded complex collections of comforting strategies, including environmental manipulation for the "comforting role of the nurse." These roles meet the patient's needs, enhancing the establishment of trust.

Comforting Strategies

Strategies are actions used by the nurse to make the patient comfortable, and are used in response to patient cues of discomfort or signals of distress. Nurses

> **TO DO 37.3. WHAT IS THE DIFFERENCE BETWEEN AN *INTERACTION* AND A *RELATIONSHIP*?**
>
> Something to think about: in the literature, theories and research focusing on nurse–patient interaction linked to literature, theories, and research about nurse–patient relationship? Why or why not?

either intentionally or intuitively assess patients for behavioral cues indicating discomfort or environmental factors (i.e., clues) contributing to the discomfort and respond with comforting strategies. Comforting strategies are developed from both the art and the science of nursing. Strategies offered by nurses may be independent, ranging from touching and talking, to interventions (e.g., positioning or giving a back rub), or may be collaborative, such as the administration of medically prescribed treatments (e.g., administering an analgesic).

Strategies may be transient (such as a tap or a sympathetic verbal response such as, "there, there") or occur over a longer duration (such as stroking or listening with empathetic silence). These comforting strategies may be premeditated or planned as a part of a nursing intervention. Alternatively, strategies may occur without the nurse's awareness (Ramos, 1992; Proctor, Morse, & Khonsari, 1996). They may be used almost reflexively, as a normal part of human and professional interaction. Strategies may be direct (that is, provided directly to the patient) or indirect (that is, provided by manipulating the environment). Examples of direct strategies are touching, talking, listening, and posturing. Indirect strategies may include providing warmth or controlling lighting or ensuring rest by limiting visitors.

Research with trauma patients and with postoperative infants (discussed previously) reveals that comfort strategies provided by nurses are patient-led (i.e., provided in response to a patient cue) and are distinct for the patient's state (Proctor, Morse, & Khonsari, 1996). For example, if the patient is perceived to be frightened or in pain, then patterns of touching and talking for a frightened patient or for a patient in pain must be provided. To treat the patient as terrified, when the patient is actually scared, escalates the patient's behaviors and is not perceived as comforting.

Some nursing strategies are learned formally as a part of nursing education, extensively described in nursing fundamentals textbooks (e.g., see Wilkinson & Treas, 2011) and are meticulously taught in introductory nursing classes. But comforting strategies are mainly acquired informally in the clinical setting by nurses observing more experienced nurses interacting with patients and providing care, and by learning by trial and error, by *doing comforting*. The provision of nursing care is interactive, and is a continuous learning process. As nurses provide care, they gain experience in which strategies are effective, which strategies are less effective, and which strategies are unwelcome, depending upon the patient's response in particular contextual situations. In this way, experience teaches nurses which strategies to use, when to use them, and with which particular patient cues and situational clues they are appropriate.

Nurses constantly assess the patient for the effectiveness and efficacy of comforting strategies. If a strategy is not "working," the nurse immediately changes the strategy. For instance, consider the research with videotaped observations of nurses comforting postoperative infants, which revealed if patterns of touch were not effective, nurses changed the type of touch sequentially from patting to stroking to rubbing usually within 10 sec or less (Solberg & Morse, 1991). However, if nurses continued with ineffective comforting strategies or persisted in using such strategies, then the infant's behavior escalated.

Compendium of Comforting Strategies

With experience, nurses develop an extensive compendium of comforting strategies. From this "bank" of comforting strategies, they develop their own individual repertoire of preferred strategies. Some are present in everyday interactions, without premeditation, as we console or commiserate. Other strategies are used thoughtfully, and with care, such as providing empathy or formal counseling strategies. Some comforting strategies are prescribed, such as administering an analgesic; some are standardized as a part of excellent nursing care, such as a massage, position change, or exercise. Some are in control of nursing but not routine, such as placing a patient on an air mattress. Some are indirect, such as controlling the environment—noise levels or the temperature.

The point is that all of these strategies enhance enduring, to help the patient get through, to reduce, minimize, or alleviate the patient's suffering. Several strategies may be used simultaneously as patterned "sets" to form unique combinations of comforting. For example, when providing comfort to trauma patients, nurses simultaneously use the Comfort Talk Register (Proctor, Morse, & Khonsari, 1996; Morse & Proctor, 1998), comforting touch, and position themselves in close proximity to the patient.

Comforting is individualized, with the nurse's actions derived from patterns of relating, unconsciously selecting or using a style of care that matches or counters the patient's discomfort, and sequentially using comforting strategies. This model is diagramed in Figure 37.1.

Backfiring of Comforting Strategies

In Chapter 36, I asked, "What if the wrong strategy is used?" and I made the case that patients were forgiving, and to apologize and try another strategy.

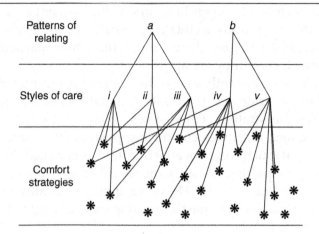

FIGURE 37.1

The derivations of nursing action.

a, b Nurses' approaches become increasingly patterned.

i, ii, iii, iv, v Individual nurse's style of care, developed from a combination of strategies and selected according to context and patient needs.

** Strategy, such as touch, verbal response, or comforting procedure.

Source: Morse, DeLuca-Havens, and Wilson (1997). Reprinted with permission.

But sometimes comforting strategies "backfire"—especially when the nurse misreads the patient and the patient's response requires something more. These are the mistakes that they may never forget and tell their visitors about. What then happens if an inappropriate comforting strategy is used?

We call the "mismanagement" of comfort, "backfiring," because the patient's comfort level escalates. The following problems have thus far been identified:

- Although well intentioned, the strategy is not comforting (see Stern & Kerry, 1996). Examples of verbal noncomforting strategies—and we are all guilty—are statements such as: *"Of course you are not going to 'throw up,'" "Just relax,"* and *"What, you've had a baby before and you don't know how to push!"*
  a. Touch may also be noncomforting, and this may happen when the part of the body touched is tender or sore, when the touch is poorly timed or unexpected, or when the touch is culturally inappropriate.
  b. Of greater concern, is using the wrong strategy: using strategies for emotional suffering (touch, sympathetic/empathetic talk, encouraging the expression of feelings) for patients who are enduring.

- *Repeating a strategy, even though it was unsuccessful the first time:* Comfort strategies must be versatile because comfort needs are individualized; strategies that may be successful with one person may not be comforting to another—as any mother who has had one infant that "settles" when his back is tickled, and another one that didn't. Repeating a failed strategy resembles victim blaming, for it appears as "What is wrong with *you* if you don't respond . . ." Such actions are useless, a waste of time, and frustrating for all.
- *Refusing to answer or to give an answer:* When a head injured patient asks repeatedly for information, the "endless loop" of questions and answers, of repeating, "You're in the hospital" or "Your family is OK," are unavoidable. The patient *cannot* recall the information that has been given—the constant repeating of requests is not intentional. The nurse responding, no matter how kindly, "I've told you that before," only escalates the patient's distress.
- *Talking over the patient's head:* Explanations, intended to prepare the patient for a painful procedure or an invasive procedure, are not comforting if they are incomprehensible. For instance, one does not say to an 11-year-old boy, "And now I'm going to catheterize you."
- *Care that is not paced:* Explanations must be given sufficiently in advance of the procedure for the patient to process the information and to psychologically prepare, to get ready to "take it." Information that is given simultaneously with the procedure is useless. Care must be paced so that one procedure is given at a time. Multiple procedures, given simultaneously, lead to assaultive care and the patient losing control.
- *Inconsistency in comforting strategies:* If the patient has a support person, that person must remain with the patient until the care is given. Ideally, that person should not be involved in the care or have other responsibilities since keeping the patient "with it," talking them through painful procedures, holding, touching, and being there will absorb the nurse's concentration; deserting or not responding will result in the instantaneous escalation of distress, particularly in children.

The aforementioned strategies, intended to comfort but causing discomfort, remove the patient's feeling of trust and feeling of safety. As the patient becomes more distressed and distraught, care is slowed and the patient's condition escalates.

These problems can be prevented by using thoughtful, sensitive care, and placing the patient needs first. These responses certainly give you a lot to think about, and rarely does a nurse make the same mistake twice.

ATTAINING COMFORT

Back to the Patient

Thus, when comforting, a nurse constantly observes the patient for cues that a comforting strategy is effective or the strategy is changed. For example, in trauma care, nurses' comfort strategies aim to keep patients in control and responsive, cooperative, and receptive to care. Despite the pain, they try to remain still, to endure, to "take it," to "bear it," and not to cry out. These patients work with staff; the patient who has completely relinquished realizes that care is necessary and submits to "whatever needs to be done." The result is that care is given quickly and safely. However, the comfort level is a dynamic continuum, and the patient's comfort level may change rapidly. Nursing assessment is continuous, and comfort strategies continually change (Morse, 2000d).

Patient Actions

Patients endure and emotionally suffer illness. They experience emotions from despair to hope and constantly respond to various symptoms and various degrees of impairment. They may fear losing who they are. These factors, along with responses to the immediate context, underlie their illness behavior. Patient actions are conceptualized in a model similar to nursing actions, as signals of discomfort (also including the cues), indices of distress, and patterns of relating.

Signals of discomfort (also including the cues)
Patients' behavioral responses to discomfort are implicitly or explicitly observable. These signals may be verbalized, they may be contextual, and they may be obtained from the report (or knowing the normative course of the disease or illness), from the patients' relatives or even from the patient in the next bed, who may be sharing the room. As noted previously, they may be observed by the nurse or verbalized in response to assessment as a complaint.

Indices of distress
Signals of distress and patient cues may cluster into indices of distress. Particular pain responses may have modes of posturing, including accompanying signs, such as facial grimacing, fever, pallor, and sweating, indicating the need for comforting as nursing an intervention.

Patterns of relating

While the indices of distress indicate comforting needs, the needs itself do not necessarily indicate the acceptance of care. The patient's personality and self-perception of the seriousness of the symptoms and discomfort will determine if he or she will accept care and, most importantly, accept that care. A patient must decide to trust the nurse, before relinquishing to care.

The nurse must "follow the patient's lead," and this strategy will facilitate the development of the relationship. The nurse usually "matches" the patient's affect: If the patient is joking, the nurse responds in a like manner; if the patient is in pain, the nurse is quiet and solicitous. Less often the nurses' affect is different from the patients: If the patient is depressed, the nurse may cajole, and so forth. With each contact between the nurse and the patient, the relationship develops and eventually evolves to one that meets the needs for both the nurse and the patient, and the patient relinquished to care.

From the patient's perspective, *attaining comfort* includes the ability to trust; be supported; to hope; to receive competent, well-paced, and synchronized care; and a medical management of the injury or illness that is bearable, the symptoms endurable, and the treatments tolerable. For instance, in the emergency department, patient comfort is not achieved until the patient *feels safe*. For the patient to *feel safe*, the nurse must demonstrate competence, caring, and vigilance by *being there*; the patient may test the nurse, learn to trust, and then *relinquish* to the care of the nurse. Yet, *feeling safe* does not alter the pain and the distress.

You are asked: "What is his comfort level?" Remember, the comfort level is actually not a level of patient comfort, but rather the level of distress and how well the pain (or whatever is causing the distress) is being tolerated (or endured). For instance, when a nurse is asked, "What is his comfort level?", the reply may be "He is tolerating it quite well"—which means to us that the patient is enduring the procedure, and it is not necessary to provide an analgesic immediately. On the other hand, the nurse may reply, "He is really scared" or "He is out of control—we really need a hand in the trauma room!" Ask yourself: How well is the pain being tolerated?

How Do Nurses Assess the Patient's Comfort Level?

Nurses consciously and subconsciously, continuously assess the patient's comfort level. There are two kinds of nursing assessment. The first is the type that is included in your basic education and continues throughout a nursing career; that is, the evaluation and interpretation of physical signs and symptoms. The second type is the assessment of the patients' comfort level, looking for patient cues and reading their signals of distress. Nurses learn how to listen to patient's complaints of discomfort, to monitor a patient's physical condition, and to intervene whenever necessary. Nurses learn from experience to assess the patient's cues and signals of distress. Nurses use perception, insight, and intuition gained from experience. Nurses respond with basic nursing care. They also respond with empathy, compathy, and sympathy, commiseration, and compassion in their selection of comforting interventions.

I observed that nurses' responses to questions such as: "How's his comfort level?" ranged from settled/comfortable to scared/afraid/distressed/agitated/terrified/out of control. Each of these categories describes clusters of behaviors displayed by patients who have differing ability to cope or endure their discomfort as signals of distress or states of discomfort. That is, comfort levels describe behavior patterns of patients who are no longer capable of cooperating with care.

Remember: The comfort level is not the amount of pain that is being experienced, but how well it is being tolerated. It enables the rapid communication of the patient's behavioral state of suffering.

THE COMFORTING INTERACTION

Despite the large amount of research on the nurse–patient interaction and relationship, this research remains fragmented, providing only partial representations of the actual nurse–patient interaction and limited perspectives on the nurse–patient relationship. Yet it is within this juncture of interaction and relationship that all the significant comforting interactions take place.[2] Recognizing the content of the interaction between the nurse and the patient and the significance and quality of the relationship established, is crucial for understanding the nature of comforting and the nature of nursing itself. Therefore, examination and reconstruction of a comprehensive model representing the nurse–patient interaction within the relationship is essential for comprehending the comfort and comforting. In developing the *Praxis Theory of Comfort and Comforting*, we will use our understanding of the comforting interactions (the components and strategies of comforting), and show how these build the relationship—or various types of nurse–patient relationships). *The type of relationship varies with the patient's need(s), the nurses' willingness to engage and to provide comfort, and in some sense, the amount of time and number of interactions.*

---

[2] The fragmentation of *interaction* and *relationship* has resulted in two separate but interrelated bodies of literature. This distinction has led, for example, to very awkward ways of discussing these concepts, and to tunnel vision and artificial delineation of the problem on the part of researchers. Authors who examine patient interaction often examine a snapshot, a scene, without considering its history or its outcomes, antecedents, or consequences—yet they pay extraordinary attention to minute detail, observing behaviors, analyzing dialogue, and noting the immediate purpose of the interaction. Researchers examining the relationship explore perceptions and interpretations attributed to the relationship, but do not, and cannot, attend to the detail described in the interaction literature. The numerous "actors"—the nurse and the patient (although the literature as a whole tends to focus on the nurse), and sometimes the family, the physician, or other health care professionals compound the problems of analysis further fragmenting the literature. In this conceptualization of comforting, I bring these perspectives together in a single, comprehensive model.

THE INTERACTIVE COMPONENTS

The comforting interaction consists of the patient cue, or a signal of distress from the patient that is perceived by the nurse, and the nurse then assesses the patient and provides a comfort strategy (Morse, DeLuca-Havens, & Wilson, 1997). The nurse subsequently observes and assesses for the effectiveness of the strategy, and, if the discomfort or distress has not been resolved, provides another comfort strategy. This cycle may be slow and deliberate, or as quick and almost subconscious within the interaction. As the comforting interactions accrue, so does the trust in the nurse–patient relationship build, and the relationship itself changes from a clinical relationship, to a therapeutic relationship, to a connected relationship (Morse, 1991b); the patient feels safe, and relinquishes to the nurse's care.

The comforting interaction is patient-led; in our observations of postoperative infants, comforting was always in response to the infant's cues. If the infant did not, or could not, "demand" a comforting strategy, it was usually not provided. For instance, because the infants were intubated, they cried silently, unable to vocalize. As a result nurses rarely used their voices to comfort intubated infants.

> Thus, the nurse provides care that is appropriate to the patient's state, and each state has a different compendium of comforting strategies. If the nurse provides the wrong strategy, then the patient's state escalates. However, the nurse immediately corrects his or her error, and changes the comforting intervention. (Morse, DeLuca-Havens, & Wilson, 1997)

How important are these comforting interventions? Did you know that the way a nurse talks to the patient while inserting a nasogastric (NG) tube affects the success of the procedure? (Morse, Penrod, Kassab, & Dellasega, 2000; Penrod, Morse, & Wilson, 1999). If the nurses use technical talk—talk that focuses solely on what the patient should do—or uses solely caring terms of endearment and is overly receptive to the patient's cues of distress and does not include instructions for the patient—the procedure will require more trials to insert the tube. The optimal way, for both patient comfort and safe insertion, is to talk to patients with a blend of technical and comfort talk, and our research has shown that when the nurse uses the optimal style of talking, the NG tube is successfully inserted with fewest trials.

THE COMPLEXITY OF PROVIDING COMFORT: THE COMFORTING RELATIONSHIP

The present model of the nurse perceiving the patient's cues and signals and using matching comforting strategies to meet the patient's needs becomes more complex and changes over time. Ideally, the nurse–patient relationship is incrementally building, and as it builds so does the nurse come to "know" the patient, just as the patient knows and trusts the nurse (Box 37.1).

BOX 37.1. THE PROCESS OF COMFORTING

- Always meet the patient as a person, at his or her level.
- A particular set of strategies works best for each situation and patient state.
- If you use the wrong strategy, apologize and use another strategy.
- Comforting strategies are often used only for a very short time—quickly and even subconsciously evaluated—and if not "working" (reducing distress/discomfort), the strategy is changed.
- Constantly re-evaluate the patient's state.

Recall that each patient does not have one nurse, but is cared for by many. Does this mean that the patient must have to build relationships with several nurses over the course of a day? Yes. And it means that each nurse must necessarily get to know several patients.

The comforting relationship evolves from the action of both the patient and the nurse. First, it evolves from how patients perceive the threat of their illness or injuries and the urgency and seriousness of their needs, and from their evaluation of nurses' competency and trustworthiness. From their response to their evaluation of the nurses, the patients' actions *as a patient* develop. Simultaneously, nurses' approaches, styles of care, and compendium of comforting strategies are particular to certain patient needs and cues. The nursing goal is to assist patients to reach an acceptable comfort level so that they may participate in or accept necessary and essential nursing care. Styles of care provide appropriate nursing strategies with which to approach individual patients and help them to accept that care. The patients' goal is to receive care that is dependable and to ensure that they will be cared for when they are in a dependent state.

Comforting is patient-led, except in exceptional situations in which the patient is compromised and cannot participate by choosing to accept or relinquish in response to the nurse, and these relationships, out of necessity, are led by the nurse. For example, when patients are unconscious and cannot verbalize their needs or when patients' condition places them at risk for self injury, nurse-led actions serve to provide for the patients' safety and comfort while maintaining their dignity.

The relationship develops and changes with every patient contact, and it may develop to a mutually satisfactory type quickly or be negotiated over a long period of time. Sometimes patients trust the nurse quickly and choose to relinquish their care to the nurse. Relinquishment may range from complete and total (e.g., "Are you a nurse?" "Yes." "Oh, thank God!") to tentative (e.g., patient holds still but constantly reminds the nurse of the pain by making pain noises). At other times, the relationship may change in a mutually and implicitly agreeable "contract" as the patient's needs and condition change throughout the course of his or her illness. Figure 37.2 shows components of the comforting relationship of the nurse and the patient, and how interactions build to form a relationship.

The time necessary for developing a relationship and for the patient to relinquish to care, and to trust the nurse, depends upon the patient's perception of the urgency of the situation. Importantly, the "fit" between the nurse and the patient, and the degree of trust acquired is also considered. However, if patient's needs are great, and life-threatening, the patient will relinquish immediately.

What Is Relinquishing for Care?

Relinquishment for care is a part of the negotiating process that occurs when the patient's trust in the comforting relationship is beginning to be established. It occurs when the patient allows, gives permission, for the nurse to do whatever is necessary (Morse, 2000d). Of course, "relinquishment" is not an all or nothing state, but is one that will change over time, and develops as the nurse–patient relationship develops. I have identified the stages of relinquishment:

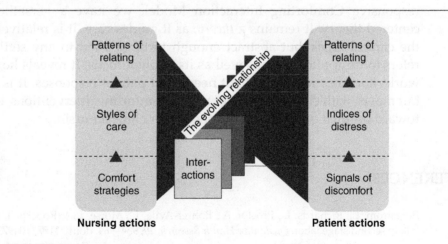

Nursing actions   **Patient actions**

FIGURE 37.2

The Comforting-Interaction Model: relinquishing to care.

Note: With each interaction, the evolving relationship develops.

Source: Morse, DeLuca-Havens, and Wilson (1997). Reprinted with permission.

1. *Forced relinquishment:* This is when the patient is reusing or objecting to care, such as when a child may be refusing an injection ("shot"). The patient does not trust the nurse; children will cry and resist.
2. *Conditional relinquishment:* Bargaining takes place between the nurse and the patient. The child may continue to protest throughout the procedure.
3. *Guarded relinquishment:* The patient lies still, cooperates, and permits treatments to be given, but there is limited trust in the nurse's care. His or her eyes monitor the care, and follow the nurse's actions. Sometimes the patient asks questions: "Why do I need that?" and "What is that pill for?" as he or she allows the nurse to proceed.
4. *Complete relinquishment:* The patient lies still, trusts the nurse, permitting treatments to be given. (Morse, 2000d). Thus, when the strategy is congruent with the patient's comfort level, the patient perceives the care as competent and necessary and is likely to readily relinquish to the procedure.

SUMMARY

As nursing care consists of many comforting interactions per patient encounter, the *Praxis*[3] *Theory of Comfort and Comforting* is a perspective for our nursing care. By combining direct and indirect comforting interactions within the responsive Comforting–Interaction Model, we have a versatile, patient-centered theory. It remains a *theory*, as it guides care. It is relatively close to the clinical areas, but abstract enough to be applied to any setting. *Praxis* refers to its applications, as well as its applied focus. It reveals how nursing works and accounts for patient needs and patient responses. It is not static, but moves with changing patient needs, comforting interventions, and works toward optimal outcomes. It is a theory for clinical nursing.

REFERENCES

Bergstrom, L., Richards, L., Proctor, A., Bohrer-Avila, L., Morse, J., & Roberts, J. (2009). Birth talk in second stage labor. *Qualitative Health Research, 19*, 954–964. doi:10.1177/1049732309338613

Morse, J. M. (1991b). Negotiating commitment and involvement in the patient–nurse relationship. *Journal of Advanced Nursing, 16*, 455–468.

---

[3] *Praxis* is the process by which a theory, lesson, or skill is enacted, practiced, embodied, or realized. "Praxis" may also refer to the act of engaging or applying, exercising, realizing, or practicing ideas (https://en.wikipedia.org/wiki/Praxis).

Morse, J. M. (1992). Comfort: The refocusing of nursing care. *Clinical Nursing Research, 1*, 91–113.

Morse, J. M. (2000b). Exploring pragmatic utility: Concept analysis by critically appraising the Literature. In B. Rodgers & K. Knafl (Eds.), *Concept development in nursing* (pp. 333–352). Philadelphia, PA: Saunders.

Morse, J. M. (2000d). On comfort and comforting. *American Journal of Nursing, 100*(9), 34–38.

Morse, J. M., & Proctor, A. (1998). Maintaining patient endurance: The comfort work of trauma nurses. *Clinical Nursing Research, 7*(3), 250–274.

Morse, J. M., Anderson, G., Bottorff, J., Yonge, O., O'Brien, B., Solberg, S., & McIlveen, K. (1992). Exploring empathy: A conceptual fit for nursing practice? *Image: Journal of Nursing Scholarship, 24*(4), 274–280.

Morse, J. M., DeLuca-Havens, G. A., & Wilson, S. (1997). The comforting interaction: Developing a model of nurse-patient relationship. *Scholarly Inquiry for Nursing Practice, 11*(4), 321–343.

Morse, J. M., Penrod, J., Kassab, C., & Dellasega, C. (2000). Evaluating the efficiency and effectiveness of approaches to nasogastric tube insertion during trauma care. *American Journal of Critical Care, 9*(5), 325–333.

Morse, J. M., Pooler, C., Vann-Ward, T., Maddox, L., Olausson, J. M., Roche-Dean, M., . . . Martz, K. (2014). Awaiting the diagnosis of breast cancer: Strategies of enduring for preserving self. *Oncology Nursing Forum, 41*(4), 350–359.

Nightingale, F. (1860/1969). *Notes on nursing. What it is and what it is not.* New York, NY: Dover.

Penrod, J., Morse, J. M., & Wilson, S. (1999). Comforting strategies used during nasogastric tube insertion. *Journal of Clinical Nursing, 8*, 31–38.

Proctor, A., Morse, J. M., & Khonsari, E. S. (1996). Sounds of comfort in the trauma center: How nurses talk to patients in pain. *Social Science & Medicine, 42*(12), 1669–1680. doi:10.1016/0277-9536(95)00298-7

Ramos, C. M. (1992). The nurse-patient relationship: theme and variations. *Journal of Advanced Nursing, 17*(4), 496–506.

Solberg, S., & Morse, J. M. (1991). The comforting behaviors of caregivers toward distressed post-operative neonates. *Issues in Comprehensive Pediatric Nursing, 14*(2), 77–92.

Stern, P. N., & Kerry, J. (1996). Restructuring life after home loss by fire. *Image: The Journal of Nursing Scholarship, 28*(1), 11–16.

Wilkinson, J. M., & Treas, L. S. (2011). *Fundamentals of nursing.* Philadelphia, PA: F. A. Davis.

Wolgast, E. H. (1992). *Ethics of an artificial person: Lost responsibility in professions and organizations.* Palo Alto, CA: Stanford University Press.

38

THE THEORY OF BECOMING RESOLUTE: GUIDING MENTAL HEALTH PRACTICE WITH SURVIVORS OF MALTREATMENT

What is your story? How would you like it to unfold?

Mental health nurses must often confront the obstacles posed by past childhood maltreatment (CM) in their adolescent and adult clients. A narrative approach, using client storytelling as an intervention is generally useful, but in complex situations, such as surviving CM, knowing what is specifically helpful, and what is not, can leave the clinician in a quandary. In this chapter, I show (a) what has worked for women survivors of CM shown in a series of studies, (b) a description of the narrative theory *Becoming Resolute* (Hall et al., 2009), followed by (c) explanation of clinical interactional strategies based on this theory.

Explicitly, the purposes of this chapter are to (a) establish marginalization as a paradigm through which to view recovery from a stigmatized condition; (b) outline the conceptual narrative threads and relationships among them in Becoming Resolute, a narratively based theory (Specter-Mersel, 2010); (c) simultaneously, ground this description in several narrative studies of women thriving post-CM; and (d) demonstrate how the theory of Becoming Resolute guides mental health practice with survivors of CM.

MARGINALIZATION AS THE PARADIGM

Marginalization is not a state of being, but rather patterns of context-specific, constantly dynamic, social structural and interpersonal changes that socially and politically peripheralize individuals and groups. The processes of marginalization are fluid in given situations, cultures, individual subjectivities, and collective experiences. These processes provide a critical paradigmatic perspective. Within this paradigm, I developed a critical feminist mid-range narrative theory of Becoming Resolute, derived from findings of a large, federally funded, interdisciplinary qualitative study of thriving in women survivors of CM (Hall et al., 2009). Becoming Resolute is context-specific to the lives of women survivors of CM, and fosters greater agency and safety, social cohesion, and thus, thriving. However, the theory is potentially applicable to many who are surviving interpersonal maltreatment and perhaps other adversities that cause complex trauma, which is not specifically amenable to approaches wherein trauma is the result of a single event or of military combat. I will explain how the practice implications are broad enough to transfer to similar contexts.

Marginalization and Narrative Voice

Hall, Stevens, and Meleis (1994) developed the concept of marginalization to guide nursing knowledge development. We theorized that persons may be marginalized due to personal characteristics, such as appearance (race, gender, body size, etc.); social status; stigmatized illness; traumatic experiences (including maltreatment); and even *association* with persons who are stigmatized as Others (Dussell, 1996; Puzan, 2003). "Others" suffer from what Bourdieu and Accardo (1999) called "sociopolitical stress." After a mental health recovery, stigma continues, showing the impact of the social environment on personal identities and how marginalized persons must strategize in everyday life to avoid further exclusion (Jenkins & Carpenter-Song, 2008).

Coping with marginalization includes the ways in which individuals and groups subsist on the edge or outside of the dominant majority group with fewer resources and increased risks (Crenshaw, 1991; Hall et al., 1994; hooks, 1984). Various theories fit within this paradigm, such as feminism(s), postcolonialism, queer theory, and critical race theory. These frameworks are best applied and researched via accessing and emphasizing the *narrative voice* of the marginalized (e.g., see Delgado & Stephancic, 2001).

Women Survivors of Maltreatment as Marginalized

Women experiencing interpersonal violence, either as children or adults, or both, are stigmatized and marginalized by: their status as women (e.g., victim blaming in the case of abuse); rejection by family of origin through humiliating treatment; not being believed when they disclose abuse; the symptoms of posttraumatic stress; and characterizations of being "damaged goods," that is, people who will never recover from such heinous experiences. The diversity and individual uniqueness of their experiences result in part from the secrecy surrounding abuse. Our study of thriving in survivors of CM revealed that survivors feel "different" because their maltreatment robbed them of a normal childhood, and they have disparate, usually negative experiences at developmental turning points, such as menarche and dating, as well as in their fleeing, being ejected, or removed by authorities from their homes as teens or young adults. Living on the streets, and even with foster caregivers, frequently results in further risks and serial abuse. The myriad aftereffects from abuse (e.g., depression, sexual dysfunction, anxiety disorders, chronic pain, self-harm) also make recovery experiences diverse. Thus, there is no "one size fits all" intervention strategy to assist people in recovery.

Intersectionality and Maltreatment

Often persons experience several forms of oppression, variably influencing their experience. For example, a woman who is Black and impoverished may experience marginalizing interactions based on gender, racialization, and socioeconomic status; this phenomenon is termed intersectionality, both a perspective on the complexities of multiple marginalized experiences and a method for analyzing them that grew out of law and postcolonial feminist scholarship (Anderson & McCormack, 2010; Cho, Crenshaw, & McCall, 2013; Crenshaw, 1991; Van Herk, Smith, & Andrew, 2011). For women survivors of CM, gender and racial bias, child status during abuse, stereotypes of abused persons, and trauma aftereffects are intersecting sources of oppression affecting them diversely.

The principles of marginalization and intersectionality can be seen in context in *narratives* of those affected. Critical race theorists and feminists have determined that narratives, including counternarratives from members of marginalized groups, are key to understanding their experiences, in view of power dynamics of the larger temporal/historical and sociocultural contexts. (Baldwin, 2013; Delgado & Stephancic, 2001; hooks, 1992). Considering these sources of inequities among the group of women survivors of CM, I hold that the life pathways of marginalized persons are best captured through narrative methodology. Likewise, narrative approaches to practice are fitting, as will be described later.

NARRATIVE AND THEORY

Narratives are historically interpretable (Bakhtin, 1981/1941), forms of expression that exhibit temporality, or quite simply, stories of social interactions, events, and their consequences over time (Tamura, 2011). Here, I am especially focused on stories of personal transitions in recovery from inter-personal trauma. Many of the general principles of transitions theory, such as the trajectory, triggers, the existence of critical points in the process, and the usefulness of debriefing apply (Meleis, 2010). Narratives are windows on transitional processes as experienced subjectively by persons.

According to Project Narrative (n.d.), narrative is a strategy via which persons make sense of the changing temporal aspects of experience. Narrative theories represent narrative structures, purposes, and consequences of events and interactions via which people make sense of the world. Although even retellings of the same story are unique, cultural influences shape common elements. In interpreting narratives it is essential to realize that in stories, time is not linear but contextual (Polkinghorne, 1988; Reissman, 2008). Stories are often not told in chronological order. Rather, events may be ordered according to priorities, meanings, emotional linkages, flashes of memory; and often vary according to the listener or the intended audience.

Theories about Narrative and Narrative Theories

In this chapter, I describe Becoming Resolute as a narratively based theory (hereafter, narrative theory). It is a theory explaining the substance of experiences narrated, not a theory *about* narrative. A narrative theory is not static and can be used in practice, to interpret, as well as to promote healing (Jolly, 2011; Saleebey, 1994). Narrative theories offer tools that enable representation of recovery goals, and frame and integrate relevant research studies (Floersch, Longhofer, Kranke, & Townsend, 2010; Lewis, 2012). They have been used to develop mental health interventions, for example, for depression and incest (Angus, 2012; Lindblom & Gray, 2010).

Much experiential information can be derived from specific linguistic constructions. Southall (2013) noted that patients often use metaphors to express experiences in palliative care. Thus, personal illness narratives warrant exploration of linguistic signs and patterns. For example, scholars have related autobiographical narratives to identity development, holding that persons integrate experiences in linguistic constructions, and form a narrative self, or selves (Crenshaw, 1991; Flaming, 2005; McAdams & Adler, 2010; Ricoeur, 1984, 1992).

Narratives and Nursing Theory

The narrative perspective is essential to nursing practice, and narrative research is just beginning to flourish in nursing science. Narrative theories (again, not referring to theories *of* narrative), however, are not common. Most nursing theories are middle range and are reasonably adaptable across similar contexts. However, even process theories that depict sequences or stages are not narrative theories if they do not connect individually specific narratives through building a core narrative that undergirds and portrays the theory. The theory of Becoming Resolute is a core narrative, and also has been further theoretically developed through identification of several component narrative strands. These strands are traceable and malleable, depicting persons' stories, and providing *guidance* to patients about how to *change their story,* moving forward out of a traumatic, stigmatizing condition, thereby fostering and enhancing recovery. Becoming Resolute is thus usable as a middle range theory. It shares characteristics of a grounded theory, but is specifically a narrative theory, wherein narrative threads are similar to but not as fixed as concepts in conventional theories. Such narrative threads are not tangled randomly, rather, identifiable interconnected patterns of these threads facilitate the construction of a singular, core narrative, such as that of Becoming Resolute.

Narrative Theory and Practice

Williams, Anderson, Barton, and McGee (2012) used culturally relevant emotional and cognitive theory to create visual narratives for use as an *intervention.* The theories were conventional, but they were used to guide development of narratives. Price (2013) described inquiry using collected client, nurse, and family caregivers' narratives and underlying discourses to *inform education* on prevention of neglect of older people. Similarly, Hsu and McCormack (2011) used narratives in translating for nursing practice with older people. My analysis of the "geography of child sexual abuse" (Hall, 1996) focused on narratives of social environmental *consequences of abuse* that permeate abused girls' family, school, and larger community, as they moved into these new spaces. Similar findings about family, home, and neighborhood were noted in a longitudinal study of bullying; thus, in both studies, *recommendations for change* were socio-environmentally rather than individually based (Bowes et al., 2009).

Policy has also been initiated in a project wherein narratives were used to *identify attributions and ideologies* about obesity (Neiderdeppe, Robert, & Kindig, 2011). Another policy change, regarding diabetes, was instituted by reducing diverse narratives of African American women to a core narrative and then using it to *persuade a wider audience* (Berline, Ako, White, & Pharris, 2011). This collective narrative can be considered a counternarrative to stigmatizing or marginalizing dominant narratives, capturing historical influences on the present (Crenshaw, 2011; Delgado & Stephancic, 2001). In the stigmatized condition of HIV infection, stories of sufferers were highly persuasive to legislators and funding agencies, and public outcry moved the science and treatment forward.

Davidson and colleagues (2010) had persons with serious mental illnesses, who had recently suffered profound losses, *collect narratives from each other*, finding that participants desired a *"map"* to find their way "back to their lives"(p. 106). Developing the theory of Becoming Resolute was akin to constructing such a map. Exemplars show diverse uses of narrative as, or in conjunction with, theory to contextually describe situations, create interventions, and influence policy.

RESEARCH UNDERPINNINGS OF THE THEORY OF BECOMING RESOLUTE

The theory of Becoming Resolute stems from a series of studies that were built upon each other, moving from a problem focus related to childhood trauma to emphasizing recovery, and thriving despite this adversity. Because I propose a new theory, I capitalize Becoming Resolute. Capitalization is not necessary in usage. Using exemplars from these narrative studies, I lay out the narrative themes developed, and refined, through the most recent study in the series (Hall et al., 2009). At this juncture I will explain the theory and then describe how Becoming Resolute is useful to mental health practice, with exemplars (Hall, 1996, 2003; Hall & Powell, 2011; Hall et al., 2009). Analyses by various members of the research team who refined the narrative threads in the major study and explicated them in the major study are included (Roman, Hall, & Bolton, 2008; Thomas & Hall, 2008).

Mental health clinicians who currently use the theory in practice provide exemplars for clinical applications of the theory that were ascertained through dialogue about several cases. Excerpts of findings from previous work provide insight into practice considerations; methodologies are not emphasized, and can be considered broadly as thematic narrative inquiry.

Specific Aims of the Major Theory-Supporting Study

Aims of the study were to (a) discover aftereffects of child maltreatment (physical, sexual, emotional/verbal abuse, and neglect) as described by adult women survivors; (b) identify self-protective, health-promoting strategies as strengths for thriving; (c) explore survivors' interactions with others as helpful, or not, in overcoming adversity; and (d) critically ascertain cultural, structural, and environmental influences on thriving post-abuse. A long-term goal was development of evidence-based interventions to improve the mental health of survivors of maltreatment.

Our team's philosophical lens was critically based, feminist interpretive (Atwater, 1998). Accordingly, we strove to create a trustworthy space for women to tell their stories (Jansen & Davis, 1998). Many findings are reported using in vivo terms. We recognized that we did not *reproduce women's voices*, but gathered practice-relevant wisdom embedded in their narratives. The research team functioned reflexively, questioning methodological decisions and findings from multiple perspectives, as in Bourdieu's (2004) construct of epistemological vigilance.

Study Definitions

CM referred to self-reported history of neglect and/or verbal, emotional, physical, and sexual violence experienced by girls less than 18 years of age. Participants defined *success* as relational satisfaction, capacity for happiness, and work achievements, and successful, protective parenting as in: "a peaceful home," "comfortable in your own skin," and "being an educated person." *Narrative* referred to text from several open-ended interviews with each participant that were intentionally focused on healing from CM, not primarily on the abuse itself.

Becoming Resolute was defined as a process of developing decisive agency and a steely willfulness in refusing to be defined by or focused on one's abuse history. It develops through social interactions; discovering, increasing, and exerting one's self-determination; recognizing the abusive past as deadly; and decentering it in one's life. Keys to this process were epiphanic moments, as well as gradual realization of a new, nonabusive social world, while strategizing to form safe relationships and living environments. Success as an outcome of Becoming Resolute was revealed in sustaining a *generally upward life trajectory* often after a "roller coaster" pattern of progress, interrupted by setbacks, followed by new insight, seeking psychotherapy (for some), and major turning points (Thomas et al., 2008).

Basic Analysis, Reflexivity, and Rigor

Multiple interviews with 35 of the 44 participants provided depth, comparisons of story versions, a prospective view over weeks or months, and coherence and credibility (Briggs, 1986; Hammersley, 1995). Rigor was ensured by the depth of a 4-year analysis, rereading of texts; interdisciplinarity; noting narrative discontinuities; contextualizing quotations within accounts; comparing within and between accounts; and iteratively raising new questions (Barthes, 1985; Kvale, 1996). Initially we considered resilience, hardiness, agency, and action potential as fitting terms for the core theme we conceptualized. Through further word comparisons and searches, we reached consensus on *resoluteness* and *Becoming Resolute* as comprehensive, appropriate terms for describing the central motif in the narratives expressing relatively greater success in recovery.

Team members conducted subanalyses: Thomas delineated life trajectories of participants (Thomas & Hall, 2008), and Roman and Bolton described relationships over the life course that promoted healing (Roman, Hall, & Bolton, 2008). The dimensions, trajectories, and relationships that were seen to be helpful provided temporal and socioenvironmental contextual information, which was then integrated with the core narrative.

Narratives of Becoming Resolute

"Resolute" and "resolve" are derived from the Latin *resolutus* and *resolvere*: to untie; to loosen back, or loosen again (Dictionary.com, 1996–2008; Language, 2006). Resolve means to divide into parts, disintegrate, clear away doubts, settle conclusively, or transform by a process (Dictionary.com, 2008). In the narratives referred to in this chapter it is clear that participants sorted out and untied their very identities from the past maltreatment they were surviving; they cleared away doubts about the deadliness of their abuse. They certainly settled for themselves who their abusers were and that abusers had acted criminally, and learned to set boundaries with them. They extricated their wills from the force of abuse dynamics, gaining ownership of their environment, their relationships, and their future as disaggregated from their past.

Synonyms of resolute as an adjective include firm, determined, and unwavering, having a fixed purpose, determined in character or ideas, and acting on decisions despite opposition (Dictionary.com, 1996–2008; Language, 2006). Descriptors of being resolute include dead-set, hell-bent, willful, courageous, brave, tenacious, undaunted, and unwavering (Thinkmap, 2005). Many of these terms were discovered to be in vivo terms, that is, gleaned from the narratives, underscoring the fit of the term resolute as the core thematic. In-depth analyses revealed *Becoming Resolute* as having six dimensions that illuminated the characteristics, actions, and interactions of the more successful participants ($n = 35$) as opposed to those struggling daily with maltreatment consequences and persistent, abusive interpersonal dynamics ($n = 9$).

NARRATIVE THREADS OF BECOMING RESOLUTE

The six dimensions have been conceptualized here as narrative threads. All of these threads were not necessarily seen in each woman's account. Rather the threads are integrated into a constructed, comprehensive core narrative; many threads were developed from the thriving survivors' accounts. Yet, also included are the positive stories embedded in accounts of the participants with static or downward-tending trajectories; all participants had some success stories to tell. In the following sections, quotes from participant accounts illustrate the six major threads of Becoming Resolute.

The six major dimensions, plus the relationships described by survivors as helpful, constituted three types of narrative threads: *supportive; centrally dynamic;* and *consequential outcomes,* which are not specifically end points, but ensuing processes associated with a major upward turn in trajectory.

SUPPORTIVE THREADS

Determined Decisiveness

Success was associated with inner determined decisiveness, the energy for change. Intrapersonally generated momentum facilitated (a) early moves into opportune roles, (b) tenacity toward goals, and (c) a sense of self-governance and leadership: "I am learning to captain my own ship." Determined decisiveness meant repeatedly and persistently trying different ways to surmount troubles, and with that, a growing sense of self-sufficiency:

> If there was, say, a whole cornfield that needed to be weeded
> with no one to help, I would tackle it all myself, even crawling
> on my hands and knees, until it was done . . . Once I put a chair
> together out of the box wrong, and I couldn't sleep . . . over and
> over I could see it in my head, and it came to me. I stayed up
> half the night fixing it right . . . and I was so pleased with
> myself for it. (Hall et al., 2009, p. 378)

Determination of this kind proved to be supportive to the central dynamics of Becoming Resolute.

Quest for Learning

The desire and persistence in gaining both general and trauma-specific knowledge was supportive of the core narrative. It referred to formal learning, such as academic achievements and upward mobility in employment. Informal learning consisted of seeking inspiring, justice-oriented experiences and stories and films of them. Successful participants grew up as book lovers; this relationship to books often became lifelong: "I walk into a library safe, surrounded by my friends [books]." Books included those with female heroines and or justice themes, including *To Kill a Mockingbird, The Count of Monte Cristo,* and *Don Quixote* (Cervantes & Smollet, 2001; Dumas, 1996; Lee, 1960). Repeatedly reviewing favorite films at low points in recovery attenuated emotional distress during these setbacks. Self-help books about abuse were mentioned, but less frequently than we expected. Currently, the availability of social media is another source of empowering stories, and possibly also information and social support. One woman found justice and compassion themes in a Biblical story and related it to the present, at the time of her interviews:

> Rahab was probably used [abused] by half the people in her
> family growing up. This was put in the Bible to say this is
> wrong, you're not supposed to do this. Her husband loved her
> enough to redeem her out of that . . . In church you don't talk
> about things like that. [But] that's where you need to talk about
> it more than any other place. (Hall et al., 2009, p. 380)

Another woman recalled a librarian who "saw something in her" (Roman et al., 2008) and helped in her quest for learning:

> She would have books for me, waiting. I could get five in a
> week . . . she would have my favorite books, "oh these just
> came in," waiting for me . . . wonderful, wonderful lady, she
> believed in me and she knew me and she knew what I liked,
> and she didn't look at my skin color. (Hall et al., 2009, p. 380)

Quest for learning supported growth and allowed identification with courageous others, as did relationships and interactions fostering Becoming Resolute. Information on relationships is included later, but can also be seen in quotations illustrating the centrally dynamic threads that are described in depth.

CENTRAL DYNAMIC THREADS OF BECOMING RESOLUTE

In particular, three threads, *facing down death, redefining abuse and abusers,* and *counter-framing perceptions* were crucial and dominant, constituting a central dynamic. At least one of these three was seen in the thriving participants' narratives. Frequently, narratives revealed that if one of these occurred, the other two of the three were triggered in turn. The reconceptualization of these major dynamic threads indicates that they were essentially tasks or actions. These were not seen linearly, or in stages. Conventional structural aspects cannot be firmly defined through narrative methods (see Figure 38.1).

Counter-Framing Perceptions

Participants described home as "hell," "nightmare house," "jungle," and "prison." This confirmed the findings of the earlier study that abuse dynamics permeated the home environment, and in fact were experienced as extending and recurring in the school and community environment (Hall, 1996). Finally, often as an adult, considering the perceptual world fostered by a terrifying and repressive situation, counter-framing was seen in gradual dawning, or, conversely, a sudden epiphany revealing that the world of

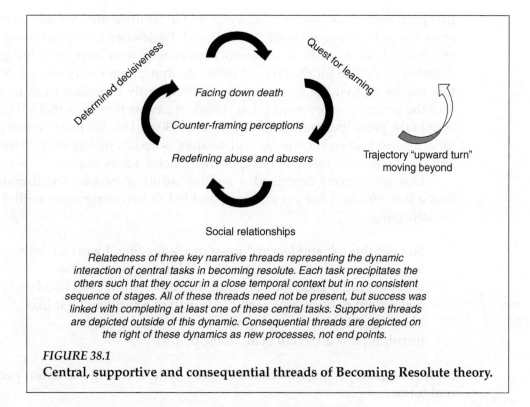

Relatedness of three key narrative threads representing the dynamic interaction of central tasks in becoming resolute. Each task precipitates the others such that they occur in a close temporal context but in no consistent sequence of stages. All of these threads need not be present, but success was linked with completing at least one of these central tasks. Supportive threads are depicted outside of this dynamic. Consequential threads are depicted on the right of these dynamics as new processes, not end points.

FIGURE 38.1

Central, supportive and consequential threads of Becoming Resolute theory.

abuse was limited, and not the only "reality." There were other ways of being in the world and socially relating. Counter-framing allowed the possibility of perceptual and actual escape, opening fissures in an otherwise "totalizing" family environment (Goffman, 1962, 1974), through alternative relationships and experiences.

Counter-framing, key to Becoming Resolute, meant reframing *against*, challenging the tenacious, negative, and hopeless perceptions trapping their victims and forming a world that abusers had normalized. Some father perpetrators were perceived outwardly as pillars of the community; many households were disguised as "perfect families." These factors made framing against, or counter to, these highly inaccurate visions of their families an uphill battle. Counter-framing fostered a new social worldview. Some remembered having returned from eating dinner at childhood friends' homes, reporting: "[We] ate food with a fork!" or "They argued without any bloodshed!" Thus, survivors were moving to a new "normal."

Counter-framing was not dependent upon, and could be impeded by, disclosure of abuse in childhood. Abuse was seldom revealed to outsiders, and childhood disclosures were commonly ineffective in stopping abuse. Women recalled being rebutted, discounted, punished, and stigmatized for breaking secrecy. One recalled childhood disclosure did force incarceration of an uncle perpetrator, but abuse ensued from another male relative. When the first perpetrator was released from prison, the family embraced him, symbolizing the girl's "insignificance." Childhood disclosures to a nonabusing parent, teacher, or another adult almost invariably were met with indignant disbelief (e.g., "He [or she] would never do that"; anger or blaming). Again, this reinforces that the abusive patterns frequently extended from families into the school environment (Hall, 1996). A caveat here was that given the ages of the participants as generally between 30 and 60, the older cohort grew up at a period when knowledge and awareness about child abuse was limited and there were few mandatory reporting policies, for example.

One participant described a sudden adult epiphanic social counterframe that affirmed her personhood, and led to becoming more willful and self-affirming:

> So I got this job and learned insurance adjusting. I worked with
> two men, and they treated me nice. If I did a good job, they
> told me I did a good job. Up until that time I didn't feel like I
> had a right to be on this earth . . . but all of a sudden, I felt like
> I had a right, I had every right to be on this earth, to be
> breathing this air. (Hall et al., 2009, p. 379)

Such relationships and experiences were key to breaking the abuse perceptual frame.

Facing Down Death

Facing down death, another central dynamic thread, meant overcoming the frightful terror of abuse by ethically seeing it for what it was: criminal, annihilative, and geared toward one's personal destruction. Participants described facing a form of existential death, or soul disintegration similar to that described by Shengold (1989) in his book, aptly titled *Soul Murder*. Children faced mortal danger in neglect/abuse and threats to kill/hurt loved ones or split the family. One father tried (unsuccessfully) to poison all of his children by lacing candy with a heavy metal. That participant described that later, while in college, she fought the sense that her (then-deceased) father's eyes were constantly watching her through windows or from behind trees. This affirms prior findings that abuse dynamics and perceptions persist into the community at large (Hall, 1996).

Participants painfully clarified such existential threats: "I don't think we [siblings] existed as people, at all, ever, at any point, in our lives, to either [parents] . . . we were pretty much nonexistent." Another woman reflected on her father's denial of her personhood for his amusement:

> His favorite thing to say to me as a little, little, girl, [was] "we
> don't want you anymore so we're gonna get rid of you and

adopt a different girl, you're no good" . . . I would burst into tears in the bathroom and be sobbing and you could hear him laughing outside. He thought that was the funniest thing in the world that he had just done. [Now I realize] he had twisted my mind into thinking that I was this horrible awful child . . . degrading [me] constantly. (Hall et al., 2009, p. 379)

Existential death was seen in daily annihilative speech from mothers, a death of caring that differentiated them from nonabused peers. Typically girls were told "you are stupid, fat, and ugly" and "You will never amount to anything, just like your father." Similarly, participants who endured an abusive marriage in adulthood faced down death from their spouses, as in this epiphanic moment:

I thought. I'm not going to be like my mother . . . taken over by a man that's so unstable. . . . stay pregnant and he's going to run around on me and leave me. So I pretended to load a gun and I pointed it at him, so desperate I had become. I told him that I would blow his head off if he didn't stop screwing with me, and for the first time, I could see a bully backing down from me. (Hall et al., 2009, p. 379)

In a few accounts, adolescent girls had threatened their abusers, for example, by wielding a baseball bat, installing a lock on their bedroom door, or threatening to report the abuse to authorities in order to stop the abuse. Participants often voiced having survived by chance. Viewing abuse as criminal and deadly ultimately evidenced to participants that since they were among the many "crime victims", it was not personal: "It could have happened to anyone," "I was in the wrong place at the wrong time."

Self-injurious behaviors were attempts to face down existential death by "living on the edge," and included suicide attempts, substance misuse, and eating disorders. One woman's suicide attempt in her 20s made her suddenly realize that she wanted to live and could change her life. One women constructed a situation that would be terrifying to her, facing deathly fear as an adult to attain mastery of it; this entailed braving a turbulent ocean on a small boat: "I told my husband, no matter what, don't help me; I have to do this."

Unfortunately those who had coped by using substances to the point of dependence added about a decade of continued struggle before a significant upward turn in their life/recovery trajectory. (Thomas & Hall, 2008).

Redefining Abusers and Family of Origin

This action makes up the third centrally dynamic thread. Becoming Resolute involved renaming perpetrators, and redrawing boundaries against perpetrators and unprotective others. This usually entailed temporarily, and sometimes permanently, separating from a destructive family of origin.

> I cut off ties, I mean you wanna be like that, you stay where you are and I'll stay where I am. It's been ugly and it's been hard because all the time I thought they loved me and all of a sudden I don't think my parents love me now or ever did. That is a hard realization when you are 36 years old. (Hall et al., 2009, p. 379)

Participants redefined and disempowered their abusers as "very sick," addicted, and criminal: as rapists, batterers, molesters, and pedophiles. Successful narratives showed strict boundaries with abusers and accomplices. By nullifying abusers' family roles, participants abated the power of abuse:

> She is not a mother, and never was, so I just call her Rita . . . we were little kids in a car. . And she'd pretend we were lost . . . . She'd get us all crying and scared . . . . That was downright damn mean. Why would you wanna scare your kids? We were scared enough for chrissake. I later figured out, so what if you get lost? You just find your way home. (Hall et al., 2009, p. 379)

Another woman redefined her abusive father as unworthy of grief:

> One of the happiest days of my life was when my father died. I couldn't believe it. It was just too good to be true . . . like somebody told me I won the lottery . . . I just couldn't believe my good fortune . . . I certainly didn't shed tears. (Hall et al., 2009, p. 379)

Redefinition led to becoming neutral toward abusers, declaring them unforgivable, or occasionally by reconciling. Alternatively, redefining oneself as adult could help to re-establish family ties:

> I said, Mom and Dad, I am 45 years old . . . I had a five hour talk with them . . . I'm still your daughter . . . I'm there for you, but you cannot treat me like a child, . . . you must respect me too. Now, I'll accept a phone call from her, but if she starts that crap, I say I'm gonna go now if you can't have a decent kind of conversation. I'm not gonna play this game. (Hall et al., 2009, p. 380)

Moving Beyond

Getting past abuse did not mean "rising above it," or transcending it. In moving beyond, a symbolic line was drawn in the life story. That was then, this is now. To move beyond was transitionally shedding the weight of an abusive past; the connection with counter-framing, as well as redefining is obvious. Moving beyond was a transition in which the new reality is clarified. Moving beyond was not moving *back* to "normal." For 36% of the participants, abuse began before age seven and was ubiquitous. There was no normality to revisit. Self-construction began at ground zero: "I would look into a mirror and there was no one."

> I had a childhood that was really lousy . . . absolutely nothing
> there. There was no emotional support, no physical support,
> there was really nothing and I somehow crawled up out of it
> and made a life for myself. (Hall et al., 2009, p. 380)

Moving beyond meant choosing not to dwell on abuse, not denying it, but avoiding disturbing memories of abuse:

> Sometimes I try to think back and I don't really remember much,
> but so what? I don't care. It doesn't matter. I remember being
> ugly. I remember kids picking on me . . . I wasn't a good student
> because I was so screwed up . . . I don't even know what I was.
> What's the point? There's no point in thinking about it if it
> makes you feel bad. Move on. (Hall et al., 2009, p. 380)

After a significant upward turn in their trajectory of healing, setbacks did not precipitate drops to "emotional ground zero," but rather to gaining traction and maintaining forward *momentum*, a term I used in a previous study of self-transitions out of abuse (Hall, 2003), and was evident here.

> Anxiety . . . tries to creep in and . . . I fight it off . . . Maybe I
> don't even need to fight it off so much as knowing I'm secure . . .
> much more secure than I was. I'm okay and I know I'm okay.
> [I've] been so good for this long, what's gonna happen now?
> (Hall et al., 2009, p. 380)

One woman said, " It was a time to learn how to get past what happened." Thus, the three types of narrative threads together served a function: to provide momentum and new insights and achievements throughout, and to move from a perception of the world as abuse-driven to a new psychic and physical environment, faced with resolve.

CLINICALLY RELEVANT FINDINGS

Psychotherapy

Finding and reviewing abuse memories were not the psychotherapy focus for the majority, and 40% chose not to have/continue an initial therapy.

Common reasons for nonengagement in therapy included feeling disbelieved or betrayed, feeling pushed to talk of abuse, feeling therapy was "talking to a blank wall," sensing therapists were focused on their *own* problems, having confidentiality broken, feeling the therapist was "stirring the pot" regarding memories, and in two cases, experiencing a therapist's serious boundary violation. Positive and negative therapy stories occurred across both, thriving versus "still struggling" accounts.

One of the few ethnic differences noted was that African American participants reported receiving opposition to therapy from otherwise supportive African American women. Mistrust of health care in this group is well warranted, as U.S. history of medical abuses shows (Washington, 2008). Nonetheless, five African American participants reported having formal therapy. Among all participants, seven spoke of the importance of the therapist as a person, versus the type of therapy practiced. One in three had positive, years-long therapy, described as "a lifeline." "Effort, love and care . . . [therapist] supported me no matter what."

Participants viewed therapists positively if they made some self-disclosure, whether or not about abuse. Helpful therapy interventions included listening to abuse accounts, assisting to end a marriage, helping to vent anger or to grieve, providing balance, "mothering," restating abuse as in the past, regarding one as unique, assigning books to read, encouraging writing/journaling, helping with adult disclosures of abuse to particular others, and even accompanying one woman to the funeral of her parent.

Nine percent essentially had no psychotherapy. Antidepressants were used at some point, positively, by about half of the participants. But narratives revealed that many of these participants did not understand the need to take this medicine continuously, versus only when they had depressive feelings. This indicates a clinical need for more explicit education about medications and their use in posttraumatic and comorbid conditions, for both patients and providers.

Disclosures of Abuse in Adulthood

Adult disclosures of CM to coworkers, friends, and partners were more successful than childhood disclosures, and were not based on the need for the listener's sympathy, reciprocity, or apology. These disclosures were milestones for the self in breaking with the past. Adult disclosures or confrontations of abusers might occur in attempts to reconnect with families of origin.

Four participants disclosed abuse in part or whole for the first time during an interview, and felt relief. After giving their accounts in the study, two women stated that they would now seek therapy, demonstrating the clinical value in telling of narratives as an intervention.

Self-Strategies

Some self-strategies were things participants spontaneously discovered that ultimately served them, such as self-hypnosis: "I found a 'place' to go," "I would be in a zone all by myself." Often women survivors reported histories of substance use and overeating. Ironically, seen in narrative contexts, these behaviors were steps *away from* interpersonal abuse and/or suicide. In the countless ways women seemed to be self-destructing, they were fighting with the only weapons they had, their ways of comforting themselves. Eventually, thrivers found healthier, more effective strategies. Addiction *treatment* precipitated the central upward turn for three women, for example. Self-strategies such as compartmentalizing, strategic memory management, helping others, and creative writing were positive strategies. (Broyles, 2006; Thomas & Hall, 2008).

Thrivers were not spared the sequelae of CM, but they exhibited persistence in surmounting problems, comparable to the "agentic" narratives reported by Polkinghorne (1996). In contrast, the participants that we identified as strugglers related narratives similar to Polkinghorne's "victimic" narratives, conveying a prevailing pessimism about ever moving beyond childhood abuse. They describe poorly bounded relationships and socially constraining fears. They had sparse social networks and reported poor outcomes of disclosures. The past was not yet behind them. They suffered from depression and poor physical health, limited self-strategies, and pronounced isolation. These women report some positive turns, such as leaving an abusive husband, but a major upward turn was not discernable in their stories. One struggler provided a description of her stalled status as "frozen in time, frozen in emotion, the ice cube that always lives in the freezer" (Hall et al., 2009 p. 381).

Supportive Relationships and Interactions in Becoming Resolute

These two aspects of the narratives were contextual, but essential, exemplifying the social environment needed to Become Resolute. All participants made reference to their interactions with others. Of course, many were negative, but here I focus on the helpful relationships (Roman et al., 2008).

Sometimes a single interaction could be instructive and motivating. One woman took cues for change in an interaction with a convenience store clerk who acted happy, friendly, and cheerful. The woman reasoned that with a menial job, the clerk still appeared confident and positive. The survivor mused, "If she can be like that, so can I." Thus, even strangers were role models.

There were two major types of relationships that fostered Becoming Resolute (Roman et al., 2008). These were preserved in vivo terms, because the exact words/phrases were repetitively found in the narratives. The first, type has already been evidenced in previous quotes, and was termed "saw something in me." Usually in childhood, a teacher, librarian, or coach, or boss, for example, verbally or otherwise showed the child that she was special in some way, and recognized as a person, making her feel known. These might be short-lived relationships, but they were often remembered and often throughout life.

The second form of relationship, usually with a lifelong friend, psychotherapist, or caring partner, was termed the "no matter what" relationship, a phrase that was repetitive, and emphasized in the narratives. After many survivors had repeated abusive relationships/partnerships in adolescence and adulthood, they remained caught in the worldview of abuse as a fact of life, with no counter-frame. Glimpses, and then breakthroughs occurred to reveal the possibility of nonabusive, mutual, egalitarian relationships. After one marriage that was abusive, it may have been a second husband who played this role. The constancy of these relationships echoed the "no matter what" theme but the content of what that signified was variable (e.g., "No matter what, he lets me yell when I am angry," "No matter what, he sticks up for me," "My therapist stood by me no matter what. She gave me her home number." [Roman et al., 2008, pp. 191–192]).

DISCUSSION OF THE STUDY FINDINGS

Findings of this study add to the literature on transcending early life trauma. The narrative motif of Becoming Resolute reflected tenacity, happiness, achievement, and relational and environmental safety, as opposed to daily struggle and isolation. Its threads are determined decisiveness, quest for learning, counter-framing, facing death, redefining abusers, and moving beyond. These dimensions are diversely contextualized, supporting evidence that survivor abuse interpretations vary greatly (Draucker, 2001). Becoming Resolute reaffirms what others have found in survivors who thrive mentally (Bonanno, 2004; Carver, 1998; Linley & Joseph, 2004; O'Leary, 1998), such as agency, reconciliation, hope, thriving, and resilience. However, resoluteness differs from resilience in some respects. Resilience has been viewed as a characteristic (Cicchetti & Rogosch, 1997), a ratio of risks and protective factors (Garmezy, 1993), an outcome (Kumpfer, 1999), and as a process involving adaptation after adversity (Luthar, Cicchetti, & Beck, 2000, p. 481). Becoming Resolute is also a process, but in narrative context the emphasis is on decisiveness and *willful steadfastness* versus *adaptation and flexibility*. The thread of facing down death, especially in acting against one's abusers, is a case in point.

Some posttraumatic growth (PTG) scholars (Cohen, Hettler, & Pane, 1998) have speculated that adversity during childhood would be less likely to precipitate PTG than adversity in adulthood. However, most participants in the study qualitatively exhibited remarkable PTG. Despite a rocky start, poor parenting, egregious maltreatment, and some unwise choices of intimate partners along the way, they ultimately achieved success in work and in relationships, including the successful parenting of their own children (Thomas & Hall, 2008). They achieved this success after suffering from multiple deleterious trauma aftereffects, including years of depression, eating disorders, posttraumatic stress, anxiety disorders, and substance misuse. In this regard, to become resolute differs from the prevalent definitions of resilience or PTG, which suggest the positive survivor suffered relatively few ill effects.

Most who were thriving at the time of the study took advantage of the changing opportunities for women wrought through the women's movement. Their determined decisiveness was most often exercised in choices that involved leaving home and/or in pursuing more education. Many left home in their teens. Several who escaped CM through marriage had to leave home a second time, if their first husband was also abusive. All but three had greater than high school educations; many returned to school at nontraditional ages. Leaving home also meant setting limits or terminating abusive relationships. All currently enjoyed adult relationships that they had *chosen*.

In comparison, those currently still struggling had few chosen relationships and they continued to have unfinished business with their childhood abusers. Several bore children very early, that is, age 13, or became involved in serious substance misuse early on. Several had been raped in adulthood, in addition to their CM. They subsequently had more serious and protracted mental and physical health problems.

Our findings support previous studies showing that college achievement is significant for abuse survivors (LeBlanc, Brabant, & Forsyth, 1996). Successes in the workplace, such as promotions and achievement of leadership positions, contributed to the pattern of steady upward progress evident in many narratives. These successes were in contrast to the economic and educational inertia described in narratives of those still struggling.

In Grossman's (1999) study of resilient women child sexual abuse survivors, moving on was associated with making sense of the abuse, school friendships, academics, working, altruism, setting boundaries, and "not focusing on problems" (Grossman, 1999). Poorman (2002) found similar resources facilitating positivity. We saw many of the same tasks identified, but also praxis of agency, justice making, and counter-framing, that is, constructing a new social reality, reflected in each one's personal transitional narrative.

The picture that participants painted of abusive families as closed systems fits with findings of constricted social maps of abused children (Kaufman, 1991). Few outside adults are available to help children view their situation in moral terms (Garbarino, 2001). Advice to children to disclose abuse to an adult was not supported in these narratives. In some accounts there were very important positive relationships with adults, but not in the role of a reporter of abuse, or as a rescuer. As one participant stated, "None of those people told anybody that I was being abused, but they told me they loved me and I was all right. That message is probably what carried me through" (Roman et al., 2008, p. 194).

NARRATIVE THREADS AND CONVENTIONAL CONCEPTS

In some respects, the study method was similar to constructing a grounded theory, yet analysis did not involve free coding or axial coding of the data, memoing, and theoretical sampling. The threads of the theory resemble conventional established concepts, and more exploration and categorical coding may now be conducted to develop the theory further. Attributes of concepts can be delineated, moving them to maturity, and linkages can be confirmed. The resultant concepts would then be bounded more clearly and relationships between concepts established. Table 38.1 classifies the threads as actions and includes one or more conventionally derived concepts that could serve as proxies for these threads, allowing for testing constructs via extant instruments.

These proxy concepts could be traced to corresponding theoretical origins and models for research and practice. Alternatively, the concepts could be combined to form new models that might be developed and tested in conventional research. Measures of the various threads, and concepts related to them, might also be constructed.

RELATIONSHIPS AMONG NARRATIVE THREADS OF BECOMING RESOLUTE

The threads of the theory are related to each other in a number of ways. Explaining these relationships clarifies the structure of the theory and points to clinical implications. Each of the central dynamics is a therapeutic task and one of the three has the capacity to trigger the other two. These threads do not occur in a consistent sequence. But, for example, facing down the existential death and mortal threat of abuse might well lead to a redefinition of abuse as criminal, and then redefinition of abusers as *not* loving parents or "friends of the family." Accomplishing these tasks may be a major turning point in breaking or countering perceptions of home and family. The survivor then relabels relationships, eschews the roles represented, and establishes protective boundaries from abusers and disordered and neglectful families of origin. Throughout, relationships and determined decisiveness constitute context and momentum to move beyond. Moving beyond signifies that central dynamic threads have led to a point of upward turn to a new normal, and no longer experiencing abuse as central to one's identity.

TABLE 38.1

Linkages Between Becoming Resolute Threads and Established Concepts

THREADS	BASIC ACTIONS	CONVENTIONAL ESTABLISHED CONCEPTS
Determined decisiveness	Thinking critically, maintaining energy for change Making choices	Momentum Willfulness Persistence Decision making
Quest for learning	Focus on school, listening to mentoring others, reading, discovering characters who triumph over oppression. Getting formal education	Mentorship Curiosity Achievement Consciousness raising Empowerment
Facing down death	Living on the edge, discovering the deadliness of abuse, fighting back against abuser.	Courage Agency Willfulness Risk taking Existential crisis
Redefining abuse/abusers	Changing one's view of abuse and abusers according to human rights and justice terms, protecting oneself and vulnerable others from continued abuse, realigning setting limits with family of origin.	Protection Advocacy Boundary setting Separation Confrontation Reconciliation
Moving beyond	Drawing temporal boundaries to see the past *as past*. Symbolically separating past from present/ future to diminish abusive worldview, Displacing abuse with personal goals and desires.	Decentering/ recentering Intrapersonal shift Desire Empowerment Transition
Relationships and Interactions	Observing others, identifying safe people, becoming known, gaining support, interacting in mutually beneficial ways, freedom to choose others	Role taking Social support Mutuality Equality Constancy
Trajectory	Situation for improving one's pathway, building, expanding horizons, making leaps, weathering difficult times, using turning points as opportunities, making an upward turn.	Context Chronology Opportunity Consequences Epiphany Hope Crisis Turning Point

These tasks to be accomplished in order to Become Resolute have clinical implications. For example in a clinical relationship over time, readiness for these tasks and therapeutic support can be assessed and even increased; sometimes the need to accomplish a task is preceded by a crisis. Although convention suggests that the "fire be turned down" during a crisis, opportunities for healing might be missed. For example, a woman might begin to realize the seriousness of her past abuse and begin a downward spiral into depression. This might be interrupted as the nurse or therapist turns the tables: "You seem to be saddened and burdened with this knowledge. Yet it can be liberating to realize that what happened to you was a violation of your human rights, your very personhood. How might things change for you in this realization if it was taken as a way to help you protect yourself?"

This then is an epiphanic experience that could shape a new social worldview as safe (a counter-framing of reality). One can protect oneself when the maltreatment and its perpetrators are reduced to their destructive and harmful actions, and the person resolves that this will not happen again. Many survivors who have this series of struggles with the nature of the abuse, regardless of the sequence of insights, seemed empowered to, for example, get their own apartments, seek education, take precautions, and re-evaluate their current relationships for signs of exploitation, establishing that they could protect themselves and their children. Thus, these three threads are dominant in the theory, and other processes and social relationships support these central threads of experience.

I illustrate another "sequence" among these threads. For example, a woman realized that her mother was aware of her abuse, and said, "Well, if he was bothering you, he would not bother me." Horrified, the woman realized this statement was inconsistent with the protectiveness that mothers should have toward their daughters. This led her to think that both of her parents were perpetrators in collusion. Her worldview was shattered, yet after some grieving she was glad to know the truth. She then decided not to have further contact with them, and this change in her perception helped her establish clear boundaries against further verbal/psychological damage from them.

BECOMING RESOLUTE: FROM THEORY TO PRACTICE

Although nurses were seldom mentioned as professionals whom participants reported having consulted, the aware nurse can adopt helpful clinical techniques and work similarly as does a psychotherapist or counselor. In this section, I often refer generically to nurses, physicians, social workers, counselors, and psychotherapists as "clinicians."

The role of therapy and therapists in adulthood recurs throughout the narratives: what worked and what did not, who helped and who did not. As others note, types of therapies and medications accessed were less important than were relationships with clinicians as persons (Lambert, 2004; Martin, Garske, & Davis, 2000). Listening, acceptance and belief were paramount characteristics in the person of the clinician for some, but not all. The most egregious behavior of a clinician was to disbelieve the woman's story of abuse. Participants appreciated the clinician "Being with and allowing for" versus breaking through their defenses to reach catharsis. Premature delving into particulars of the abuse and pushing to confront abusers was not helpful. These actions were more successfully self-determined, with the clinician in an affirming role; the impetus came from the client.

Many participants who used therapy found affirmation and evidence of *the clinician's investment and trust in the client*, as powerful. Several clinicians were described as being "no matter what" persons. This reflects a psychiatric model of interpersonal connection as an ethic (Runions, 1984). It also reflects feminist postcolonial articulation of healing as liberation, based on a "face-to-face" response to the other (Kirkham & Anderson, 2002; Levinas, 1985; Stocker, 2005). This is also congruent with the tenets of relational-cultural therapy (Walker, 2004), based in the feminist "self-in-relation" theory of the psychology of women (Miller, 1976), and is consonant with McCullough's (2006) explanation of discipline in engagement as needed for treating chronic depression.

Childhood Therapeutics

The study provided little data on successful clinical intervention during childhood. Disclosure was not always helpful for our participants, despite the prevailing view that this is protective. One school counselor disbelieved a girl's disclosure, and the advice of a teacher to another girl was simply to lock her door at night. Several teachers or counselors talked with parents about supporting their children, but little change occurred. Again, it was a different time when women now 50 to 60 years old were children. Nevertheless, childhood disclosure should be viewed from the child's framing of it, considering contingencies, choice of listener, and the probable response *to* the child (Staller & Nelson-Gardell, 2005). Even today, disclosures can initiate an investigation and removal of children and placement in foster care, but often have little impact on the supportiveness of the home environment. Mandatory reporting should be supplemented by offering genuine care and regard for children, to provide a glimpse of nonabusive social worlds, and help counter-frame a child's distorted assumptive views of the world at large.

Assessments and Safety Nets

History of CM should be assessed in those who are suicidal and included in psychological autopsies of completed suicides (Shahtahmasebi, 2005). As shown in our data, depression is virtually universal in CM survivors; 98% had depression and half reported attempted suicide. Although therapy initiated an upward turn in many trajectories, medications and hospitalizations maintained ballast for many. Hospitalization was seen as a lifesaver in some cases, important in the healing process, although it caused a serious setback, for instance, when a participant's family was prematurely brought to the inpatient unit for a "confrontation" about the abuse. Clinicians should provide pharmacologic safety nets as CM survivors become depressed and as they undertake tough steps in healing, especially facing down the deadliness of abuse, redefining it, and realizing that life is larger than the abuse framework.

Thus, a clinician might note the client's focus on one of these threads and try to push that realization into self-protective action. Many clinicians may already realize many of the insights this study provided and have used its indications in their practice; however, the data and the constructed theory are a source of evidence, supportive confidence, and authority in making even bolder moves with clients. The following are clinical principles with exemplars, through which one can apply the theory of Becoming Resolute.

CLINICAL PRINCIPLES TOWARD BECOMING RESOLUTE

Clinical principles in approaching women survivors of interpersonal maltreatment involve (a) dialogic engagement; (b) maintaining a narrative focus; (c) decreasing stigma and marginalization; and (d) exploring, explaining, and reinforcing the tasks of Becoming Resolute as the theory guiding the clinician. I have constructed these principles with the assistance of Dr. Jill Powell, a PhD level psychiatric nurse clinician who uses these principles in her practice with forensic, acutely ill, and chronically ill mental health patients, most of whom have a history of trauma, and experience stigma as psychiatric patients, among other, marginalizing characteristics, such as race, gender, SES, sexual orientation, and gender identity. I also consulted with Clifton Tennison, MD, a community-based psychiatrist. Both were involved in data analysis on the team in the large thriving study (Hall et al., 2009).

What follows are some examples of narratively based interventions, which are mostly verbal interactions. They are geared to help abuse survivors, and potentially others surviving similar adversity, to move in the direction of Becoming Resolute, by using crises as turning points, and acknowledging movement toward a more empowered stance in one's life story. These clinical approaches are not listed in a particular order, because the tasks of Becoming Resolute do not flow in a linear way:

- *Elicit stories*. Understand that a goal of intervention is to first understand clients' stories that reveal identities, worldviews, and life experiences over time. Second, conversation starters should elicit narrative information. An opening could be: "What was happening when things started to fall apart?" Or it might be "How did things get better after you had been through so much?", "Tell me about someone who helped you get through?", "Who has stood in your way?", and "What happened then?" These are questions based on a narrative understanding of the client and of relationships, including the therapeutic one. Notice that questions are intentionally vague, versus precise.

- Interpret the narratives as told as ways of connecting experiences in some *personal narrative logic*, without derailing the dialogue with linearly ordered facts. It is *often not helpful* to say, "Did that really happen?" or even, "When did this occur?" Instead, one might ask, "What happened next?" Or, "What led up to that?" Remember, in this approach clinicians are working in the context of narrative time, which is nonlinear. Instead, incidents and interactions are connected by priorities, consequentiality, audience, and associations shown in the meanings attributed to them by clients.

- *Explore experiences of marginalization*, and intersecting sources of oppression, and specific stigma regarding being an abuse survivor. Affirm the validity of these experiences. Avoid minimization of sexism, racism, heterosexism, and so on because it may be that these sources of social trauma outweigh the aftereffects of CM, or just as likely, that the two are entangled intersectionally. An invitation might be, "Can you recall a time when you felt discriminated against, or singled out in a negative way?"

- Be aware that *problems such as substance misuse may still be active*, yet they may be allaying worse problems, such as suicidality and trauma setbacks. Assess on an individual basis whether this use seems to be for relief, or has become a problem in itself. Provide suggestions on replacing substances with other supports. *Avoid withdrawing therapy until the client is clean and sober.* In a previous study (Hall, 2003) a participant who had experienced childhood and adulthood abuse related how she overcame a daily habit of alcohol and cocaine use by integrating with a new church community at the same time. "I would come home every evening and stop at the drug man for a rock, and the liquor store. At the same time I was going to church. I did this for a year. Finally I realized I didn't need the vodka and the drugs any more." Intuitively, she had constructed a layered foundation for stopping her substance habits. Confrontational approaches are not recommended as trauma-informed care.

- *Provide support and media* to aid in the quest for learning. Ask about favorite stories. Suggest films and books with justice themes. Support, and even challenge clients to further their education, whether via technical programs, online coursework, or advanced degrees, emphasizing the self-sufficiency and economic independence that they enable.

- *Provide authority* for taking a route to Becoming Resolute. In another actual clinical encounter a patient who was feeling rather hopeless stated, "When I was young there was a choir leader who put me in the front row and said 'you are very good at harmonizing.' She knew I was really good at something." The clinician responded: "Did you know that there is research that supports that people recovering from abuse who have had this kind of relationship, when someone saw something special in them, have a good chance of becoming successful in achievements and relationships." The woman was quite buoyed up from her hopeless outlook and felt permission to progress.

In a recent case, a nurse clinician advocating narrative interventions (Hall & Powell, 2011) decided to give a copy of the major article on Becoming Resolute (Hall et al., 2009) to a person with cancer, who was feeling hopeless, but who was not an abuse survivor. Despite the technical language in the research article, on the next visit the client was excited and felt affirmed, stating, "This is it! This article describes how I can survive my struggle with cancer." Thus, there is indication that the study and the theory emergent from it resonate with those struggling with other adversities.

- See the therapeutic process as a means to help clients to *change their life/ recovery story*. Good questions are "How do you want your life to go from here? Where are you headed? How can we change directions?" Less effective questions, by contrast are "What is your five year plan?" or "What are your goals for this week?" The latter calls for exiting the story to put together a plan, insinuating that the client is somewhat "on her own" and that there is a correct answer to the question. Even an opener such as "Well, what is your story?" can be on target, yet sincere and lighthearted.

- *Recognize crises as opportunities*, when interpreted through the threads of Becoming Resolute. A dire event may signal a collapse in the abusive frame of reference. This is (reasonably) appropriate for counter-framing; the clinician can acknowledge this as a past worldview. "That is the way things used to go for you; sounds like it is changing. Tell me about how you came to this new realization." Reinforce, validate, the changed perception: "This makes everything clearer to me. What is clearer to you about the world around you?"

- *Note changes in the trajectory and assist with interpretation.* "Three years ago, what seemed to be happening was that everyone around you was abusive in some way. That certainly has changed. What has happened since that turning point for you?" "What is happening to make you more optimistic?" "You have definitely turned a crisis into an opportunity by separating from those who were not respecting you. Now it is your choice whether to see them or interact with them."

- *Refer to Becoming Resolute as a core narrative and acknowledge it:* "You have learned to protect yourself, make your own decisions and get your own place to live. That is excellent. It shows you no longer focus on what others did *to* you, but on exerting your *own will*. Research shows that is the major hurdle after an abusive past, or traumatizing relationship. You are becoming a resolute person. This is the big story."

- Ascertain what is *happening in the present*, by eliciting habitual narratives: "How are you getting through things now?" "Tell me what a normal day is like for you." "What happened yesterday? Is that usual for you?" Elicit stories relevant to Becoming Resolute. "Tell me about how you are taking (or would like to take) ownership of your life" "What has been the heart and soul of struggle for you?"

- In negative times when abuse memories predominate, *support the client to face down death.* "What happened was brutal and unfair. You were not respected as a child, as person with basic rights. When you break it down, you weren't supposed to survive this stuff. To you, did it seem, overall, to be a life or death situation?" This allows the client to express the egregiousness of the abuse, but does not disempower. Although it may be initially upsetting, it reinforces the reality of abusive power dynamics against a child as being unjust and wrong. This may be anathema in some conventional therapies, wherein the clinician follows the rationale that emphasizing the brutality of abuse will create more anxiety, precipitate a setback, and make the client feel helpless. We saw this as a crucial moment in healing, and worth the risk, despite that admitting victimhood can be a low point. The central issue is that it can be a major turning point, as the theory has outlined.

- *Invite the client to redefine abusive others by drawing comparisons.* "Tell me about when people who were supposed to take care of you did not do so." "You said your stepfather was a 'tyrant.' How did you see him then, and what about now?" "You have told me about how your mother talked to you as a child. Was that how it should have been?" "Tell me about a time when you heard someone else talk with their mother that was different from your experience." If the abusive dynamics are not perceived to have changed, the clinician might say, "Tell me how he continues to hurt you. Is it exactly the same as in the past? I see some differences." This focuses on the differences between perceptions of childhood and adulthood, and helps the client see subtle indicators that the perpetrator is not as important in the survivor's life, and not in the same powerful role, as (he or she) formerly was. This is using the narrative uniqueness of each story as a way to help the client differentiate matters. The two stories, of childhood and adulthood will have distinctions that can be pointed out. "These stories of then and now might on the surface seem simply as the 'same old, same old,' but what are some differences?"

- *Note rituals, symbols, and progress in moving beyond.* Increasingly people are getting tattoos and piercings to signify things about themselves and their lives, for example (Hall & Powell, 2011). Seeing this as symbolic, one might say, "What does your tattoo mean to you? What led you to get it?" Similarly an opening here might be, "When you wrote that letter to your mother about how she talked to you as an adolescent, did you feel a change?" "I'm curious. Did your visit to the mountains have special meaning to you?

What happened?" After an epiphany, the clinician might say, "You have turned an important corner here. I bet things will get better from now on." This is a way to both acknowledge and give permission to see the line between then and now, and to not turn back on the journey in Becoming Resolute. Likewise, the clinician may help clients to create rituals that divide their personal story into "then" and "now," emphasizing the division. Some clients who have a history of abuse have found ways to symbolically separate from their past. This could entail something simple, like burning some object from the past; or it might be more complex, such as moving to a new apartment or a new city. "How might you move beyond a life where abuse seems to be taking up too much space in your life? What would symbolize for you that the old life is gone, and the next phase has begun?"

- When appropriate, *allow the relationship with the client to equalize* in terms of power dynamics by nonspecific self-disclosure. This does not mean disclosing past interpersonal violence specifically and so on; that might be perceived as focusing on your own problems. You might say, "The truth is, I have found that I often don't have the answers for myself. It can make me feel sad and helpless, even ashamed." "I have been a mental health nurse for years, but I can be wrong about people, too. I often stumble. And it hurts to realize I too can be taken advantage of."

- *Encourage reflection on strengths and positive relationships.* "How did you meet your partner/spouse? Did you have good vibes about [him or her]? How has it been since then?" "Do you find that it is easier to make friends now that you have learned so much about what makes you feel respected?" "Your story shows your determination, and even stubbornness, is one of your most useful qualities. Have you always had that strength?" How do you use it to your advantage?"

- *Limit setbacks.* The movement toward Becoming Resolute took many narrative and chronological configurations (Thomas & Hall, 2008), and often proceeded in fits and starts. There were setbacks and re-emergences of trauma symptoms. However, setbacks did not have to be shattering if the survivor grabbed on, and kept from falling back to a traumatized, devastated condition. Thus, clinicians should reinforce forward movement and traction by acknowledging that the setback has occurred, while inoculating the client against a serious collapse: "This was a huge blow to you, and there is no getting around that. But you are in charge of your own story. How can we work to regain your footing here, based on all of the progress you have made? You have made amazing progress." Be aware that during setbacks, sometimes a safety net of extra therapy sessions or supportive medication may be in order.

- *Psychopharmacologic recommendations* are not within my scope of knowledge, at least from a prescriptive point of view. Therefore I asked my clinician colleague, Powell, to provide some insights. Traumatic stress from complex interpersonal abuse often produces an aftermath that involves many mental health problems and dynamics, such as anxiety (posttraumatic stress disorder [PTSD], panic, phobias, including social phobias); depression; and self-harm, including cutting and eating disorders. These should be assessed for, and medications may be appropriate to decrease symptoms and suffering, even if the problems are not totally eliminated. Anti-anxiety agents, for example, might be used short term during a period of panic or flashbacks, and then discontinued when these problems pass, as they usually do. Sleep medications might be necessary at these times as well. Antidepressants and mood stabilizers would be used long term for those with mood problems, especially until the client has gotten to a place of traction in her recovery journey.

Medications should be integrated into the recovery narrative, as in "This medicine is for anxiety and stress from the rough spot you are going through. Experience and research shows this decreases over time, but this way the hard time may be shortened, and you can rest."

Instructions about how the drugs work, and whether they are to be taken regularly or on an as needed basis should be clear, and reinforced often. A mistake is to see only the past trauma, and not the person in front of the clinician, whose mental health situation has evolved over time. Another mistake is to assume all problems originate from the trauma itself. Because of stigma, abuse permeates the image of the person, and sometimes causes the clinician to have a myopic view, versus understanding the dynamics and human costs of marginalization and having a holistic and "curious" framework for assessment and treatment. There may be comorbid conditions such as clinical depression, bipolar disorder, PTSD and/or thought disorders. It may help to separate discussion of the trauma from teaching about medications, for example, since traumatic tress interferes with learning.

The research I have conducted about maltreatment indicates interventions must be tailored creatively. For example, it may be counterintuitive that although some participants found individual therapy and silent group art therapy useful, many stated that support groups with other abuse survivors were problematic. However, several participants stated that in talk groups others' accounts of trauma would trigger memories of one's own abuse, throwing one backward in the trajectory when this was not desired nor perceived as helpful.

THE STORY FROM HERE

These suggestions for dialogic interventions are based on a foundation of research and supported theoretically by considering a core narrative as a healing framework. The clinical approaches are often not conventional, and yet it seems clear from the major study findings that "breaking the rules," though not the boundaries, often was highly affirming and perceived as caring and respectful. Undoubtedly, experienced clinicians have intuitively used the approaches described here, but research offers supporting evidence for them. With the theory of Becoming Resolute, there is reassurance and further guidance that there is empirical and conceptual "sense" to those interventions and therapeutic standpoints.

Practice is often described as an art. However, this does not mean that creative, narrative approaches cannot be evidence-based. Arguably, narratives are not the stuff of conventional verifiable evidence. But, consider that mental health involves the use of medications whose exact mode of action often has not been fully explained, and yet their treatment value is indisputable. Likewise, it is difficult to separate the person of the clinician from the mode of therapy used, but the practice still yields palpable results. I have proposed that clinicians can (a) assume that survivors of abuse, and those needing mental health care are marginalized (b) proceed with a narrative general approach, and (c) keep a specific narrative theory in mind. They can frame treatment on an appropriate form of evidence for the context, which is the clinician–client relationship, itself a narrative in the making.

I have suggested proxy, conventional, established concepts for the narrative threads of Becoming Resolute, representing linkages that enable further development and forms of theorizing toward more structure and measurability. The relationships among the narrative threads have been identified and depicted in a diagram. More conventional theorizing would involve searches for concept analyses of these threads and established theories depicting relationships among several of the proxy concepts in conventionally articulated mid-range theory. Undoubtedly, a "new theory" would not correspond exactly to the narrative theory but could facilitate quantitative or mixed-method intervention research. Another potential area for development is a broadening of the term "concept" to accommodate the fluid nature and boundaries of narrative threads so as to use them *as concepts.*

Articulation of how a narrative theory works and promises to continue to be effective in moving clients along the road *of* recovery is a step toward developing interventions that are not necessarily grounded in "real" time, but are comprehensible in experiential time.

The next steps are not fully clear, and scrutiny of this theory-to-practice explanation is in order. There is a way forward. I welcome continuing dialogue on the theory of Becoming Resolute. I believe additional therapeutic approaches can be framed on this narrative theory and, over time, more narratively based conceptualizations might be derived from core narratives of *other* recovery and transitional life processes, especially in the realm of illness and trauma narratives. As narrative research increases, more narrative theories will be available to guide clinical practice. So begins a new story, a new direction for nursing science.

NOTE

Portions of this chapter are adapted from Hall, J. M., Roman, M. W., Thomas, S. P., Travis, C. B., Powell, J., Tennison, C. R., . . . McArthur, P. M. (2009). Thriving as becoming resolute in narratives of women surviving CM. *American Journal of Orthopsychiatry, 79*(3), 375–386. With permission.

REFERENCES

Anderson, E., & McCormack, M. (2010). Intersectionality, critical race theory, and American sporting oppression: Examining black and gay male athletes. *Journal of Homosexuality, 57*(8), 949–967. doi:10.1080/00918369.2010.503502

Angus, L. (2012). Toward an integrative understanding of narrative and emotion processes in emotion-focused therapy of depression: Implications for theory, research and practice. *Psychotherapy Research, 22*(4), 367–380.

Atwater, M. M. (1998). Science literacy through the lens of critical feminist interpretive framework. *Journal of Research in Science Teaching, 35,* 375–377.

Bakhtin, M. (1981/1941). *The dialogical imagination: Four essays* (M. Holquist & C. Emerson, Trans.). Austin, TX: University of Texas Press.

Baldwin, C. (2013). *Narrative social work: Theory and application.* Bristol, UK: The Policy Press.

Barthes, R. (1985). *The grain of the voice: Interviews 1962–1980* (L. Coverdale, Trans.). Berkeley, CA: University of California Press.

Berline, P., Ako, V., White, P., & Pharris, M. D. (2011). Patterns in the lives of African American women with diabetes. *Nursing Science Quarterly, 24*(3), 227–236. doi:10.1177/0894318411409423

Bonanno, G. A. (2004). Loss, trauma, and human resilience: Have we underestimated the human capacity to thrive after extremely aversive events? *American Psychologist, 59*(1), 20–28.

Bourdieu, P. (2004). *Science of science and reflexivity*. Chicago, IL: University of Chicago.

Bourdieu, P., & Accardo, A. (1999). *The weight of the world: Social suffering in contemporary society*. Stanford, CA: Stanford University Press.

Bowes, L., Arseneault, L., Maughan, B., Taylor, A., Caspi, A., & Moffitt, T. E. (2009). *Journal of the American Academy of Child and Adolescent Psychiatry, 48*(5), 545–553.

Briggs, C. L. (1986). *Learning how to ask: A sociolinguistic appraisal of the role of the interview in social science research*. Cambridge: Cambridge University Press.

Broyles, T. J. (2006). *Facing down death and moving beyond: Strategies utilized by female survivors of childhood maltreatment* (Unpublished doctoral dissertation). University of Tennessee, Knoxville, TN.

Carver, C. S. (1998). Resilience and thriving: Issues, models and linkages. *Journal of Social Issues, 54*(2), 245–266.

Cervantes, M. de., & Smollett, T. (2001). *The history and adventures of the renowned Don Quixote de la Mancha*. New York, NY: Modern Library.

Cho, S., Crenshaw, K. W., & McCall, L. (2013). Toward a field of intersectionality studies: Theory, applications and praxis. *Signs: Journal of Women in Culture and Society, 38*(4), 785–810.

Cicchetti, D., & Rogosch, F. A. (1997). The role of self-organization in the promotion of resilience in maltreated children. *Development and Psychopathology, 9*(4), 797–815.

Cohen, L. H., Hettler, T. R., & Pane, N. (1998). Assessment of posttraumatic growth. In R. G. Tedeschi, C. L. Park, & L. G. Calhoun (Eds.), *Posttraumatic growth: Positive changes in the aftermath of crisis* (pp. 23–42). Mahwah, NJ: Erlbaum.

Crenshaw, K. W. (1991). Mapping the margins: Intersectionality, identity politics and violence against women of color. *Stanford Law Review, 43*(6), 1241–1299.

Crenshaw, K. W. (2011). Twenty years of critical race theory: Looking back to move forward. *Connecticut Law Review, 1253*, 1–85.

Davidson, L., Shaw, J., Wellborn, S., Mahon, B., Sirota, M., Gilbo, P., . . . Pelletier, J. (2010). "I don't know how to find my way in the world": Contributions of user-led research to transforming mental health practice. *Psychiatry, 73*(2), 101–113.

Delgado, R., & Stephancic, J. (2001). *Critical race theory: An introduction*. New York, NY: New York University Press.

Dictionary.com. (2008). *Dictionary.com Unabridged* (v. 1.1). Retrieved from http://goo.gl/KrK4nu

Draucker, C. B. (2001). Learning the harsh realities of life: Sexual violence, disillusionment, and meaning. *Health Care for Women International, 22*(1–2), 67–84.

Dumas, A. (1996). *The count of monte cristo*. New York, NY: Modern Library.

Dussell, E. (1996). *The underside of modernity: Apel, Ricoeur, Taylor and the philosophy of liberation*. Atlantic Highlands, NJ: Humanities Press International.

Flaming, D. (2005). Becoming a nurse "It's just who I am." *Journal of Medical Ethics; Medical Humanities, 31*, 95–100. doi:10, 1136/jmh.2005-000202

Floersch, J., Longhofer, J. L., Kranke, D., & Townsend, L. (2010). Integrating thematic, grounded theory and narrative analysis: A case study of adolescent psychotropic treatment. *Qualitative Social Work, 9*(3), 407–425.

Garbarino, J. (2001). An ecological perspective on the effects of violence on children. *Journal of Community Psychology, 29*(3), 361–378.

Garmezy, N. (1993). Children in poverty: Resilience despite risk. *Psychiatry, 56,* 27–136.

Goffman, E. (1962). *Asylums: Essays on the social situations of mental patients and other inmates.* Chicago, IL: Aldine Publishing Company.

Goffman, E. (1974). *Frame analysis: An essay on the organization of experience.* Cambridge, MA: Harvard University Press.

Grossman, F. K. (1999). *With the phoenix rising: Lessons from ten resilient women who overcame the trauma of childhood sexual abuse.* San Francisco, CA: Jossey-Bass.

Hall, J. M. (1996). Geography of childhood sexual abuse: Women's narratives of their childhood environments. *Advances in Nursing Science, 18*(4), 29–47.

Hall, J. M. (2003). Positive self-transitions in women child abuse survivors. *Issues in Mental Health Nursing, 24,* 647–666. doi:10.1080/01612840305325

Hall, J. M., & Powell, J. (2011). Understanding the person through narrative. *Nursing Research and Practice, 2011,* 1–10. doi:10.1155/2011/293837

Hall, J. M., Roman, M. W., Thomas, S. P., Travis, C. B., Powell, J., Tennison, C. R., . . . McArthur, P. M. (2009). Thriving as becoming resolute in narratives of women surviving CM. *American Journal of Orthopsychiatry, 79*(3), 375–386. doi:10.1037/a0016531

Hall, J. M., Stevens, P. E., & Meleis, A. I. (1994). Marginalization: A guiding concept for valuing diversity in nursing knowledge development. *Advances in Nursing Science, 16*(4), 23–41.

Hammersley, M. A. P. (1995). *Ethnography: Principles in practice.* London, UK: Routledge.

hooks, b. (1984). *Feminist theory: From margin to center.* Boston, MA: South End Press.

hooks, B. (1992). *Black looks: Race and representation.* Boston, MA: South End Press.

Hsu, M. Y., & McCormack, B. (2011). Using narrative inquiry with older people to inform practice and service developments. *Journal of Clinical Nursing, 21,* 841–849. doi:10.1111/j.1365-2702.2011.03851.x

Jansen, D. D., & Davis, D. R. (1998). Honoring voice and visibility: Sensitive topic research and feminist interpretive inquiry. *Affilia, 13,* 289–311.

Jenkins, J. H., & Carpenter-Song, E. A. (2008). Stigma despite recovery: Strategies for living in the aftermath of psychosis. *Medical Anthropology Quarterly, 22*(4), 381–409.

Jolly, R. (2011). Witnessing embodiment: Trauma, narrative and theory at the limit in field research and in the classroom. *Australian Feminist Studies, 26*(69), 297–317.

Kaufman, J. (1991). Depressive disorders in maltreated children. *Journal of the American Academy of Child and Adolescent Psychiatry, 30,* 257–265.

Kirkham, S. R., & Anderson, J. M. (2002). Postcolonial nursing scholarship: From epistemology to method. *Advances in Nursing Science, 25,* 1–17.

Kumpfer, K. L. (1999). Factors and processes contributing to resilience: The resilience framework. In M. D. Glantz & J. L. Johnson (Eds.), *Resilience and development: Positive life adaptations. Longitudinal research in the social and behavioral sciences* (pp. 179–224). New York, NY: Kluwer Academic/Plenum.

Kvale, S. (1996). *InterViews: An introduction to qualitative research interviewing.* Thousand Oaks, CA: Sage.

Lambert, M. (Ed.). (2004). *Bergin and Garfield's handbook of psychotherapy and behavior change* (5th ed.). New York, NY: Wiley.

Language. (2006). *The American heritage dictionary of the english language.* Retrieved from http://goo.gl/jy0Y1S

LeBlanc, J. B., Brabant, S., & Forsyth, C. J. (1996). The meaning of college for survivors of sexual abuse: Higher education and the older female college student. *American Journal of Orthopsychiatry, 66*(3), 468–473.

Lee, H. (1960). *To kill a mockingbird* (Book Club ed.). Philadelphia, PA: Lippincott.

Levinas, E. (1985). *Ethics and infinity: Conversations with Philippe Nemo* (R. A. Cohen, Trans.). Pittsburgh, PA: Duquesne University Press.

Lewis, B. (2012). Recovery, narrative theory and generative madness. In A. Rudnick (Ed.), *Recovery of people with mental illness: Philosophical and related perspectives.* Oxford: Oxford University Press.

Lindblom, K. M., & Gray, J. J. (2010). Relationship closeness and trauma narrative detail: A critical analysis of betrayal trauma theory. *Applied Cognitive Psychology, 24*(1), 1–19.

Linley, P. A., & Joseph, S. (2004). Positive change following trauma and adversity: A review. *Journal of Traumatic Stress, 17*(1), 11–21.

Luthar, S. S., Cicchetti, D., & Becker, B. (2000). The construct of resilience: A critical evaluation and guidelines for future work. *Child Development, 71*, 543–562.

Martin, D., Garske, J., & Davis, M. (2000). Relation of the therapeutic alliance with outcome and other variables: A meta-analytic review. *Journal of Consulting and Clinical Psychology, 68*, 438–450.

McAdams, D. P., & Adler, J. M. (2010). Autobiographical memory and the construction of a narrative identity: Theory, research and clinical implications. In J. E. Maddux & J. Tangney (Eds.), *Social psychological foundations of clinical psychology* (pp. 3–50). New York, NY: Guilford.

McCullough, J. P. (2006). *Treating chronic depression with disciplined personal involvement: Cognitive behavioral analysis system of psychotherapy.* New York, NY: Springer Publishing.

Meleis, A. I. (2010). *Transitions theory: Middle range and situation-specific theories in nursing research and practice.* Philadelphia, PA: J. B. Lippincott.

Miller, J. B. (1976). *Toward a new psychology of women (Work in progress, No).* 12. Wellesley, MA: Stone Center Working Paper Series.

Niederdeppe, J., Robert, S. A., & Kindig, D. A. (2011). Qualitative research about attributions, narratives, and support for obesity policy. *Preventing Chronic Disease: Public Health Research, Practice and Policy, 8*, 1–8.

O'Leary, V. E. (1998). Strength in the face of adversity: Individual and social thriving. *Journal of Social Issues, 54*(2), 425–446.

Polkinghorne, D. E. (1988). *Narrative knowing and human sciences.* Albany, NY: SUNY Press.

Polkinghorne, D. E. (1996). Transformative narratives: From victimic to agentic life plots. *American Journal of Occupational Therapy, 50*, 299–305.

Poorman, P. B. (2002). Perceptions of thriving by women who have experienced abuse or status-related oppression. *Psychology of Women Quarterly, 26*, 51–62.

Price, B. (2013). Using narratives and discourses in neglect-prevention training. *Nursing Management, 20*(3), 28–36.

Puzan, E. (2003). The unbearable whiteness of being (in nursing). *Nursing Inquiry, 10*(3), 193–200.

Reissman, C. K. (2008). *Narrative methods for the human sciences*. Thousand Oaks, CA: Sage.

Ricouer, P. (1984). *Time and narrative* (Vol. 1, K. McLaughlin & D. Pellar, Trans.). Chicago, IL: Chicago University Press.

Ricouer, P. (1992). *Oneself as another* (K. Blamey, Trans.). Chicago, IL: Chicago University Press.

Roman, M. W., Hall, J. M., & Bolton, K. S. (2008). Nurturing natural resources: The ecology of interpersonal relationships in women who have thrived despite childhood maltreatment. *Advances in Nursing Science, 31*(3), 184–197.

Runions, J. E. (1984). Whatsoever things are true: Ways, means and values in modern psychiatry. *Canadian Journal of Psychiatry, 293,* 223–227.

Saleebey, D. (1994). Culture, theory and narrative: The intersection of meanings in practice. *Social Work, 39*(4), 351–359.

Shahtahmasebi, S. (2005). Suicide in New Zealand. *Scientific World Journal, 5,* 527–534.

Shengold, L. (1989). *Soul murder: The effects of childhood abuse and deprivation*. New Haven, CT: Yale University Press.

Southall, D. (2013). The patient's use of metaphor within a palliative care setting: Theory, function and efficacy. A narrative literature review. *Palliative Medicine, 27*(4), 304–313.

Spector-Mersel, G. (2010). Narrative research: Time for a paradigm. *Narrative Inquiry, 20*(1), 204–224.

Staller, K. M., & Nelson-Gardell, D. (2005). "A burden in your heart": Lessons of disclosure from female preadolescent and adolescent survivors of sexual abuse. *Child Abuse & Neglect, 29*(12), 1415–1432.

Stocker, S. (2005). The ethics of mutuality in feminist relational therapy. *Women and Therapy, 28,* 1–15.

Tamura, E. H. (2011). Narrative history and theory. *History of Education Quarterly, 51*(2), 150–157.

Thinkmap, I. (2005). *Visual thesaurus*. Retrieved January 14, 2005, from http://www.visualthesaurus.com

Thomas, S. P., & Hall, J. M. (2008). Life trajectories of female child abuse survivors thriving in adulthood. *Qualitative Health Research, 18,* 149–165. doi:10.1177/1049732307312201

Van Herk, K. A., Smith, D., & Andrew, C. (2011). Examining our privileges and oppressions: Incorporating an intersectionality paradigm into nursing. *Nursing Inquiry, 18*(10), 29–39.

Walker, M. (2004). *How relationships heal*. New York, NY: Guilford.

Washington, H. A. (2008). *Medical apartheid: The dark history of medical experimentation on Black Americans from colonial times to the present*. New York, NY: Anchor.

Williams, B., Anderson, A. A., Barton, K., & McGee, J. (2012). Can theory be embedded in visual interventions to promote self-management? A proposed model and worked example. *International Journal of Nursing Studies, 49,* 1598–1609. Retrieved from http://dx.doi.org/10.1016/j.ijnurstu.2012.07.005

SECTION X

POSTFACE

Data don't generate theory—only researchers do that.
—Mintzberg (1979, p. 584)

THE MYTH OF A THEORY BASE

> *Theories, derived from qualitative research, languish in libraries and in*
> *journals, separated from patient care by the infamous research-practice.*
> —Morse (2016, Chapter 1, p. 1)

I begin this chapter with a complaint from Chapter 1 (p. 1). Why do our theories languish, unadmired, after we have gone to so much trouble? Only last week an editor, who was accepting one of our articles, wrote:

> *The Implications section is also in need of further clarification and*
> *enlargement. While you suggest that empathy should be withheld by*
> *health care providers? This is counter intuitive and needs further*
> *exploration. Most of our readers are going to be shocked by this*
> *assertion – and I think that the succinct discussion of this is in your*
> *manuscript does not do the assertion any justice.*

Dear Editor: This is old knowledge that should be known: Publishing is not enough to ensure dissemination. I wrote it in two articles in 1992. The first, Morse et al. (1992), was published in a U.S. internationally distributed journal [*Journal of Nursing Scholarship*] and reprinted in French in a second journal; and the second article (Morse, Bottorff, Anderson, O'Brien, & Solberg, 1992) was published on the other side of the Atlantic, in the *Journal of Advanced Nursing (JAN)*, and in 2006, got a second chance when it was reprinted in the JAN's 30th Anniversary Issues as the "Best of . . . ."

According to Google Scholar (December, 2015), the first article has been cited 176 times, the second has been cited 144 times, and the 2006 reprint 69 times. But apparently that is not enough to move it generally into practice.

It seems that there is a vast amount of knowledge "out there"—more than we can ever absorb. Whereas we used to complain that clinicians did not

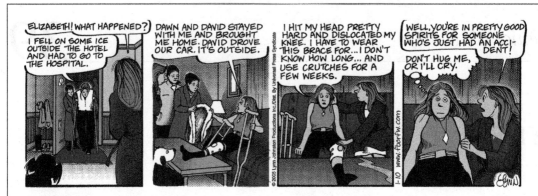

FIGURE 39.1

An example of the nontherapeutic use of empathetic touch.

Source: For Better or for Worse, ©2005 Lynn Johnson Productions. Distributed by Universal UClick. Reprinted with permission. All rights reserved.

read, now it seems that it is not possible even for academics (or even for students, who read all the time) to keep up to date. We have far too much research for traditional ways of dissemination to actually disseminate it. Publishing in a "good" journal (high impact, targeted to the right audience) is not going to be adequate to make a noticeable impact.

How much evidence is needed?

Why is it that the public seems to already know about empathy, that which we have not yet articulated formally in our practice? Even in comic pages we find examples of the nontherapeutic use of empathic touch (Figure 39.1).

I am not certain that I have the answer. But, in this chapter, we consider the important subject of dissemination, along with "worth." In this volume (Chapter 23) we considered the question of proof, of knowing what and how we know, so we can decide if the materials we are researching should be prioritized for practice. But there is still a problem if our solid and useful work is still not making the bedside. In this chapter, we consider why our present system of researchers "presenting and publishing" is not working, and why our models of dissemination in high impact journals have virtually no clinical impact.

DISSEMINATION OR DISSIPATION?

Green (2001) noted that for articles in public health this process took 17 years before a change was adopted into practice. This time frame in itself is interesting, as you and I know that students are taught not to search more than 10 years back in the indexes (and some say only 5 years). A minor problem here is that such instructions come from borrowing the values of medicine and bench science (where knowledge is incremental and published mainly in journals) to social sciences (where knowledge expands laterally, does not "expire," and is often to be found in longer monographs). Things of interest to social scientists (e.g., interactions and social behaviors) are similar nowadays to those 35 years ago, so let us read more Goffman. If we believe that anything published more than 10 years ago is of no use, then we, as a discipline, will be in great trouble, reinventing the wheel and, like busy hamsters, running nowhere. Worse, we will be ignoring and devaluing the contributions of those who came before.

Now, reconsider the numbers of articles published in 2014. Of course, these were not equally "valuable" or "useful." Which ones were more useful or needed, either clinically or for research or education? Which ones made a greater contribution? Were they data-based (and what kind of data?) or critical, or summaries, or theoretical? Did they address education, clinical issues, populations, health or illness, care practices, evaluation, policy, or ethics?

We have to select what we read, and what we research, and what we cite.

Some publications "take off" and are highly cited, whereas others dissipate and remain unnoticed and forgotten. And, as an editor I cannot tell which ones will make a difference, nor predict how influential an article will be.

THE PROBLEM OF DISSEMINATION

Why Dissemination Fails

We drill into our students that we should disseminate by publishing articles in high impact journals (publish "*once*, for goodness sake"; "do not plagiarize yourself" we are tell them), and wait for the miraculous adoption processes of dissemination to occur. Other researchers may be excited to read your insights, and immediately apply for grants to build on your work. Some may cite you, skeletal synopses may appear in clinical journals for those too busy to read the original, your work may take on a distorted life of its own on the Internet, and be tweeted, and students may immediately pick up your work. Unfortunately, this "picking up" is not likely.

Why is this unrealistic? How many articles appeared in nursing journals in 2015?

Why Ideas Fail (Mehta, 2014, pp. 26–29) claims that innovators do not attend to the human factors inherent in change. Whereas his list was developed for innovations in engineering, I apply his list to the attempted changes as we publish ideas in nursing.

We must ask ourselves several hard questions about the proposed change.

- *Is it desirable?* Change, and changing the way one does something, is simply a bother, a "pain in the neck." Habit is comfortable. Consider the difficulties infection control nurses have in getting people to wash their hands. Thus, to have one's ideas accepted, those who are adopting the change must really want to do it, whatever "it" is.
- *Does it meet every need?* It is possible that the recommended innovation is not perceived to be a good fit for every clinical situation or client's every need in the new setting.
- *Is it pretty?* The innovation has to be desired, attractive, and appealing not only to clinicians, but also to patients.
- *Who is going to "champion" it?* A change must have a champion: someone prepared to teach, to incorporate it into the policy manual, and to supervise and evaluate.
- *Is it socially acceptable?* The innovation must fit into the regulations regarding patient care, such as privacy regulations, dignity and respect, as well as Food and Drug Administration Guidelines, and other such regulations.
- *Is it feasible?* It will not be a feasible intervention if it increases patient caseload or has a negative impact on the time of patient care.
- *Is it a strong or powerful enough intervention to make a difference?* I call this the "dose theory of dissemination." Borrowing a term from experimental design, "dose" means to ensure that the intervention is adequate to make a measurable difference when evaluated. The intervention must be adequately strong to make a difference, or the intervention may be trialed or piloted, inaccurately demonstrating that the intervention makes no difference. This may be particularly problematic for behavioral interventions, which are often difficult to describe in writing, to measure with the prerequisite rigor, and are easier to model.
- *Is it visible?* All who should be interested in the intervention must be able to see the article when it is published. My computer says that there are 23,232 peer-reviewed journals; 43,353 full text online journals; and 193 available in my library (and 104 nursing journals now listed on the ISI *Web of Knowledge*). This volume is problematic, as researchers are discouraged from "double publishing," and indeed, if we were to adopt such a habit, it would increase the volume of new research and subsequently increase the problem of being swamped with literature. Yet, we know from advertising theory that repeated exposure leads to more effective retention. It is probable that one 15-page publication is not

enough to grab the attention of an adequate number of clinicians to implement a finding, and we do not know what those attention-grabbing factors are. One possible solution is the publication of synopses, as published by *Evidence Based Nursing*. Or else "do more" meta-analyses, meta-syntheses, and work on theoretical coalescence.

- *Are the instructions adequate?* Maybe the descriptions in the 15-page article are too thin/scant to describe the intervention properly. Frequently, researchers "split" their findings into several articles to overcome this problem. While this gives researchers additional "publication credit," it poses the risk that readers may not be aware of the other related articles in the set, which are now separated and published in other journals. And their theory loses its coherence. Thus knowledge is scattered, and implementation is more difficult. So this fragmentation probably weakens the impact of the research.

- *Do you **really** have a problem?* Sometimes, change is recommended inappropriately: Something that is suitable and beneficial for one group of patients, is sometimes recommended for all, and sometimes the problem is not serious enough or large enough to warrant the effort of making a change.

Perhaps these questions should become review criteria for those who are responsible for implementing change in clinical practice.

TO DO 39.1. DISCUSS THE IMPORTANCE OF REPLICATION IN QUANTITATIVE RESEARCH

In relation to accepting, altering, or rejecting the theory, concepts, and operationalization of those concepts in the original study. Why must the theoretical foundation of the research be constantly re-examined? Think of examples in which theoretical foundation has been faulty, and jeopardized in subsequent research.

Dissemination Through Education

The basic problem is that researchers have no control over the acceptance and use of their products. But perhaps there is one other thing to try.

Dissemination through education appears to be a promising, albeit slow way to implement change. The idea is to ensure the content from research is included in basic nursing texts, or in this case, even more advanced texts, so that students read and learn the innovations as a part of their basic education.

Later, when they graduate and move into practice, they may take the innovative practices and models of care with them.

Wearing my other hat, I study patient falls. This research has been going on since about 1990, is applied and useful, yet I am stunned at the quality of information, or even its absence, in basic texts about patient falls. The *Morse Fall Scale* (MFS) has taken on a life of its own in the Internet, has become distorted, invalidated, popularized, and trivialized (Morse, 2006). Something is wrong with this picture.

Dissemination Using Policy Change

To dictate change through policy change is the most effective way to bring about such change. Major behavioral changes, such as banning smoking and the mandatory use of seatbelts and child seats, have been achieved through legislation, combined with penalties for noncompliance. When change is simply recommended or suggested, it is ineffective, as I am reminded every time I see a motorcyclist, zooming past my car, with hair blowing in the breeze. Helmets for motorcyclists are not regulated in the state of Utah; policy and legislation override evidence.

Another problem is that many minor changes are implemented in individual hospitals through policy manuals, rather than through research channels, and recommending and formalizing the change in a journal article. Perhaps the evidence-based movement will correct this problem, although it introduces another problem—what exactly is evidence?[1]

How Will the Findings Be Implemented

If implementing a technical procedure is hard, implementing theory or theoretical finding is doubly difficult. By implementing our research, we are asking people to actually think differently. I have argued that they must have the new conceptualization not only accessible, but have time to read, comprehend, and understand; and most of all, a desire to *do*.

But there is another problem: a theory per se is not a tangible product. Although it may provide understanding, that understanding may or may not be translated into action. The theory may or may not change care. Is it a visible? Measurable?

In this volume, we have tried to suggest ways that theory may be converted into a tangible product. Developing such products as assessment guides means additional responsibility for the researchers; they must take the research one step further, beyond the stage that the project is usually finished.

---

[1] Back to my fall research: I notice that single items have been removed from the MFS, and adopted in a mix-and-match mode to create "evidence-based" homemade fall scales for use in some hospitals. Researchers with little knowledge of metrics do not understand that such borrowing from a copyright scale is not only impolite, but an invalid strategy.

But even so, it still involves waiting to see if the research is noticed and implemented once the work is "done."

The second approach is for the researcher, or another research team, to develop and implement an applied research project—actually developing a project that will test the efficacy of the change. Such a project will bring the research one step closer to more general use. The results of the program testing the implementation will be published this time in a clinical or specialty journal, bringing them again to the attention of clinicians.

The third approach is for the hospital or clinic to adopt the changes as a procedure, even arranging for re-evaluation. This would be a wonderful start, but remember, again, it is *local* utilization, the recalculation of validity of the MFS is a futile practice given the fall interventions in place (see Morse, 2006), and is still a long way from general adoption into practice.[2]

How Theory Actually Disseminates

Elsewhere (Morse, 2012) I noted that knowledge develops slowly and in clusters. It is rare that a seminal study leapfrogs to a position of influence and remains as a milestone, as for instance, the introduction of empathy into nursing from Carl Rogers's (1956) address to the American Nurses Association (ANA) convention in 1956. If a study does have impact, I am not certain why one particular study is constantly cited, rather than another. The fact remains, that no matter how important you think your dissertation is, once it is published, it will probably make its mark by adding strength incrementally to a number of similar studies conducted by other authors, rather than being cited singly as a seminal study.

This is generally how all knowledge develops, although sometimes a cluster of studies may go "off course" and need to be corrected. Most studies fall into a black hole or die in mediocrity, ignored or forgotten. Look at the number of times your articles have been cited—a humbling task—and this is usually an indicator of use by other researchers, rather than by clinicians.

TO DO 39.2. HOW MANY ARTICLES WERE PUBLISHED IN NURSING JOURNALS IN 2015?

Look it up and let me know.

How? Use the Thompson Reuters "Web of Knowledge" for Nursing. Add the *Numbers of articles* column. Nice number, eh?

Discuss publication statistics. What is an impact factor? How do you identify a journal you would like to publish in?

Now think about this. How can we possibly integrate and use this knowledge effectively and efficiently. Who should be responsible?

---

[2] This problem does not occur in medicine. Consider the equivalent Appearance, Pulse, Grimace, Activity and Respiration (APGAR) scale (for newborn assessment) or Glasgow Coma Scale. These scales of equivalent type to the MFS remain in use, unchallenged, and intact in medicine.

Nevertheless, the *course* of knowledge adoptions for qualitative and quantitative research is different. First, we examine the course of qualitative theory or knowledge.

The Accrual of Qualitative Knowledge

There are eight phases, or levels of development, of qualitative inquiry (Morse, 2012), from the first exploratory studies of the phenomenon to the implementation of an intervention (see Table 39.1). Most qualitative health research studies are conducted at Level 1; hence, the adage that "qualitative studies go nowhere." This may be true for many studies, but if you consider these studies to be a part of a whole, then this "nowhere hypothesis" is not entirely correct—they do eventually contribute to the whole.

When examining Table 39.1, note that the studies at the various levels are not conducted in a stepwise, linear direction. An investigator may start at Level 2 and then, because he or she realizes that he or she does not have adequate description, conduct a Level 1 study; alternatively, he or she may start at Level 3. The important point is that rarely does a study include several levels at once, or include information for Levels 3, 4, and 5 in the same study.

Level 1: Identification of Significant Concepts

Level 1 studies explore phenomena that appear interesting, that need *describing*. They may target something that appears problematic, therapeutic, difficult, or simply interesting. The researcher may elect to use any qualitative method that *provides thick description* (hopefully the most appropriate according to the question and other factors): ethnography, grounded theory, phenomenology, narrative inquiry, and so forth. Their goal is primarily to see what is going on.

Although these studies are generally descriptive, data will be synthesized, and the results may include a minor, lower level theory. Some themes or concepts will have been identified. Some of these concepts may be common and obvious, and others will be new, named, described, and delineated. Hopefully the researcher will have linked his or her findings with the literature, but this, unfortunately, is an uncommon occurrence.

Level 2: Delineation and Description of the Anatomy of the Concept

At Level 2, the researcher has identified the major concept of interest, and the purpose of inquiry is to develop it further. The concept may be a *lay concept* (one that is used in everyday language, such as dignity, privacy, care, or suffering) or a *scientific concept* (one that has been identified in the process of doing research and defined operationally). The researcher uses methods according to what is known about the concept and its level of maturity (Morse, Mitcham, Hupcey, & Tasón, 1996), which range from the methods of concept

TABLE 39.1
The Phases of Development for Qualitative Nursing Research, from Exploring a Phenomenon to Application.

LEVEL	CONTRIBUTION TO KNOWLEDGE DEVELOPMENT
Level 1	Identification of significant phenomena Careful description of the phenomenon enables the concept(s) to emerge as "interesting" or "significant" within the context being described.
Level 2	Delineation and description of the anatomy of the concept Inquiry targets the concept, using various methods of concept identification or analysis to describe the anatomy of the concept.
Level 3	Examination of the concept in different situations Researchers now focus on the concept as it appears in different contexts or situations.
Level 4	Exploring the relationship of the concept of interest with other co-occurring concepts Examination is undertaken of the co-occurrence or interaction of the concept of interest with other concepts in a particular setting.
Level 5	Synthesizing knowledge The literature about the concept is synthesized to identify common attributes and to remove the "noise" (i.e., the "mock" attributes or those associated with one set of particular circumstances).
Level 6	Model and theory development Model building begins by examining and identifying internal processes, mechanisms, and their linkages. The strength and interactions of the attributes and the therapeutic interaction of the concept are important. The internal mechanisms and the interrelationships of the attributes are explored, usually using grounded theory (Forbes et al., 1999; Morse & Doberneck, 1995).
Level 7	Assessment and measurement Quantitative researchers may develop questionnaires and instruments to measure the concept, to determine its prevalence epidemiologically, to test the qualitative model, and to test emerging hypotheses.
Level 8	Clinical application and evaluation of outcomes The concept has now matured and is used formally in therapy, both quantitatively, as for instance, in assessments (Martin & Stermac, 2010), and qualitatively, as a framework for practice or interventions.

Source: Morse (2012). Reprinted with permission of Sage Publications.

analysis, such as those suggested by Rodgers and Knafl (2000), to qualitative methods that enable description and delineation of the concept. From such an inquiry, the attributes (characteristics), boundaries, antecedents, and consequences are identified and delineated. Ideally, researchers can now agree on the nature of the concept, and the inquiry can move forward.

Level 3: Examination of the Concept in Different Situations

Researchers conducting studies at this level commence their study by targeting the concept, rather than the phenomenon, and waiting for the concept to emerge inductively in the process of data collection. They therefore seek to study caregiving, bereavement, resilience, or whatever, in a certain group or situation. The selected concept provides the terms for the literature search, whereas the context of the study is of secondary importance. The researchers are using the information about the concept—what is known about its boundaries, attributes, antecedents, and consequences—to plan ahead. In their study, they will be looking for differences in the *form* of the concept according to characteristics of the participants (gender, ethnicity, and so forth) in individual or family groups. The form of the concept is important for qualitative health research, perhaps changing in participants with different medical conditions, symptoms, or health problems. Conditions that we frequently see investigated recently are participants with HIV/AIDS, sexually transmitted diseases, chronic conditions such as diabetes and arthritis, and spinal cord injuries.

These studies provide important information on two levels. First, attributes that remain consistent in the concept in various situations are probably true attributes, a part of the concept. Second, those attributes that change in strength, but remain in the concept, and are altered because of context, provide significant information as the research moves toward constructing theory.

Level 4: Exploring the Relationship of the Concept With Other Co-Occurring Concepts

Studies become more complex—and more representative of reality—when the researcher examines more than one concept in a single setting. The researcher must ask: Are these concepts independent? Do they co-occur? How do the interactions between two concepts change when they merge or they separate? Do they run parallel or intersect? And, when examining concepts in another culture, is the concept altered or changed, and if so how? Are the attributes the same or different? These questions are important, for if the concept changes form, it is not a culturally universal concept. Further, as the concept responds to conditions within the context, new forms of the concept may appear. For instance, in the previously discussed context of hope in the heart transplant unit, where participants have only one chance at a transplant (and the alternative is death), the form of hope becomes "hoping for a chance for a chance" (Morse & Doberneck, 1995). The stakes are very high, and those in this situation are very aware that they are hoping against hope.

Level 5: Synthesizing Knowledge

By this time, there have been many studies conducted on the concept, and it is moving toward maturity. Once the concept has been described in many qualitative studies in various contexts, researchers should consider conducting a meta-synthesis. Researchers have enough data (i.e., studies of the various types described in the previous chapters), from enough perspectives, to determine that the conceptual attributes (or characteristics) will be present in every case. Because we know that variations in the strength or the role of the attributes give rise to different forms of the concept, it should be relatively easy at this point to identify the types or forms of the concept(s) of interest. The outcomes of meta-synthesis, then, should be a higher level of abstraction and with consensus on labels and definitions for the concept.

Level 6: Model and Theory Development

Qualitative researchers begin model building by examining and identifying internal processes and mechanisms and their linkages. This may take place within a project in the course of data collection or by using the literature as data, extending from a meta-analysis.

At this point, concepts are more than labels to a qualitative researcher. We are interested in the strength and interactions of the attributes, and what the concept does therapeutically. As collections of behaviors, concepts are not static, but change their form to fit a particular situation. Exploring the process of development and utilization of the concepts, researchers explore the internal mechanisms and the interrelationships of the attributes, usually using grounded theory. Researchers examine studies exploring how the concept is used—how it is manipulated and supported by nurses and physicians in the provision of care, by relatives in interactions or lay caregiving, and by the patient within his or her cultural context—thereby leading to solid, mid-range theory.

This process may be extended to explore how the concept links with other concepts and how attributes and the boundary of the concept link as shared attributes of another concept. Concepts are "opened," and the common or shared characteristics are where the two concepts join. We study how concepts change during trajectories (i.e., process), and how the strength and ordering of attributes change as, for instance, the researcher moves through the process, focusing on the concepts and hence developing an emerging theory.

Level 7: Assessment and Measurement

By this stage, quantitative researchers may have become interested in the concept, developing questionnaires and instruments to measure the concept to determine its prevalence in the population epidemiologically, and designing quantitative experiments to test emerging hypotheses. The concept will find its way into conceptual frameworks, or itself be considered a conceptual framework, and will be "opened" so that its attributes form the framework.

Level 8: Clinical Application and Evaluation of Outcomes

Ever since the advent of evidence-based medicine, clinical application and utilization is becoming a formal research task in which clinical problems are identified and appropriate research-based interventions, selected to solve the particular problem, are deliberately applied and evaluated. Then, if they pass this particular test, they are adopted into practice. Interestingly, this process of evaluation tends to be done on a case-by-case, hospital-by-hospital, or unit-by-unit basis, rather than in the coordinated and funded manner of medicine.

To summarize, decades of work by many research teams working relatively independently form a foundation from which concepts are identified, theories are developed and generalized, and insights and interventions are developed to improve practice. However, that process of conducting research and building knowledge is not sequential, but rather haphazard. Researchers follow their own research programs, their own disciplinary agendas, and their personal interests, and they respond to funding calls and clinical opportunities. And as qualitative researchers, we teach our students to be skeptical of the work of others and to value and prioritize principles of induction. All of this slows down the progression of knowledge development.

The Accrual of Quantitative Research

First, remember that the products of qualitative and quantitative research are quite different. The most usual outcome of qualitative research is theory; the outcome of quantitative research is usually a product: a scale or an instrument; population-based data that may be used as rates or norms, efficacy information on the improvement of treatments or therapies or programs, and so forth. Quantitative theory is hidden beneath these products, but is crucial for guiding what they become, and ultimately how they inform care.

Recall that quantitative research uses *scientific concepts*, which are created according to the needs of a particular research program, and these concepts are operationalized according to the limitations of available measures. For instance, coping (Lazarus, 1966) and social support (Cobb, 1976) were scientific concepts developed by quantitative researchers and were operationally defined to meet the needs of subsequent research. Scientific concepts are rarely introduced into the literature without first being brought to the level of research. However, in the next phase, quantitative frameworks and theories are sometimes developed and published—perhaps because they are commonsense frameworks for organizing data, or perhaps because they have a mathematical basis, such as Einstein's theory of relativity.

One major difference with quantitative research, especially in experimental design, is in the significance of replication: Research should be replicated by the investigator and also by others; methods must be transparent and clear, and results are available to all. Quantitative research moves

---

TABLE 39.2
The Phases of Development for Quantitative Nursing Research, from Exploring a Phenomenon to Application.

Level 1	Identification of a significant problem Conduct of study
Level 2	Replication of the study by the investigator
Level 3	Replication of the study by others
Level 4	Replication in different populations; comparison of males and females; socioeconomic groups; populations with different illnesses. Extending the intervention
Level 5	Synthesizing knowledge Conducting a meta-analysis
Level 6	Development of clinical protocols, and interventions
	Clinical application and evaluation of outcomes The concept has now matured and is used formally in therapy, both quantitatively, as for instance, in assessments (Martin & Stermac, 2010)

---

forward in a stepwise fashion, replicating the research in different populations, extending the research intervention, and modifying and strengthening the model (as shown on Table 39.2).

Level 1: Developing a Scientific Concept

A researcher has a particular problem, which cannot be addressed by currently available theories and concepts. The researcher names the phenomenon, develops a theory around the phenomenon, and creates the significant concept(s) and theorizes the relationships between these concepts. The concepts are defined, and means to measure the theoretical concepts are developed. At this point, the researcher develops a hypothesis to demonstrate the theory.

The investigator then conducts a pilot study, and from the results of the pilot study revises the operational definitions, improves the measures (or introduces others), and conducts a second study. The circular process of testing (by conducting a study) and improving the measure or adjusting the operational definitions continues until the researcher is satisfied, and conducts a major study. This process cannot be taken lightly, for if the results are not promising, the researcher must consider: Is the theory incorrect? Are the concepts adequate? Are the definitions representative? Is the operationalization of the concepts correct? Is there disjuncture between the operationalization and the measures? Note this model fits research from exploratory studies to experimental designs. This is the part of the study that involves creative thinking, and it is on this theory development that the entire project rests. Note, however, that once the measures have been created, the neutral stance of the investigator, ensured by blinding, means that the theory and theoretical thinking do not enter the research process, until the analysis is completed. Qualitative researchers, on the other hand, must constantly use and test theory and theoretical assumptions in the process of conducting the research. Thus, the use of theory in the conduct of research is the major difference between qualitative and quantitative research.

Level 2: Replication

Once the study has performed well for the investigator, he or she then replicates it from scratch on another sample. Note that qualitative studies do not replicate at the end of the study, as it interferes with induction, and invalidates the results.

Level 3: At This Point the Study Is Published, and Other Researchers, Interested in the Results, Replicate the Study and Compare Their Results

This process of validation is extremely important.

TO DO 39.3. DISCUSS THE IMPORTANCE OF REPLICATION IN *QUANTITATIVE* RESEARCH

A clinician is implementing a new intervention. Must or should the clinician practicing evidence-based practice know the theory on which his or her intervention is based?
Why or why not?

Level 4: Replication and Expansion of the Findings in Other Populations

Other investigators now noticing the significance of the emerging research area seek funding to conduct replications in other populations and groups to make certain that the theory continues to perform well. These results are published and form a nice group of complementary studies.

Level 5: Meta-Analyses

Quantitative meta-analyses differ from qualitative meta-analyses, in that researchers collect all of the studies that have addressed similar hypotheses, but often in different populations. Of course, there is some variation in how these studies have performed, so the investigator analyzes all of the *effects* to determine the overall effectiveness across all studies of the intervention.

Level 6: Clinical Application and Evaluation

Clinical protocols are developed for the interventions and programs are set up. Data are collected to evaluate these programs, and the efficacy of the interventions is again tested, and the results disseminated. At this point the interventions become embedded in standard practice.

A new phase is emerging in evidence-based practice, in which the interventions are tested every time they are implemented in a clinical area.

SUMMARY

Scholarship has changed dramatically over the past two decades. There has been a surge of new journals, many of them open source. Nursing research has exponentially increased, although I argued it was "exceeding demand." I do not think the problems in the implementation of nursing research are worse than those of other disciplines.

Research accrues in distinct patterns, according to whatever is being studied, how much information is available, and the methods used. Given that nursing is a relatively newcomer to research, advances in knowledge are rapid and measurable. Although there are difficulties in dissemination, we are aware of those problems and are addressing them. We may still be classified as a new discipline, but we are moving toward maturity.

REFERENCES

Cobb, S. (1976). Social support as a moderator of life stress. *Psychosomatic Medicine, 38*(5), 300–314.

Forbes, D. A., King, K. M., Kushner,K. E., Letourneau, N. L., Myrick, A. F., & Profetto-McGrath, J. (1999). Warrantable evidence in nursing science. *Journal of Advanced Nursing, 29*, 373–379.

Green, L. (2001). From research to "best practices" in other settings and populations. *American Journal of Health Behavior, 25*, 165–178.

Lazarus, R. A. (1966). *Psychological stress and the coping process*. New York, NY: McGraw-Hill.

Martin, K., & Stermac, L. (2010). Measuring hope: Is hope related to criminal behavior in offenders. *Offender Therapy and Comparative Criminology, 54*(5), 693–705.

Mehta, K. M. (2014). Why ideas fail. *The Penn Stater, 101*(3), 26–29.

Morse, J. M. (2006). The safety of safety research: The case of patient fall research. *Canadian Journal of Nursing Research, 38*(2), 74–88.

Morse, J. M. (2016). *Analyzing and conceptualizing the theoretical foundations of nursing* (p. 1). New York, NY: Springer Publishing.

Morse, J. M., & Doberneck, B. M. (1995). Delineating the concept of hope. *Image: Journal of Nursing Scholarship, 27*(4), 277–285.

Morse J. M., Mitcham, C., Hupcey J. E., & Tasón, M. C. (1996). Criteria for concept evaluation. *Journal of Advanced Nursing, 24*, 385–390.

Morse, J. M. (2012). *Qualitative health research: Creating a new discipline.* Walnut Creek, CA: Left Coast Press.

Morse, J. M., Anderson, G., Bottorff, J., Yonge, O., O'Brien, B., Solberg, S., & McIlveen, K. (1992). Exploring empathy: A conceptual fit for nursing practice? *Image: Journal of Nursing Scholarship, 24*(4), 274–280.

Morse, J. M., Bottorff, J., Anderson, G., O'Brien, B., & Solberg, S. (1992/2006). Beyond empathy. Expanding expressions of caring. *Journal of Advanced Nursing, 17*, 809–821. (Reprinted, *53*[1], 75–87)

Mintzberg, H. (1979). An emerging strategy of "direct" research. *Administrative science quarterly, 24*, 582–589.

Rodgers, B. L., & Knafl, K. A. (2000). Concept analysis: An evolutionary view. In B. L. Rodgers & K. A. Knafl (Eds.), *Concept development in nursing* (pp. 77–117). Philadelphia, PA: Saunders.

Rogers, C. (1956). A counseling approach to human problems. *American Journal of Nursing, 56*, 994–997.

BIBLIOGRAPHY

Acheson, D. (1998). *Independent inquiry into inequalities in health.* Retrieved from http://webarchive.nationalarchives.gov.uk/20130107105354/http://www.archive.official-documents.co.uk/document/doh/ih/contents.htm

Agar, M. (2011). *Method to my madness.* Michael Agar Ethnoworks LLC. Retrieved from http://www.ethknoworks.com

Aiken, L. H., Clarke, S. P., Sloane, D. M., Sochalski, J. A., Busse, R., Clarke, H., . . . Alexander, K. (2013). Social determinants of methadone in pregnancy: Violence, social capital, and mental health. *Issues in Mental Health Nursing, 34*, 747–751. doi:10.3109/01612840.2013.813996

Aiken, L. H., Sermeus, W., Van den Heede, K., Sloane, D. M., Busse, R., McKee, M., . . . Kutney-Lee, A. (2012). Patient safety, satisfaction, and quality of hospital care: Cross sectional surveys of nurses and patients in 12 countries in Europe and the United States. *British Medical Journal, 344*, e1717. doi:10.1136/bmj.e1717

American Nurses Association. (2001). *Code of ethics for nurses with interpretative statements.* Retrieved from http://goo.gl/gDn2Nu

Andrykowski, M. A., Carpenter, J. S., Studts, J. L., Cordova, M. J., Cunningham, L. L., Beacham, A., . . . McGrath, P. (2002). Psychological impact of benign breast biopsy: A longitudinal, comparative study. *Health Psychology, 21*(5), 485–494.

Bagarozzi, D. A. (2011). A closer look at couple collusion: Protecting the self and preserving the system. *The American Journals of Family Therapy, 39*, 390–403. doi:10.1080/01926187.2011.575633

Bambra, C., Gibson, M., Sowden, A., Wright, K., Whitehead, M., & Petticrew, M. (2010). Tackling the wider social determinants of health and health inequalities: Evidence from a systematic review. *Journal of Epidemiology & Community Health, 64*, 284–291. doi:10.1136/jech.2008.082743

Barnard, H. R. (2011). *Research methods in anthropology: Qualitative and quantitative approaches* (5th ed.). Maryland, MD: AltaMira Press.

Barroso, J., & Sandelowski, M. (2001). In the field with the beck depression inventory. *Qualitative Health Research, 11*(4), 491–504. doi:10.1177/104973201129119271

Barton, F., Miltin, D., Mulholland, C., Hardoy, A., & Stern, R. (2007). Integrated approaches to address the social determinants of health for reducing health inequity. *Journal of Urban Health, 84*(Suppl. 1), 164–173. doi:10.1007/s11524-007-9173-7

Bebeau, M. J., & Brabeck, M. M. (1989). Ethical sensitivity and moral reasoning among men and women in the professions. In M. M. Brabeck (Ed.), *Who cares? Theory, research, and educational implications of the ethic of care* (pp. 144–163). New York, NY: Praegar.

Becker, V. (1983). A conceptualization of a concept. *Nursing Paper, 15*(2), 51–58.

Belcher, J. R., Greene, J. A., McAlpine, C., & Ball, K. (2001). Considering pathways into homelessness: Mothers, addictions, and trauma. *Journal of Addictions Nursing, 13*, 199–208.

Blas, E., & Kurup, A. S. (2010). *Equity, social determinants and public health programmes.* Geneva, Switzerland: World Health Organization. Retrieved from http://goo.gl/NZulQm

Bloch, J. R. (2011). Using geographical information systems to explore disparities in preterm birth rates among foreign-born and U.S.-born Black mothers. *Journal of Obstetric, Gynecological & Neonatal Nursing, 40*, 544–554. doi:10.1111/j.1552-6909.2011.01273.x

Bonnefoy, J., Morgan, A., Kelly, M. P., Butt, J., & Bergman, V. (2007). *Constructing the evidence base on the social determinants of health: A guide.* Retrieved from http://goo.gl/6EXWVC

Bourgois, P., Prince, B., & Moss, A. (2004). The everyday violence of hepatitis C among young women who inject drugs in San Francisco. *Human Organization, 63*, 253–264.

Braverman, P. (2006). Health disparities and health equity: Concepts and measurement. *Annual Review of Public health, 27*, 167–194.

Braverman, P., Egerter, S., & Williams, D. R. (2011). The social determinants of health: Coming of age. *Annual Review of Public Health, 32*, 381–398. doi:10.1146/annurev-publhealth-031210-101218

Brewer, N. T., Salz, T., & Lillie, S. E. (2007). Systematic review: The long-term effects of false-positive mammograms. *Annals of Internal Medicine, 146*(7), 502–510.

Brofenbrenner, U. (1977). Toward an experimental ecology of human development. *American Psychologist, 32*, 513–531.

Brunner, E., & Marmot, M. (2006). Social organization, stress, and health. In M. Marmot & R. G. Wilkinson (Eds.), *Social determinants of health* (2nd ed., pp. 6–29). Oxford, UK: Oxford University Press.

Bubela, N., Galloway, S., McKinnon, A., Nagel, L., Pringle. D., Ross, E., & Shamian, J. (1990). The patient learning needs scale: Reliability and validity. *Journal of Advanced Nursing, 15*(10), 1181–1187.

Butterfield, P. G. (1990). Thinking upstream: Nurturing a conceptual understanding of the social context of health behaviour. *Advances in Nursing Science, 12*, 1–8.

Butts, J. B., Rich, K. L., & Fawcett, J. (2012). The future of nursing: How important is discipline-specific knowledge? A conversation with Jacqueline Fawcett. *Nursing Science Quarterly, 25*(2), 151–154. doi:10.1177/0894318412437955

Canadian Nurses Association. (2005). *Social determinants of health and nursing: A summary of the issues. CNA backgrounder.* Retrieved from http://www.cna-aiic.ca/BG8_Social_Determinants

Canadian Nurses Association. (2008). *Code of ethics for registered nurses.* Ottawa: Author. Retrieved from http://www.cna-aiic.ca/Code_of_Ethics_2008

Canadian Nurses Association. (2010). *Social justice . . . a means to and end, an end in itself* (2nd ed.). Ottawa: Author. Retrieved from http://www.cna-aiic.ca/Social_Justice

Canadian Nurses Association. (2013). *Position statement: Social determinants of health.* Retrieved from http://www.nanb.nb.ca/PDF/CNA_Determinants_of_Health_E.pdf

Canales, K. K., & Bowers, B. J. (2001). Expanding conceptualizations of culturally competent care. *Journal of Advanced Nursing, 36*(1), 102–111. doi:10.1046/j.1365-2648.2001.01947.x

Cassem, N. H., & Hackett, T. P. (1977). Psychological aspects of myocardial infarction. *Medical Clinics of North America, 61,* 711–721.

Cavendish, R., Konecny, L., Mitzeliotis, C., Russo, D., Luise, B. K., Lanza, M., . . . Bajo, M. A. M. (2003). Spiritual care activities of nurses using nursing interventions classification (NIC) labels. *International Journal of Nursing Terminologies and Classifications, 14,* 113–124.

Centers for Disease Control and Prevention. (2010). *Establishing a holistic framework to reduce inequities in HIV, viral hepatitis, STDs, and tuberculosis in the United States.* Atlanta, GA: U.S. Department of Health and Human Services, Centers for Disease Control and Prevention. Retrieved from http://www.cdc.gov/socialdeterminants/docs/SDH-White-Paper-2010.pdf

Chase, S. K. (2001). Response to "The Concept of Nursing Presence: State of the Science." *Scholarly Inquiry for Nursing Practice: An International Journal, 15,* 323–327.

Chen, C. C., David, A., Thompson, K., Smith, C., Lea, S., & Fahy, T. (1996). Coping strategies and psychiatric morbidity in women attending breast assessment clinics. *Journal of Psychosomatic Research, 40*(3), 265–270.

Chopoorian, T. J. (1986). Reconceptualizing the environment. In P. Moccia (Ed.), *New approaches to theory development in nursing* (pp. 39–54). New York, NY: National League for Nursing.

Commission on the Social Determinants of Health. (2008). *Closing the gap in a generation: Health equity through action on the social determinants of health. Final Report of the Commission on Social Determinants of Health.* Geneva, Switzerland: World Health Organization. Retrieved from http://goo.gl/3x0ek9

Community Health Nurses Association of Canada. (2008). *Canadian community health nursing standards of practice.* Retrieved from http://goo.gl/s6laZz

Corwin, E. J., Meek, P., Cook, P. F., Lowe, N. K., & Sousa, K. (2012). Shape shifters: Biological phenomena in symptom research. *Nursing Outlook, 60*(4), 191–197.

Coward, D. D. (1991). *Correlates of self-transcendence in women with advanced breast cancer.* Ann Arbor, MI: University of Arizona

Coward, D. D. (1997). Constructing meaning from the experience of cancer. *Seminars in Oncology Nursing, 13*(4), 248–251.

Cox, T. (2008). Scraping sounds and disgusting noises. *Applied Acoustics, 69,* 1195–1204. doi:10.1016/j.apacoust.2007.11.004

Crighton, A., Robertson, A., Gordon, C., & Farrant, W. (1997). *Health care a community concern? Developments in the organization of Canadian health care services.* Calgary: University of Calgary.

Dahlgren, G., & Whitehead, M. (2006). *Levelling up Part 2: European strategies for tackling social inequities in health.* Geneva, Switzerland: World Health Organization. Retrieved from http://goo.gl/fODFWN

Daniels, M. (2001). On transcendence in transpersonal psychology. *Transpersonal Psychology Review, 5*(2), 3–11.

Davidson, L., Shaw, J., Wellborn, S., Mahon, B., Sirota, M., Gilbo, P., . . . Pelletier, J. (2010). "I don't know how to find my way in the world": Contributions of user-led research to transforming mental health practice. *Psychiatry, 73*(2), 101–113.

DeGuzman, P. B., & Kulbok, P. A. (2012). Changing health outcomes of vulnerable populations through nursing's influence on neighbourhood built environment: A framework for nursing research. *The Journal of Nursing Scholarship, 44,* 341–348. doi:10.1111/j.1547-5069.2012.01470.x

Dickoff, J., & James, P. (1968). A theory of theories: A position paper. *Nursing Research, 17*(3), 197–203.

Doornbos, M. M., Zandee, G. L., DeGroot, J., & De Maagd-Rodriguez, M. (2013). Using community-based participatory research to explore social determinants of women's mental health and barriers to help-seeking in three urban, ethnically diverse, impoverished, and underserviced communities. *Archives of Psychiatric Nursing, 27,* 278–284. doi:10.1016/j.apnu.2013.09.001

Drageset, S., & Lindstrøm, T. C. (2005). Coping with a possible breast cancer diagnosis: Demographic factors and social support. *Journal of Advanced Nursing, 51*(3), 217–226.

Dysart-Gale, D. (2010). Social justice and social determinants of health: Lesbian, gay, bisexual, transgendered, intersexed and queer youth in Canada. *Journal of Child and Adolescent Psychiatric Nursing, 23,* 23–28. doi:10.1111/j.1744-6171.2009.0023.x

Ellsworth, W., & Maxwell, R. (Producers). (1952). *Adventures of superman* [Television series].

Epp, J. (1986). *Achieving health for all: A framework for health promotion.* Ottawa: Minister of Supply and Services Canada.

Eppler, M. J., & Mengis, J. (2011, July). *Drawing distinction: The visualization of classification in qualitative research* (=mcm working paper, No. 2/2011). St. Gallen: mcm institute, University of St. Gallen. Retrieved from www.knowledge-communication.org

Eriksson, K. (2006). *The suffering human being.* Chicago, IL: Nordic Studies.

Etches, V., Frank, J., Di Ruggiero, E., & Manuel, D. (2006). Measuring population health: A review of the indicators. *Annual Review of Public Health, 27,* 29–55. doi:10.1146/annurev.publhealth.27.021405.102141

Eva, G., & Paley, J. (2004). Numbers in evidence. *The British Journal of Occupational Therapy, 67*(1), 47–49.

Fawcett, J. (1984b). *Analysis and evaluation of conceptual models of nursing.* Philadelphia, PA: F. A. Davis.

Fawcett, J., & DeSanto-Madeya, S. (2013). *Contemporary nursing knowledge: Analysis an evaluation of nursing models and theories* (3rd ed.). Philadelphia, PA: FADavis.

Federal/Provincial/Territorial Advisory Committee on Population Health. (1994). *Strategies for population health: Investing in the health of populations.* Ottawa: Minister of Supplies and Services. Retrieved from http://goo.gl/ZyRgMJ

Fellowes, J. (2010). *Downton Abbey* (UK Edition). United Kingdom: PBS/Carnival Film & Television.

Ferguson, E. J. (1978). *Protecting the vulnerable adult: A perspective on policy and program issues in adult protective services.* Ann Arbor, MI: The University of Michigan/Wayne State University.

Field, P. A., & Marck, P. B. (1994). *Uncertain motherhood: Negotiating the risks of the childbearing years.* Thousand Oaks, CA: Sage.

Fink, A. M. (2009). Toward a definition of health disparity: A concept analysis. *Journal of Transcultural Nursing, 20,* 349–357. doi:10.1177/1043659609340802

Flaskerud, J. H., & Nyamathi, A. M. (2002). Guest editorial: New paradigm for health disparities needed. *Nursing Research, 51,* 139.

Frank, J. W., & Mustard, J. F. (1994). The determinants of health from a historical perspective. *Daedalus, 123,* 1–19. Retrieved from http://www.jstor.org/stable/20027264

Gagnon, A. J., Carnevale, F., Mehta, P., Rousseau, H., & Stewart, D. E. (2013). Developing population intervention with migrant women for maternal-child health: A focused ethnography. *BMC Public Health, 13,* 471–484. doi:10.1186/1471-2458-13-471

Geering, J. (2012). *Social Science methodology* (2nd ed.). New York, NY: Cambridge.

Germain, C. P. H. (1979). *The cancer unit: An ethnography.* Philadelphia, PA: Lippincott Williams & Wilkins.

Giddens, J., & Brady, D. (2007). Rescuing nursing education from content saturation: A case for a concept-based curriculum. *Journal of Nursing Education, 46*(2), 65–69.

Gilje, F. (1992). Being there: An analysis of the concept of presence. In D. A. Gaut (Ed.), *The presence of caring in nursing.* New York, NY: National League for Nursing.

Gillis, A., & MacLellan, M. A. (2013). Critical service learning in community health nursing: Enhancing access to cardiac screening. *International Journal of Nursing Education Scholarship, 10,* 63–71. doi:10.1515/ijnes-2012-0031

Glaser, B. G. (1992). *Basis of grounded theory analysis.* Mill Valley, CA: Sociology Press.

Goffman, E. (1963). *Stigma: Notes on a spoiled identity.* New York, NY: Simon & Schuster.

Gottlieb, L., & Rowat, K. (1987). The McGill model of nursing: A practice-derived model. *Advanced in Nursing Science, 9*(4), 51–56.

Graham, H. (2004). Social determinants and their unequal distribution: Clarifying policy understandings. *The Milbank Quarterly, 82,* 101–124.

Greene, J. A., Ball, K., Belcher, J. R., & McAlpine, C. (2003). Substance abuse, homelessness, developmental decision-making and spirituality: A women's health issue. *Journal of Social Work Practice in the Addictions, 3,* 39–56.

Griffin, A. P. (1980). Philosophy and nursing. *Journal of Advanced Nursing, 5,* 261–272.

Haase, J. E., Leidy N. K., Coward, D. D., Britt, T., & Penn, P. E. (2000). Simultaneous concept analysis: A strategy for developing multiple interrelated concepts. In B. L. Rodgers & K. A. Knafl (Eds.), *Concept development in nursing: Foundations, techniques, and applications* (pp. 209–229). Philadelphia, PA: W. B. Saunders.

Halloran, E. J. (1995). *A virginia henderson reader: Excellence in nursing.* New York, NY: Springer Publishing.

Hamilton, N., & Bhatti, T. (1996). *Population health promotion: An integrated model of population health and health promotion.* Retrieved from http://www.phac-aspc.gc.ca/ph-sp/php-psp/index-eng.php#toc

Hanna, D. R., & Roy, C. (2001). Roy adaptation model and perspectives on the family. *Nursing Science Quarterly, 14*(1), 10–13.

Happ, M. B. (2013). Qualitative research program for the care of ventilator-dependent ICU patients. In C. T. Beck (Ed.), *Routledge international handbook of qualitative research* (pp. 86–102). New York, NY: Routledge/Taylor & Francis.

Harmer, B., & Henderson, V. (1939). The principles and practice of nursing. *The American Journal of Nursing, 39*(12), 1407.

Harrison, K. M., & Dean, H. D. (2011). Use of data systems to address social determinants of health: A need to do more. *Public Health Reports, 53,* 1–5. Retrieved from http://www.jstor.org/stable/41639296

Hatton, D. C., Kleffel, D., Bennett, S., & Gaffrey, E. A. N. (2001). Homeless women and children's access to health care: A paradox. *Journal of Community Health Nursing, 18,* 25–34.

Haugan, G., Rannestad, T., Hammervold, R., Garåsen, H., Hammervold, R., & Espnes G. A. (2012). The self-transcendence scale: An investigation of the Factor structure among nursing home patients. *Journal of Holistic Nursing, 30,* 147–159.

Hawkins, S. F., & Morse, J. (2014). The praxis of courage as a foundation for care. *Journal of Nursing Scholarship, 46*(4), 263–270.

Henderson, V. (1964). The nature of nursing. *The American Journal of Nursing, 64*(8), 62–68.

Henderson, V. (1978). The concept of nursing. *Journal of Advanced Nursing, 3,* 113–130.

Herschbach, P., Keller, M., Knight, L., Brandl, T., Huber, B., Henrich, G., & Marten-Mittag, B. (2004). Psychological problems of cancer patients: A cancer distress screening with a cancer-specific questionnaire. *British Journal of Cancer, 91*(3), 504–511.

Hertzman, C., Frank, J., & Evans, R. G. (1994). Heterogeneities in health status and the determinants of population health. In R. G. Evans, M. L. Barer, & T. R. Marmor (Eds.), *Why are some people healthy and others not? The determinants of health of populations* (pp. 67–92). New York, NY: Aldine de Gruyter.

Hill, R. P. (1991). Homeless women, special possessions, and the meaning of "home:" An ethnographic case study. *Journal of Consumer Research, 18,* 298–310.

Hinshaw, A. S. (1979). Problems in doing research. *Western Journal of Nursing Research, 1,* 319–324. doi:10.1177/019394597900100410

Hislop, T. G., Harris, S. R., Jackson, J., Thorne, S. E., Rousseau, E. J., Coldman, A. J., . . . Olivotto, I. A. (2002). Satisfaction and anxiety for women during investigation of an abnormal screening mammogram. *Breast Cancer Research and Treatment, 76*(3), 245–254.

Homer, S. (1988). Intersubjective co-presence in a caring model. In *Caring and nursing explorations in the feminist perspective* (pp. 166–180). Denver, CO: Center for Human Caring, University of Colorado Health Sciences Centre.

Huey, L., & Quirouette, M. (2010). "Any girl can call the cops, no problem": The influence of gender on support for the decision to report criminal victimization within homeless communities. *British Journal of Criminology, 50,* 278–295.

Hume, D. (1960). *A treatise on human nature.* In L. A. Selby-Bigge (Ed.), [Reprinted from the original in three volumes]. Oxford, UK: Oxford University Press.

Hunt, J., Raffertty, A., & Shamian, J. (2001). Nurses' reports on hospital care in five countries. *Health Affairs, 20*(3), 43–53. doi:10.1377/hlthaff.20.3.43

Illich, I. (1995). Pathogenesis, community and the quality of public health. *Qualitative Health Research, 5*(1), 7–14.

Im, E.-O., & Meleis, A. I. (1999). Situation-specific theories: Philosophical roots, properties, and approach. *Advances in Nursing Science, 22*(2), 11–24.

Institute for Population and Public Health. (2014). *Canadian Institutes for Health Research*. Retrieved from http://www.cihr-irsc.gc.ca/e/13777.html

International Council of Nurses. (2012). *The ICN code of ethics for nurses*. Geneva, Switzerland: Author. Retrieved from http://goo.gl/zvX3Lk

International Organization for Standardization. (1985). *Information Processing* (ISO 5807). Retrieved from www.iso.org/iso/home.htm

Intraspec.ca. (2010). *Homeless in Canada*. Retrieved from http://goo.gl/Y9wA5e

Irvine, L., Elliott. L., Wallace, H., & Crombie, I. K. (2006). A review of major influences on current public health policy in developed countries in the second half of the 20th century. *The Journal of the Royal Society for Health promotion, 126,* 73–78. doi:10.1177/1466424006063182

Iwamitsu, Y., Shimoda, K., Abe, H., Tani, T., Okawa, M., & Buck, R. (2005). The relation between negative emotional suppression and emotional distress in breast cancer diagnosis and treatment. *Health Communication, 18*(3), 201–215.

Jackson, J., McGibbon, E., & Waldon, I. (2013). Racism and cardiovascular disease: Implications for nursing. *Canadian Journal of Cardiovascular Nursing, 23*(4), 12–18.

Jackson, S. F., Birn, A.-E., Fawcett, S. B., Poland, B., & Schultz, J. A. (2013). Synergy for health equity: Integrating health promotion and social determinants of health approaches in and beyond the Americas. *Revista Panamericana de Salud Pública, 34,* 473–480.

Janesick, V. J. (2000). The choreography of qualitative research design: Minuets, improvisations, and crystallization. In N. K. Denzin & Y. S. Lincoln (Eds.), *Handbook of qualitative research* (2nd ed., pp. 379–399). Thousand Oaks, CA: Sage Publications.

Johnson, D. E. (1959). A philosophy of nursing. *Nursing Outlook, 61*(11), 63–66.

Johnson, J. L., & Morse, J. M. (1990). Regaining control: The process of adjustment following myocardial infarction. *Heart and Lung, 19*(2), 126–135.

Josephson, R., & Josephson, G. (1996). *Abductive inference: Computation, philosophy, technology*. New York, NY: Cambridge University Press.

Kawachi, I., Subreamanian, S. V., & Almeida-Filho, N. (2002). A glossary for health inequalities. *Journal of Epidemiology & Community Health, 56,* 647–652. Retrieved from http://jech.bmj.com/content/56/9/647.full

Kelly, M. P. (2010). The axes of social differentiation and the evidence base on health equity. *Journal of the Royal Society of Medicine, 103,* 266–272. doi:10.1258/jrsm.2010.100005

Kelly, M. P., Bonnefoy, J., Morgan, A., & Florenzano, F. (2006). *The development of the evidence base about the social determinants of health*. World Health Organization. Retrieved from http://goo.gl/7UktQw

Kelly, M. P., Morgan, A., Bonnefoy, J., Butt, J., Bergman, V., & The Measurement and Evidence Knowledge Network. (2007). *The social determinants of health: Developing and evidence base for political action*. Final Report to World Health Organization Commission on the Social Determinants of Health from the Measurement and Evidence Knowledge Network. Retrieved from http://goo.gl/6TbnDR

Kneipp. S. M., & Drevdahl, D. J. (2003). Problems with parsimony on research on social determinants of health. *Advances in Nursing Science, 26,* 162–172.

Knowlden, V. (1988). Nurse caring as constructed knowledge. In *Caring and nursing explorations in the feminist perspective* (pp. 318–339). Denver, CO: Center for Human Caring, University of Colorado Health Sciences Centre.

Krieger, N. (2001). A glossary for social epidemiology. *Journal of Epidemiology and Community Health, 55,* 693–700. Retrieved from http://goo.gl/jy0Y1S

Krumeich, A., & Meershoek, A. (2014). Health in global context: Beyond the social determinants of health? *Global Health Action, 7,* 23506. Retrieved from http://dx.doi.org/10.3402/gha.v7.23506

Kuhn, T. S. (1970). *The structure of scientific revolutions* (Postscript, 2nd ed., pp. 174–210). Chicago, IL: The University of Chicago Press.

Kunyk, D., & Olson, J. K. (2001). Clarification of conceptualizations of empathy. *Journal of advanced nursing, 35*(3), 317–325.

Lalonde, M. (1974). *A new perspective on the health of Canadians: A working document.* Ottawa, ON, Canada: Government of Canada.

Lathrop, B. (2013). Nursing leadership in addressing the social determinants of health. *Policy, Politics, & Nursing Practice, 14,* 41–47. doi:10.1177/1527154413489887

Levine, M. (1996). The conservation principles: A retrospective. *Nursing Science Quarterly, 9,* 38–41.

Levine, M. E. (1995). The rhetoric of nursing theory. *Image Journal of Nursing Scholarship 27*(1), 11–17.

Li Ka-shing. (n.d.). Retrieved from BrainyQuote.com: http://www.brainyquote.com/quotes/quotes/l/likashing173343.htm

Lightsey, D., McQueen, D., & Anderson, L. (2005). Health promotion in the USA: Building a science-based health promotion policy. In A. Scriven & S. Garman (Eds.), *Promoting health: Global perspectives* (pp. 266–278). New York, NY: Palgrave MacMillan.

LoBiondo-Wood, G., & Haber, J. (2014). *Nursing Research: Methods and critical appraisal* (8th ed.). St Louis, MO: Mosby.

Loseke, D. E. (2013). *Methodological thinking: Basic issues in social research design.* Thousand Oakes, CA: Sage.

MacDonald, S. E., Newburn-Cook, C. V., Allen, M., & Reuter, L. (2013). Embracing the population health framework. *Nursing Inquiry, 20,* 30–41. doi:10.1111/nin.12017

MacFarlane, A., & O'Reilly-de Brún, M. (2012). Using a theory-driven conceptual framework in qualitative health research. *Qualitative Health Research, 22*(5), 607–618. doi:10.1177/1049732311431898

Mahony, D., & Jones, E. J. (2013). Social determinants of health in nursing education, research and health policy. *Nursing Science Quarterly, 26,* 280–284. doi:10.1177/08943/84/3489186

Mao, A., Yang, T., Bottorff, J. L., & Sarbit, G. (2014). Personal and social determinants sustaining smoking practices in rural China: A qualitative study. *International Journal for Equity in Health, 13,* 12.

Marck, P. B., Field, P. A., & Bergum, V. (1994). A search for understanding. In P. A. Field & P. B. Marck (Eds.), *Uncertain motherhood: Negotiating the risks of the childbearing years* (pp. 268–298). Thousand Oaks, CA: Sage.

Margolis, E., & Laurence, S. (1999). *Concepts: Core readings.* Cambridge, MA: MIT Press.

Marmot, M. (2001). From black to acheson: Two decades of concern with inequalities in health. A celebration of the 90th birthday of Professor Jerry Morris. *International Journal of Epidemiology, 30,* 1165–1171. doi: 10.1093/ije/30.5.1165

Marmot, M. (2010). *"Fair societyhealthy lives" (The Marmot Review)*. UCL Institute of Health Equity. Retrieved from http://www.instituteofhealthequity.org/projects/fair-society-healthy-lives-the-marmot-review

Marmot, M., & Wilkinson, R. G. (Eds.). (2006). *Social determinants of health* (2nd ed.). Oxford: Oxford University Press.

Martz, C., & Morse, J. M. (2016). The changing nature of guilt in family caregivers: Living through care transitions of parents at the end of life. *Qualitative Health Research*. doi:10.1177/1049732316649352

Maslow, A. H. (1971). *The farther reaches of human nature*. New York, NY: Penguin.

Mason, D. J. (1999). Nursing science: Who cares? [Editorial]. *American Journal of Nursing, 99*, 7.

Maxwell, J. R., Bugbee, M. E., Wellisch, D., Shalmon, A., Sayre, J., & Bassett, L. W. (2000). Imaging-guided core needle biopsy of the breast: Study of psychological outcomes. *The Breast Journal, 6*(1), 53–61.

McCullagh, M., Lusk, S. L., & Ronis, D. L. (2002). Factors influencing use of hearing protection among farmers: a test of the Pender health promotion model. *Nursing Research, 51*(1), 33–39.

McGibbon, E., Etowa, J., & McPherson, C. (2008). Health care access as a social determinant of health. *The Canadian Nurse, 104*(7), 23–27.

McKenna, H. P. (1997). *Nursing theories and models*. New York, NY: Psychology Press.

McKeown, T. (1976). *The modern rise of population*. New York, NY: Academic Press.

McKeown, T. (1979). *The role of medicine: Dream, mirage, or nemesis?* (2nd ed.). Oxford: Basil Blackwell.

Medlin, D. L. (1989). Concepts and conceptual structure. *American Psychologist, 44*, 1469–1481.

Meecham, G. T., Collins, J. P., Moss-Morris, R. E., & Petrie, K. J. (2005). Who is not reassured following benign diagnosis of breast symptoms? *Psycho-Oncology, 14*, 239–246.

Mohnkern, S. M. (1992). *Presence in nursing: Its antecedents, defining attributes and consequences* (Unpublished doctoral dissertation). University of Texas, Austin, TX.

Morse, J. M. (2016). *The essentials of qualitatively-driven mixed-method designs*. New York, NY: Routledge.

Morse, J. M., Harrison, M., & Prowse, M. (1986). Minimal breastfeeding. *Journal of Obstetric Gynecologic and Neonatal Nursing, 15*(4), 333–338.

Muntaner, C., Ng, E., & Chung, H. (2012). *Better health: An analysis of public policy and programming focusing on the determinants of health and health outcomes that are effective in achieving the healthiest populations*. Ottawa, Canada: Canadian Health Services Research Foundation. Retrieved from http://goo.gl/ktcO4P

Musil, C. M., Jones, S. L., & Warner, C. D. (1998). Structural equation modelling and its relationship to multiple regression and factor analysis. *Research in Nursing & Health, 21*(3), 271–281.

National Collaborating Centre for Determinants of Health. (2012). *Determinants of health*. Retrieved from http://www.nccah-ccnsa.ca/en

National Forum on Health. (1996). *What determines health?* Ottawa, Canada: Minister of Public Works and Government Services Canada.

National League for Nursing. (1970). *Theory development: What, why and how.* New York, NY: National League for Nursing.

New Zealand Nurses Organization. (2011). *Closing the gap: How nurses can help achieve health access and equality* [Position statement]. Retrieved from http://www.nzno.org.nz

Olsson P., Armelius K., Nordahl G., Lenner P., & Westman G. (1999) Women with false positive screening mammograms: how do they cope? *Journal of Medical Screening 6*(2), 89–93.

Orlando-Pelletier, I. J. (1990). *The dynamic nurse/patient relationship: Function, process and principles.* New York, NY: National League for Nursing.

Orne, R. M. (1993). The meaning of survival: The early aftermath of a near-death experience. *Research in Nursing & Health, 18,* 239–247.

Osswald, R., & Petersen, W. (2002, July). Induction of classifications from linguistic data. In *Proceedings of the 15th European Conference, ECAI* (Vol. 2, pp. 75–84). Amsterdam, NL: ISO Press.

Park, E. J. (2005). Self-sacrifice, self-transcendence and nurses' professional self. *Nurse Philosophy, 6*(4), 247–254

Parse, R. R., & Pelto, P. (2013). *Applied ethnography: Guidelines for field research.* Walnut Creek, CA: Left Coast Press.

Paterson, J. G., & Zderad, L. T. (1988). *Humanistic nursing.* New York, NY: National League for Nursing.

Pauly, B. M. (2013). Challenging health inequities: Enacting social justice in nursing practice. In J. L. Storch, P. Rodney, & R. Starzomski (Eds.), *Towards a moral horizon: Nursing ethics for leadership and practice* (pp. 430–447). Toronto, ON, Canada: Pearson.

Pawlowski, T. (1980). Concepts with family meanings in the humanities. In T. Pawłowski (Ed.), *Concept formation in the humanities and the social sciences* (pp. 23–54). Dordrecht, Holland: D. Reidel.

Pawson, R. (2006). Digging for nuggets: How "bad" research can yield "good" evidence. *International Journal of Social Research Methodology, 9,* 127–142.

Pederson, A., Rootman, I., & O'Neill, M. (2005). Health promotion in Canada: Back to the past or towards a promising future? In A. Scriven & S. Garman (Eds.), *Promoting health: Global perspectives* (pp. 255–278). New York, NY: Palgrave MacMillan.

Pelto, P. (2013). *Applied ethnography: Guidelines for field research.* Walnut Creek, CA: Left Coast Press.

Pender, N. (1982). *Health promotion in nursing practice.* Appleton-Century Crofts.

Pender, N. J., Barkauskas, V. H., Hayman, L., Rice, V. H., & Anderson, E. T. (1991). Health promotion and disease prevention: Toward excellence in nursing practice and education. *Nursing Outlook, 40*(3), 106–12.

Pender, N. J., Bar-Or, O., Wilk, B., & Mitchell, S. (2002). Self-efficacy and perceived exertion of girls during exercise. *Nursing Research, 51*(2), 86–91.

Pender, N. J., Walker, S. N., Sechrist, K. R., & Frank-Stromborg, M. (1990). Predicting health-promoting lifestyles in the workplace. *Nursing research, 39*(6), 326–332.

Pender, N. J., Walker, S. N., Sechrist, K. R., & Frank-Stromborg, M. (1988). Development and testing of the Health Promotion Model. *Cardio-Vascular Nursing, 24*(6), 41.

Pender, N., Murdaugh, C. L., & Parsons, M. A. (2011). *Health promotion in nursing practice* (6th ed.). Boston, MA: Pearson.

Porter, D. (2006). How did social medicine evolve, and where is it heading? *PLoS Medicine, 3*(e399), 1667–1672. doi:10:1371/journal.pmed.00

Porter, L., Redfern, S., Wilson-Barnett, J., & Le May, A. (1986). The development of an observation schedule for measuring nurse-patient touch, using an ergonomic approach. *International Journal of Nursing Studies, 23*(1), 11–20. doi:10.1016/0020-7489(86)90034-9

Priss, U. (2004). *Linguistic approaches to formal concept analysis.* The First International Conference on Formal Concept Analysis. Retrieved from http://goo.gl/eMb3M5

Project Narrative. (n.d.). *What is narrative theory?* Retrieved from http://projectnarrative.osu.edu/about/what-is-narrative-theory

Public Health Agency of Canada. (2013). *What makes Canadians healthy or unhealthy?* Retrieved from http://goo.gl/vUQDdY

Putt, A. M. (1971). *General systems theory applied to nursing.* Boston, MA: Little, Brown.

Quint, J. (1967). *The nurse and the dying patient.* New York, NY: Macmillan.

Ramsden, I. (1993). Kawa Whakaruruhau—Cultural safety in nursing education in Aotearoa (New Zealand). *Nursing Praxis in New Zealand, 8*(3), 4–10.

Raphael, D. (2010). *About Canada: Health and illness.* Nova Scotia: Fernwood Publishing.

Raphael, D. (2011). A discourse analysis of the social determinants of health. *Critical Public Health, 2*, 221–236. doi:10.1080/09581596.2010.485606

Raphael, D. (Ed.). (2004). *Social determinants of health: Canadian perspectives.* Toronto, Canada: Canadian Scholars' Press Inc.

Ratner, P. A., Bottorff, J. L., Johnson, J. L., & Hayduk, L. A. (1994). The interaction effects of gender within the health promotion model. *Research in Nursing & Health, 17*(5), 341–350.

Ravitch, S. M., & Riggan, M. (2012). *Reason and rigour: How conceptual frameworks guide research.* Thousand Oaks, CA: Sage.

Registered Nurses Association of Ontario. (2013). *Fairer societies for better health equity.* Retrieved from http://goo.gl/KBDPfg

Remler, D. K., & Van Ryzin, G. G. (2011). *Research methods in practice: Strategies for description and causation.* Thousand Oaks, CA: Sage.

Resolute. (1996–2008). *Your Dictionary.com.* Retrieved February 25, 2008, from http://www.yourdictionary.com/resolute

Respress, B. N., Morris, D. L., Lewin, L. C., & Francis, S. A. (2013). Social determinants of adolescent depression: An examination of racial differences. *Issues in Mental Health Nursing, 34*, 539–549. doi:10.3109/01612840.2012.758206

Reutter, L., & Kushner, K. E. (2010). Health equity through action on the social determinants of health: Taking up the challenge in nursing. *Nursing Inquiry, 17*, 269–280.

Rew, L. (2004). Beyond concept analysis in holistic nursing [Editorial]. *Journal of Holistic Nursing, 22*(2), 95–96.

Richards, L., & Morse, J. M. (2012). *Readme first for a user's guide to qualitative inquiry.* Thousand Oaks, CA: Sage.

Roche, E. (1978). Principles of categorization. In E. Roche & B. Lloyd (Eds.), *Cognition and categorization* (pp. 27–28). Hillside, NJ: Erlbaum.

Ronis, D. L., Hong, O., & Lusk, S. L. (2006). Comparison of the original and revised structures of the health promotion model in predicting construction workers' use of hearing protection. *Research in Nursing & Health, 29*(1), 3–17.

Royal College of Nursing. (2012). *Health inequalities and the social determinants of health* [Position statement]. Retrieved from http://goo.gl/Xmcs5S

Samuels-Denis, J. (2006). Relationship among employment status, stressful life events, and depression in single mothers. *Canadian Journal of Nursing Research, 38,* 59–80.

Sandelowski, M. (2002). Visible humans, vanishing bodies, and virtual nursing: Complications of life, presence, place, and identity. *Advances in Nursing Science, 24*(3), 58–70.

Sasano, P., & Morse, J. M. (2006). *What is a patient's comfort level? Defining a nursing concept* (Unpublished paper). University of Alberta, Canada.

Satcher, D. (2010). Commentary: Include a social determinants of health approach to reduce health inequities. *Public Health Reports, 125*(Suppl. 4), 6–7. Retrieved from http://www.jstor.org/stable/41434913

Savenstedt, S., Zingmark, K., & Sandman, P. O. (2004). Being present in a distant room: Aspects of teleconsultations with older people in a nursing home. *Qualitative Health Research, 14,* 1046–1057.

Scambler, G., & Hopkins, A. (1990). Generating a model of epileptic stigma: The role of qualitative analysis. *Social Science & Medicine, 30,* 1287–1194.

Schlegal, F. V. (1991). *Philosophical fragments* (p. 27). Minnesota, MN: University of Minnesota Press.

Scriven, A. (2005). Promoting health: A global context and rationale. In A. Scriven & S. Garman (Eds.), *Promoting health: Global perspectives* (pp. 1–13). New York, NY: Palgrave MacMillan.

Scriven, A., & Garmin, S. (Eds.). (2005). *Promoting health: Global perspectives.* New York, NY: Palgrave MacMillan.

Segall, A., & Fries, C. J. (2011). *Pursuing health and wellness.* Oxford, UK: Oxford University Press.

Shengold, L. (1989). *Soul murder: The effects of childhood abuse and deprivation.* New Haven, CT: Yale University Press.

Sherwood, G. D. (1997). Meta-synthesis of qualitative analyses of caring: Defining a therapeutic model of nursing. *Advanced Practice Nursing Quarterly, 3,* 32–42.

Singer, P. (2000). *Writings on an ethical life.* New York, NY: Ecco.

Smith, A. C., & Kleinman, S. (1989). Managing emotions in medical school: Students' contacts with the living and the dead. *Social Psychology Quarterly, 52*(1), 56–69.

Smith, J. (1999). *Patient education practice: A study of patient's perceptions* (Unpublished report). University of Utah Hospitals and Clinics, Salt Lake City, UT.

Social Determinants of Health Alliance (SDHA). (2013). Retrieved from http://socialdeterminants.org.au

Solar, O., & Irwin, A. (2010). *A conceptual framework for action on the social determinants of Health. Social determinants of health discussion. Paper 2 (Policy and Practice).* Retrieved from http://goo.gl/xkq6Cv

Solberg, S. M. (2006). Researching the social determinants of women's health. *Canadian Journal of Nursing Research, 38*, 169–174.

Solberg, S. M., Canning, P., & Buehler, S. (2008). Changing patterns of household food consumption in rural communities of Atlantic Canada. In C. C. Parish, N. J. Turner, & S. M. Solberg (Eds.), *Resetting the kitchen table: Food security, culture, health, and resilience in coastal communities* (pp. 161–175). New York, NY: Nova Science Publishers Inc.

Spradley, J. P. (1980). *Participant observation.* New York, NY: Holt, Rinehart, Winston

Spradley, J. P. (1999). *You owe yourself a drunk: An ethnography of urban nomads.* Long Grove, IL: Waveland Press.

Srinivasan, S., & Williams, S. D. (2014). Transitioning from health disparities to a health equity research agenda: The time is now. *Public Health Reports, 129*(Suppl. 2), 71–76.

Srof, B. J., & Velsor-Friedrich, B. (2006). Health promotion in adolescents: A review of Pender's health promotion model. *Nursing Science Quarterly, 19*(4), 366–373.

Substance Abuse and Mental Health Services Administration. (2004). Characteristics of homeless female admissions to substance abuse treatment: 2002. *The DASIS Report.* Retrieved September 3, 2010, from http://goo.gl/dQNWgW

Taylor, J. B. (2008). *Stroke of insight.* TED. Retrieved from http://goo.gl/fl72ow

Taylor, S. G., & Renpenning, K. (2011). *Self-care science, nursing theory and evidenced-based practice.* Philadelphia, PA: Springer Publishing.

Thagard, P. (2005). What is a medical theory? *Studies in Multidisciplinarity, 3,* 47–62.

Thorne, S., Canam, C., Dahinten, S., Hall, W., Henderson, A., & Kirkham, S. R. (1998). Nursing's metaparadigm concepts: Disimpacting the debates. *Journal of Advanced Nursing, 27*(6), 1257–1268.

Torrance, H. (2013). The practice of educations and social research. *International Review of Qualitative Research, 8*(3), 323–336.

Townsend, P., Davidson, N., & Whitehead, M. (Eds.). (1992). *Inequalities in health: The Black Report and the Health Divide.* New York, NY: Penguin

Trickett, E. M., & Chung, D. (2007). Brickbats and bouquets: Health services, community and police attitudes and the homeless experiences of women 45 years and over living in rural South Australia. *Rural Social Work and Community Practice, 12,* 5–15.

Turrell, G., Oldenburg, B., McGuffog, I., & Dent, R. (1999). *Socioeconomic determinants of health: Towards a national research program and a policy and intervention agenda.* Canberra, Australia: Queensland University of Technology, School of Public Health/Ausinfo. Retrieved from socialdeterminants.org.au

U.S. Department of Health and Human Services. (2010). *Healthy people 2020 framework.* Retrieved from http://www.healthypeople.gov/2020/TopicsObjectives2020/pdfs/HP2020_brochure_with_LHI_508.pdf

United Nations. (2000). *General Assembly: United Nations Millennium Declaration.* Retrieved from http://www.un.org/en/ga/search/view_doc.asp?symbol=A/RES/55/2

University of British Columbia Nursing Framework. (2003). Retrieved from January 10, 2014 http://goo.gl/3OqcHj .

Vaclavik, J. M. (1999). *Health, illness, and homeless women: A phenomenological study.* (Unpublished doctoral dissertation). Denton: Texas Woman's University.

Villarruel, A. M., Bigelow, A., & Alvarez, C. (2014). Integrating the 3Ds: A nursing perspective. *Public Health Reports, 129,* 37–44. Retrieved from http://goo.gl/84kpJU

Viseltear, A. J. (1984). Milton C. Winternitz and the Yale Institute of Human Relations: A brief chapter in the history of social medicine. *The Yale Journal of Biology and Medicine, 57,* 869–889. Retrieved from http://goo.gl/ufwzlU

Vygotsky, L. (1962). *Thought and language* (E. Hanfmann & G. Walker, Trans.). Cambridge, MA: MIT Press.

Walker, S. N., Sechrist, K. R., & Pender, N. J. (1987). The health-promoting lifestyle profile: Development and psychometric characteristics. *Nursing Research, 36*(2), 76–81.

Weaver, K. (2007) Ethical sensitivity: state of the science and needs for further research. *Nursing Ethics, 14,* 141–155.

Weed, M. (2005). "Meta interpretation": A method for the interpretive synthesis of qualitative research [53 paragraphs]. *Forum Qualitative Sozialforschung / Forum: Qualitative Social Research, 6*(1), Art. 37. Retrieved from http://goo.gl/a1bKgy

Whitehead, M., & Dahlgren, G. (2006). *Levelling up (Part 1): A discussion paper on concepts and principles for talking about social inequities in health.* Retrieved from http://goo.gl/2HfdcE

Wilkinson, R. G., & Marmot, M. (Eds.). (2003). *Social determinants of health: The solid facts* (2nd ed.). Copenhagen: The Regional Office for the World Health Organization. Retrieved from http://goo.gl/ehmm20

Wilson. J. (1963/1969). *Thinking with Concepts.* New York, NY: Cambridge University Press.

World Health Organization. (1978). *Declaration of Alma-Ata International conference on primary health care, Alma-Ata, USSR.* Retrieved from http://www.who.int/publications/almaata_declaration_en.pdf

World Health Organization. (1986). *The Ottawa Charter for Health Promotion.* Retrieved from http://www.who.int/health promotion/conference/previous/ottawa/en/index.html

World Health Organization. (2011). *Rio Political Declaration on Social Determinants of Health.* Retrieved from http://www.who.int/sdhconference/declaration/Rio_political_declaration.pdf

World Health Organization. (2014). *What are the social determinants of health?* Retrieved from http://www.who.int/social_determinants/sdh_definition/en

Zderad, L. T. (1970). Empathy—From cliché to construct. In C. M. Norris (Ed.), *Proceedings of the third nursing theory conference, Kansas City* (pp. 46–75). Kansas City, KS: University of Kansas Medical Centre Department of Nursing Education.

POSTFACE: THE (R)EVOLUTION OF NURSING

Before I refuse to take your questions, I have an opening statement...
—Ronald Reagan

Actually, this revolution in nursing is making me dizzy. It has been very exciting to be on the fringes, watching. I am filled with admiration of the main actors, many of whom are tenacious, still trying to get it right. For us. For all.

But now it is over to you . . .

Where will it go?

We are living in the "technologicalization" of care: check marks on a computer screen; soon by automatic tracking of care, of the nurse and the patient. (Oh, yes. Some have already started video monitoring patients.) The world of the iPatient.

Will this be followed by the mechanization of care . . . ?

Nursing theory has now grown way beyond Fawcett's metaparadigmatic concerns and the nursing frameworks of the 1970s and 1980s. We must stop considering nursing theory as something limited to the frameworks of nursing practice, discussed in Chapter 2. We have started to develop useful concepts and decent theory that targets nursing's concerns, and, best of all, started to use them. At the same time, nursing also has much to offer other disciplines. I have another worry: that the transdisciplinary movement will absorb what is uniquely nursing's "domain."

Maybe it is time to remove those fences.

Nursing theory is the conceptualization of nursing concepts and theories that come from nursing philosophy, nursing practice, and all of nursing research, both qualitative and quantitative. Considered together, nursing has created a vast array of nursing theory: a cohesive body of knowledge that is growing faster than any of us may comprehend.

And it is finally making a difference.

INDEX